Essentials of
MEDICINE
for DENTAL Students

Essentials of MEDICINE for DENTAL Students

FOURTH EDITION

Anil K Tripathi
MD FRCP (London) FRCP (Glasgow) FRCP (Ireland) FAMS
FICP FIACM FISHTM Fellow NIH (USA) WFH Fellow (UK)

Professor and Head
Department of Clinical Hematology
King George's Medical University
Lucknow, Uttar Pradesh, India

Former Director
Dr RML Institute of Medical Sciences
Lucknow, Uttar Pradesh, India
email: *tripathiak2010@hotmail.com*

Kamal K Sawlani
MD FICP

Professor
Department of Medicine
King George's Medical University
Lucknow, Uttar Pradesh, India
email: *kksawlani@gmail.com*

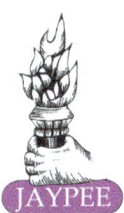

JAYPEE BROTHERS MEDICAL PUBLISHERS
The Health Sciences Publisher
New Delhi | London

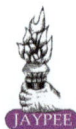

Jaypee Brothers Medical Publishers (P) Ltd

Headquarters

Jaypee Brothers Medical Publishers (P) Ltd
EMCA House, 23/23-B
Ansari Road, Daryaganj
New Delhi 110 002, India
Landline: +91-11-23272143, +91-11-23272703
+91-11-23282021, +91-11-23245672
Email: jaypee@jaypeebrothers.com

Corporate Office

Jaypee Brothers Medical Publishers (P) Ltd
4838/24, Ansari Road, Daryaganj
New Delhi 110 002, India
Phone: +91-11-43574357
Fax: +91-11-43574314
Email: jaypee@jaypeebrothers.com

Overseas Office

J.P. Medical Ltd
83 Victoria Street, London
SW1H 0HW (UK)
Phone: +44 20 3170 8910
Fax: +44 (0)20 3008 6180
Email: info@jpmedpub.com

Website: www.jaypeebrothers.com
Website: www.jaypeedigital.com

© 2022, Jaypee Brothers Medical Publishers

The views and opinions expressed in this book are solely those of the original contributor(s)/author(s) and do not necessarily represent those of editor(s) of the book.

All rights reserved. No part of this publication may be reproduced, stored or transmitted in any form or by any means, electronic, mechanical, photocopying, recording or otherwise, without the prior permission in writing of the publishers.

All brand names and product names used in this book are trade names, service marks, trademarks or registered trademarks of their respective owners. The publisher is not associated with any product or vendor mentioned in this book.

Medical knowledge and practice change constantly. This book is designed to provide accurate, authoritative information about the subject matter in question. However, readers are advised to check the most current information available on procedures included and check information from the manufacturer of each product to be administered, to verify the recommended dose, formula, method and duration of administration, adverse effects and contraindications. It is the responsibility of the practitioner to take all appropriate safety precautions. Neither the publisher nor the author(s)/editor(s) assume any liability for any injury and/or damage to persons or property arising from or related to use of material in this book.

This book is sold on the understanding that the publisher is not engaged in providing professional medical services. If such advice or services are required, the services of a competent medical professional should be sought.

Every effort has been made where necessary to contact holders of copyright to obtain permission to reproduce copyright material. If any have been inadvertently overlooked, the publisher will be pleased to make the necessary arrangements at the first opportunity.

Inquiries for bulk sales may be solicited at: jaypee@jaypeebrothers.com

Essentials of Medicine for Dental Students

First Edition: 2006

Second Edition: 2011

Third Edition: 2017

Fourth Edition: **2022**

ISBN: 978-93-5465-126-7

Preface to the Fourth Edition

It is with great pleasure and gratification that we are now presenting the next edition. Basic and translational researches in medical sciences are adding new knowledge every year and hence practice of medicine is likely to change rapidly. Therefore our resolve is to offer new edition of the book at short intervals in order to keep readers well updated.

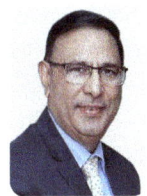

Our principal aim has been to provide the subject material in clear, simple, concise, and affable manner, which is beneficial to students and practitioners alike. We have updated the text according to the most recent literature and guidelines. Additional pictures and tables have been added to make the reading more easy and comfortable. Recently introduced newer drugs for various diseases such as hypertension, diabetes mellitus, HIV, blood cancers, hepatitis C, etc., have also been included. The 2020 has been the year of great predicament and challenges for humankind posed by COVID 19 pandemic. A section is dedicated to the management of COVID 19 as well.

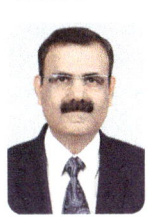

Previous editions of the book have been widely read and appreciated all over India. We have received valuable comments and advice from experts and readers and tried to incorporate their suggestions in this edition.

Any work done is never perfect and there is always a room for improvement. This is possible only with the continued feedback which we are looking forward from our esteemed readers.

Anil K Tripathi
Kamal K Sawlani

Preface to the First Edition

Over the years, a customized and concise textbook of *General Medicine* for dental students and dental practitioners has been much awaited. Students need a textbook that is easily readable, concise and in accordance with the prescribed curriculum.

The primary objective of this book is to provide basic and practical information on the pertinent topics that will enable the reader to understand and improve his/her diagnostic and therapeutic skills. Special attempt has been made to make the book succinct without compromising on the required details.

The chapters are chosen according to the Dental Council of India guidelines. However, additional chapters on other important subjects, such as HIV/AIDS, malaria, stroke, and pleural diseases, have also been included. Emphasis has been given on the clinical methods including history taking and physical examination which are described in the beginning of each system. This will make a wholesome reading without much need to go for other books on clinical methods.

Each chapter contains relevant "Multiple choice questions" and "Fill in the blanks" to help the reader self-assess their knowledge. In addition, a "Model test paper" is also provided at the end of the book which will enable the readers to prepare for the competitive entrance tests.

The essence of learning general medicine by dental students is in applying the concept and knowledge while they deal with patients suffering from various medical disorders. In such endeavor, each chapter is followed by a section "Implications on dental practice", which describes how the presence of medical disorders affect the management decisions.

While the book is intended primarily for dental undergraduate and postgraduate students, this should also be useful for medical students and practitioners.

Although every attempt has been made to avoid any error or controversy, shortcomings are inevitable. Readers are requested to offer their valuable comments and suggestions that will be of great help in improving the next edition.

Anil K Tripathi
Kamal K Sawlani

Acknowledgments

We owe to our family members particularly Mrs Sushma Tripathi, Dr Tanya Tripathi, Dr Vanchha Tripathi and Dr Kriti Tripathi for their constant support and encouragement without which the task could never have been possible.

We are immensely thankful to our colleagues from King George's Medical University: Dr Sandeep Saxena, Professor, Department of Ophthalmology, for providing images of diabetic retinopathy, Dr SP Verma, Associate Professor, Department of Clinical Hematology and Dr Tanmay Tiwari, Associate Professor, Department of Anesthesia for helping us in updating the chapters on Hematology and Preoperative Evaluation respectively.

We are also thankful to Dr Ritu Karoli, Additional Professor of Medicine, Dr Abhilash Chandra, Additional Professor in Nephrology, Dr S Namrata Rao, Associate Professor in Nephrology, Dr Hemant Kumar, Associate Professor in Respiratory Medicine, Dr RML Institute of Medical Sciences, Lucknow for their contributions.

We are indebted to Dr Deepak Verma and Dr Deepak Sharma, Residents in the Department of Medicine, King George's Medical University for their help in writing on COVID 19 and providing photographs.

We are truly indebted to our teachers, students and patients, who have been constant source of inspiration and learning. We acknowledge the contributions of various experts and readers who provided us with their valuable comments and suggestions.

We are very grateful to the whole team of M/s Jaypee Brothers Medical Publishers (P) Ltd, New Delhi, India, who helped and guided us: Shri Jitendar P Vij (Group Chairman), Mr Ankit Vij (Managing Director), Mr MS Mani (Group President), Dr Madhu Choudhary (Publishing Head–Education), Ms Pooja Bhandari (Production Head), Ms Sunita Katla (Executive Assistant to Group Chairman and Publishing Manager), Ms Samina Khan (Executive Assistant to Publishing Head–Education), Dr Sneha Kashyap (Development Editor), Mr Rajesh Sharma (Production Coordinator), Ms Seema Dogra (Cover Visualizer), Mr Deepak Saxena (Typesetter), Ms Geeta Srivastava (Proofreader), Mr Gopal Kirola (Graphic Designer) and their team members, for all their support to work in this project and make it a success. Without their cooperation, we could not have completed this project.

Contents

CHAPTER 1 Clinical Methods — 1
- History 1
- Physical Examination 3
- Scheme of the General Examination 13
- Frequently Used Terms 13

CHAPTER 2 Gastrointestinal System — 16
- Symptoms and Signs of Gastrointestinal Diseases 16
- Stomatitis and Oral Ulcers 21
- Gingival Hyperplasia 23
- Dysphagia 23
- Gastritis 25
- Peptic Ulcer 26
- Diarrhea, Dysentery and Food Poisoning 28
- Malabsorption 31
- Implications on Dental Practice 33

CHAPTER 3 Hepatobiliary System — 35
- Liver: Structure and Function 35
- Jaundice 37
- Acute Hepatitis 39
- Acute Viral Hepatitis 39
- Chronic Hepatitis 43
- Cirrhosis of Liver 47
- Portal Hypertension 48
- Upper Gastrointestinal Bleeding 49
- Hepatic Encephalopathy 49
- Ascites 51
- Hepatomegaly 52
- Splenomegaly 53
- Implications on Dental Practice 53

CHAPTER 4 Hematological System — 55
- Anemia 55
- Iron Deficiency Anemia 57
- Megaloblastic Anemia 59
- Aplastic Anemia 61
- Hemolytic Anemia 62
- Anemia of Acute Blood Loss 64
- Leukemia 64
- Acute Leukemias 64
- Lymphomas 70
- Multiple Myeloma 73
- Normal Hemostasis 74
- Platelet Disorders 76
- Von Willebrand Disease 78
- Coagulation Disorders 78
- Splenomegaly 81
- Lymphadenopathy 82
- Implications on Dental Practice 83

CHAPTER 5: Cardiovascular System — 86

- Symptoms and Signs of Cardiovascular Diseases   86
- General Examination   87
- Cardiac Examination   90
- Investigations   90
- Acute Rheumatic Fever   91
- Rheumatic Valvular Heart Disease   92
- Aortic Stenosis (AS)   95
- Aortic Regurgitation (AR)   96
- Infective Endocarditis   97
- Hypertension   100
- Ischemic Heart Disease/Coronary Artery Disease   108
- Stable Angina   109
- Unstable Angina   110
- Acute Myocardial Infarction or STEMI   112
- Heart Failure   114
- Acute Pulmonary Edema (Cardiogenic)   119
- Congenital Heart Disease   120
- Syncope   122
- Arrhythmia   124
- Bradyarrhythmias   124
- Tachyarrhythmias   127
- Implications on Dental Practice   130

CHAPTER 6: Respiratory Diseases — 133

- Symptoms   133
- Examination   135
- Investigations   137
- Pneumonia   138
- Lung Abscess   141
- Bronchiectasis   142
- Bronchial Asthma   143
- Chronic Obstructive Pulmonary Disease   147
- Cor Pulmonale   151
- Pulmonary Eosinophilia   152
- Pulmonary Embolism   153
- Tuberculosis   156
- Respiratory Failure   163
- Pleural Diseases   164
- Pneumothorax   165
- Interstitial Lung Disease   167
- Lung Cancers (Bronchogenic Carcinoma)   168
- Swine Influenza A (H1N1)—"Swine Flu"   171
- Implications on Dental Practice   171

CHAPTER 7: Renal Diseases — 175

- Structure and Functions of Normal Kidneys   175
- Syndromes in Nephrology   175
- Investigations In Renal Disease   176
- Nephrotic Syndrome   176
- Acute and Rapidly Progressive Glomerulonephritides   180
- Acute Kidney Injury   181
- Chronic Kidney Disease   184
- Renal Replacement Therapy   186
- Implications on Dental Practice   186

CHAPTER 8: Nervous System — 188

- Examination of Cranial Nerves   188
- Examination of a Comatose Patient   194
- Epilepsy   196
- Meningitis   200
- Headache   204
- Facial Pain   207

- Facial Nerve Palsy 209
- Cerebrovascular Diseases 211
- Implications on Dental Practice 212

CHAPTER 9 Endocrine and Metabolic Disorders 215
- Thyroid Disorders 215
- Calcium Metabolism 219
- Parathyroid Disorders 221
- Pituitary Gland 222
- Diabetes Mellitus 227
- Implications on Dental Practice 237

CHAPTER 10 Infections 240
- Measles (Rubeola) 240
- Mumps 241
- Rubella (German Measles) 242
- Chickenpox (Varicella) and Herpes Zoster (Shingles) 243
- Herpes Simplex 245
- Infectious Mononucleosis 247
- Diphtheria 249
- Enteric Fever (Typhoid Fever) 250
- Gonorrhea 251
- Syphilis 252
- Amebiasis 255
- Malaria 256
- Human Immunodeficiency Syndrome (HIV)/Acquired Immunodeficiency Syndrome (AIDS) 259
- COVID-19 268
- Implications on Dental Practice 271

CHAPTER 11 Medical Emergencies in Dental Practice 274
- Postural Hypotension (Orthostatic Hypotension) 275
- Syncope 275
- Hypertensive Crisis 276
- Acute Pulmonary Edema 276
- Chest Pain 277
- Asthmatic Attack 277
- Airways Obstruction 278
- Hyperventilation 278
- Seizures 278
- Stroke (Cerebrovascular Accident) 279
- Anaphylaxis 280
- Hypoglycemia 280
- Adrenal Crisis 281
- Excessive Bleeding 281
- Dental Procedures in Pregnant Women 281
- Cardiopulmonary Resuscitation 281

CHAPTER 12 Critical Care 283
- Shock 283
- Acute Respiratory Distress Syndrome 288
- Cardiovascular Collapse 289
- Cardiac Arrest 290
- Cardiopulmonary Resuscitation 290

CHAPTER 13 Anaphylaxis and Drug Allergy 293
- Anaphylaxis 293
- Drug Allergy 295
- Implications on Dental Practice 297

CHAPTER 14 Nutrition 298
- Diet and Nutrition 298
- Protein Energy Malnutrition 299
- Obesity 300
- Vitamins 301
- Implications on Dental Practice 308

CHAPTER 15	**Preoperative Evaluation**	**310**

- Medical History 310
- Physical Examination 311
- Airway Examination 311
- Modified Mallampati Classification 311
- Preoperative Laboratory Tests 312
- Risk Assessment 312

Test Paper *315*
Answers *322*
Reference Laboratory Values *326*
Index *329*

Theory Syllabus

1. **Aims of Medicine**
   Definitions of Signs, Symptoms, Diagnosis, Differential Diagnosis, Treatment and Prognosis.

2. **Gastrointestinal and Hepatobiliary Systems**
   Core Topics (Must Know)
   - Stomatitis and Oral Ulcers
   - Gingival Hyperplasia
   - Dysphagia
   - Gastritis
   - Peptic Ulcer
   - Jaundice
   - Acute Viral Hepatitis
   - Cirrhosis of Liver
   - Ascites
   - Hepatomegaly

   Collateral Topics (Desirable to Know)
   - Diarrhea
   - Dysentery
   - Amebiasis
   - Malabsorption

3. **Cardiovascular System**
   Core Topics (Must Know)
   - Acute Rheumatic Fever
   - Rheumatic Valvular Heart Disease
   - Infective Endocarditis
   - Hypertension
   - Ischemic Heart Disease
   - Congestive Heart Failure
   - Acute Pulmonary Edema
   - Congenital Heart Disease
   - Common Arrhythmias

4. **Respiratory System**
   Core Topics (Must Know)
   - Pneumonia
   - Chronic Obstructive Pulmonary Disease (COPD)
   - Pulmonary Tuberculosis
   - Bronchial Asthma

   Collateral Topics (Desirable to Know)
   - Lung Abscess
   - Bronchiectasis
   - Pleural Diseases (Pleural Effusion, Pneumothorax)
   - Lung Cancer

5. **Hematology**
   Core Topics (Must Know)
   - Anemias
   - Bleeding and Clotting Disorders
   - Leukemias
   - Lymphomas
   - Agranulocytosis
   - Splenomegaly
   - Oral Manifestations of Hematological Disorders
   - Lymphadenopathy

6. **Renal System**
   Core Topics (Must Know)
   - Acute Nephritis
   - Nephrotic Syndrome

   Collateral Topics (Desirable to Know)
   - Renal Failure

7. **Central Nervous System**
   Core Topics (Must Know)
   - Facial Nerve Palsy
   - Facial Pain including Trigeminal Neuralgia
   - Epilepsy
   - Headache including Migraine

   Collateral Topics (Desirable to Know)
   - Meningitis
   - Examination of Comatose Patient
   - Examination of Cranial Nerves

8. **Infections**
   Core Topics (Must Know)
   - Enteric Fever (Typhoid Fever)
   - Human Immunodeficiency Virus (HIV)/ Acquired Immunodeficiency Syndrome (AIDS)
   - Herpes Zoster
   - Herpes Simplex
   - Syphilis
   - Diphtheria

   Collateral Topics (Desirable to Know)
   - Infectious Mononucleosis
   - Measles (Rubeola)
   - Mumps
   - Rubella (German Measles)
   - Malaria

9. **Endocrinal System**
   Core Topics (Must Know)
   - Diabetes Mellitus
   - Thyroid Disorders (Hypothyroidism, Thyrotoxicosis)
   - Calcium Metabolism
   - Parathyroid Disorders
   - Pituitary Gland (Acromegaly)

   Collateral Topics (Desirable to Know)
   - Addison's Disease
   - Cushing's Syndrome

10. **Nutrition**
    Core Topics (Must Know)
    - Avitaminosis

    Collateral Topics (Desirable to Know)
    - Balanced Diet and Nutrition
    - Protein-Energy Malnutrition

11. **Critical Care**
    Core Topics (Must Know)
    - Syncope
    - Cardiac Arrest
    - Cardiopulmonary Resuscitation (CPR)
    - Shock

    Collateral Topics (Desirable to Know)
    - Acute Left Ventricular Failure (LVF)
    - Adult Respiratory Distress Syndrome (ARDS)

12. **Emergencies in Dental Practice**
    - Myocardial Infarction
    - Status Epilepticus
    - Status Asthmaticus
    - Syncope
    - Anaphylaxis
    - Bleeding
    - Arrhythmia

13. **Anaphylaxis and Drug Allergy**
    - Anaphylaxis
    - Drug Allergy

List of Abbreviations

Drug Administration

bd	twice daily
IM	intramuscular
IV	intravenous
od	daily, once a day
qid	four times a day
q4h	every four hours
SC	subcutaneous
SL	sublingual
stat	immediately
tid	three times a day, alternative tds

Units

cm	centimeter(s)
d	per day
dL	deciliter(s)
fL	femtoliter(s)
g	gram(s)
a	hour(s)
hrly	hourly
Hg	mercury
IU	international unit(s), alternative U
Kg	kilogram(s)
L	liter(s)
mcg (µg)	microgram(s)
µL	microliter(s)
mEq	milliequivalent(s)
mg	milligram(s)
mL	milliliter(s)
mm	millimeter(s)
mmol	millimole(s)
min	minute(s)
pg	picogram(s)

CHAPTER 1

Clinical Methods

Clinical methods form the basis of the approach to a patient by which a proper diagnosis is achieved. The skill of a clinician depends on his knowledge of theoretical as well as practical aspects of the clinical methods. This skill is acquired and refined with experience. Symptoms are the complaints that the patient tells whereas signs are elicited by the examiner.

HISTORY

History is the physician's abstraction of certain facts developed in the course of the patient's interview and arranged in a manner that facilitates diagnosis.

Proper history is important for making a correct diagnosis. A careful evaluation by competent clinicians reveals that 82% of diagnoses are made by history, 9% by physical examination and 9% by the laboratory tests. A history is not simply a collection of facts. It must also contain information. Facts are the true statements made by the patient, while information consists of facts arranged in useful manner. A general format is followed while taking a history of the patient. The contents of history are recorded in the patient's version and no part in the history should be distorted or omitted. However, the focus and contents may vary from patient to patient and also with the experience of the clinician.

The standard format used for history taking is as follows:
- Patient's details (name, age, sex, marital status, occupation, address).
- Presenting complaints with duration.
- History of present illness.
- History of past illnesses.
- Treatment history.
- Personal history.
- Family history.
- Menstrual history (in females).

Presenting Complaints

This is also known as chief complaints. The patient is asked about the main problems for which he has come to the doctor. These main symptoms/problems are listed in a chronological order (noted in the order of their appearance). Generally the patient is allowed to tell by himself. Leading questions are avoided. The list should not be too long.

History of Present Illness

The patient is then asked to narrate individual symptoms in details. Once this is over, leading questions are asked to clarify certain points or associations related to different symptoms. For example, if the patient is complaining of pain, details should be recorded about the site, severity, character, radiation, duration and timing, relieving and aggravating factors.
- *Site:* The exact site of pain is noted. Whether it is localized or diffuse pain.
- *Severity:* Does the pain interfere with routine daily activities or keep the patient awake at night? Is the patient in severe agony or is he shouting?
- *Character:* Description of character of pain such as burning, stabbing, pricking, colicky, and dull ache are helpful. Colicky pain is the waxing and waning type of pain and may cause the patient to roll about. Colicky pain suggests obstruction of hollow structure like intestine, ureter or common bile duct.
- *Timing and duration:* When does it start and when does it stop?
- *Relieving factors and aggravating factors:* Cardiac pain occurs on exertion and is relieved by rest and nitrates. Pain of duodenal ulcer is relieved by eating. Musculoskeletal pain may be relieved by change in the posture and by

ESSENTIALS OF MEDICINE FOR DENTAL STUDENTS

Table 1.1: Characteristics of chest pain in stable angina.

Site of the pain	Retrosternal or precordial
Character	Squeezing, constricting, piercing, feeling of heaviness or pressure
Precipitating factors	Physical exertion, cold exposure, heavy meals, emotional stress, anemia, thyroid disease, vivid dreams (nocturnal angina)
Associated features	Feeling of impending death, breathlessness, apprehension, nausea, vomiting
Relieving factors	Rest, sublingual nitroglycerin
Radiation	Left shoulder, both arms, jaw, neck
Duration	Typically 2–10 minutes (>30 minutes suggests infarction)

Table 1.2: Common symptoms in various systemic disorders.

General
- Fever
- Weight loss/Weight gain
- Weakness
- Bodyache
- Headache

Respiratory system
- Cough
- Sputum
- Hemoptysis
- Dyspnea
- Chest pain
- Wheezing

Cardiovascular system
- Chest pain
- Dyspnea
- Orthopnea
- Palpitation
- Edema
- Cough

Gastrointestinal system
- Anorexia
- Nausea
- Vomiting
- Heart burn
- Dysphagia
- Diarrhea
- Constipation
- Jaundice
- Pain in abdomen
- Vomiting of blood (hematemesis)
- Blood in stool (hematochezia, malena)

Hematological system
- Pallor
- Weakness
- Fever
- Dyspnea
- Bleeding
- Lymph gland enlargement

Urinary system
- Dysuria
- Hematuria
- Polyuria
- Oliguria
- Anuria
- Retention

Nervous system
- Headache
- Seizures
- Stroke
- Altered sensorium

simple analgesics. Anginal pain is relieved by sublingual nitrates. Pain can be radiating or referred. Radiating pain travels along with some anatomical part such as ureteric colic while referred pain is because of same dermatomal supply. History should include progression of symptoms. Negative history is also important

The typical anginal (ischemic) pain is described in **Table 1.1**.

Symptoms pertaining to different systems are asked. Important symptoms regarding disorders of various systems are given in **Table 1.2**.

History of Past Illness

A detailed account is noted about any illness which occurred in the past. A disease or symptom which has occurred in the past could be a part of the present disease process or related to the present problem.

For example, a patient with liver cirrhosis may give a history of jaundice or blood transfusion.

History of chronic illnesses like tuberculosis, diabetes mellitus, hypertension, stroke, epilepsy, coronary artery disease and autoimmune disorders should be asked.

Treatment History

The details of medications taken are noted. History of any adverse effects of drugs is also asked. It is imperative to know what drugs the patient is taking currently so that drug interactions may be avoided. The history of intake of certain drugs may help in knowing the cause of disease. For example, steroids and NSAIDs can cause gastric erosion and hematemesis.

History of previous hospitalizations, prolonged treatment, history of allergic/hypersensitivity reactions should be noted. Many drugs are available over the counter without any proper prescription. Self-administration of drugs, herbal remedies, alternative medicines to be recorded.

It is noted whether the patient has been compliant or not. If not, the reason for the drug noncompliance is discussed.

Personal History

The patient is asked about the consumption of alcohol, tobacco or smoking. His occupation should also be noted.

Personal history includes dietary history, appetite, work pattern, bowel and bladder habits and addiction. Addiction is stated only when person is physically and psychologically dependent on something. Diet is important as it can lead to various deficiency disorders and malnutrition. Vitamin B_{12} deficiency is more common in vegans. Diet having inadequate fibers leads to constipation. Consumption of khesari dal can lead to lathyrism. Hobbies such as pets, exposure to birds can cause hypersensitivity pneumonitis. Sedentary lifestyle is associated with obesity and metabolic disorders. Shift duties lead to anxiety, depression and insomnia. Stress can predispose to hypertension, diabetes and coronary artery disease.

Certain occupations are associated with a higher incidence of a particular disease, e.g., persons working in a silica factory are prone to develop silicosis. A history of stress at home and office should also be recorded. Financial status of the patient is also an important fact to be noted in the history.

Lower socioeconomic status is associated with increased prevalence of malnutrition and infectious diseases because of poor hygienic practices, illiteracy and overcrowding.

Family History

Any history of genetic disorders in the family is enquired about. Any history of similar illness in other family members and cause of death of immediate relative should be recorded. History of hypertension, diabetes mellitus, tuberculosis, cardiovascular diseases, and bleeding diathesis in other family members should be noted.

Family history is also important for environmental factors. Communicable diseases get transmitted in close contacts and family members.

Menstrual History

Women should be asked about menstruation. Regularity of the cycle, duration of cycle, and amount of bleeding are noted. Age of menarche and dysmenorrhea is also recorded. Obstetric history is also important. Obstetric history includes number of pregnancies, abortions, stillbirths and children alive. Osteoporosis is very common in postmenopausal females. Many drugs are contraindicated or avoided during pregnancy. Migraine can be triggered by menstruation and heart failure may become worse during pregnancy. Excessive bleeding during menstruation (menorrhagia) may be due to bleeding disorder and amenorrhea can occur in certain diseases.

PHYSICAL EXAMINATION

- Proper physical examination needs cooperation of the patient
- The patient should be comfortable and relaxed
- The nature and need of such an examination should be explained to him
- Examination is performed in a quiet and well-lit room. Day light is always better as skin color may look different from actual in artificial light
- Examination is carried out as gently as possible
- Physician should stand on right side of the patient
- Part to be examined has to be adequately exposed.

The examination is carried out in a routine manner. However, the information from the history may suggest which part or system should be particularly examined in greater detail.

The examination is customarily divided into general and systemic examination. **Systemic examination is described in specific chapters.**

General Physical Examination

General examination of the patient starts even as the history is being taken. A standard scheme should be followed to avoid any omissions. Points that should be noted are given in **Table 1.3**.

Physician should have stethoscope, measuring tape, thermometer, torch, sphygmomanometer, tuning fork, cotton wool and patellar hammer for examination.

Mental and Emotional Status

History taking and simple observations can assess the mental, emotional status and intelligence of the patient. State of consciousness is noted.

- In *a confusional state*, the patient is subdued, drowsy and physically inactive. He is also disoriented about time, place and person
- *Delerium* is a confusional state accompanied by agitation, hallucination and illusion. These always indicate disease of the nervous system
- *Stupor* state is lesser degree of altered consciousness from which patient can be awakened by vigorous stimuli.
- *Coma* is a deep sleep-like state from which the patient cannot be aroused. The patient does not respond to external stimulus or to inner needs
- In *dementia*, there is a loss of previously acquired intellectual functions but in the absence of impairment of

Table 1.3: Points for general physical examination.

- Mental and emotional state
- Built of the body
- Facial expression
- Temperature
- Pulse
- Blood pressure
- Respiration
- Anemia
- Jaundice
- Cyanosis
- Oral cavity and throat
- Neck veins
- Thyroid
- Lymphadenopathy
- Clubbing
- Peripheral edema
- Skin and mucous membrane

consciousness. Memory is the most common intellectual function lost in dementia.

Facial Expression

Mask like facies is found in Parkinsonism. The look is apathetic in hypothyroidism. Patient of Grave's disease has startled expression while those with anxiety or mania may have agitated look.

Built of the Body

This can be assessed by general inspection. The physique may be short, tall, obese, muscular, thin or asthenic.
- Dwarfism is found in hypopituitarism, hypothyroidism, and achondroplasia
- Height is increased in Marfan's syndrome and hyperpituitarism (gigantism)
- Weight loss may occur in malnutrition, malabsorption, thyrotoxicosis, chronic infections (tuberculosis), diabetes mellitus, malignancies, depression, anxiety, and anorexia nervosa. Weight loss despite normal or increased food intake suggests diabetes mellitus, thyrotoxicosis or malabsorption
- Weight gain may occur due to hypothyroidism or fluid retention.

The most widely used method to measure obesity is body mass index (BMI). BMI is calculated as weight in kg divided by the square of height in meters (kg/m^2). According to Indian consensus guidelines, BMI of 18.5–22.9 is normal, 23–24.9 is overweight and above 25 is obesity **(Table 1.4)**. Abdominal obesity (increased waist-hip ratio: >0.9 in females, >1.0 in males) is an important risk factor for coronary artery disease.

Temperature

Temperature is measured with a thermometer. Thermometer is placed in the mouth or in the axilla in adults, while it is placed in the fold of the groin with thigh flexed or in the rectum in case of small children.
- Mouth temperature is 0.5°C higher than that of groin or axillae. Rectal temperature is about 0.4°C (0.7°F) higher than mouth temperature
- The evening (pm) temperature may be up to 0.5°C or 0.9°F higher than the morning (am) temperature in normal persons
- The maximum normal is 37.2°C (98.9°F) at 6 am and 37.7°C (99.9°F) at 4 pm
- A fever of more than 41.5°C (106.7°F) is known as *hyperpyrexia*. A temperature less than 35°C (95°F) is called *hypothermia*.

The causes of hypothermia are severe hypothyroidism, water emersion and exposure to cold weather.

The fever may be continued, remittent or intermittent. These classical patterns of fever are less commonly seen due to early initiation of treatment with antipyretics and antibiotics.

Chill is sensation of cold which is associated with most of the cases of fever. Rigor is piloerection associated with severe shivering.
- Fever, which at no time touches the normal and does not fluctuate more than 1°C during 24 hours is called *continued* fever.
- When the daily fluctuation in the temperature is more than 2°C, the fever is of the *remittent* type.
- Fever, which occurs only for several hours during 24 hours is called *intermittent fever*. Intermittent fever can be quotidian (occurs daily), tertian (occurs on alternate days) or quartan (occurs every third day). Infection with *P. falciparum* causes intermittent quotidian fever, *P. vivax* and *P. ovale* cause tertian fever and *P. malariae* causes quartan fever.

Step ladder pattern of fever is found in enteric fever, saddleback in dengue and Pel-Ebstein type in Hodgkin's disease. Pel-Ebstein fever is cyclic fever where there is equal duration of febrile and afebrile period (3–10 days).

Pulse

Arterial pulse should be examined mainly for following things:
- Rate.
- Rhythm.
- Volume.
- Character.
- Radiofemoral delay.
- Synchronicity.

The rate and rhythm are assessed by palpating the radial artery **(Fig. 1.1)**. The character of the pulse is better assessed by palpating the carotid artery **(Fig. 1.2)**. Carotid pulses should not be palpated simultaneously. Other peripheral arteries like brachial, popliteal, posterior tibial and dorsalis

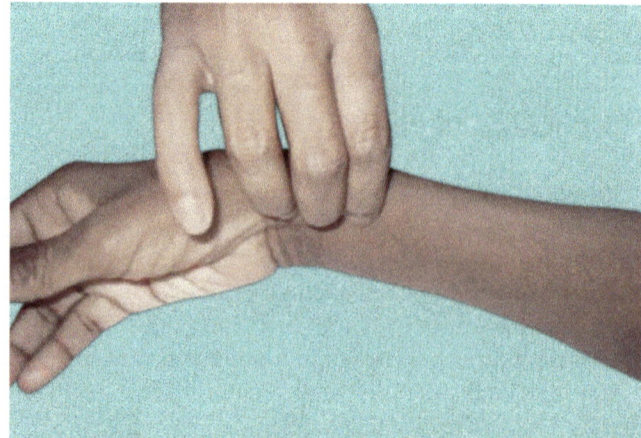

Fig. 1.1: Palpation of the radial artery; the forearm of the patient is in semiprone position with wrist semiflexed.

Table 1.4: Body mass index values (kg/m^2).	
• Normal	18.5–22.9
• Overweight	23.0–24.9
• Obesity	more than 25

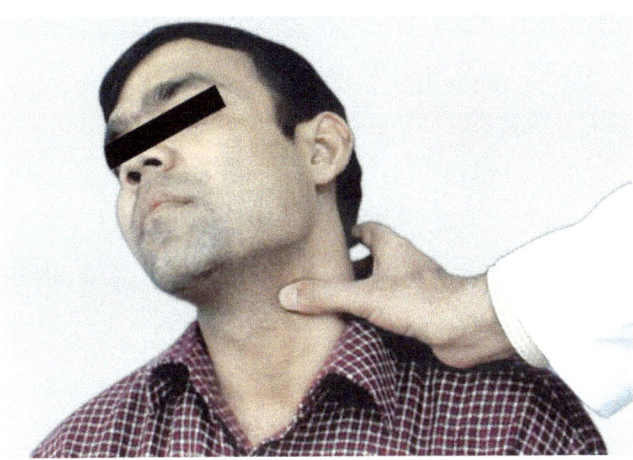

Fig. 1.2: Palpation of the left carotid artery with the right thumb.

Table 1.5: Causes of pulse rate abnormalities.

Bradycardia
- Raised intracranial pressure
- Heart blocks
- Sinus node disease
- Cholestatic jaundice
- Hypothyroidism
- Drugs (beta blockers, verapamil, digoxin)
- Athletes

Tachycardia
- Fever
- Exercise
- Anxiety
- Thyrotoxicosis
- Anemia
- Tachyarrhythmias
- Shock
- Drugs (theophylines, beta agonists, anticholinergics)

pedis can also be palpated. The pulse may be *absent or weak* in obstruction in the proximal part of the artery due to thromboembolism and atherosclerosis.

Rate: The *pulse rate* is determined by counting it for at least 30 seconds. The normal pulse rate varies from 60–100 per minute **(Table 1.5)**.

- Bradycardia is defined as pulse rate <60/min. Important causes are raised intracranial pressure, heart blocks and sinus node disease, cholestatic jaundice, hypothyroidism and drugs (beta blockers, verapamil, digoxin). Bradycardia may also be present in athletes
- Tachycardia(pulse rate >100/min) occurs due to fever, exercise, anxiety, thyrotoxicosis, anemia, tachyarrhythmias, shock and drugs
- Pulse is slower than would be expected from the height of fever in typhoid fever *(relative bradycardia).*

Rhythm: Normally the rhythm of the pulse is regular. An *irregular rhythm* is seen in atrial fibrillation (irregularly irregular) and frequent ectopic beats (regularly irregular).

Character:
- Low volume pulse is noted in shock and heart failure. A low volume and slow rising pulse *(parvu set tardus)* is found in aortic stenosis (AS)

- A large bounding pulse (hyperkinetic pulse, high volume) is seen in hyperkinetic states (anemia, fever, anxiety, thyrotoxicosis, beri beri, Paget's disease, exercise), patent ductus arteriosus, ventricular septal defect, and aortic regurgitation (AR)
- *Bisferiens pulse* which has two systolic peaks is found in mixed lesion of AS and AR
- Alternating strong and weak pulse *(pulsus alternans)* is present in severe left ventricular failure
- Normally, there is a fall in systolic arterial pressure of <10 mmHg during inspiration. An accentuation in this phenomenon can lead to weakening or disappearance of pulse during inspiration *(paradoxical pulse)*. This is found in cardiac tamponade and obstructive airway disease.

Radiofemoral delay: The femoral pulse is weak and delayed as compared with the radial pulse *(radiofemoral delay)* in coarctation of aorta.

Blood Pressure

Blood pressure (BP) is measured with the help of a sphygmomanometer.
- BP should be measured in both arms and also in the lower limb. In coarctation of aorta, the arterial pressure in the upper limb is much higher than in the lower limbs
- Patient and doctor should not talk during the blood pressure measurement
- Patient should not sit crossed legged
- The patient should be sitting at ease and must not be having distended urinary bladder at the time of blood pressure measurement
- The cuff should be applied closely to the upper arm; it should not be loose or tight. The lower border of the cuff must be one inch (2.5 cm) above the cubital fossa
- The instrument should be placed at the same level as the cuff on the patient's arm and the observer's eye
- The standard cuff width for adults is 12.5 cm. The size of cuff is also important since a small cuff may record false high blood pressure
- The blood pressure must be recorded when the patient is resting quietly as anxiety, exertion, excitement, smoking and intake of coffee and tea within last half an hour will give rise to false readings
- In elderly and patients on drugs (for hypertension), BP should be recorded in standing and lying down position to detect the occurrence of postural hypotension.

Initially the assessment of systolic BP is made by palpatory method. The radial or brachial artery is palpated while the cuff is inflated to raise pressure about 30 mmHg above the level at which radial/brachial pulse disappears The stethoscope is placed over the brachial artery and cuff is deflated slowly **(Figs. 1.3A and B)**. The level at which Korotkoff sounds appear (phase 1) is the systolic pressure and the level at which they disappear completely (phase 5) is the diastolic pressure. When the *pulse pressure* (the difference between systolic and diastolic blood pressure) is increased as

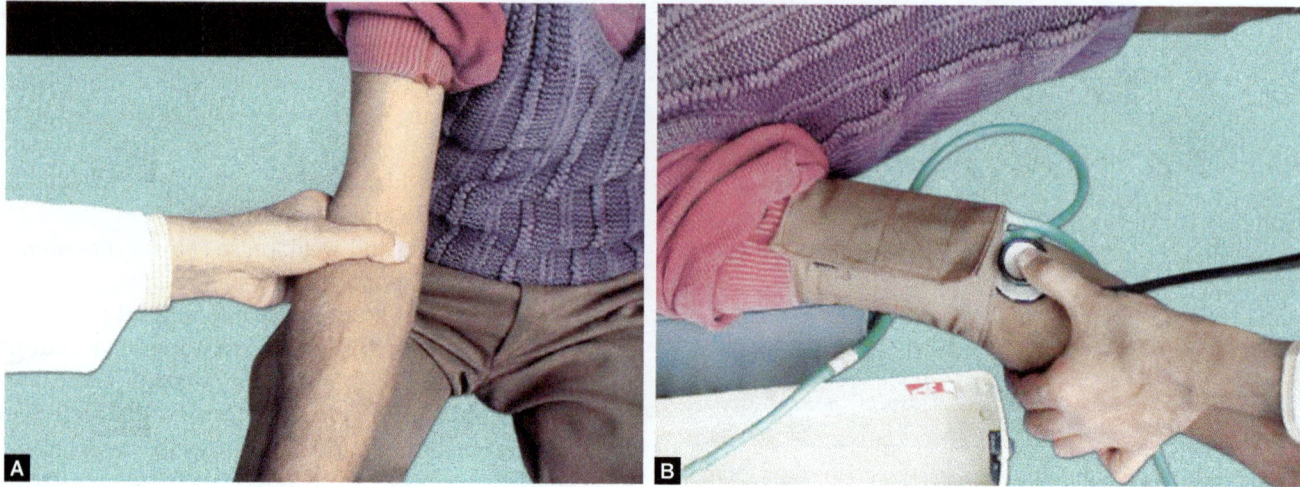

Figs. 1.3A and B: (A) Localization of brachial artery; (B) Measurement of blood pressure; Note the position of cuff and the stethoscope.

in cases with hyperdynamic circulation (aortic regurgitation, pregnancy, thyrotoxicosis, anemia, arteriovenous fistula) the sounds may not disappear completely even at 0 level. In such cases the level at which sounds become suddenly muffled (phase 4) is taken as diastolic blood pressure. Mean arterial blood pressure is diastolic blood pressure +1/3 of pulse pressure.

Auscultatory gap or silent gap: In occasional patient of hypertension after initial appearance of korotkoff sounds (phase 1) that depicts systolic blood pressure, there is disappearance of sounds and as the cuff further deflated sounds reappear and finally disappear that marks diastolic pressure.

The patient is said to be hypertensive if the systolic BP is >140 mmHg and/or diastolic BP is >90 mmHg **(Table 1.6)**. Sometimes the blood pressure recorded by the clinician at clinic or hospital is high while normal readings are obtained at home or when BP is measured under casual circumstances. This is known as *white coat hypertension* and is the result of the anxiety upon visiting a physician or a hospital.

Orthostatic or postural hypotension is characterized by fall in systolic blood pressure of >20 mmHg and >10 mmHg in diastolic blood pressure within 3 minutes of standing from supine position in absence of any antihypertensive treatment. It suggests defects of autonomic nervous system.

Jugular Venous Pulse

It provides an estimate of central venous pressure and hence it denotes volume status and cardiac function of patient **(Fig. 1.4)**. Pulsations and pressure in internal jugular vein in the neck are noted between the two heads of sternocleidomastoid **(Fig. 1.5)**. Fluctuations in right atrial pressure during the cardiac cycle generate a pulse that is transmitted backwards into the jugular veins.

- *Venous vs arterial pulsation:* Venous pulsations must be differentiated from carotid artery pulsations. Venous pulsations are better seen while arterial pulsations are better palpable. The upper level of venous pulsation varies with the change in posture and phases of respiration
- Pressure at the root of the neck causes disappearance of venous pulsations
- It is measured in semi-recumbent position, at sternal angle a vertical scale is placed and in the neck uppermost

Table 1.6: Classification of blood pressure for adults (>18 years) based on office blood pressure measurement.

Category	Systolic blood pressure (mmHg)	Diastolic blood pressure (mmHg)
Normal	<130	<85
High-normal BP	130–139	85–89
Hypertension	>140	>90
Stage 1	140–159	90–99
Stage 2	>160	>100

Note: Blood pressure values are based on the average of two or more readings taken at each of two or more visits after an initial screening. When systolic and diastolic values fall into different categories, the higher category should be selected for classification.

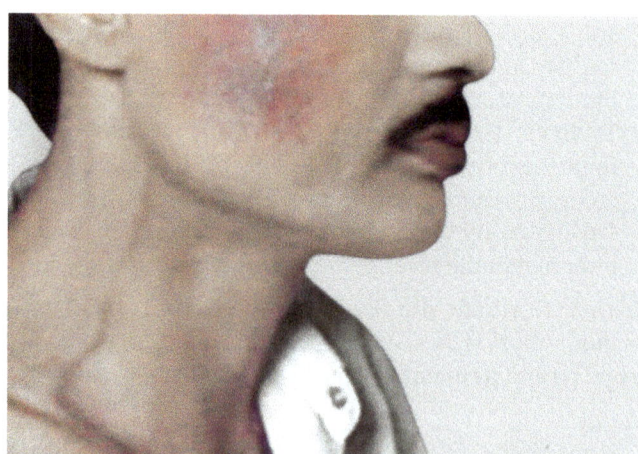

Fig. 1.4: Prominent jugular vein.

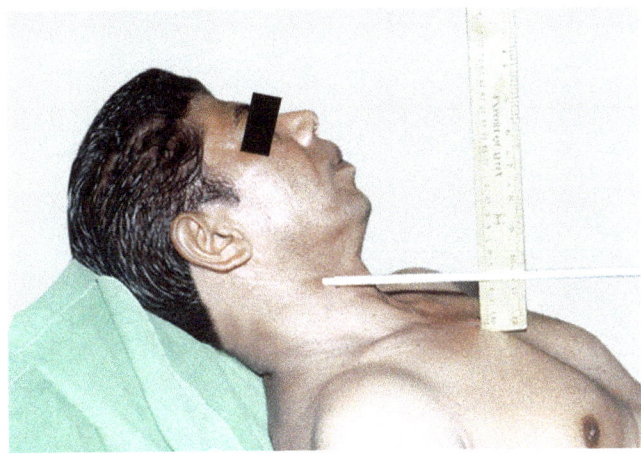

Fig. 1.5: How to measure JVP in a patient.

level of pulsations are noted with the help of horizontal scale. Normal JVP in health should be <3–4 cm of water (H_2O), 1.36 cm H_2O = 1.0 mmHg
- Jugular veins are distended and pulsatile in congestive heart failure and pericardial effusion. Neck veins are also distended in cases of mediastinal tumors and retrosternal goiter but these are not pulsatile
- Normally there is fall in the jugular venous pressure (JVP) during inspiration. There may be a paradoxical rise in the JVP during inspiration in constrictive pericarditis and cardiac tamponade (*Kussmaul's sign*).

Hepatojugular reflex: It is elicited by firm compression over right hypochondrium for 30 seconds. In normal individuals JVP will increase to less than 3 cm and falls even when pressure is continued. In patients with impending heart failure, JVP remains elevated.

The venous pulse has three positive waves a, c, and v and two negative waves or descents x and y. The a wave is due to atrial contraction. This is followed by x descent (due to descent of tricuspid valve ring) which is interrupted by a small c wave. The v wave is due to passive filling of blood from veins into the right atrium during ventricular systole. This is followed by y descent due to rapid flow of blood from the right atrium to the right ventricle when the tricuspid valve is open **(Fig. 1.6)**.

The "a" wave is absent in atrial fibrillation, while it is prominent in tricuspid stenosis (TS). Prominent "y" descent is seen in tricuspid regurgitation.

Respiration

Normal rate of respiration is 12–16 per minute in adults. The causes of fast breathing (tachypnea) are given in **Table 1.7**. Dyspnea is an abnormally uncomfortable awareness of breathing. This could be due to respiratory diseases, cardiac diseases, anemia, acidosis and psychogenic. Dyspnea, orthopnea and paroxysmal nocturnal dyspnea are described in detail in Chapters 5 and 6.
- Noisy breathing may occur due to obstruction of the respiratory passages at various levels. Obstruction at

Table 1.7: Causes of tachypnea.

- Recent exertion
- Anxiety
- Fever
- Metabolic acidosis
- Hysterical overbreathing
- Pulmonary and cardiac conditions causing hypoxia
- Cerebral disturbance

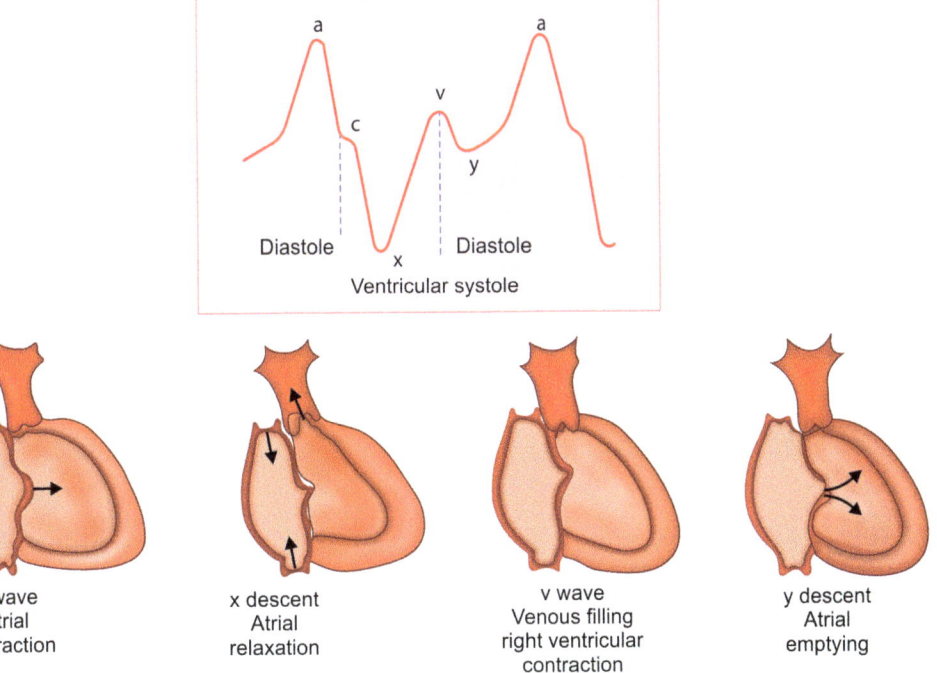

Fig. 1.6: Wave forms of jugular venous pulse.

the level of larynx and trachea causes inspiratory stridor and obstruction in bronchi and bronchioles produces wheezing
- Rapid and deep respiration (Kussmaul's breathing) is present in metabolic acidosis, while rapid shallow breathing is a feature of restrictive lung disease
- Cheyne-Stokes respiration is characterized by cyclical waxing and waning of rate and depth of respiration intervened with periods of apnea. It is observed in narcotic overdose and severe left heart failure.

Pallor

- The presence of pallor depends on the thickness and quality of the skin, amount of blood in the capillaries and quality of the blood in the capillaries
- The evidence of pallor is looked at palpebral conjunctiva and mucous membrane of the mouth (**Figs. 1.7 and 1.8**). Other sites are nail bed and palmar creases (**Fig. 1.9**)
- If the color of the palmar crease becomes pallor than the surrounding area, it is suggestive of severe anemia
- Generalized pallor is present in anemia. Pallor can also be found in hypopituitarism, thick or opaque skin, and

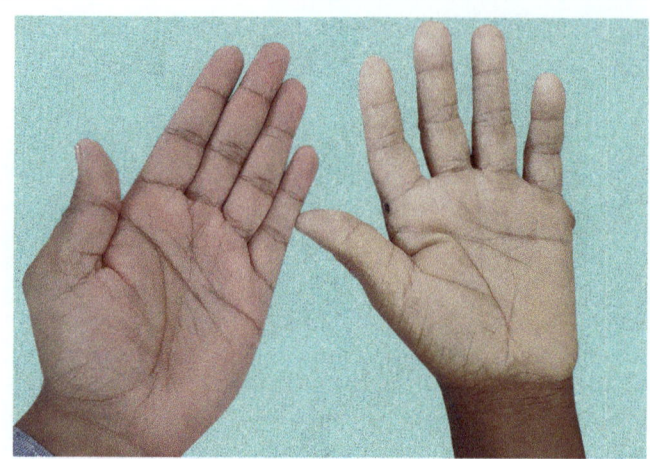

Fig. 1.9: Pallor of the palm; compare with palm of normal person (left).

diminished capillary blood flow as in shock, syncope, left heart failure.

Jaundice

A yellowish discoloration of the skin and mucous membrane due to deposition of bilirubin is known as jaundice (icterus). The deposition of bilirubin in tissues occurs when the serum bilirubin level is raised (hyperbilirubinemia). Sclerae have a high affinity for bilirubin due to their rich elastin content. (For details, see Chapter 3).
- The normal total serum bilirubin level is 0.3–1.0 mg/dL. Jaundice is clinically apparent in sclera when the bilirubin level is raised above 3 mg/dL (**Fig. 1.10**)
- The clinical detection of jaundice is difficult in artificial light. Hence, it should be examined preferably in day light. Besides sclera, other sites to be looked for the evidence of jaundice are mucosa of oral cavity underneath the tongue and skin
- Yellow discoloration of the skin can also occur in *carotenemia* (carotenoderma) and exposure to *quinacrine or phenols*. Sclera is typically not involved in carotenemia. Carotenemia is more prominent on palms and soles and nasolabial folds.

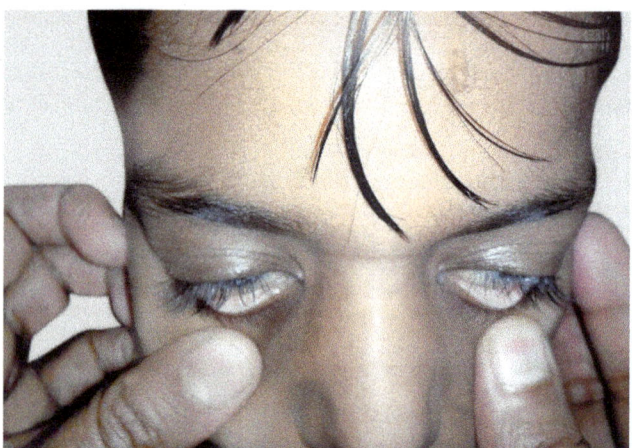

Fig. 1.7: Palpebral conjunctiva showing pallor.

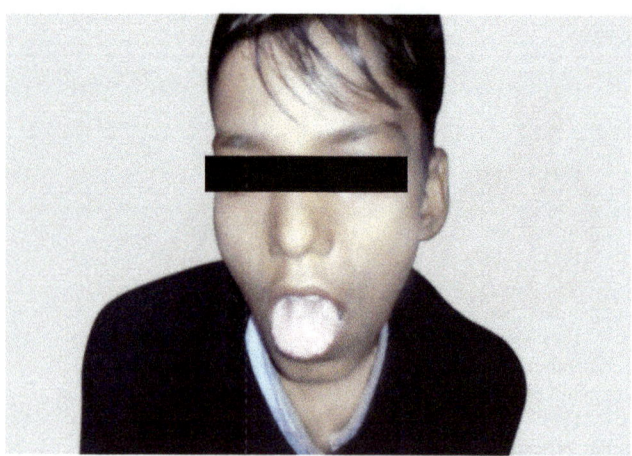

Fig. 1.8: Pallor visible at tongue.

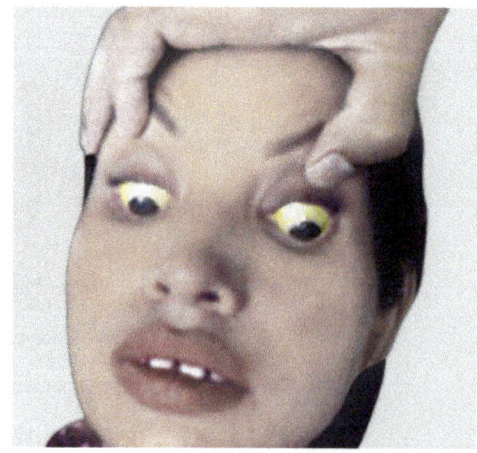

Fig. 1.10: Jaundice visible over sclera.

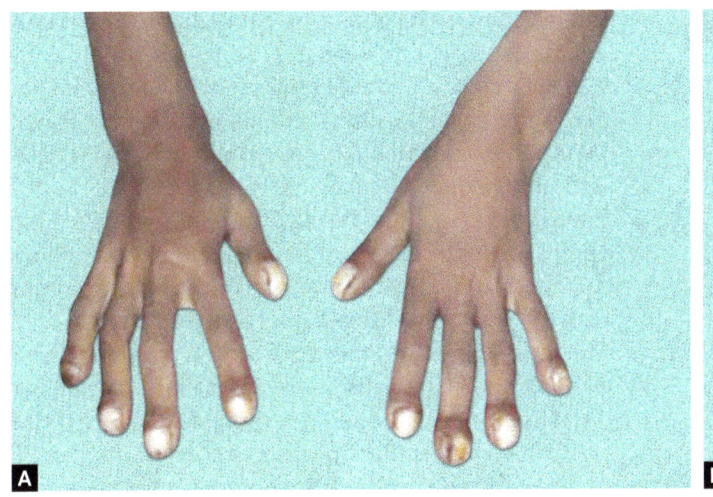
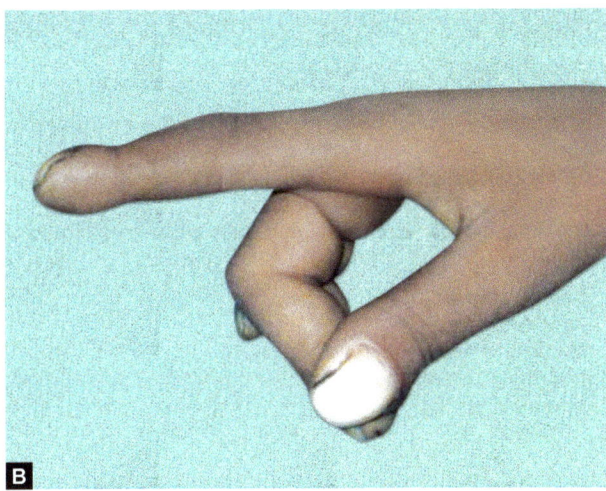

Figs. 1.11A and B: (A) Marked digital clubbing; (B) Severe clubbing (drumstick appearance).

Clubbing

The enlargement of the distal portion of the fingers and toes, due to proliferation of connective tissues, is known as clubbing **(Fig. 1.11A)**. The clubbing is graded as follows:
- *Grade I:* There is thickening of tissues at the nail base
- *Grade II:* In addition to the features of grade I, the angle between nail base and the adjacent skin fold of the finger is obliterated. There is reduction in the space between thumb nails when placed in apposition as an angle of greater than 180° between the nail and nail-fold is lost *(Schamroth's window test)*
- *Grade III:* In addition to the features of grade I and grade II, the shape of the nail becomes convex in both horizontal and vertical directions. In severe cases there is bulbous enlargement of the distal segment of the fingers (drumstick appearance) **(Fig. 1.11B)**
- *Grade IV:* Along with the clubbing, there may be swelling above the wrist and ankles due to periostitis of long bones *(hypertrophic osteoarthropathy)*.

The exact mechanism of clubbing is clearly not known. However, it is thought to be due to some humoral substances leading to increased vascularity in the nail bed.

Clubbing may be present since birth (congenital), or acquired. Acquired causes of clubbing are given in **Table 1.8**.

Cyanosis

Cyanosis is bluish discoloration of the skin and mucous membrane caused by an increased quantity of reduced hemoglobin (>4 g%) in superficial blood vessels. The bluish discoloration can also be seen in methemoglobinemia and sulfhemoglobinemia where the patient is cyanosed, but not breathless. A cherry red discoloration is caused by carboxyhemoglobin in carbon monoxide poisoning (not true cyanosis).

Cyanosis is looked for at lips, nail beds, malar area, ear lobes and mucous membrane of the oral cavity **(Fig. 1.12)**.

Table 1.8: Causes of clubbing.

Respiratory diseases
- Chronic suppurative lung diseases
  - Lung abscess
  - Bronchiectasis
  - Empyema
- Bronchogenic carcinoma
- Mesothelioma (pleural neoplasm)
- Pulmonary tuberculosis
- Fibrosing alveolitis

Cardiac diseases
- Congenital cyanotic heart diseases
  - Fallot's tetralogy
  - Eisenmenger syndrome
- Subacute bacterial endocarditis

Gastrointestinal diseases
- Inflammatory bowel diseases
  - Ulcerative colitis
  - Crohn's disease
- Hepatic cirrhosis

Idiopathic

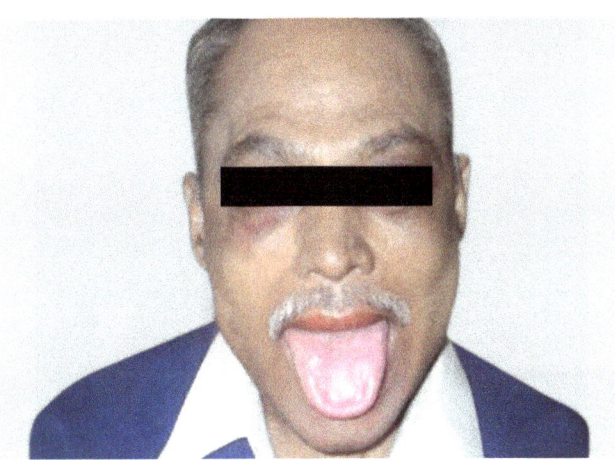

Fig. 1.12: Central cyanosis.

Table 1.9: Causes of cyanosis.

Central cyanosis
- High altitude
- Respiratory diseases (COPD, extensive pneumonia, pulmonary edema, massive pulmonary embolism)
- Cardiac diseases (congenital cyanotic heart diseases, Eisenmenger syndrome, heart failure)
- Abnormal hemoglobin (methemoglobinemia, sulfhemo globinemia)

Peripheral cyanosis
- Cold exposure
- Heart failure (reduced cardiac output)
- Arterial obstruction
- Venous obstruction

Cyanosis is classified into central and peripheral types (**Table 1.9**).

- The imperfect oxygen saturation or abnormal hemoglobin derivatives lead to *central cyanosis*, which is seen in both the mucous membrane (tongue) and skin and also nail beds of the limbs. The extremities are warm.
- *Peripheral cyanosis* is due to excessive extraction of oxygen from the capillaries when the flow of blood is slow. The extremities are cyanosed and cold, while mucous membrane of the oral cavity and tongue are spared. Warming of the cyanotic extremity may increase blood flow and abolish peripheral (but not central) cyanosis. Improvement in oxygenation will reduce central cyanosis while peripheral cyanosis will be unaffected.
- Cyanosis due to heart failure is of *mixed type*, both central and peripheral. Differential cyanosis involves only lower extremities and not present in upper and is seen in cases of patent ductus arteriosus with reversal of shunt (**Fig. 1.13**).

Edema

Edema is the presence of an excess of fluid in interstitial space causing swelling of the tissues.

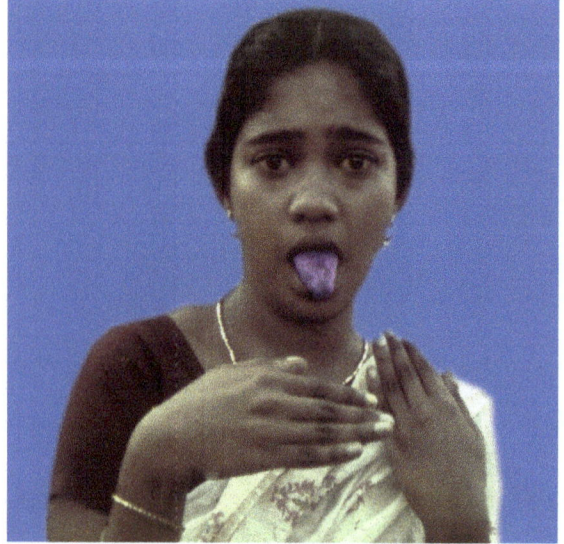

Fig. 1.13: Patient with differential cyanosis and central cyanosis.

- Edema may be localized or generalized. Generalized edema is known as anasarca, in which the fluid may also accumulate in the pleural cavity (hydrothorax) and peritoneal cavity (ascites). Edema over feet is known as pedal edema. It can be unilateral or bilateral (**Fig. 1.14**). Causes of pedal edema are given in **Table 1.10**.
- Edema may be of the pitting or non-pitting type. Pitting edema means formation of an indentation or pit following the application of firm pressure for a sustained period over the area of swelling (**Figs. 1.15A and B**).

The mechanisms of edema can be described as follows:
- The hydrostatic pressure in vascular system and tissue colloid oncotic pressure tend to drive fluid from the vascular to the extravascular space. On the contrary, colloid oncotic pressure maintained by plasma proteins in the vascular system and hydrostatic pressure in the interstitial fluid promote the movement of fluid in the vascular compartment. The development of edema is a result of the imbalance between these "Starling forces". For example, the edema in congestive heart failure is due to an increase in the vascular hydrostatic pressure. A decrease in the plasma colloid oncotic pressure is the cause of edema in hypoalbuminic states like nephrotic syndrome,

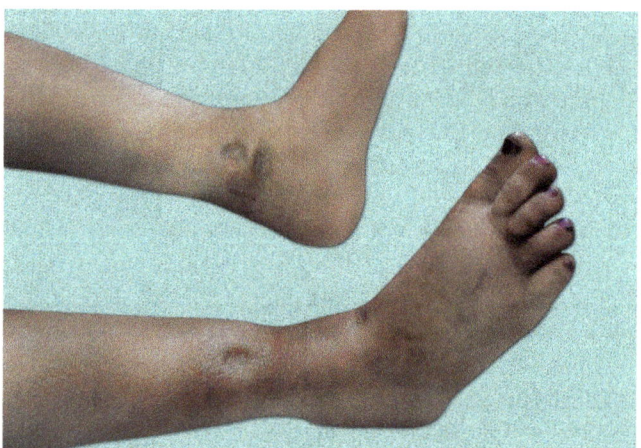

Fig. 1.14: Bilateral pedal edema.

Table 1.10: Causes of pedal edema.

Bilateral pedal edema
Pitting type
- Congestive heart failure
- Nephrotic syndrome, acute nephritis
- Liver cirrhosis
- Malnutrition
- Epidemic dropsy
- Drugs (calcium channel blockers, NSAIDs, steroids)

Non-pitting type
- Myxedema

Unilateral edema
- Filariasis
- Thrombophlebitis
- Cellulitis
- Trauma
- Regional lymph node resection

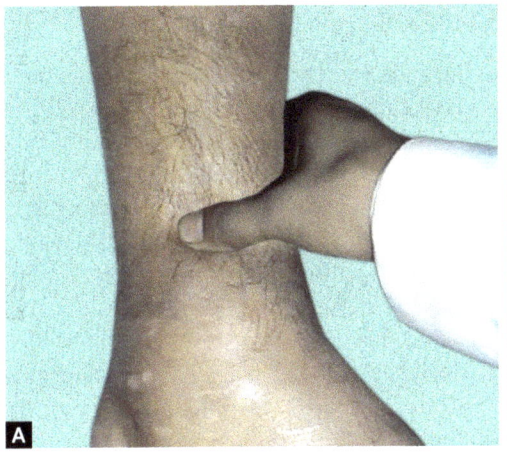
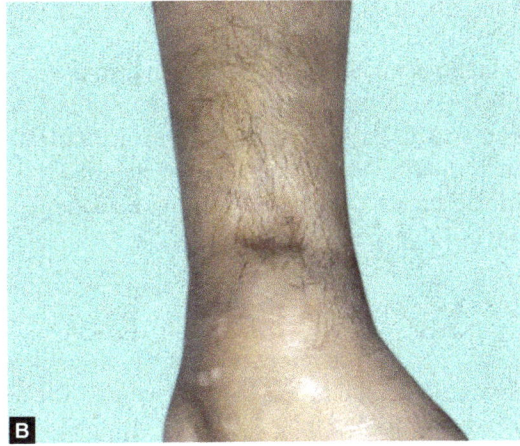

Figs. 1.15A and B: (A) Pressure applied over edematous limb; (B) Pitting edema.

malnutrition and liver disease. The edema is of the pitting type.
- Edema may result from damage to the capillary endothelium which causes exudation of fluid and protein due to increased permeability. Injury to capillary endothelium may occur due to drugs, infections and trauma. Capillary permeability is also increased in hypersensitivity reactions. This type of edema is usually localized, non-pitting and may be accompanied by other signs of inflammation.
- In many forms of edema, the effective arterial blood volume is reduced. This in turn initiates physiological mechanisms to restore the volume by renal salt and water retention, which further adds up to the edema. Compensatory physiological responses are activation of rennin-angiotensin-aldosterone system, and increased secretion of vasopressin.

Edema generally appears first over the periorbital area and is more marked in the mornings, in nephrotic syndrome and acute nephritis (see **Fig. 7.1**). In heart failure, the edema is more marked during the evenings and present over the ankles and dorsum of the feet. In these conditions, edema may become generalized later on. In bedridden patients, the edema first appears in the presacral region.

Localized edema in a single limb is generally due to either venous or lymphatic obstruction. For example, edema of the leg may occur due to thrombosis of the popliteal or femoral vein. Compression of axillary vein due to malignant lymph nodes may cause edema of the arm.

Lymphatic obstruction due to resection of regional lymph nodes or in filariasis leads to non-pitting edema. Generalized non-pitting edema is found in myxedema.

Lymph Nodes

Palpation of lymph nodes is an important part of general examination (**Fig. 1.16**). Lymph nodes are examined for:
- Size
- Number
- Texture
- Tenderness

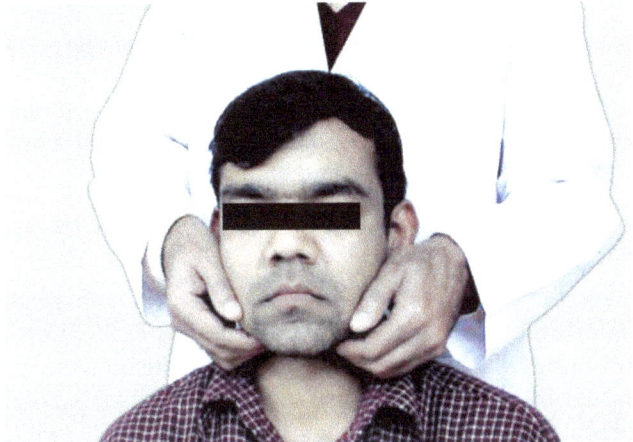

Fig. 1.16: Palpation of the submandibular lymph nodes.

- Mobility
- Signs of inflammation over the nodes.

Important groups of lymph nodes which must be examined are submental, submandibular, preauricular, postauricular, cervical (anterior and posterior chains), supraclavicular, axillary and inguinals. For other details, see Chapter 4.

Nails

- Koilonychia: Spoon shaped nails (iron deficiency)
- Leukonychia: White nails (hypoalbuminemia)
- Beau's lines: Transverse ridges due to temporary arrest of nail growth
- Splinter hemorrhages: Infective endocarditis
- Onycholysis: Separation of nail from nail bed (thyrotoxicosis, psoriasis).

Examination of Hand

- Warm sweaty hands: Anxiety, hyperthyroidism
- Cold, dry hands: Hypothyroidism
- Large fleshy hands: Acromegaly
- Delayed relaxation of hands: Myotonic dystrophy
- Deformities: Rheumatoid arthritis.

Halitosis

Halitosis is an unpleasant odor or smell emerging from the mouth or nostrils that is detected by the patient or others. It is also referred as bad breath, breath malodor, puppy breath, and dragon mouth. About 35% of world population is suffering from bad breath problem. Important causes of halitosis are given in **Table 1.11**.

Types of Halitosis

- *Physiologic bad breath:* This affects all normal healthy persons and is caused by anaerobic bacterial overgrowth mainly on the tongue deep in the papillae.
- *Pathologic bad breath:* Occurs due to oral infections including carious teeth.
- *Halitophobia:* Some patients may complain of bad breath in spite of treatment being given to them. It may be due to psychiatric illness.
- *Transitory bad breath:* This type occurs after consumption of certain foods like garlic, onions and certain medications. It usually lasts for hours/days.

Pathophysiology of Halitosis

Anaerobic bacteria are responsible for bad breath. These bacteria are abundantly present in the oral cavity, tonsils and throat. Bacteria react with food, medications in the presence of acidic environment and produce volatile sulphur compounds (VSC) such as hydrogen sulphide (HS) which smells like rotten eggs, methyl mercaptans (smells like gym. socks), putrescine and cadverin (smells like old garbage).

Table 1.11: Causes of halitosis.

Dental causes
- Dental decay—caries, exposed teeth
- Gum diseases
- Oral infections—abscess
- Oral cancer
- Xerostomia (dry mouth)
- Mouth breathing habit
- Tongue coating

Medical causes
- Sinus infections, cough and cold
- Allergies, post-nasal drip
- Lung abscess
- Diabetic ketoacidosis (sweet and fruity)
- Renal failure (ammoniacal, urinary)
- Hepatic failure (fishy, mousy)
- Hiatus hernia
- Menstruation
- Medications

Miscellaneous
- Certain foods—fish, dairy products, garlic, eggs
- Smoking
- Alcohol
- Stress
- Certain professions
- High protein diets (Atkins diet)

Foods Causing Bad Breath

- *Sugars:* Bacteria cause breakdown of sugar and produce acidic environment.
- *Dense proteins/milk products:* Cheese, yoghurt, ice cream stay on the tongue and between teeth. Anaerobic bacteria break down the proteins and produce VSC.
- *Acidic foods:* Anaerobic bacteria multiply very fast in acidic medium and produce high levels of VSC. Acidic foods include coffee, tomato juice, citrus fruit juices, aerated drinks.
- *Onion, garlic, cabbage:* When taken raw, smell comes from mouth because of sulphur compounds present in them.

Examination/Tests for Halitosis

Scientifically proven ways to check breath:

- *Using Halimeter:* It measures the concentration of sulphides in the breath. Reading above 75 ppb (parts per billion) indicates bad breath.
- *Using bad breath detective:* It measures the amount of VSC coming from the tongue by simply swabbing the back of tongue and placing it into the test tube that comes with bad breath detective.
- Other methods used to detect halitosis are as follows:
  - Lick the back surface of hand, let it dry and smell after 15–20 seconds.
  - Use floss interdentally and smell it.
  - If the back surface of tongue is whitish it indicates that person has bad breath.
  - If friends, colleagues and relatives, move away or offer mint, while person is talking to them.

Myth about Halitosis

Bad breath comes from stomach is myth. There is no open tube connecting the stomach or intestines to mouth as there are valves, sphincters and muscles, etc., that keep digested food at its place.

Tongue and Bad Breath

Tongue is responsible for almost 85% of bad breath that comes from the mouth. Tongue has glossy surface so the food gets accumulated here and bacteria utilize the food to produce the VSC. Tongue cleaning is more effective than brushing in stopping bad breath. Tongue cleaning reduces oral bacteria thereby decreasing chances of bad breath and plaque formation. It also improves taste sensitivity and quality.

Treatment of Bad Breath

Treatment of bad breath is possible if the cause is removed. It can be done in multiple visits to dental clinic (fresh breath clinics). It includes following:

- Thorough dental and oral checkup
- Medical history to rule out any medical cause
- Dietary analysis and counseling
- Bad breath testing using halitometer
- Oral hygiene instructions and techniques.

Mouth wash: Sugar, saccharin and alcohol containing mouth washes should be avoided. Alcohol causes dryness of mouth. Special mouthwashes are used which release oxygen that kills the anaerobic bacteria.

Xylitol chewing gums: Sugar free xylitol chewing gums are also useful.

SCHEME OF THE GENERAL EXAMINATION

General Physical Examination:
- General appearance
- Mental state
- Built
- Height and weight
- Decubitus

Vitals:
- Pulse
  - Rate and rhythm (radial)
  - Character and volume (carotids)
  - Symmetry
- Blood pressure
- Temperature
- Respiration.

Eyes:
- Exophthalmos, ptosis, eye movements
- Conjunctiva—pallor, icterus
- Pupils—size, reaction to light and accommodation.

Face: Symmetry, puffiness, cyanosis, parotid gland.

Oral cavity: Odor, lips, tongue, teeth, gum, buccal mucous membrane.
- Lips: Color, eruption
- Teeth: Denture, other abnormalities
- Gums: Swelling, bleeding, inflammation, ulcers
- Tongue: Color, appearance, ulcers
- Buccal mucosa: Color, ulcers.

Pharynx: Tonsils, oropharynx.

Neck:
- JVP
- Thyroid
- Lymph nodes (cervical).

Upper limbs:
- Nails: Clubbing, koilonychia, pallor, cyanosis
- Pulse
- Blood pressure
- Lymph nodes (axillary).

Lower limbs:
- Edema of feet, ankles

FREQUENTLY USED TERMS

Certain terms are frequently used in clinical medicine. These have profound effects on presentations. Some important terms are defined below.

Diagnosis

Diagnosis is an act or process of identifying or determining the nature of a disease by way of examination and assessment of the symptoms and signs.

Diagnosis is an art wherein scientific methods are applied to the elucidation of problems presented by a patient. A concept is formed about the site, etiology, pathology and organ dysfunctions which constitutes the patient's disease.

Diagnosis provides a firm basis for the treatment and prognosis of the individual patients.

Clinical Diagnosis

Diagnosis made by bedside methods without the help of laboratory tests.

Differential Diagnosis

The recognition of a particular condition from amongst others which closely resemble it in certain aspects.

Prognosis

Prognosis is a considered opinion of the probable development and outcome of the disease based upon all the relevant available facts of the case.

Treatment

Treatment is the course of action adopted to deal with illness and control of the patient.

Illness

Illness is defined by the totality of effects, predicaments, and repercussions of the disease, deformity, or circumstances produced in the patient.

SELF ASSESSMENT

Multiple Choice Questions

1. Rate and rhythm of the pulse is best appreciated by palpating:
   A. Brachial artery   B. Radial artery
   C. Popliteal artery   D. Femoral artery
2. Following is not true in pulsus paradoxus:
   A. Found in cardiac tamponade
   B. Disappears during expiration
   C. Inspiratory fall in blood pressure
   D. May be present in bronchial asthma

3. Following conditions are associated with bradycardia, *except*:
   A. Hypothyroidism B. Athletes
   C. Hypotensive shock D. Raised intracranial tension
4. Edema in both lower limbs can occur in:
   A. Filariasis B. Cellulitis
   C. Nephrotic syndrome D. Popliteal vein thrombosis
5. Cyanosis in CHF is of following type:
   A. Central
   B. Peripheral
   C. Both, central and peripheral
   D. Not found
6. Which of the following is not matched correctly:
   A. Pulsus *Parvu set tardus*— aortic stenosis
   B. Pulsus besferiens—severe mitral stenosis
   C. Water hammer pulse—aortic regurgitation
   D. Hyperkinetic pulse—thyrotoxicosis
7. Clubbing can be found in the following, *except*:
   A. Bronchiectasis B. Lung abscess
   C. Pneumonia D. Bronchogenic carcinoma
8. Yellowish discoloration of sclera and skin occurs in the following:
   A. Carotinemia B. Hyperbilirubinemia
   C. Quinacrine ingestion D. Both A and B
   E. All of the above
9. Cyanosis is seen in:
   A. Fallot's tetralogy B. Methemoglobinemia
   C. Sulfhemoglobinemia D. All of the above
10. All of the following is true in peripheral cyanosis, *except*:
    A. It improves on warming
    B. Best seen in oral mucous membrane
    C. Occurs in cases with low cardiac output
    D. May occur following exposure to cold
11. Following is not matched properly:
    A. CHF _____ pedal edema
    B. Thyrotoxicosis _____ tachycardia
    C. High arterial CO_2 _____ cyanosis
    D. Orthopnea _____ mitral stenosis
12. Early morning periorbital edema suggests the disease of following system:
    A. Cardiac B. Renal
    C. Hepatic D. All of the above
13. "a" wave in JVP is absent in:
    A. Pericardial tamponade B. Complete heart block
    C. Atrial fibrillation D. Hypotension
14. Distended but nonpulsatile neck veins are found in:
    A. Right heart failure B. Tricuspid stenosis
    C. Mediastinal tumor D. Constrictive pericarditis
15. JVP is best examined in:
    A. External jugular vein B. Internal jugular vein
    C. Subclavian vein D. Any one of the above
16. Sweet fruity odor is found in the oral cavity in case of:
    A. Renal failure
    B. Hepatic failure
    C. Diabetic ketoacidosis
    D. All of the above
17. Blood pressure is generally measured by auscultating over following artery:
    A. Radial artery B. Brachial artery
    C. Carotid artery D. Any of the above
18. The diastolic BP corresponds best with:
    A. First appearance of Korotkoff sound
    B. Disappearance of Korotkoff sound
    C. Muffling of Korotkoff sound
    D. In between appearance and disappearance of korotkoff sound
19. The following can be measured by sphygmomanometer and palpating the artery:
    A. Systolic blood pressure
    B. Diastolic blood pressure
    C. Both
    D. None
20. In coarctation of aorta, following is true:
    A. BP in lower limbs is higher than in upper limbs
    B. BP is equal in lower and upper limbs
    C. BP in upper limb is higher than in lower limbs
    D. BP is generally not recordable in upper limbs
21. Cyanosis is accompanied with clubbing in the following, *except*:
    A. Eisenmenger's syndrome
    B. Fallot's tetralogy
    C. Interstitial lung disease
    D. Conditions with peripheral cyanosis
22. Clubbing may be present in the following, *except*:
    A. Lung cancer B. Crohn's disease
    C. Infective endocarditis D. Left to right cardiac shunts
23. Unilateral lower limb edema is present in all of the following conditions, *except*:
    A. Deep vein thrombosis B. Filariasis
    C. Trauma D. Nephrotic syndrome
24. Clubbing can be present in all of the following conditions, *except*:
    A. Mesothelioma
    B. Subacute bacterial endocarditis
    C. Lung abscess
    D. Bronchial asthma
25. Paradoxical rise in JVP during inspiration is seen in:
    A. Constrictive pericarditis
    B. Mitral stenosis
    C. Superior vena cava obstruction
    D. Cor-pulmonale
26. Kussmaul's breathing is present in:
    A. Metabolic acidosis B. Respiratory acidosis
    C. Metabolic alkalosis D. Respiratory alkalosis
27. If the blood pressure recorded at the clinic or hospital is high, while normal readings are obtained at home; this phenomenon is called:
    A. Masked hypertension
    B. White coat hypertension
    C. Labile hypertension
    D. Uncontrolled hypertension
28. Following is not properly matched:
    A. Clubbing_____Fallot's tetralogy
    B. Cyanosis_____pulmonary edema
    C. Eisenmenger's syndrome_____cardiac shunts with left to right flow
    D. Pulmonary osteoarthropathy_____lung cancer.
29. Differential cyanosis is seen in:
    A. PDA with reversal B. VSD with reversal
    C. ASD with reversal D. Coarctation of aorta

Fill in the Blanks

1. Radiofemoral delay is found in _____.
2. Pulsus alternans is present in _____.
3. Cyanosis appears when amount of reduced Hb exceeds _____ g/dL.
4. Rise in JVP during inspiration in constrictive pericarditis is called _____ sign.
5. Prominent Y descent in JVP is seen in _____.
6. Bradycardia is defined as pulse rate less than _____ per minute.
7. Tachycardia is defined as pulse rate more than _____ per minute.
8. Normal respiratory rate in adults is _____ per minute.
9. Regularly irregular pulse is found in _____.
10. Fishy mousy odor in the oral cavity suggests _____.
11. Cherry red discoloration of skin is found in _____.
12. Waxing and waning respiration with intervening periods of apnea is called _____.
13. Step ladder pattern of fever is present in _____.
14. Pel Epstein fever is seen in _____.

CHAPTER 2

Gastrointestinal System

SYMPTOMS AND SIGNS OF GASTROINTESTINAL DISEASES

The gastrointestinal (GI) system extends from the mouth to the anus. The symptoms arising from GI tract diseases are complex and varied. Some important symptoms are:
- Abdominal pain
- Nausea and vomiting
- Heart burn
- Altered bowel habits (diarrhea, constipation)
- Abdominal distension
- Bleeding (hematemesis and melena)
- Dysphagia (difficulty in swallowing)
- Odynophagia (painful swallowing)
- Loss of appetite.

Symptoms

Abdominal Pain

Causes of abdominal pain are given in **Table 2.1**. Some important causes of abdominal pain are:
- Appendicitis
- Gallstones
- Liver abscess
- Pancreatitis
- Peptic ulcer
- Intestinal obstruction
- Renal stones
- Gynecological diseases.

The extra-abdominal diseases like myocardial infarction, pneumonia, herpes zoster and spinal diseases may present with abdominal pain.

The points to be noted in relation to the abdominal pain are site, nature, severity, radiation, time of onset, aggravating and relieving factors.

Table 2.1: Causes of abdominal pain.

Local causes:
- Appendicitis
- Perforation of appendix
- Gallstones
- Cholecystitis
- Peptic ulcer
- Perforation of ulcer
- Pancreatitis
- Intestinal obstruction
- Ureteric obstruction
- Pyelonephritis
- Mesenteric ischemia
- Pelvic inflammatory disease
- Cystitis
- Liver abscess
- Hepatitis
- Splenic infarction

Referred pain:
- Acute myocardial infarction
- Lower lobe pneumonia
- Empyema
- Pleurodynia
- Pneumothorax
- Testicular torsion

Miscellaneous:
- Diabetic ketoacidosis
- Porphyria
- Herpes zoster
- Spinal cord or nerve root compression
- Lead poisoning
- Angioneurotic edema
- Functional/psychiatric disorder

Site: The pain may be localized or generalized. Localized pain in epigastrium may be due to peptic ulcer disease, acute pancreatitis while right hypochondrial pain occurs in liver and gallbladder diseases like hepatitis and cholecystitis **(Table 2.2)**.

Table 2.2: Causes of localized abdominal pain.	
Site of pain	Diseases
Epigastrium	Peptic ulcer, acute pancreatitis, gastritis, GERD
Right hypochondrium	Hepatitis, cholecystitis, liver abscess, subdiaphragmatic abscess
Right lower quadrant	Appendicitis, tubo-ovarian disease, inguinal hernia, ectopic pregnancy, renal stone
Left lower quadrant	Diverticulitis, tubo-ovarian disease, inguinal hernia, ectopic pregnancy, renal stone
Periumbilical	Bowel obstruction, early appendicitis
Hypogastrium	Cystitis

Generalized abdominal pain is found in gastroenteritis, bowel obstruction, mesenteric ischemia, metabolic diseases (diabetes, porphyria), and peritonitis.

Nature: The nature could be colicky or a diffuse dull ache. Colicky pain is spasmodic in nature with episodes of pain lasting for a few seconds or even up to minutes intervening with pain free periods. This is typical of bowel obstruction, ureteric obstruction or bile duct obstruction. Diffuse severe abdominal pain is found in peritonitis.

Radiation: The pain due to ureteric stone starts in lumbar region and radiates to groin. In acute pancreatitis, pain may radiate to the back. Diseases of right hypochondrial region may cause radiation of pain to right shoulder.

Relieving and aggravating factors: Pain of gastric ulcer increases after meals while early morning pain is present in duodenal ulcer. Pain of peptic ulcer disease is relieved on taking antacids. Pain due to peritonitis increases on abdominal movements, palpation, coughing and sneezing. The patient with peritonitis prefers to lie quietly in bed.

Nausea and Vomiting

Nausea is a feeling of need to vomit. Nausea and vomiting due to gastrointestinal causes are generally associated with abdominal pain. Vomiting and nausea may also be due to causes such as pregnancy, medications, toxins, infections, central nervous system disorders and motion sickness **(Table 2.3)**.

Table 2.3: Causes of nausea and vomiting.	
Abdominal causes	Extra-abdominal causes
• Intestinal obstruction • Pyloric obstructions • Gastroenteritis • Gastroesophageal reflux • Gastroparesis • Cholecystitis • Pancreatitis • Hepatitis • Appendicitis • Biliary colic • Ureteric colic • Abdominal irradiation	• Motion sickness • Labyrinthitis • Myocardial infarction • Increased intracranial pressure • Psychiatric illnesses • Drugs • Pregnancy • Uremia • Ketoacidosis

Heart Burn

Heart burn is the burning pain in the epigastrium, chest and neck due to the reflux of acid into the esophagus. There may be sour eructation or a bitter taste in the mouth. The pain can be confused with angina. Heart burn occurs more frequently when the patient lies flat in bed or bends forward.

Altered Bowel Habits

Altered bowel habits include constipation and diarrhea.
- Constipation is referred by patients as incomplete evacuation of stool, passage of hard stools, defecation with straining, or infrequent defecation (less than 3 times a week). The common causes of constipation are intestinal obstruction, medications, motility disorders and hypothyroidism **(Table 2.4)**
- Passage of unformed and liquid stools and/or increased frequency of stools is called diarrhea. Acute diarrhea generally occurs due to infections. Chronic diarrhea (of more than 4 weeks) raises the possibility of inflammatory bowel diseases and malabsorption.

Abdominal Distension

- Generalized distension of the abdomen may occur due to fat, fluid, flatus, feces or fetus **(Fig. 2.1)**. Flatulence (excessive wind) usually represents functional bowel disease where large amount of air is swallowed. Certain foods may also produce flatulence.
- Localized distension may result from organ enlargement (liver, spleen, kidneys and ovary) or small bowel obstruction **(Fig. 2.2)**.

GI Bleeding

Bleeding may occur in the upper or lower gastrointestinal tracts.
- Upper GI bleeding (bleeding from esophagus, stomach and duodenum) commonly presents with hematemesis or melena. *Hematemesis* is vomiting of blood or "coffee grounds" material while *melena* is foul smelling, black

Table 2.4: Causes of constipation.
• Painful hemorrhoids • Anal fissure • Colonic obstruction • Irritable bowel syndrome • Drugs (calcium channel blockers, antidepressants, opiates, iron, anticholinergic) • Hypercalcemia • Hypothyroidism • Diabetes • Pregnancy • Parkinsonism • Spinal cord injury • Depression • Low fiber intake • Low fluid intake

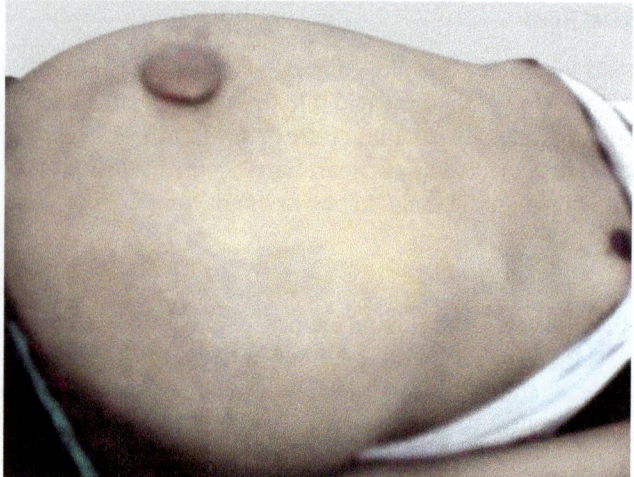

Fig. 2.1: Massive ascites with umbilical hernia.

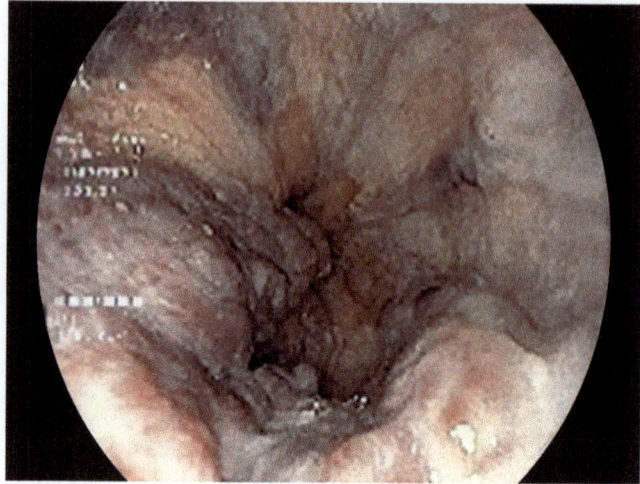

Fig. 2.3: Endoscopic view of esophageal varices.

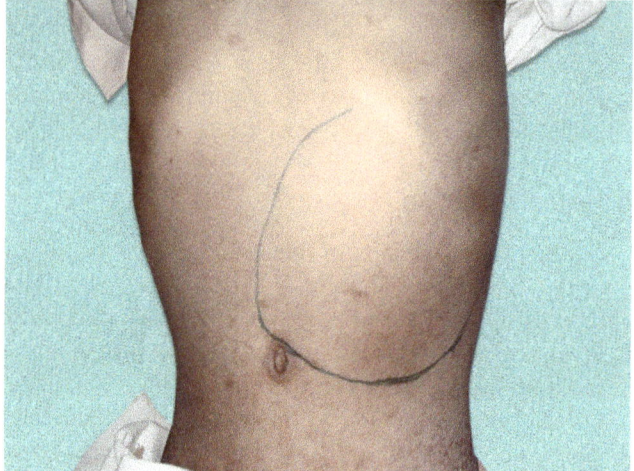

Fig. 2.2: Localized abdominal distension due to splenomegaly.

Table 2.5: Causes of GI bleeding.	
Causes of upper GI bleeding	**Causes of lower GI bleeding**
• Peptic ulcer • Esophageal varices • Gastroduodenal erosions • Neoplasms • Mallory-Weiss tears • Vascular ectasia	• Hemorrhoids • Anal fissure • Diverticula • Neoplasm • Colitis • Inflammatory bowel disease • Ischemia of colon • Radiation

tarry stools. Melena indicates that blood has remained in GI tract for some time (at least 14 hours). Common causes of upper GI bleeding are peptic ulcer, variceal rupture **(Fig. 2.3)**, erosive gastritis, gastric neoplasm and Mallory-Weiss tear **(Table 2.5)**.

- Passage of bright red blood in stool (*hematochezia*) indicates lower GI bleeding (small intestine and colon), arising below the ligament of Treitz. Common causes of lower GI bleeding are hemorrhoids, anal fissures, neoplasms, diverticula, inflammatory bowel diseases, infections and ischemia of the colon **(Figs. 2.4A and B)**. Massive upper GI bleeding may present as *hematochezia* if blood does not remain in the bowel for long time.
- Occult GI bleeding refers to bleeding that is not visible but can be identified by a positive fecal occult blood test. Chronic blood loss of < 100 mL/day may not cause any

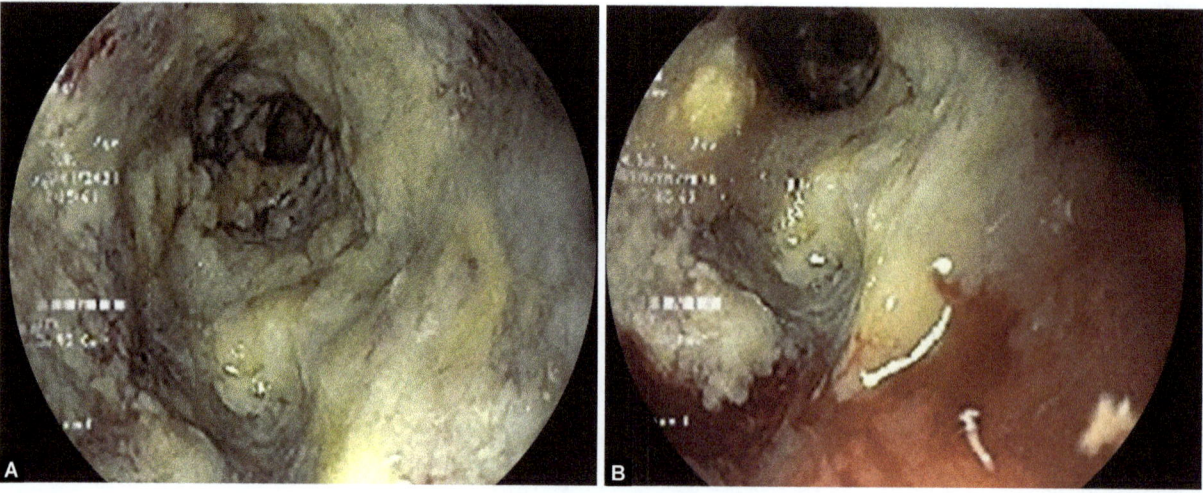

Figs. 2.4A and B: Endoscopic view of carcinoma rectum.

change in appearance of stools although it may present as iron deficiency anemia.

Dysphagia

Difficulty in swallowing may occur due to problem in oropharynx (oropharyngeal dysphagia) or in the esophagus (esophageal dysphagia).

Odynophagia

Odynophagia is a painful swallowing that may limit oral intake. It usually occurs in erosive disease of oropharynx or esophagus. Common causes are esophagitis due to candida, herpes virus and CMV. Corrosive injury and drug induced ulcers may also cause odynophagia.

Other Symptoms

- *Hiccups* can arise due to distension or irritation of the upper GI tract. However, they may also occur because of non-GI causes.
- *Weight loss, anorexia and fatigue* are non-specific manifestations and can be seen in malignancy, malabsorption, inflammatory and psychiatric conditions.
- *Dyspepsia* generally refers to symptoms of upper abdominal discomfort, bloating, belching, burning, fullness, early satiety, nausea and vomiting. This is usually benign and occurs due to overeating, high fat diet, alcohol, coffee and medicines. Dyspepsia may be the symptom of peptic ulcer or gastric cancer. Functional or non-ulcer dyspepsia is the most common cause of chronic dyspepsia. In this condition no obvious organic cause is found.

General Examination

Certain features in general examination are important and should be recorded **(Table 2.6)**.

One should look for the presence of jaundice, signs of chronic liver disease (spider nevi, palmer erythema, gynecomastia, testicular atrophy, parotid swelling), clubbing (seen in inflammatory bowel disease, cirrhosis), edema, anasarca and anemia. Scratch marks (pruritus) may suggest cholestasis. Assessment of nutritional status particularly about weight loss is an important in chronic malabsorption, chronic liver disease, malignancies and severe protein loss.

Left supraclavicular lymph node (Virchow node) and umbilical nodule (Sister Mary Joseph nodule) may be present in cases of metastatic gastric adenocarcinoma

Careful examination of lips, teeth, gums, tongue and buccal mucosa is performed for the presence of glossitis, bald tongue, ulcers, cheilitis and angular stomatitis.

Abdominal Examination

The examination of the abdomen should be performed in a systemic manner. This includes inspection, palpation, percussion and auscultation. Procedure should be clearly explained to the patient.

Inspection

The patient should be supine and the abdomen should be adequately exposed. The inspection should be performed under proper lighting conditions. Following points should particularly be noted;
- *Shape of the abdomen:* The abdomen may be distended or sunken (scaphoid). The generalized distension of the abdomen may occur due to fat, fluid, flatus, feces or fetus. Localized distension could be due to organ enlargement or small bowel obstruction. Sunken abdomen is seen in starvation and malignancy.
- *Umbilicus:* Umbilicus is everted and horizontal in ascites. Umbilical hernia may occur in massive ascites **(Fig. 2.1)**.
- *Movements of the abdominal wall:* Movements of abdominal wall are absent in peritonitis. Visible pulsations can be seen normally in thin persons or can also be due to aortic aneurysms. Visible peristalsis may be present in gastric outlet obstruction and small bowel obstruction.
- *Prominent veins:* Prominent superficial veins may be present in inferior vena cava obstruction **(Fig. 2.5)** or portal hypertension (caput medusae).

Table 2.6: Important clinical features on general examination.	
Diseases	Features on examination
Chronic liver disease (CLD)	Spider nevi, palmer erythema, gynecomastia, parotid swelling, testicular atrophy
Inflammatory bowel disease	Clubbing
Obstructive jaundice	Scratch marks
Iron and vitamin deficiency	Angular stomatitis, oral ulcers
Malignancy, malabsorption, CLD	Cachexia
Gastric carcinoma	Virchow node (Left supraclavicular lymphadenopathy) Abdominal nodule (Sister Mary Joseph nodule)

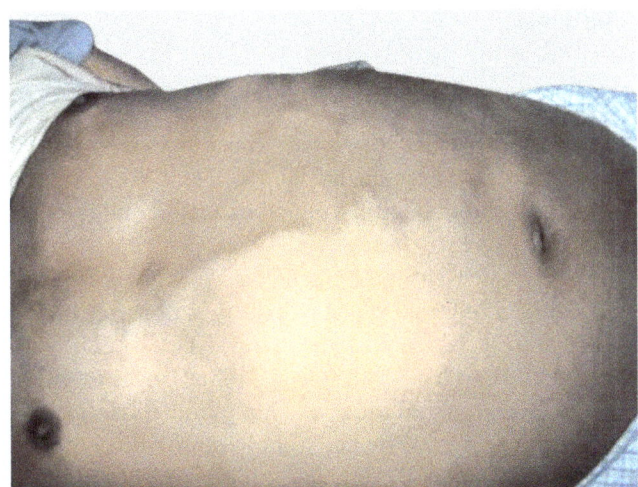

Fig. 2.5: Prominent veins over abdomen.

ESSENTIALS OF MEDICINE FOR DENTAL STUDENTS

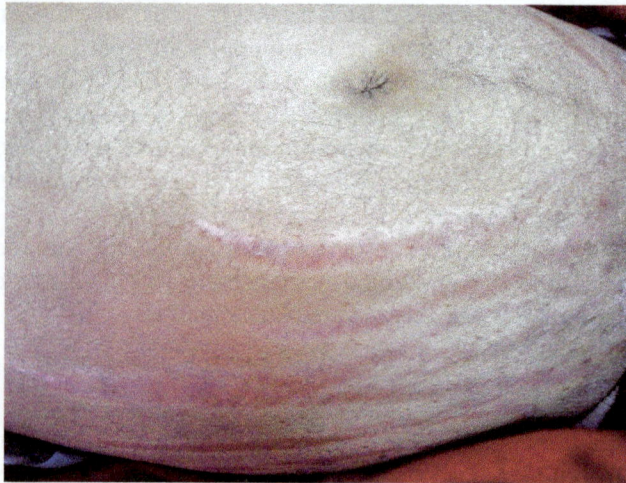

Fig. 2.6: Purple striae.

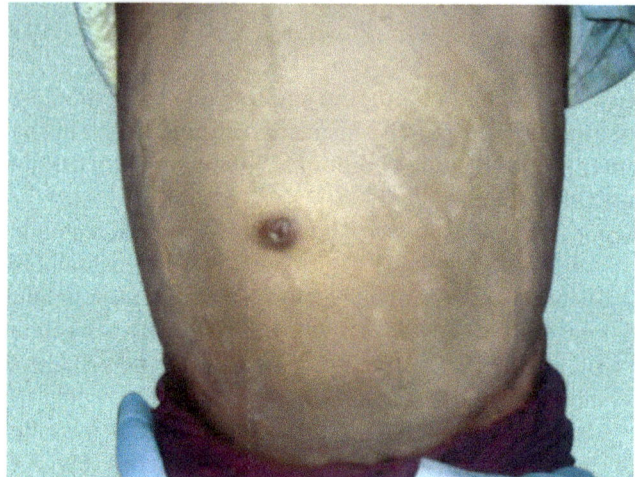

Fig. 2.7: Abdominal stria in a patient with ascites.

Features of enlarged liver:
» Enlarged liver is palpable in the right hypochondrium **(Fig. 2.8)**.
» It moves with respiration.
» Fingers cannot be insinuated between the costal margin and the lump.
» The upper border of the liver should also be demarcated by percussion in order to assess the size (see hepatomegaly in Chapter 3).

Features of enlarged spleen:
» Enlarged spleen is palpable in the left hypochondrium **(Fig. 2.9)**.
» It moves with respiration
» Fingers cannot be insinuated between the costal margin and the lump.
» A notch is felt at the medial border of the spleen.
» This is not palpable bimanually.

Features of enlarged kidney:
» Enlarged kidney may be palpable in lumbar region
» This is bimanually palpable.
» Colonic band of resonance is present anterior to the kidney lump.

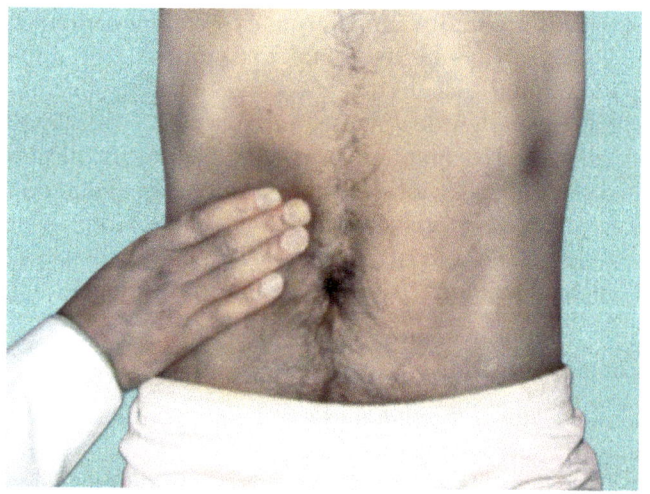

Fig. 2.8: Palpation of the liver.

- *Skin:* Skin over the abdomen is shiny and smooth in marked distension. Purple striae are seen in Cushing's syndrome **(Fig 2.6)**. Striae atrophica or gravidorum are pink or white linear marks produced by gross stretching of abdomen as in ascites and pregnancy **(Fig. 2.7)**.
- *Inspection* of groin, genitalia and hernial sites should also be done.

Palpation

- The patient is asked to bend the knees to relax abdominal muscles and to breathe deeply.
- The palpation begins anti-clockwise from left iliac fossa.
- The palpation should be gently performed with warm hands. Initially superficial palpation is done to find out tender areas, which are to be examined in the end.
  - Organs such as liver, spleen, kidneys, ovaries, uterus and urinary bladder are palpated to detect any enlargement. Further details about the enlarged organs like size, surface, borders, consistency, and tenderness are noted.

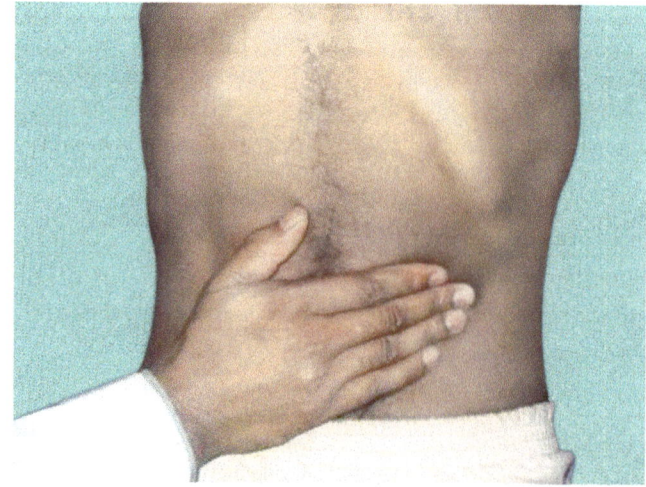

Fig. 2.9: Palpation of the spleen.

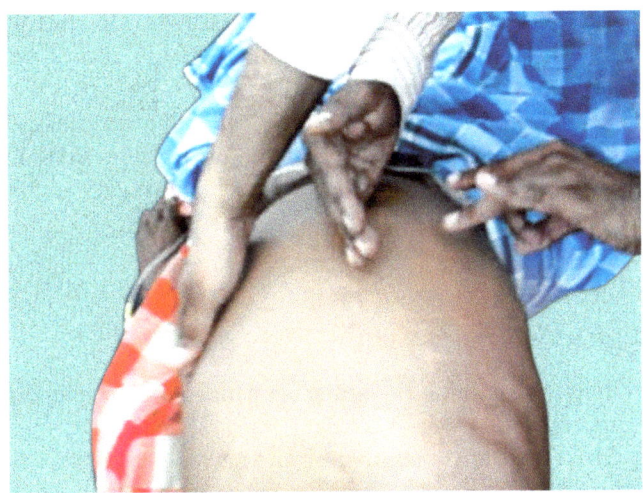

Fig. 2.10: Method to elicit fluid thrill.

» Kidney lump is ballotable (it can be pushed from the one hand to the other).
- Any area showing tenderness or rigidity should be noted. *Murphy's sign* may be present in acute cholecystitis, which is tenderness in right upper quadrant with arrest of inspiration due to pain.
- *Fluid thrill* detects the presence of free fluid in the abdomen (ascites). An assistant is asked to put the side of hand in the midline of the abdomen. Examiner places one hand flat in the lumbar region of one side and taps the opposite lumbar region with other hand. A wave or thrill is felt by the hand held flat in the other lumbar region **(Fig. 2.10)**. The assistant's hand does not allow the transmission of impulse through the abdominal wall. Fluid thrill is a sign of tense and massive ascites.

Percussion

The normal note of the abdominal percussion is tympanitic (resonant). Percussion is useful in confirming the enlargement of liver and spleen and detecting fluid in the peritoneal cavity (ascites).

Shifting dullness: Shifting dullness is a sign of moderate ascites and may be absent when the ascites is tense. Percussion is performed in supine patient from the midline of the abdomen toward the flank till dullness is detected **(Figs. 2.11A and B)**. Keeping the hand on the abdomen in the same position (at the point of dullness), patient is rolled laterally to the opposite side. Percussion is repeated after a minute from flank toward the umbilicus. In case of fluid (as in ascites), the previously dull point at flank becomes resonant because of shifting of fluid towards the umbilicus. To confirm, the test is repeated on the other side of the abdomen.

Auscultation

The bowel sound is exaggerated in small bowel obstruction. These may be absent in paralytic ileus. Vascular bruit may be heard in case of stenosis or aneurysm of the vessels.

STOMATITIS AND ORAL ULCERS

The inflammation of oral mucosa is called *stomatitis*. This can lead to disruption of mucosa leading to ulcers **(Fig. 2.12)**. Important causes of stomatitis/oral ulcers are given in **Table 2.7**.

Recurrent aphthous ulcers and herpes simplex ulcers are among the commonest causes of oral ulcers.

Angular Stomatitis (Cheilosis)

Cheilosis is characterized by the presence of cracks or fissures at the corners of the mouth. Important causes are:
- Ill fitting dentures (in elderly)
- Severe iron deficiency
- Vitamin B complex deficiency
- Candidiasis.

Aphthous Ulcer (Ulcerative Stomatitis, Canker Sore)

- Ulcerative stomatitis is a common condition.

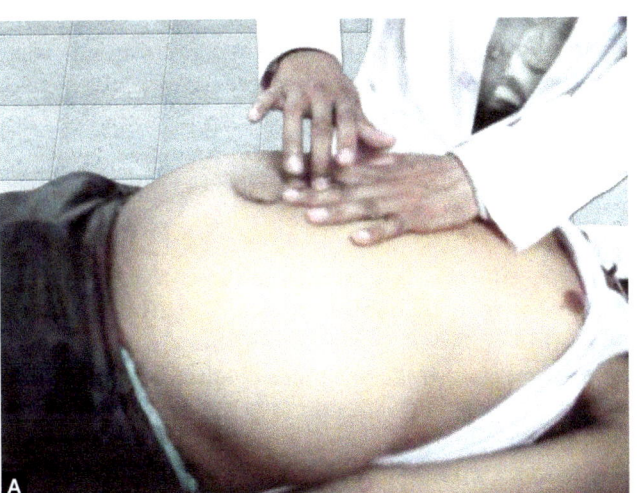 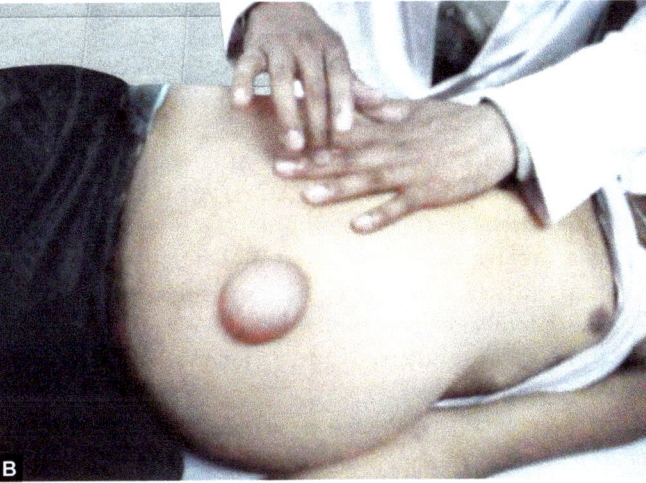

Figs. 2.11A and B: Method to elicit shifting dullness: (A) Supine position and (B) Lateral position.

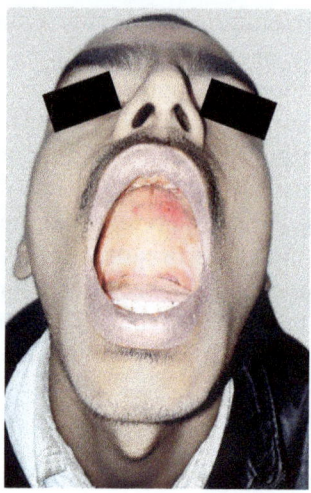

Fig. 2.12: Oral ulcer.

Table 2.7: Causes of oral ulcers.
Aphthous ulcer (ulcerative stomatitis)
Infections: • Viral (Herpes, CMV, EBV, HIV) • Fungal (Candida) • Bacterial (Vincent's infection, syphilis)
Dermatological: • Pemphigus, pemphigoid, lichen planus
Drugs: • Chemotherapy drugs • Erythema multiforme, Stevens-Johnson syndrome
Systemic diseases: • Behçet's syndrome, SLE
Nutritional: • Vitamin deficiency (Vitamin B and C), iron deficiency
Neoplasia: • Squamous cell carcinoma, leukemia, Kaposi's sarcoma
Gastrointestinal: • Crohn's disease, celiac disease
Traumatic: • Dentures
Chemical or thermal burns: • Corrosives, hot liquids

- Etiology is unknown (idiopathic), however, human herpes virus-6 has been associated with this condition. Stress is an important predisposing factor.
- Aphthous ulcers are recurrent single or multiple, superficial painful lesions with central yellow gray slough surrounded by erythematous borders.
- These involve non-keratinized oral mucosa such as buccal mucosa, labial mucosa, floor of the mouth, soft palate, lateral and ventral tongue.
- The painful stage lasts for 7–10 days followed by complete healing within a week.
- Size of the ulcers is generally less than 1 cm, however it can be larger. In cases with large and persistent ulcers, biopsy is needed to differentiate them from other causes such as carcinoma, erythema multiforme, herpes simplex, pemphigus, pemphigoid, Behçet's disease and inflammatory bowel disease.
- Local anesthetic gel or mouth washes give symptomatic relief. Topical steroids (triamcinolone or fluocinonide) can accelerate healing. Severe cases may need a course of oral prednisolone.

Vincent's Infection (Necrotizing Ulcerative Stomatitis, Trench Mouth)

- These are painful, sloughing deep ulcers which primarily involve gums.
- There is severe inflammation and necrosis of gingiva with bleeding.
- It may be associated with halitosis, fever and cervical lymphadenopathy.
- The causative organisms are fusiform bacilli and spirochetes.
- Malnutrition, poor oral hygiene and immunosuppression (such as AIDS, chemotherapy) predispose to this condition.
- Treatment includes debridement and hydrogen peroxide mouth wash. Antibiotic (penicillin) is helpful in acutely ill patients.

Herpetic Stomatitis

- Herpetic stomatitis or gingivostomatitis is caused by herpes simplex virus (HSV) type I and rarely by HSV type 2.
- This occurs mainly in children and young adults.
- Lesions involve lips and oral mucosa. Labial lesions are in the form of vesicles that rupture and crust **(Figs. 2.13A and B)**. Intraoral vesicles are very painful and they rapidly ulcerate.
- There may also be fever, malaise, halitosis and cervical lymphadenopathy.
- Labial lesions are common in recurrent herpes simplex (herpes labialis).
- Lesions usually heal within 10–14 days.
- Topical or oral antiviral (acyclovir, valcyclovir, famciclovir) drugs enhance healing in severe cases. Daily acyclovir may be needed to prevent recurrent herpetic lesions, particularly in immunocompromised cases.

Oral Candidiasis

Candida albicans is normal mouth commensal. It can produce thrush in babies, diabetics, patients on corticosteroids or broad spectrum antibiotics and immunosuppressed states (AIDS, cancer chemotherapy). This can involve any part of the mouth **(Fig. 2.14)**. Oral candidiasis can present in following forms:

- *Pseudomembranous type (thrush):* Creamy white curd-like patches are seen over erythematous mucosa. These

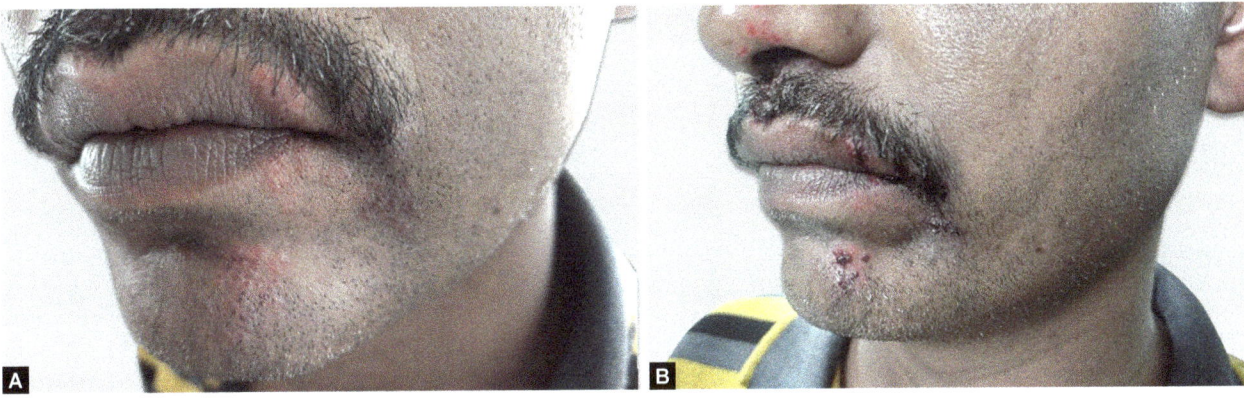

Figs. 2.13A and B: (A) Herpes labialis; (B) Herpes labialis; crusting of lesions.

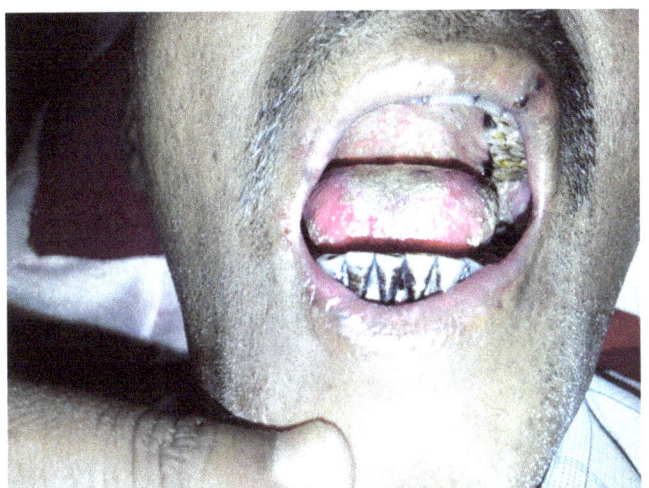

Fig. 2.14: Oral candidiasis.

can be easily scraped and reveal raw bleeding surface. Painful deglutition (odynophagia) suggests pharyngeal and esophageal involvement.
- *Erythematous type:* These are flat, red, sore areas in the oral cavity.
- *Candidal leukoplakia:* There is non-removable white thickening of mucosal epithelium due to candida.
- *Angular cheilitis:* Sore fissures at the corner of the mouth can be caused by candida.

Diagnosis: The diagnosis can be made clinically and is confirmed by the demonstration of spores and mycelia on KOH wet preparation or biopsy of the lesion.

Treatment: Clotrimazole lozenges or nystatin mouth washes are effective in oral candidiasis. Ketoconazole (200–400 mg oral daily) or fluconazole (200 mg oral daily) is given for 1–2 weeks in oroesophageal candidiasis in immunocompromised patients. Itraconazole is given in refractory cases.

Nutritional Deficiency

Swollen bleeding gums and ulcers are common in vitamin C deficiency. Deficiency of vitamin B complex (B_2, B_{12}, folic acid) can cause glossitis, oral ulceration and cheilosis. Cheilosis, glossitis and dysphagia are also found in iron deficiency cases.

Hematological Diseases

All forms of leukemia, particularly acute myelomonocytic leukemia can produce oral ulcers, gingival swelling and bleeding. Oral ulcers are also found in agranulocytosis (see in Chapter 4). Mucositis and ulcers are complications of chemotherapy and radiation therapy.

GINGIVAL HYPERPLASIA

Gingival hyperplasia is swelling or enlargement of gingiva. Apart from oro-dental causes, gingival swelling can be manifestation of systemic diseases. Hence, understanding various systemic causes of gingival hyperplasia is very important.

Gingival swelling can be:
a. Generalized
b. Localized

Important causes of generalized gingival swelling are scurvy (Vitamin C deficiency), acute myeloid leukemia and drugs (phenytoin, cyclosporine and calcium channel blockers). Causes of gingival hyperplasia are given in **Table 2.8**.

Diagnosis can be made by proper history including drug intake and the underlying features of causative disease. Hematological investigations can rule out the presence of leukemia.

Treatment includes management of underlying cause and withdrawal of offending drug.

DYSPHAGIA

Dysphagia is defined as difficulty in swallowing. Odynophagia is painful swallowing while phagophobia is fear of swallowing or refusal to swallow.

Classification

Dysphagia is divided into following types:
- *Oropharyngeal dysphagia:* There is problem in transferring food from mouth to the esophagus. This is associated with nasal regurgitation and pulmonary aspiration during swallowing. The causes of oropharyngeal dysphagia can be

Table 2.8: Causes of gingival hyperplasia.

Generalized gingival hyperplasia
Acquired
- Acute myeloid leukemia (M4 and M5 type)
- Vitamin C deficiency
- Drugs: Phenytoin, cyclosporine, calcium channel blockers (nifedipine, verapamil, diltiazem, amlodipine), sodium valproate, tranexamic acid
- Wegener's disease (strawberry gums)

Congenital
- Mucopolysaccharidosis
- Primary amyloidosis
- Hereditary gingival fibromatosis

Localized gingival hyperplasia
Acquired
- Lymphomas
- Multiple myeloma
- Squamous cell carcinoma
- Kaposi sarcoma
- Pregnancy
- Sarcoidosis
- Wegener's disease
- Giant cell epulis (primary hyperparathyroidism)

Congenital
- Fabry's syndrome
- Tuberous sclerosis
- Sturge-Weber angiomatosis

Table 2.9: Causes of oropharyngeal dysphagia.

Mechanical
- Oropharyngeal tumors
- Post-surgical/radiation changes
- Zenker's diverticulum
- Retropharyngeal abscess/mass
- Thyroid disorders
- Plummer-Vinson syndrome
- Inflammatory lesions

Motor
- Brain injury, cerebral palsy, parkinsonism, stroke
- Rabies, tetanus
- Cranial nerve palsy, Guillain-Barre syndrome
- Myasthenia gravis, botulinum toxin
- Myositis, myopathies

Table 2.10: Causes of esophageal dysphagia.

Mechanical
- Esophageal cancer
- Peptic stricture
- Inflammatory esophagitis
- Schatzki's ring (lower esophageal mucosal ring)
- Posterior mediastinal mass
- Aortic aneurysm

Motor
- Achalasia
- Scleroderma
- Diffuse esophageal spasm

---

subgrouped into (a) mechanical and (b) motor dysphagia. Important causes are given in **Table 2.9**.
- *Esophageal dysphagia:* Difficulty in swallowing the food down the esophagus. Patients with mechanical obstruction complain of dysphagia mainly for solids whereas those with motility disorders have dysphagia for both solids and liquids. Causes are given in **Table 2.10**. **Figures 2.15A to C** show a case of esophageal carcinoma.

Odynophagia

Odynophagia is a painful swallowing that may limit oral intake. Important causes are infectious esophagitis due to candida, herpes, or CMV **(Fig. 2.16)**. It can also be due to corrosive injury (due to caustic ingestion) or pill-induced ulcers (pill esophagitis).

Diagnosis

Following investigations are helpful in making the diagnosis:
- Endoscopy (esophagogastroscopy)
- Video esophagography
- Barium esophagography
- Esophageal manometry
- Esophageal pH recording
- Imaging studies (CT scan)
- Specific tests to rule out neuromuscular disorders.

Treatment

General
- Modification of diet
- Enteral feeding through a gastrostomy tube

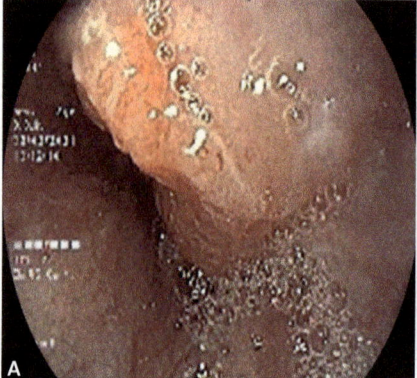
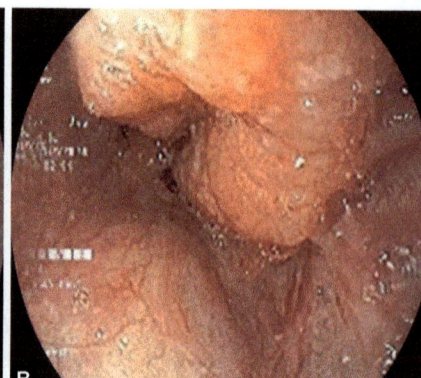
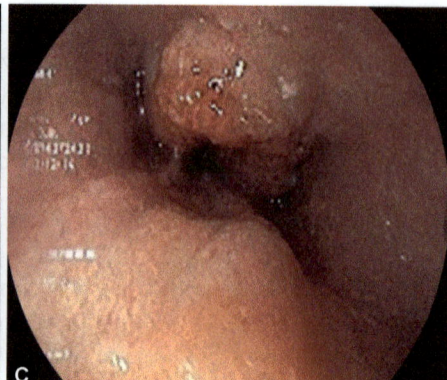

Figs. 2.15A to C: Carcinoma esophagus.

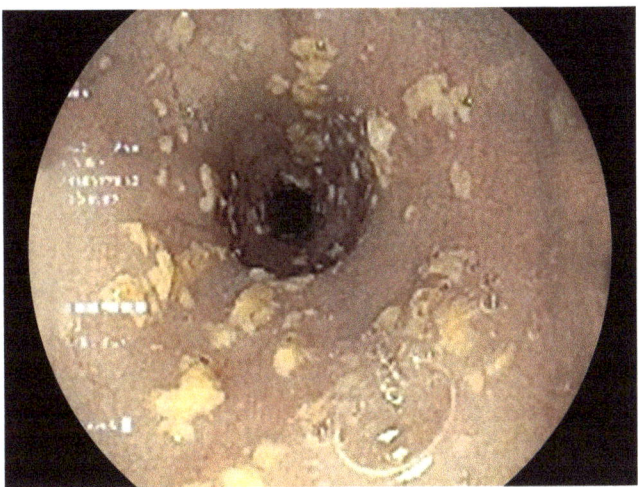

Fig. 2.16: Endoscopic view of esophageal candidiasis.

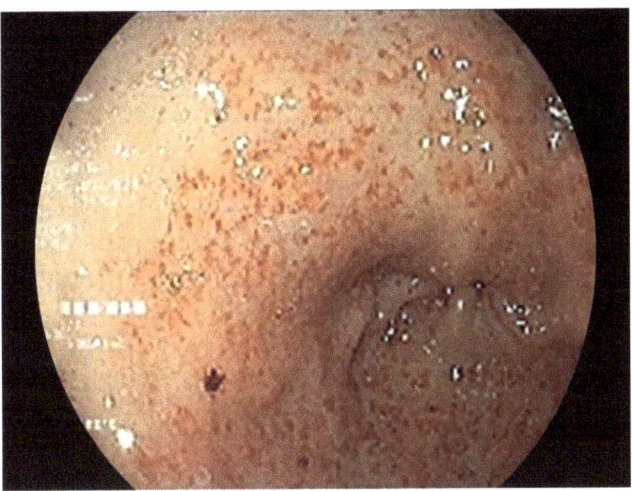

Fig. 2.17: Multiple gastric erosions.

- Endoscopic removal of obstructing food bolus in acute dysphagia
- Nutrition counseling.

Medical

- Proton pump inhibitors (for mucosal inflammation in reflux disease)
- Antimicrobial agents (infectious esophagitis)
- Viscous lidocaine solution for symptomatic relief
- Anticholinergic medications in cases with drooling of saliva and oropharyngeal dysphagia.

Endoscopic Therapy

- Esophageal dilatation
- Esophageal stent placement
- Pneumatic dilatation of lower esophageal sphincter (LES) for achalasia.
- Botulinum toxin injection to LES in achalasia.

Surgical

Laparoscopic myotomy in achalasia.

GASTRITIS

Gastritis is a histological diagnosis characterized by inflammation of the gastric mucosa.

Acute Erosive and Hemorrhagic Gastritis

Acute gastritis is usually erosive and hemorrhagic. Important causes of erosive and hemorrhagic gastritis are:
- Drugs (aspirin, NSAIDs)
- Alcohol
- Stress due to severe illness
- Congestive gastropathy due to portal hypertension.

Stress ulceration in patients with head trauma is called *Cushing's ulcer* and in severe burns, *Curling's ulcer*. Stress injury is not characterized by inflammation, thus the term 'gastritis' is a misnomer.

Erosive gastritis is usually asymptomatic. It may present with anorexia, nausea, vomiting and abdominal pain. Hematemesis and melena are most important manifestations of erosive gastritis.

Diagnosis is made by endoscopy which reveals superficial hemorrhages and erosions **(Fig. 2.17)**. Biopsy may be required to differentiate it from peptic ulcer and cancer.

Management

- The treatment of acute gastritis consists of administration of sucralfate suspension (1 g 4-6 hrly) and H_2 receptor antagonist (ranitidine 150 mg twice daily, famotidine 20 mg twice daily) or proton pump inhibitors (omeprazole 20 mg once daily, esomeprazole 40 mg once daily, rabeprazole 20 mg once daily, pantoprazole 40 mg once daily, lansoprazole 30 mg once daily, dexlansoprazole 30 mg once daily).
- The consumption of alcohol and drugs [Non-steroidal anti-inflammatory drugs (NSAIDs)] should be avoided.
- Stress gastritis can be prevented by the administration of sucralfate, H_2 receptor antagonist or proton pump inhibitor in critically ill patients.

Acute Gastritis Due to Infections

A variety of infections can lead to acute inflammatory changes in the gastric mucosa. This presents as sudden onset of epigastric pain, nausea and vomiting.

H. pylori infection can lead to acute gastritis which generally progresses to chronic gastritis.

Acute bacterial infections (aerobic and anaerobic bacteria) can lead to progressive life-threatening necrotizing gastritis (phlegmonus gastritis). The treatment includes antibiotics and emergency gastrectomy.

Herpes simplex virus, CMV and candida can cause gastritis in immunocompromised patients such as AIDS.

Chronic Gastritis

Histologically chronic gastritis is characterized by chronic inflammation with predominant infiltration by lymphocytes and plasma cells. The early stage of chronic gastritis is superficial gastritis. This is followed by the stage of atrophic gastritis. The final stage is gastric atrophy. The subsequent development of metaplasia may be precancerous. The two main types of chronic gastritis are autoimmune gastritis and *H. pylori* related chronic gastritis.

Autoimmune Gastritis (Type A Gastritis)

- This is characterized by the involvement of fundus and body of the stomach, *sparing antrum*.
- Circulating autoantibodies are found against parietal cells and intrinsic factor.
- This type of gastritis is generally asymptomatic. However, it may be associated with vitamin B_{12} deficiency *(pernicious anemia)*.
- Features of other *autoimmune involvement* (such as thyroid disease) may be present.
- There is four-fold increase in the incidence of gastric cancer, hence follow up endoscopy is suggested.
- The treatment of pernicious anemia includes regular parenteral B_{12} supplementation.

Helicobacter pylori Gastritis (Type B Gastritis)

- *H. pylori* is the most common cause of chronic gastritis.
- The incidence of *H. pylori* gastritis increases with age.
- Initially, the antrum is predominantly involved, later pangastritis occurs.
- The majority of patients are asymptomatic with no sequelae.
- It is associated with peptic ulcer disease, with a 2-6 fold increase in the risk of *gastric adenocarcinoma* and low grade B-cell gastric lymphoma (MALT lymphoma).
- Eradication of *H. pylori* is often recommended. Regular follow up endoscopy is needed.
Patients with peptic ulcer disease and MALT (mucosa associated lymphoid tissue) lymphoma are tested and treated for *H. pylori*. Antibiotics are given to treat *H. pylori* (see peptic ulcer).

Uncommon Types of Gastritis

Other types of gastritis are granulomatous gastritis (tuberculosis, sarcoidosis, candidiasis, syphilis, Crohn's disease), eosinophilic gastritis and lymphocytic gastritis.

PEPTIC ULCER

Peptic ulcer is defined as the presence of ulcer in the lower esophagus, stomach and duodenum. The ulcer is a breach in the mucosa due to an imbalance between mucosal defensive factors and luminal factors such as acid and pepsin. A break in the mucosal surface of more than 5 mm and depth to the submucosa are characteristics of an ulcer.

Duodenal ulcer is more common than gastric ulcer and occurs at younger age group (30-55 years) as compared to gastric ulcer (55-70 years).

Etiology

The common etiological factors of peptic ulcer are:
- *H. pylori* infection
- NSAIDs (Non-steroidal anti-inflammatory drugs)
- Smoking
- Acid hypersecretory states (Zollinger-Ellison syndrome).

Multiple factors may be responsible for the ulcer in a particular patient. Whatever the cause, the common abnormality is an imbalance between mucosal defensive factors and the aggressive factors (acid, pepsin).

H. pylori Infection

H. pylori infection is a very common and important factor in the etiology of peptic ulcer. The prevalence of *H. pylori* infection is around 75% in duodenal ulcer and 30-60% in gastric ulcer. The infection leads to a state of hypergastrinemia, increased gastric acid secretion and decreased duodenal bicarbonate secretion. These factors result in patches of gastric metaplasia in the duodenal bulb. Colonization of theses patches by *H. pylori* subsequently causes inflammation and formation of duodenal ulcer. The gastric ulcer in *H. pylori* infection occurs predominantly due to reduced gastric mucosal resistance.

NSAIDs-induced Ulcers

The chronic use of NSAIDs is more commonly associated with gastric ulcer than duodenal ulcer. Users of NSAIDs are also more likely to suffer from serious ulcer-related complications. These drugs reduce prostaglandins synthesis in the gastric mucosa by inhibiting enzyme cyclooxygenase 1 (COX-1). Prostaglandins play an important role in the gastric cytoprotection and repair. Drugs which selectively inhibit COX-2 at the site of inflammation (valdecoxib, celecoxib, etoricoxib) without affecting COX-1 activity are less likely to cause gastric ulcer.

Smoking, Diet and Other Risk Factors

Smokers are more likely to develop peptic ulcers and related complications. The healing of the ulcer and response to therapy are diminished in smokers.

There is no association of any specific diet, alcohol or caffeine with the formation of ulcers, although certain foods can cause dyspepsia. Chronic obstructive lung disease, chronic kidney disease, coronary artery disease, obesity, old age and tobacco use are risk factors for development of peptic ulcer **(Table 2. 11)**.

Table 2.11: Risk factors for peptic ulcer disease.

- *Helicobactor pylori*
- NSAIDs
- Chronic obstructive lung disease
- Chronic kidney disease
- Coronary artery disease
- Obesity
- Diabetes
- Old age
- Tobacco use

Clinical Features

- Recurrent abdominal pain is the most common symptom.
- Pain is localized to epigastrium and is burning or gnawing type. It may be dull aching, vague or described as hunger pain. Pain in duodenal ulcer is relieved by taking meals and antacids whereas pain in gastric ulcer may increase after meals. Nocturnal pain (at 3-4 am) usually indicates duodenal ulcer.
- Nausea and weight loss are commonly present in gastric ulcer.
- Physical examination may be normal or may reveal epigastric tenderness in uncomplicated peptic ulcer. Complications of peptic ulcer are given in **Table 2.12**.

Constant pain not relieved by food or antacids suggests penetration. Severe pain (acute abdomen) may occur in case of perforation of peptic ulcer. Melena or hematemesis occurs in case of bleeding. Peptic ulcer is the most common cause of upper GI bleeding.

Investigations

- Endoscopy is the investigation of choice for the diagnosis of peptic ulcer **(Figs. 2.18 and 2.19)**. Biopsy of

Table 2.12: Complications of peptic ulcer.

- GI hemorrhages
- Perforation
- Ulcer penetration (into pancreas, liver)
- Gastric outlet obstruction

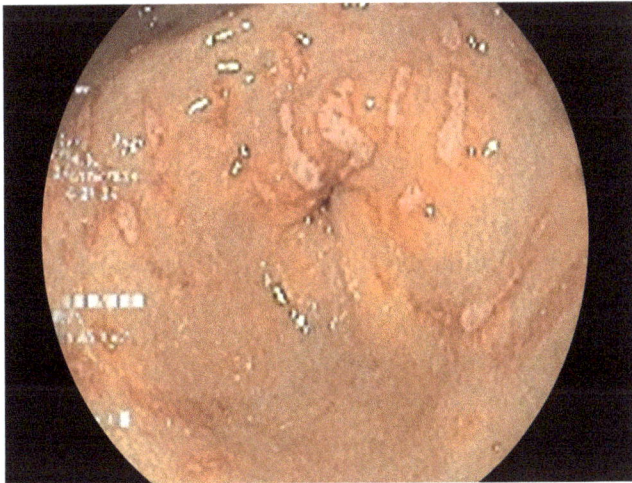

Fig. 2.18: Multiple antral ulcers.

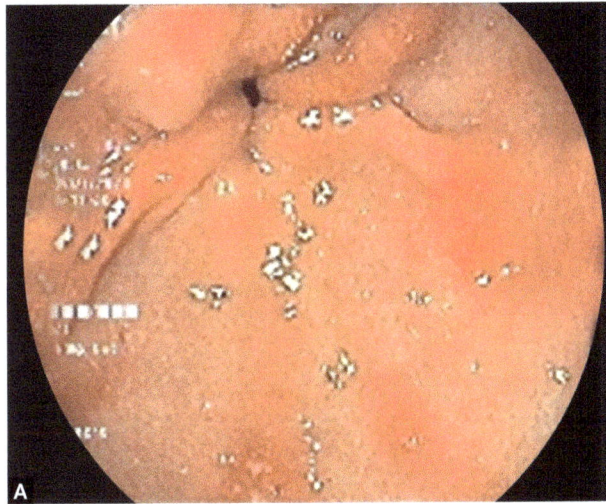
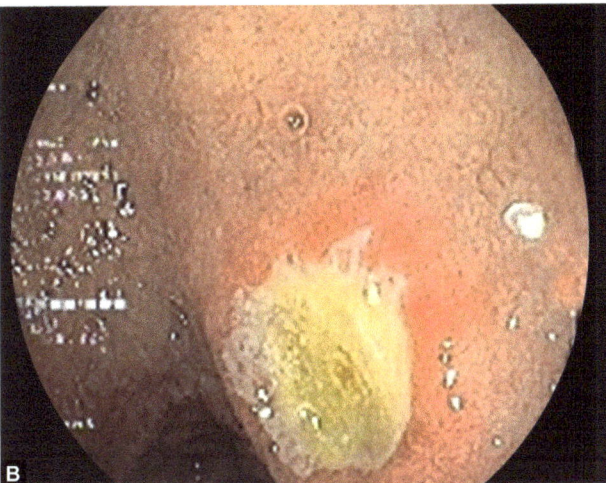

Figs. 2.19A and B: (A) Antral ulcers; (B) Duodenal ulcer.

the lesion is needed to detect malignancy and *H. pylori* infection.
- Barium studies of the upper GI tract done earlier are not generally needed as it is less sensitive to detect ulcers.
- Abdominal CT imaging may be required to detect complications of peptic ulcer disease such as perforation, penetration and gastric outlet obstruction.
- *H. pylori* infection can be diagnosed by noninvasive tests like serology, fecal antigen assay and urea breath test. Rapid urease test, histology and culture can be performed upon the biopsy sample.
- There may be anemia. Stool may be positive for occult blood. Leukocytosis suggests complications such as penetration or perforation.

Treatment

General Measures

- No specific dietary restriction is needed.
- Meals should be taken at regular intervals.
- Smoking or tobacco in any form should be stopped completely.
- Drugs like aspirin and NSAIDs must be avoided.

Medical Treatment

The medical treatment of peptic ulcer can be divided into three categories:
1. Acid neutralizing or inhibitory drugs
2. Mucosal protective agents
3. Eradication of *H. pylori*.

Acid Neutralizing or Inhibitory Drugs

- *Antacids:* These are commonly a mixture of aluminium hydroxide and magnesium hydroxide. Antacids are used in the initial phase of treatment because they provide rapid relief.
- H_2 *receptor antagonist:* Ranitidine (300 mg daily) or famotidine (40 mg daily) in single or divided dosage can cause healing of the ulcer in 85% cases in 6–8 weeks.
- *Proton pump inhibitor (PPI):* These agents are preferred over H_2 receptor antagonists because of superior efficacy. The healing of the ulcer occurs in over 90% cases in case of gastric ulcer in 8 weeks and in case of duodenal ulcer in 4 weeks. Agents used are omeprazole or rabeprazole 20 mg, lansoprazole 30 mg, dexlansoprazole 30–60 mg, esomeprazole or pantoprazole 40 mg daily half an hour before breakfast.

Mucosal Protective Agents

Protective agents (sucralfate, bismuth, misoprostol) promote ulcer healing by enhancing the mucosal defensive mechanism. However, these are not used as the first line therapy in active ulcers because other agents (PPI and H_2 receptor blockers) are more efficacious and better tolerated.
- Sucralfate (1 g 4 times daily) is used in addition to other drugs in refractory ulcers.
- Bismuth containing compounds are given along with antibiotics to eradicate *H. pylori*.
- Misoprostol is used to prevent ulcers due to NSAIDs.

H. pylori Eradication Therapy

Eradication of *H. pylori* is achieved with treatment in 85–90% cases. Successful eradication reduces the recurrence of ulcer. Following regimens are used for the treatment:
- *Standard triple drug therapy:* Amoxycillin 1 g twice daily plus clarithromycin 500 mg twice daily plus PPI twice a day
- *Bismuth containing quadruple therapy:* Tetracycline 500 mg four times daily plus bismuth subsalicylate 262 mg two tablets/bismuth subcitrate 120–400 mg orally four times daily plus metronidazole 500 mg twice daily plus PPI twice a day
- *Non-bismuth containing quadruple therapy:* Amoxycillin 1 g twice daily plus clarithromycin 500 mg twice daily plus metronidazole 500 mg twice daily plus twice a day PPI.

PPI: Omeprazole or rabeprazole 20 mg, lansoprazole 30 mg, pantoprazole 40 mg twice a day.

Quadruple drug therapy is preferred if clarithromycin resistance is >15%.

Duration: Treatment with anti-*H pyori* therapy is given for 14 days and PPI is continued for further 4–6 weeks if ulcer is large or complicated.

Treatment of NSAIDs-induced Ulcers

- Treatment of active ulcer due to NSAIDs includes immediate withdrawal of the offending agent and administration of PPI or H_2 receptor antagonist. All such patients should also be tested for *H. pylori* infection. If positive, eradication therapy should also be given.
- Preventive treatment with PPI or misoprostol is required in high risk patients on NSAIDs such as age >60 years, history of ulcer disease, concurrent therapy with corticosteroids, anti-platelets or anticoagulants and serious underlying medical illness. Use of COX-2 selective NSAIDs reduces injury to the gastric mucosa.

Certain PPI interfere with the conversion of clopidogrel into active metabolite, hence in such case, H2 receptor antagonists should be preferred.

Treatment of Bleeding due to Peptic Ulcer

- Stabilization of hemodynamic condition
- Restore the intravascular volume by the blood transfusion
- Intravenous PPI by continuous infusion; pantoprazole (80 mg bolus followed by 8 mg per hour) for 72 hours in high risk cases.
- Oral PPI is given in low risk cases.
- Endoscopic therapy: Injection of epinephrine, cauterization of vessel by heater probe, application of endoclip are helpful in arrest of bleeding from ulcers.
- Intra-arterial embolization is done in cases with persistent bleeding.

Surgical Treatment

- Emergency surgery is performed in case of perforation and persistent hemorrhage.
- Elective surgery is done in gastric outflow obstruction and recurrent ulcer despite medical treatment.

DIARRHEA, DYSENTERY AND FOOD POISONING

Diarrhea is defined as passage of stool weighing more than 200–250 g. Practical definition is passage of liquid or unformed stools at an increased frequency. Normal frequency varies from 1–3/day to once in 3 days.

Approximately 9–10 L of fluid enters the small intestine daily. The majority of this fluid is absorbed in the small intestine and only about 1.5 L enters the colon. Fluid absorption also occurs in the colon and normally only 100–200 mL fluid is excreted daily in the stool.

Diarrhea is classified into:
- Acute (< 2 weeks)
- Persistent (2-4 weeks)
- Chronic (> 4 weeks).

Acute Diarrhea

Acute diarrhea is caused mainly by infections (90%). It may also be caused by drugs, ischemia, toxins and other conditions. Causes of acute diarrhea are given in **Table 2.13**.

Incubation Period

The incubation period varies from few hours to days. It is few hours (1-6 hrs) in case of preformed toxin-induced diarrhea while 12-24 hours in infective diarrhea.

Pathogenic Mechanisms

Pathogens can cause diarrhea via various mechanisms. These are described as below:
- *Toxin production:* Bacterial toxins either preformed or produced in the gut can cause diarrhea. Such toxins are exotoxins and include enterotoxins, cytotoxins, and neurotoxins. Enterotoxins disturb normal secretory mechanisms and cause profuse watery diarrhea whereas cytotoxins lead to inflammatory diarrhea by causing destruction of mucosal cells. Some bacteria produce exotoxins with both enterotoxin and cytotoxin activities. Neurotoxins produced by *S. aureus* and *B. cereus* act on the nervous system to produce vomiting.
- *Invasion:* Inflammatory diarrhea or dysentery results from the invasion and destruction of mucosal cells by *Shigella* or Enteroinvasive *E. coli*. Intraepithelial multiplication and spread to adjacent cells also occurs.
- *Penetration: Salmonella typhi* and *Yersinia enterocolitica* penetrate intestinal mucosa and multiply in Peyer's patches or intestinal lymph nodes. They disseminate from these lymph nodes and cause fever.

Clinical Manifestations

- Fever, abdominal pain and bloody diarrhea (dysentery) suggest inflammatory type such as sheigellosis, salmonellosis, amoebiasis, *C. difficile* and Entero-hemorrhage *E. coli.*
- Watery non-bloody diarrhea with nausea, vomiting and abdominal bloating is indicative of noninflammatory diarrhea caused by toxin producing bacteria, giardia or viruses **(Table 2.13)**.

The diarrhea may be profuse leading to dehydration.
  - Thirst, dry mouth, decreased sweating, oliguria and mild weight loss suggest mild dehydration.
  - Orthostatic hypotension, sunken eyes, sunken fontanelles in infants and loss of skin turgor indicate moderate dehydration.
  - Severe dehydration may result in hypotension, tachycardia, altered sensorium and shock.

Investigations

Stool examination is the basic investigation. This may reveal ova or parasites, fecal leukocytes and increased fecal lactoferrin, blood and mucus. Presence of blood, mucus and increased fecal lactoferrin suggests inflammatory diarrhea. Microbiological investigations include culture for viral and bacterial pathogens and immunoassays for toxins.

Lower GI endoscopy and biopsy of the intestine may be needed in cases with persistent diarrhea and non-infectious diarrhea. Upper GI endoscopy and duodenal aspirate examination may also be required.

Dysentery

Dysentery is defined as diarrhea due to acute inflammation of the large intestine characterized by the presence of blood and mucus in the stool. The two main types of dysentery are *bacillary dysentery* and *amebic dysentery*. Important causes of bacillary dysentery are shigella, enteroinvasive *E. coli* (EIEC), and *Yersinia enterocolitica*. Amebic dysentery is caused by *E. histolytica*.

Table 2.13: Causes of acute diarrhea.

Infectious
Viral
- Rotavirus
- Norwalk agents
- Cytomegalovirus*

Bacterial
1. Preformed toxin
    - *S. aureus*
    - *B. cereus*
    - *Clostridium perfringens*
2. Enterotoxin induced
    - Enterotoxigenic *E. coli* (ETEC)
    - *Vibrio cholerae*
3. Cytotoxin production*
    - Enterohemorrhagic *E. coli* (EHEC)
    - *Clostridium difficile*
4. Mucosal invasion*
    - *Shigella*
    - *Campylobacter jejuni*
    - *Salmonella*
    - Enteroinvasive *E. coli* (EIEC)
    - *Yersinia enterocolitica*

Protozoal
- *Entamoeba histolytica**
- *Giardia lamblia*
- *Cryptosporidium*

Non-infectious
- Diverticulitis
- Inflammatory bowel disease (Ulcerative colitis, Crohn's disease)
- Metabolic (DKA, carcinoid)
- Sepsis
- Drugs (NSAIDs, antibiotics)
- Ischemic colitis

* Causes associated with inflammatory diarrhea.

Clinical features of dysentery include diarrhea, fever, abdominal pain and tenesmus. Stools are usually small and contain blood or purulent material. The colon is tender to palpate. Diagnosis depends on stool examination and culture.

Food Poisoning

- Food poisoning is gastroenteritis of infective or non-infective origin.
- The important infective causes are *S. aureus, salmonella, B. cereus* and *E. coli.*
- Non-infective causes are allergy to sea foods, fish or fungal toxins **(Table 2.14)**.
- The presentation is in the form of vomiting, diarrhea or both which usually occurs within 1–48 hours of consumption of contaminated drinks or food.
- The incubation period is short (from minutes to hours) in case of noninfective causes or due to ingestion of food with preformed toxins.
- The concurrent occurrence of illness in more than one member of the family, group or institution suggests the possibility of food poisoning.

Investigations

The stool, vomitus or suspected food should be sent for culture. The tests for the presence of specific toxins should also be performed.

Management

Most cases are mild and do not require specific therapy. However evaluation and treatment are required in:
- Profuse diarrhea
- Bloody stools
- Presence of fever
- Severe abdominal pain
- Duration of more than 48 hours without improvement
- Elderly
- Immunocompromised patients.

Fluid and Electrolyte Management

Fluid and electrolyte management is the cornerstone in the treatment of diarrhea. In most cases with non-inflammatory diarrhea, no treatment is required except adequate rehydration. The disease is mostly self limiting. The patient is advised to take fluids orally to maintain hydration and electrolytes. *Oral rehydration solutions* (ORS) are available for fluid and electrolyte replacement. This usually contains 3.5 g of sodium chloride, 2.5 g of sodium bicarbonate, 1.5 g of potassium chloride and 20 g of glucose to be dissolved in one liter of water. In severe dehydration in infants and elderly, intravenous fluids are required.

Diet

Liquids, semisolids, soft and easily digestible foods are permitted, while the intake of milk, high fiber, fat, caffeine and alcohol is to be avoided.

Antimotility/Antisecretory Agents

Antimotility/antisecretory agents are used in noninflammatory diarrhea and avoided if diarrhea is bloody and there is fever.
- Antimotility/antisecretory agents such as codeine phosphate, loperamide and bismuth subsalicylates may be used to reduce the frequency and fluidity of stools.
- Racecadotril is a newer antisecretory agent useful in acute watery diarrhea.
- Diphenoxylate should be avoided in acute diarrhea.

Antimicrobial Agents

Antibiotics are not used routinely even in inflammatory diarrhea which is generally self-limiting. However, empirical antibiotics are given in patients with fever, bloody diarrhea, tenesmus and in elderly or immunocompromised patients.
- The antibiotics include fluoroquinolones (ciprofloxacin 500 mg, ofloxacin 400 mg or norfloxacin 400 mg twice daily) for 5–7 days. Alternatively, doxycycline 100 mg twice daily or trimethoprim-sulfamethoxazole 160/800 mg twice daily may be used.
- Metronidazole, tinidazole, ornidazole or nitazoxanide can empirically be given if giardiasis or amebiasis is suspected.
- Specific antimicrobial treatment is needed in shigellosis, cholera, salmonellosis, traveller's diarrhea, *C. difficile* infection. Rifaximin 200 mg three times daily or azithromycin 500 mg once daily for 3 days is indicated in non-inflammatory traveller's diarrhea.

Table 2.14: Causes of food poisoning.

Infective
Toxin mediated
- S. aureus (1–6 H)*
- C. perfringens (8–16 H)
- C. botulinum
- E. coli (EHEC, ETEC) (>16 H)
- Bacillus cereus (1–6, 8–16 H)
- Vibrio cholerae (>16 H)

Non-toxin mediated
- Salmonella (>16 H)
- Shigella (>16 H)
- Campylobacter jejuni (>16 H)
- Bacillus anthracis
- Listeria monocytogenes
- Viruses (rotavirus)

Non-infective
Allergic
- Shellfish, strawberries

Non-allergic
- Fish (Ciguatoxin, scombotoxin)
- Fungi (Amanita phalloides)
- Chemicals, metals

*Incubation period in hours.

Chronic Diarrhea

Diarrhea lasting for more than 4 weeks is known as chronic diarrhea. It is mostly caused by noninfectious causes. A number of pathologic mechanisms can lead to chronic diarrhea **(Table 2.15)**.

Secretory Diarrhea

This is due to alteration in fluid and electrolyte transport across the mucosa. Watery, large volume diarrhea which persists on fasting is characteristic. Important causes include medications (laxatives), hormone-mediated (VIPoma, Carcinoid), villous adenoma and bile salt malabsorption.

Osmotic Diarrhea

Osmotic diarrhea occurs when an ingested nutrient is not absorbed and drags fluid along with it. This type of diarrhea ceases on fasting. Osmotic laxatives (antacids, lactulose, sorbitol) and carbohydrate malabsorption, lactase deficiency are important causes of osmotic diarrhea.

Treatment: Treatment of chronic diarrhea depends on the cause. Antibiotics are useful in tropical sprue. Avoidance of lactose intake is recommended in lactose intolerant patients. However, fluid and electrolyte management is important in all such cases.

MALABSORPTION

Disorders of digestion and diminished absorption of dietary nutrients (one or more) are referred as malabsorption

TABLE 2.15: Causes of chronic diarrhea.

Inflammatory causes
- Ulcerative colitis
- Crohn's disease
- Malignancies (lymphoma, adenocarcinoma)

Chronic infections
- Giardia, Entamoeba
- AIDS related
    - Cytomegalovirus
    - Microsporidium (Enterocytozoon bieneusi), cryptosporidium
    - Isospora belli (Cytoisospora belli)

Motility disorders
- Diabetes
- Hyperthyroidism
- Irritable bowel syndrome

Osmotic diarrhea
- Medications (Lactulose, sorbitol)
- Lactose intolerance

Secretory diarrhea
- Medications
- VIPoma
- Carcinoid
- Zollinger-Ellison syndrome
- Villous adenoma

Factitious diarrhea
- Laxatives
- Magnesium containing antacids

Malabsorption syndromes

Table 2.16: Causes of malabsorption.

Intraluminal maldigestion
Pancreatic enzyme deficiency
- Chronic pancreatitis
- Pancreatic carcinoma
- Cystic fibrosis

Reduced bile acids
- Liver diseases
- Intestinal bacterial overgrowth (fistula, blind loop)
- Decreased enterohepatic circulation (ileal resection, Crohn's disease)

Mucosal defects
- Intestinal resection
- Infiltration, inflammation or infection of mucosa
    - Crohn's disease
    - Celiac sprue
    - Tropical sprue
    - Whipple's disease
    - Giardiasis
    - Lymphoma
- Genetic diseases (lactase deficiency)

Impaired nutrient uptake
- Lymphatic obstruction (lymphoma, lymphangiectasia)
- CHF, pericarditis

Miscellaneous
- Diabetes mellitus
- Hyperthyroidism
- Hypoparathyroidism

syndromes. Various diseases with varied etiologies can lead to malabsorption and may present with different clinical manifestations.

Normal digestion and absorption may be divided into three phases and malabsorption can result from abnormalities in one or more of these phases **(Table 2.16)**.

Intraluminal Phase

There is inadequate hydrolysis and solubilization of dietary nutrients (protein, fat and carbohydrates) leading to malabsorption. This is mainly due to insufficient bile or pancreatic enzymes. The important causes are pancreatic diseases, biliary obstruction, cholestatic liver diseases and decreased enterohepatic circulation of bile salts.

Mucosal Phase

The damage to the intestinal epithelium or resection of a part of small intestine diminishes the surface area for absorption. The brush border enzyme defects may also lead to malabsorption.

Absorptive Phase

Lymphatic obstruction prevents proper uptake and transport of absorbed lipoproteins and chylomicrons. Increased pressure in lymphatics may cause leakage of absorbed nutrients back into the intestinal lumen leading to steatorrhea and protein loosing enteropathy.

The deficiency of any specific nutrient and its manifestations depend on the site and extent of the intestinal involvement. Iron, folic acid and calcium are absorbed in the proximal intestine while vitamin B_{12} and bile salts are absorbed in the ileum. For example, the disease of terminal ileum may lead to vitamin B_{12} deficiency and involvement of proximal small intestine may cause iron deficiency.

Clinical Manifestations

Diarrhea and weight loss despite normal dietary intake should prompt one to evaluate the patients for malabsorption. In most patients, there is steatorrhea that is an increase in excretion of more than 7 g per day fat in the stool. Bulky, pale and offensive stool which floats on water is characteristic of steatorrhea. Malabsorption syndromes should be considered in the differential diagnosis of chronic diarrhea.

Diarrhea may result due to following pathogenetic mechanisms:
- *Osmotic diarrhea:* It occurs due to decreased absorption of dietary nutrients. It improves on prolonged fasting.
- Nonabsorbed fatty acids in cases of steatorrhea interfere with intestinal ion transport leading to diarrhea.
- *Secretory diarrhea:* It occurs due to increased intestinal fluid and electrolytes secretion in response to exotoxins or increased gut hormones (VIP). The diarrhea does not improve on fasting.

Other features are abdominal distension, cramps in abdomen and presence of undigested food in stool. Increased flatus formation occurs due to bacterial fermentation of unabsorbed carbohydrates. Symptoms related to specific deficiency of minerals, vitamins or other nutrients can also be present. Weakness, lethargy and malaise may also be present **(Table 2.17)**.

Investigations

Routine laboratory studies: Tests are performed to detect any nutrient deficiency (one or many). These tests reveal malabsorption of particular nutrient/nutrients but do not establish the cause. Some important tests are given in **Table 2.18**.

TABLE 2.17: Pathologic basis of symptoms of malabsorption.	
Symptoms/Signs	Malabsorbed nutrients
Anemia	Iron, folic acid, Vitamin B_{12}
Bleeding	Vitamin K, Vitamin C
Glossitis, stomatitis	Iron, folic acid, Vitamin B_{12}, Vitamin A
Night blindness, xerophthalmia	Vitamin A
Tetany, paresthesia	Calcium, magnesium, potassium
Bone pain	Calcium, Vit D, protein
Neuropathies	Vitamin B_{12} and Vitamin B_1
Dermatitis	Vitamin A, zinc, essential fatty acids
Azotemia, hypotension	Fluid and electrolytes
Edema	Protein
Muscle wasting	Protein
Bleeding gums	Vitamin C

TABLE 2.18: Routine blood tests in malabsorption.	
Complete blood count	Anemia (iron, folate and cobalamin deficiency)
General blood picture • Microcytic • Macrocytic	Iron deficiency Folate and cobalamin deficiency
Prothrombin time	Vitamin K deficiency
Total serum protein and albumin	Protein malabsorption
Alkaline phosphatase	Vitamin D deficiency
Serum carotene	Vitamin A deficiency
Serum cholesterol	Fat malabsorption
Serum iron, folate, cobalamin	Iron, folate, cobalamin malabsorption
Serum calcium	Calcium or Vitamin D

Specific Tests

- *Fecal fat estimation:* This is a reliable test to confirm steatorrhea and fat malabsorption. Sudan III stain may show an increase in the stool fat. Quantitative estimation of fat in the stool is more reliable and sensitive. A 72 hours stool collection, while the patient is on a defined diet, is used for fat estimation. Excretion of more than 10 g fat per day suggests fat malabsorption.
- *Schilling test:* This is useful in the diagnosis of cobalamin malabsorption and its cause. Cobalamin metabolism and absorption depends on the normal gastric, pancreatic and ileal functions. Cobalamin malabsorption may occur in pernicious anemia, chronic pancreatitis, achlorhydria and bacterial overgrowth. Schilling test can be used to assess the functional status of these organs and to determine the pathological processes responsible for malabsorption. Radio-labeled cobalamin (1 mg ^{58}Co) is given orally and its excretion in urine is measured. One mg cobalamin is administered intramuscularly to saturate hepatic binding sites so that all radio-labeled cobalamin is excreted in the urine. The test is abnormal if less than 10% of the radio-labeled cobalamin is excreted in the urine in 24 hours. If the test is abnormal, it is repeated by giving radio-labeled cobalamin in combination with intrinsic factor or pancreatic enzymes. It may also be repeated after a 5 days course of antibiotics. This will help in differentiating the various defects responsible for malabsorption of cobalamin.
- *D-Xylose test* is performed to detect carbohydrate malabsorption. 25 g D-Xylose is given orally and its excretion is measured in urine. Excretion of less than 4.5 g in 5 hours is indicative of malabsorption.
- *Upper GI endoscopy and biopsy of small intestinal mucosa*: This is essential for the diagnosis of conditions

like tropical sprue, celiac sprue, Whipple's disease and Crohn's disease.
- *Radiological assessment* of the small intestine with barium contrast is helpful in evaluation of structural abnormalities.
- *Pancreatic exocrine functions* are assessed in patients with steatorrhea.
- *Serological studies:* Autoantibodies are detected in some conditions such as celiac sprue and pernicious anemia.

Treatment

- Deficient nutrients are replaced.
- Specific therapy depends on the cause:
  – Gluten diets (wheat, barley) should be avoided in celiac sprue.
  – Tropical sprue is treated with tetracycline and folic acid for 6 months.
  – Cotrimoxazole double strength tablet daily is given for 1 year in Whipple's disease.
  – A one to two week course of antibiotics (fluoroquinolone, tetracycline, metronidazole) is given in malabsorption due to bacterial overgrowth.
  – Milk products are avoided in lactase deficiency.

IMPLICATIONS ON DENTAL PRACTICE

- Patients with gastric acid reflux may develop foul taste (dysgeusia), increased dental sensitivity, dental erosion and pulpitis. Such patients should be treated in semisupine position. Proton pump inhibitors and antacids are administered before the procedure.
- Oral manifestations in peptic ulcer disease are rare. However, regurgitation of gastric acid may lead to dental erosion, particularly at the palatal aspect of maxillary teeth.
- Use of aspirin and NSAIDs should be avoided in patients with history of peptic ulcer disease. Paracetamol can be used safely. Antacids may interfere with the absorption of antibiotics. Hence, patients are advised to take antibiotics 2 hours before or after the ingestion of antacids.

SELF ASSESSMENT

Multiple Choice Questions

1. The most common extraintestinal complication of amebiasis is:
   A. Lung abscess
   B. Liver abscess
   C. Brain abscess
   D. Subdiaphragmatic abscess
2. Complications of peptic ulcer include all, *except*:
   A. Perforation
   B. Hemorrhage
   C. Gastric outlet obstruction
   D. Gallstones
3. All the following organisms can cause bloody diarrhea, *except*:
   A. *Yersinia enterocolitica* B. *Shigella*
   C. *Giardia lamblia* D. *Entamoeba histolytica*
4. All the following are common causes of hematemesis, *except*:
   A. Esophageal varices B. Peptic ulcer
   C. Pernicious anemia D. Mallory-Weiss tears
5. Stress ulcer may occur in:
   A. Head injury B. Trauma
   C. Burns D. All the above
6. Hunger pain is found in:
   A. Duodenal ulcer B. Gastric ulcer
   C. Gastric carcinoma D. Esophageal diseases
7. Most common cause of hematemesis is:
   A. Variceal bleed B. Peptic ulcer
   C. Carcinoma stomach D. Gastric erosions
8. Peptic ulcer is etiologically related to:
   A. *H. pylori* infection
   B. Opioid analgesics
   C. Increased consumption of tea, coffee and spicy food
   D. All the above
9. Following is used to prevent NSAIDs-induced peptic ulcer:
   A. Sucralfate B. PPI
   C. H_2 blockers D. Steroid
10. *H. pylori* infection can cause:
    A. Gastritis
    B. Peptic ulcer
    C. Adenocarcinoma of stomach
    D. All the above
11. Erosive and hemorrhagic gastritis can occur in:
    A. Alcohol
    B. Patients with head injury
    C. Patients with severe burns
    D. All the above
12. Black tarry stools usually suggest:
    A. Upper GI bleeding B. Lower GI bleeding
    C. Amoebic dysentery D. Bacterial dysentery
13. Schilling test is used for the diagnosis of:
    A. Folate deficiency B. Cobalamin deficiency
    C. Protein malabsorption D. Fat malabsorption
14. Vitamin B_{12} absorption occurs in:
    A. Duodenum and jejunum
    B. Large intestine
    C. Stomach
    D. Ileum
15. Treatment of choice in patients with acute watery diarrhea is:
    A. Antimotility agents
    B. Antibiotics
    C. Rehydration therapy
    D. Antispasmodic agents
16. Murphy's sign is present in:
    A. Acute cholecystitis B. Acute appendicitis
    C. Acute diverticulitis D. Acute salpingitis
17. Hematochezia is present in which of the following conditions:
    A. Colon carcinoma B. Peptic ulcer
    C. Esophageal varices D. Barret's esophagus
18. Gingival hyperplasia is a feature of:
    A. Acute myeloid leukemia
    B. Acute lymphoid leukemia

ESSENTIALS OF MEDICINE FOR DENTAL STUDENTS

   C. Chronic myeloid leukemia
   D. Chronic lymphoblastic leukemia
19. **"Strawberry Gums" are seen in:**
   A. Lymphoma
   B. Multiple myeloma
   C. Wegener's disease
   D. Squamous cell carcinoma
20. **Odynophagia is usually a feature of:**
   A. Achalasia cardia
   B. Gastritis
   C. Esophageal candidiasis
   D. Esophageal diverticulitis

Fill in the Blanks

1. Coffee ground emesis or vomiting of dark, altered blood with clots is known as _____.
2. Large, bulky stools which float in water are suggestive of _____.
3. Shifting dullness is a sign of _____.
4. Stress ulcers in patients after head injury are known as _____ ulcers.
5. Stress ulcers in patients with burns are known as _____ ulcers.
6. Iron absorption occurs in _____.

CHAPTER 3

Hepatobiliary System

LIVER: STRUCTURE AND FUNCTION

The liver is the largest organ of the body. It is situated in the right hypochondrium under the diaphragm. Anatomically it is divided into right and left lobes. It has dual blood supply, 80% comes from the portal vein and the remainder from the hepatic artery. Two-third of the mass of the liver is constituted by hepatocytes. Other important cell types are Kupfer cells (RE system), stellate cells (Ito or fat storing cells) and endothelial cells. Histologically the liver is composed of lobules with portal areas at the periphery and central vein in the center of the lobule.

The liver has numerous functions necessary for good health. The main functions can be classified into following groups:
- *Synthetic function:* Liver is the site for the synthesis of albumin, coagulation factors, carrier proteins, hormones and growth factors. Almost all coagulation factors (except factor VIII) are synthesized in the liver. The synthesis of factors II, VII, IX, X requires Vitamin K.
- *Metabolic functions:* Liver is an important site for the metabolism of carbohydrates, proteins and lipids. It also metabolizes drugs, alcohol and bilirubin. Ammonia is metabolized in the liver into urea.
- *Excretory functions:* The bile and its contents (bile acid, bile salts) are synthesized and excreted by the liver.
- *Storage functions:* Liver is the storage site for vitamins (A, D, B_{12}, folate and K) and minerals (iron and copper). Iron is stored in the form of ferritin and hemosiderin.

Liver Function Tests

The liver has numerous functions and no single test is enough to assess all its functions. However, certain tests are performed to assess some of the main functions of the liver (serum albumin, serum bilirubin and prothrombin time) while other tests indicate the severity of damage

Table 3.1: Liver function tests.

Tests to assess excretory function	Serum bilirubin Urine bilirubin Blood ammonia
Tests to assess synthetic function	Serum albumin Coagulation factors: • Prothrombin time (PT), International normalized ratio (INR) • Activated partial thromboplastin time (aPTT) Others: • α-1 antitrypsin • α-fetoprotein • ceruloplasmin
Serum enzymes Indicate either damage to hepatocytes or cholestasis	Aminotransferases: • Alanine aminotransferase (ALT) or serum glutamic pyruvic transaminase (SGPT) • Aspartate aminotransferase (AST) or serum glutamic-oxaloacetic transaminase (SGOT) Alkaline phosphatase (ALP) Serum 5'nucleotidase Gamma glutamyl transpeptidase (GGT)

(aminotransferases) or obstruction to bile flow (alkaline phosphatase) **(Table 3.1)**.

Tests to Assess Excretory Functions

- *Serum bilirubin:* The normal level of serum total bilirubin is 0.3–1.0 mg/dL. It is present in two forms, unconjugated (0.2–0.7 mg/dL) and conjugated bilirubin (0.1–0.3 mg/dL). A rise in the level of conjugated bilirubin suggests liver or biliary tract disease. Isolated elevation of unconjugated bilirubin is rare in liver disease and it indicates hemolysis.
- *Urine bilirubin:* Conjugated bilirubin (not the unconjugated bilirubin) is excreted in the urine when the plasma level of conjugated bilirubin is raised. Hence, the presence of bilirubin in the urine suggests liver disease.

- *Blood ammonia level:* Blood ammonia level may be raised in severe hepatic dysfunction and hepatic encephalopathy. It may also be high due to portal shunting in portal hypertension.

Tests to Assess Synthetic Functions

- *Serum albumin:* Albumin is exclusively synthesized in the liver. The normal value of serum albumin is 3.5–5.5 g/dL. It has a long half life of about 20 days, therefore a low serum albumin suggests chronic liver disease.
- *Coagulation factors:* The half life of most coagulation factors is short; factor VII has the shortest half life (six hours). Hence, measurement of prothrombin time (PT) is helpful in the diagnosis and the prognosis of acute parenchymal liver disease. Prothrombin time may also be prolonged in obstructive jaundice due to vitamin K malabsorption. Correction of PT after administration of vitamin K suggests vitamin K deficiency.
- *Miscellaneous:* Other tests used to measure synthetic functions of the liver include serum levels of α-1 antitrypsin, α-fetoprotein and ceruloplasmin.

Serum Enzymes

The liver contains thousands of enzymes. Many are present in the serum in very low quantity. The elevation of these enzymes in the serum indicates either damage to hepatocytes or cholestasis.

- *Aminotransferases:* Serum alanine aminotransferase or serum glutamic pyruvic transaminase (ALT or SGPT) and aspartate aminotransferase (AST or SGOT) are raised in acute liver cell injury. The normal serum levels of ALT and AST are 0–35 Unit/L. However, its elevation does not correlate with the severity of the disease. A rise in ALT is more specific to liver cell injury since AST can also be raised in other conditions such as diseases of myocardium, skeletal muscles, kidneys and brain. The ratio of serum AST to ALT is less than one in viral hepatitis whereas it is greater than two in alcoholic liver disease. They are usually not significantly elevated in obstructive jaundice.
- *Alkaline phosphatase:* A significant rise in serum alkaline phosphatase (ALP) suggests cholestasis (obstruction in the bile flow). It may be mildly raised in other liver diseases. The normal serum level is 30–120 units/L. Alkaline phosphatase is also present in other body tissues like bone, intestine, placenta and leukocytes.
- *Serum 5'nucleotidase and gamma glutamyltranspeptidase (GGT)* are also raised in cholestasis. Hence, a concomitant rise in serum 5'nucleotidase or gamma glutamyltranspeptidase (GGT) along with ALP suggests hepatic origin of alkaline phosphatase.

Imaging Techniques

- *Ultrasonography:* It is useful to screen for the evidence of intrahepatic or extrahepatic cholestasis and gallstones (Figs. 3.1A and B). In addition, it can detect liver cysts, abscesses and masses. Biopsy of a lesion can be done under ultrasonographic monitoring. Ultrasonography may also detect portal hypertension (dilated portal vein, ascites, splenomegaly and collateral vessels).
- *CT scan and MRI:* These are useful in the evaluation of parenchymal liver disease. Contrast enhancement can be used to differentiate the nature of space occupying lesions. With MRI, vessels can be visualized without use of IV contrast.
- *Endoscopic retrograde cholangiopancreatography (ERCP) and Percutaneous transhepatic cholangiography (PTC):* These help in the detection of the cause, location and the extent of the biliary obstruction. ERCP can be used for therapeutic interventions such as stone extraction from common bile duct and for placing a stent. Magnetic resonance cholangiopancreatography (MRCP) is a sensitive and noninvasive technique of visualizing the biliary tree.

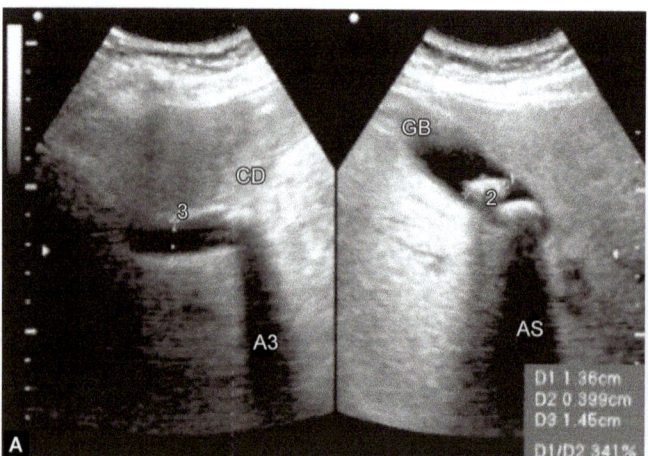
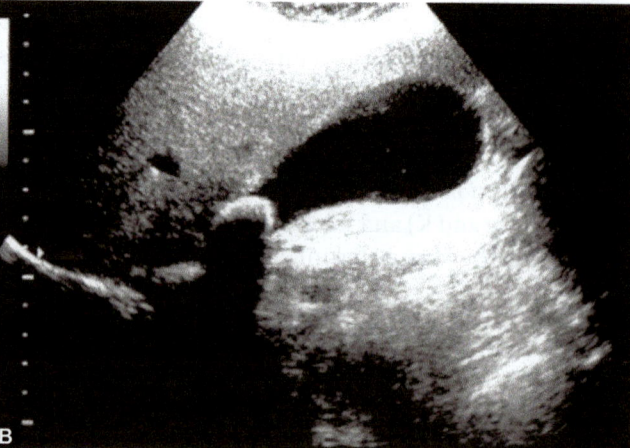

Figs. 3.1A and B: (A) Ultrasound showing stones in the gallbladder; (B) Ultrasound showing impacted stone in the neck of gallbladder.

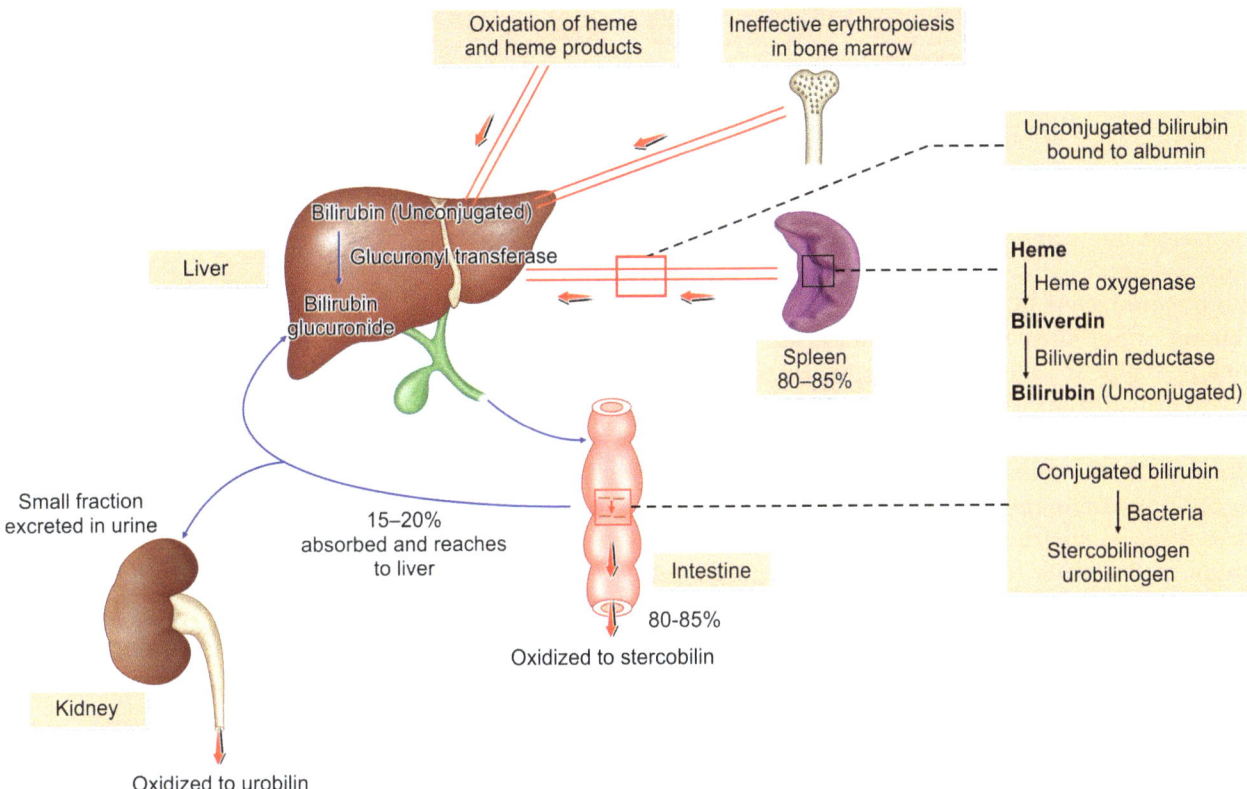

Fig. 3.2: Bilirubin metabolism.

Liver Biopsy

Biopsy is a definitive method to diagnose the cause and severity of hepatocellular diseases. This is usually done through percutaneous route. Transjugular route can be used in patients with ascites or a risk of bleeding.

■ JAUNDICE

A yellowish discoloration of the skin and mucous membrane due to deposition of bilirubin is known as jaundice (icterus). The deposition of bilirubin in tissues occurs when the serum bilirubin level is raised (hyperbilirubinemia).
- The normal total serum bilirubin level is 0.3–1.0 mg/dL. With the use of Van den Bergh's method, it has been shown that up to 30% of the total bilirubin (0.3 mg/dL) may be the conjugated or direct reacting type. However, newer techniques have shown that in normal individuals, almost all bilirubin in the serum is unconjugated.
- Sclerae have a high affinity for bilirubin due to their rich elastin content. Jaundice is clinically apparent in sclera when bilirubin level is raised above 3 mg/dL.
- The clinical detection of jaundice is difficult in artificial light. Hence, it should be examined preferably in day light.
- Other sites to be looked for the evidence of jaundice are mucosa of oral cavity underneath the tongue and skin.
- Urine is dark yellow in color due to excretion of conjugated bilirubin.
- Yellow discoloration of the skin can also occur in carotenemia (carotenoderma) and exposure to quinacrine or phenols. Sclera is typically not involved in carotenemia.

Bilirubin Metabolism

- Bilirubin is a product of heme metabolism. The breakdown of old red blood cells in the reticuloendothelial system (primarily spleen and liver) leads to the release of heme **(Fig. 3.2)**. Heme is further metabolized into biliverdin and subsequently to bilirubin. About 70–80% of bilirubin is derived from this mechanism. The rest comes from the breakdown of premature erythroid cells in bone marrow (ineffective erythropoiesis) and the catabolism of myoglobin and cytochromes.
- This insoluble bilirubin binds reversibly and noncovalently to albumin (unconjugated or indirect bilirubin) and is transported to the liver where it is detached from albumin and is taken up by hepatocytes.
- In hepatocytes, the bilirubin is solubilized by conjugation to glucuronic acid that yields bilirubin monoglucuronide and diglucuronide (conjugated or direct bilirubin). This reaction is catalyzed by the enzyme UDP-glucuronyl transferase.
- Conjugated bilirubin is then transported to the duodenum via bile. Colonic bacteria metabolize the conjugated bilirubin into stercobilinogen which may be further oxidized to stercobilin. Stercobilinogen and stercobilin are excreted in stool. A small amount of stercobilinogen is absorbed to reach the liver through portal system and is re-excreted into the bile. A fraction escapes liver uptake

Table 3.2: Urinary findings in different types of jaundice.

Urine findings	Hemolytic	Hepato-cellular	Obstructive	Normal
Urobilinogen	+++	++	–	+
Bilirubin	–	++	++	–

and passes into urine as urobilinogen and its oxidized form, urobilin.
- The unconjugated bilirubin, because it is bound to albumin, is not filtered through kidneys and therefore does not appear in urine. Hence, in unconjugated hyperbilirubinemia (as in hemolysis), bilirubin is absent in the urine (acholuric jaundice). However, urobilinogen is increased in the urine. The presence of bilirubin in urine suggests predominant conjugated hyperbilirubinemia (liver disease, obstructive jaundice). Urobilinogen is absent in the urine in cases of obstructive jaundice because bilirubin is not available in the intestine to be metabolized into stercobilinogen **(Table 3.2)**.

Types of Jaundice

Jaundice is classically divided into two broad types, unconjugated hyperbilirubinemia and conjugated hyperbilirubinemia.

Unconjugated hyperbilirubinemia: This is characterized by predominantly high levels of serum unconjugated bilirubin.
- The color of urine is normal as there is no bilirubin.
- The jaundice is generally mild (serum bilirubin <6 mg/dL).
- Additionally patients may have anemia and splenomegaly.
- The raised unconjugated bilirubin (>20 mg/dL) can lead to central nervous system manifestations in neonates (kernicterus).
- Liver transaminases and alkaline phosphatase are normal.

Unconjugated hyperbilirubinemia may result either from overproduction of bilirubin or from impaired hepatic uptake or conjugation of bilirubin. **Table 3.3** shows the clinical and laboratory features in different types of jaundice.
- *Overproduction of bilirubin (prehepatic):* This may occur in hemolytic disorders such as hereditary spherocytosis, sickle cell anemia, G6PD deficiency, paroxysmal nocturnal hemoglobinuria and autoimmune hemolytic anemia. Other causes include ineffective erythropoiesis, hemolytic reaction and resolution of hematoma.
- *Impaired hepatic metabolism:* The hepatic uptake of bilirubin is impaired because of some drugs (like rifampicin and probenecid) and in Gilbert's syndrome. The conjugation of bilirubin is impaired in Gilbert's syndrome and Criggler-Najjar syndromes because of decreased activity of the enzyme, glucuronyl transferase.

Most neonates develop mild rise in unconjugated bilirubin because of incompletely developed hepatic

Table 3.3: Features of different types of jaundice.

	Prehepatic (Hemolytic)	Hepatic (Hepatocellular)	Posthepatic (Obstructive)
History	Recurrent jaundice, positive family history, anemia	Prodrome: fever, anorexia, nausea	Pain in abdomen, may be recurrent
Skin color	Lemon yellow	Yellow	Dark yellow
Pruritus	Absent	Occasional (early phase)	Present
Spleen	Enlarged	Occasional	Not enlarged
Gallbladder	Not palpable	Not palpable	May be palpable
Feces	Normal	Pale (if cholestasis)	Pale
Urine color	Colorless, yellow on standing (Urobilinogen)	Dark (Bilirubin and urobilinogen)	Very dark (High bilirubin)
Tests for hemolysis	Positive	Negative	Negative
Serum bilirubin	Unconjugated (<6 mg/dL)	Mixed	Conjugated
ALT (SGPT)	Normal	Increased (+++)	Minimally increased (+)
Alkaline phosphatase	Normal	Minimally high (+)	High (+++)
Serum albumin	Normal	Low (in chronic disease)	Normal
Prothrombin time	Normal	Prolonged	Prolonged (correctable with vitamin K)
Important causes	Hemolysis, Gilbert's syndrome	Viral hepatitis, Drugs, Alcohol	Gallstones, Carcinoma pancreas

functions *(physiologic neonatal jaundice)*. Marked elevation of unconjugated bilirubin in premature infants can lead to kernicterus.

Gilbert's syndrome, an autosomal dominant disorder, is a common disorder with mild jaundice. Conjugation of bilirubin is also impaired due to decreased activity of glucuronyl transferase enzyme. Serum bilirubin is generally less than 6 mg/dL. No treatment is required.

Criggler-Najjar syndromes are characterized by complete absence of activity of glucuronyl transferase (Type I) or reduced activity of the enzyme (Type II). The jaundice is severe and death occurs early in type I Criggler-Najjar syndrome. Most patients with type II Criggler-Najjar syndrome survive up to adulthood.

Conjugated Hyperbilirubinemia: Serum conjugated bilirubin is raised in inherited conditions such as Dubin-Johnson syndrome and Rotor syndrome, hepatocellular diseases and cholestatic conditions.
- *Dubin-Johnson and Rotor syndromes:* These are rare inherited disorders characterized by asymptomatic jaundice due to altered excretion of bilirubin in the bile

ducts. The liver transaminases and alkaline phosphatase levels are normal.
- *Hepatocellular diseases:* The bilirubin uptake, conjugation and its transport to bile canaliculi can all be affected due to parenchymal liver disease. Besides conjugated bilirubin, unconjugated bilirubin may also be raised. Levels of amino transferases (ALT, AST) are raised out of proportion to alkaline phosphatase. Clinical features of hepatocellular jaundice are given in the **Table 3.3**. Causes of hepatocellular jaundice are given in **Table 3.4**.
- *Cholestatic jaundice (Obstructive jaundice):* This type of jaundice results from the obstruction in the bile flow which may be intrahepatic or extrahepatic. Clinical features of cholestatic jaundice are given in the **Table 3.3**. Causes of obstructive jaundice are given in **Table 3.5**.
    - Conjugated bilirubin enters into blood and appears in urine.
    - The stool becomes pale due to reduced formation of stercobilinogen in the intestine.
    - Retention of bile salts leads to its deposition in the skin and severe pruritus (itching). Patients usually have scratch marks on skin.
    - Reduced availability of bile in the intestine may lead to malabsorption of fat and fat soluble vitamins (vitamin K and vitamin D). This may result in bleeding diasthesis and osteomalacia.
    - Serum alkaline phosphatase is raised out of proportion as compared to aminotransferases.

ACUTE HEPATITIS

Acute hepatitis can be mainly caused by viral infections, alcohol and drugs. Important causes are given in **Table 3.6**. Acute viral hepatitis is described below in detail.

ACUTE VIRAL HEPATITIS

Acute viral hepatitis is a systemic viral infection characterized by the predominant involvement of liver. It is caused by one of the specific hepatitis viruses. Rarely, other viruses may also cause hepatitis particularly in immunocompromised host **(Table 3.7)**.

Infection by any of the viruses mentioned in the **Table 3.7** results in similar clinical features, which may vary from asymptomatic anicteric presentation to fulminant hepatic failure. The infection due to HBV, HCV, and HDV can lead to chronic hepatitis, cirrhosis and hepatocellular carcinoma.

Pathology

The pathological features are generally the same in all types of hepatitis.
- Acute hepatitis is characterized by generalized mononuclear cell infiltration, hepatic cell damage (swelling and necrosis), Kupffer cell hyperplasia and variable degree of cholestasis.
- The hepatocytes are swollen and granular. Hepatic cells undergo acidophilic degeneration. These are called Councilman bodies.
- More severe damage leads to the collapse of the reticulin framework bringing the central vein and portal tracts closer. This is known as *bridging or subacute hepatic necrosis*.
- Wide spread massive hepatic necrosis occurs in fulminant hepatitis.

Hepatitis A

Hepatitis A virus (HAV) is a RNA virus of the picornavirus family.
- The transmission is by the feco-oral route. An epidemic can occur due to contamination of food and drinking

Table 3.4: Causes of hepatocellular jaundice.

Viral hepatitis: A, B, C, D, E, EBV, CMV
Alcohol
Drugs: Isoniazid, paracetamol
Toxins: Vinyl chloride, Amanita phalloides
Metabolic: Wilson's disease
Immune: Autoimmune hepatitis

Table 3.5: Causes of obstructive jaundice.

Intrahepatic
- Hepatitis
- Primary biliary cirrhosis
- Drugs: Chlorpromazine, anabolic steroids, contraceptives

Extrahepatic
- Stone in bile duct
- Sclerosing cholangitis
- Neoplasms of gallbladder and pancreas
- Compression by enlarged lymph nodes

Table 3.6: Important causes of acute hepatitis.

- Viral hepatitis
- Alcohol
- Drugs (INH, rifampicin, phenytoin, methyldopa)
- Autoimmune hepatitis
- Weil's disease (leptospirosis)
- Toxins (CCl4, yellow phosphorus, Amanita phalloides)
- Wilson's disease
- Hemochromatosis

Table 3.7: Causes of viral hepatitis.

Specific hepatitis viruses
- Hepatitis A virus (HAV)
- Hepatitis B virus (HBV)
- Hepatitis C virus (HCV)
- Hepatitis D virus (HDV)
- Hepatitis E virus (HEV)

Other viruses
- Cytomegalovirus
- Epstein Barr virus
- Herpes simplex virus
- Yellow fever virus

water by HAV. Poor sanitation and overcrowding facilitate its spread.
- Infected persons excrete the virus in their feces about two weeks before the onset and during the first two weeks of illness. Rarely, the HAV can also be transmitted by blood and via the sexual route.
- The incubation period of HAV infection is about 4 weeks (15-45 days).
- Infection and subsequent immunity occurs usually in childhood.
- Mortality is low and fulminant hepatitis is uncommon.
- There is no carrier state and chronic hepatitis does not occur.

Diagnosis: Anti-HAV of IgM type is useful for the diagnosis of acute hepatitis A. Anti-HAV of IgG type appears later and indicates previous infection and immunity **(Table 3.8)**.

Table 3.8: Hepatitis A serology.

Stage	Test
Acute	IgM anti-HAV antibody +
Recovered	IgG anti-HAV antibody +
After vaccination	IgG anti-HAV antibody +

Hepatitis B

Hepatitis B virus (HBV) is a DNA virus.
- It is transmitted through infected blood and blood products or by sexual contact. Infected mother can transmit infection to the child at delivery (vertical transmission). Tattooing and acupuncture can also spread the disease.
- Incubation period is generally 30-180 days.
- High-risk groups for HBV infection include staff and patients of hemodialysis center, physicians, surgeons, dentists, paramedical staff and persons working in laboratory and blood bank.
- Patients are infectious during the incubation period and the illness and as long as they are positive for HBsAg.
- Fulminant hepatitis can occur in less than 1% patients. Acute infection can progress to the chronic phase in about 1-10% adults and 90% children who have acquired the infection from the mother at birth. Cirrhosis may develop in 15-20% patients with chronic HBV infection after 5-20 years. Hepatocellular carcinoma may also occur. The risk is higher when infection is acquired in early life.

Diagnosis: HBV has a number of antigens. The three important antigens are hepatitis B surface antigen (HBsAg), core antigen (HBcAg) and hepatitis e antigen (HBeAg). The various HBV antigens and antibodies at various stages of illness are presented in **Table 3.9**.
- Appearance of Hepatitis B surface antigen (HBsAg) in serum is the first evidence of infection **(Fig. 3.3)**. It normally persists for 3-4 weeks but can persist upto 6 months. After disappearance of HBsAg, antibody against

Table 3.9: Hepatitis B serology.

Stage	ALT/AST	HBsAg	Anti-HBs antibody	HBeAg	Anti-Hbe antibody	IgM anti-HBc antibody	IgG anti-HBc antibody	HBV DNA
Acute	++++	+	-	+	-	+	-	High load
Resolved Acute HBV	N	–	+	-	+	-	+	Nil
Chronic	+++	+	-	+	-	-	+	High load
Chronic	++	+	-	-	+	-	+	High
After vaccination	N	–	+	-	-	-	-	Nil

(ALT: alanine aminotransferase; AST: aspartate aminotransferase; HBc: Hepatitis B core antigen; HBe Ag: Hepatitis B e antigen; HBsAg: Hepatitis B surface antigen)

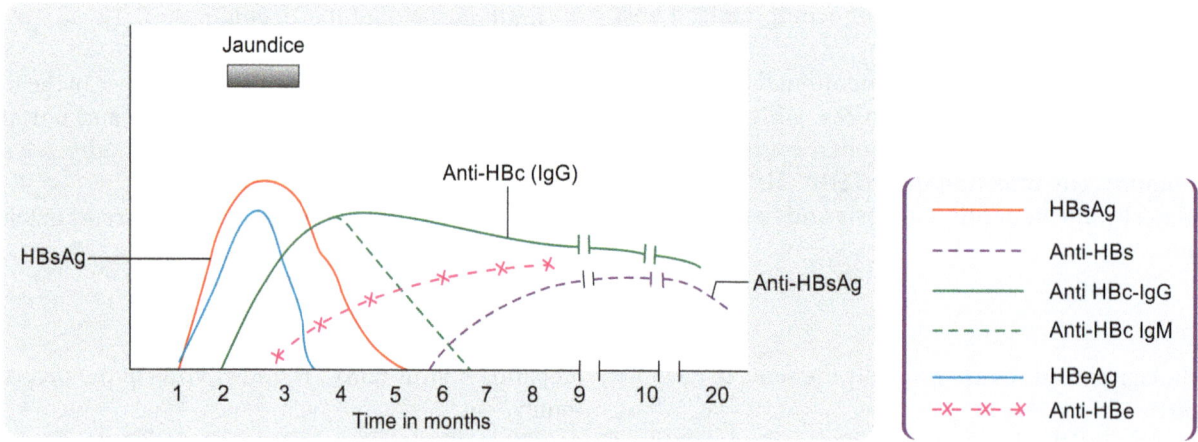

Fig. 3.3: Serological findings in acute viral hepatitis B.

HBsAg (Anti-HBs) appears and persists for years and confers immunity. Presence of Anti-HBs antibody means either previous infection or vaccination.
- The HBcAg is not found in the blood. However, antibody to it (anti-HBc) appears early during the illness. Presence of IgM anti-HBc indicates acute infection and IgG anti-HBc suggests chronic infection (when HBsAg is positive) or recovery (when anti-HBs is positive).
- The presence of HBeAg indicates active viral replication and high degree of infectivity. Anti-HBe appears as HBeAg disappears and its presence suggests low level of viral replication and decreased infectivity (seroconversion).
- The presence of HBV DNA in the serum runs parallel with HBeAg. However, it is a more sensitive and precise marker of viral replication and infectivity.

Hepatitis C

Hepatitis C virus (HCV) is a RNA virus and the only member of genus Hepacivirus of the Flaviviridae family. Six genotypes of HCV have been identified.
- The route of transmission is parenteral (transfusion of blood and blood products, IV drug abuse). Sexual and vertical spread is less common than in hepatitis B infection. In the past it was responsible for 90% of post-transfusion hepatitis.
- Incubation period is about 15–160 days.
- Acute HCV infection is usually subclinical. Chronic infection occurs in 70–80% cases. Cirrhosis and hepatocellular carcinoma can also occur.
- Extrahepatic manifestations like vasculitis, arthritis, glomerulonephritis and cryoglobulinemia may occur.

Diagnosis: HCV contains several antigens leading to antibody formation which are used in its diagnosis. The antibody is not protective and does not confer immunity. The most commonly used screening tests detect anti-HCV. These antibodies generally appear late and thus identify chronic infection. PCR test can detect HCV-RNA in the serum 1–2 weeks after infection and is used for the confirmation of diagnosis and for the monitoring of therapy **(Table 3.10)**.

Hepatitis D

Hepatitis D virus (HDV) is a RNA-defective virus.
- It requires HBV for replication and causes hepatitis only in the presence of hepatitis B infection.

Table 3.10: Hepatitis C serology.

Stage	Test
Acute (Tests may be negative)	HCV Nucleic acid test + HCV RNA + Anti-HCV antibody +
Chronic	Anti-HCV antibody + HCV RNA +
Recovered	Anti-HCV antibody + HCV RNA −

Table 3.11: Hepatitis D serology (HBV infection markers are also present).

Stage	Test
Acute	IgM anti-HBV antibody +
Chronic	IgG anti-HDV antibody + HDV Ag +
Recovered	IgG anti-HDV antibody +

- HDV infection can occur simultaneously with HBV (co-infection) or it can cause infection in patients suffering from chronic hepatitis B (superinfection).
- Chronic HBV infection superimposed with HDV can rapidly progress to cirrhosis.

Diagnosis: The diagnosis is made by detecting antibody to hepatitis D antigen (anti-HDV) or by finding HDV-RNA in serum **(Table 3.11)**.

Hepatitis E

Hepatitis E virus (HEV), a RNA virus, spreads by feco-oral route. It leads to water borne epidemics of hepatitis.
- The clinical features are similar to HAV infection.
- Incubation period is about 14–60 days.
- It does not cause chronic infection.
- Acute fulminant hepatic failure occurs at high frequency if the hepatitis occurs during pregnancy and is associated with high mortality.

Diagnosis: The diagnosis is made by detecting anti-HEV antibodies, IgM type during early phase and IgG type after recovery **(Table 3.12)**.

Clinical Features of Acute Hepatitis

The clinical features of acute hepatitis may be described under various stages:
- *Prodromal phase:* Development of jaundice is usually preceded by a prodromal phase during which nonspecific systemic symptoms like anorexia, nausea, vomiting, headache, fatigue, malaise, myalgia and arthralgia may occur. There may be distaste for smoking. Low grade fever is common in hepatitis A and E. There may be mild pain in the right upper abdomen.
- *Icteric phase:* Many patients with acute hepatitis may never become icteric (Anicteric hepatitis). Prodromal symptoms usually diminish with the onset of clinical jaundice. Patients may notice dark urine and yellowish discoloration of eyes and skin. Clay-colored stool and pruritus suggest cholestasis.

Table 3.12: Hepatitis E serology.

Stage	Test
Acute	IgM anti-HEV antibody +
Chronic	Not seen generally
Recovered	IgG anti-HEV antibody +

c. *Recovery phase:* The icteric phase is followed by an improvement in general symptoms and a diminution of jaundice. Complete clinical and biochemical recovery occurs within 1-2 months in hepatitis A and E and 3-4 months in the majority of patients with hepatitis B. In about 5% cases recovery is delayed.
d. *Signs:* The sclera is yellow and the skin may show scratch marks due to pruritus. Tender hepatomegaly is present in more than 50% cases. Splenomegaly and lymphadenopathy may occur in 10-20% cases.

Complications

The most feared complication of acute hepatitis is fulminant hepatitis. It is primarily seen in hepatitis B and D, hepatitis E during pregnancy and rarely in hepatitis A. Relapsing jaundice and cholestasis may complicate hepatitis A. A serum sickness like syndrome (arthralgia, rash, angioedema) may occur in hepatitis B. Extrahepatic complications are seen in hepatitis B and C. Important complications are given in **Table 3.13**.

Investigations

- During the early phase of hepatitis, there is significant (>400 units/L) increase in the plasma ALT and AST.
- This is followed by the rise in serum bilirubin level. However, in anicteric hepatitis, the rise in ALT and AST is not associated with any rise in bilirubin.
- High alkaline phosphatase level suggests cholestasis.
- Serum albumin concentration is normal.
- Prolongation in prothrombin time (PT) is a reliable indicator of severe liver damage and correlates with the prognosis.
- The total leukocyte count is normal or low. There may be relative lymphocytosis.
- Serological tests (as mentioned above) are performed to identify the cause of hepatitis.

Differential Diagnosis

Viral hepatitis should be differentiated from drug-induced hepatitis and alcoholic hepatitis. Important causes of acute hepatitis are given in **Table 3.6**.

Table 3.13: Complications of acute hepatitis.

Hepatic
- Acute fulminant hepatitis
- Relapsing hepatitis
- Cholestatic hepatitis
- Chronic hepatitis
- Cirrhosis
- Hepatocellular carcinoma

Extrahepatic
- Aplastic anemia
- Henoch-Schönlein purpura
- Glomerulonephritis
- Papular acrodermatitis
- Myelitis and neuropathy
- Arthritis
- Cryoglobulinemia

- History of alcoholism and intake of hepatotoxic drugs should be noted.
- Other viruses (CMV, EBV, Herpes simplex) can lead to acute hepatitis and can be diagnosed by appropriate serological tests.
- The presence of Kayser-Fleischer (KF) ring in the cornea and low serum ceruloplasmin are indicative of Wilson's disease.
- Serum ferritin is very high in hemochromatosis.

Treatment

- Physical activity is restricted. However, bed rest is recommended only in severe cases.
- A high calorie diet is recommended. A good protein intake should be encouraged. The contents of the diet should be palatable and according to the wish and acceptability of the patient. Hospitalization and intravenous fluid (10% glucose) are indicated if oral intake is not adequate or there is marked nausea and vomiting.
- Drugs which are hepatotoxic or those that are metabolized in the liver should be avoided.
- Alcohol intake should be avoided.
- Bile salt sequestering agent (cholestyramine) reduces pruritus in cases with cholestasis.
- Patients with features of severe hepatic failure such as alteration in mental status (hepatic encephalopathy) and prolonged PT/bleeding should be hospitalized.
- No specific therapy is recommended for acute viral hepatitis except in acute HCV infection. Subcutaneous interferon alpha was shown to reduce the rate of chronicity in acute HCV hepatitis. Recently oral direct acting drugs (sofosbuvir and ledipasvir) have been shown to prevent chronic hepatitis in patients with acute heptitis C.
- Liver transplantation may be required in cases with acute fulminant hepatic failure.

Prevention of Viral Hepatitis

- The prophylaxis for HAV and HBV are available. However, currently no prophylaxis is available against HCV and HEV. HDV is prevented by taking prophylactic measures against HBV.
- Improvement in sanitation and provision for safe drinking water are helpful in preventing waterborne infections like hepatitis A and E. A thorough hand washing is mandatory after bowel movements and before taking meals.
- Careful handling and disposal of used needles, use of safe blood and blood products and universal work precautions help in prevention of hepatitis B, D and C.

Hepatitis A

Active immunization: Hepatitis A vaccine (formalin inactivated vaccine) is given intramuscularly followed by a booster dose at 6-12 months. The dose is 1440 ELU for adults and half the dose for the children. Travellers to endemic area should receive it at least 4 weeks before the date of travel. This is also recommended for patients with chronic hepatitis B or C to prevent hepatitis A infection.

Passive immunization: Immune serum globulin is administered intramuscularly in the dosage of 0.02 mL/kg to the contacts soon after the exposure or traveler visiting endemic areas.

Hepatitis B

Pre-exposure prophylaxis:
- Recombinant vaccines containing HBsAg are available.
- The standard regimen in adults is 20 µg IM in the deltoid region at 0, 1 and 6 months. For rapid immunity a schedule of 0, 1, 2 and 12 months is followed. Children need half the dose (10 µg) while immunocompromized patients need 40 µg.
- Vaccine is particularly indicated in those at high risk of getting HBV infection **(Table 3.14)**.
- HBV vaccination is integrated in the Universal Immunization Programme (UIP) in India.

Post-exposure prophylaxis:
- This is given to nonvaccinated persons or persons who are vaccinated but have anti-HBS antibody titer of <10 mIU/mL (non-responders), and exposed to HBV through mucous membrane, breaks in the skin such as accidental needle-stick injury or through sexual contact **(Table 3.15)**
- If person has been infected with HBV infection earlier, no prophylaxis is recommended as they are immune to reinfection.
- This is also indicated for newborn infants of HBsAg positive mothers and in individuals who had sexual contact with persons with HBV infection.
- A dose of 0.06 mL/kg hepatitis B immunoglobulin (HBIG) is given intramuscularly as soon as possible.
- Active immunization with vaccine is also initiated simultaneously if the person is unvaccinated. These are injected at different sites.
- In persons who have completed two full courses of vaccination and still have anti-HBS antibody titer of <10 mIU/mL, two dosage of HBIG is recommended at interval of one month.

Prognosis

- Clinical recovery is generally complete in 3–6 weeks. However, laboratory recovery may be delayed. Overall mortality is less than 1%.
- Hepatitis A patients recover completely without progressing to chronic liver disease. Some patients may have relapses up to one year.
- The mortality rate in hepatitis B is low but rises higher if superimposed with hepatitis D infection.
- Acute hepatitis is less severe and more likely to be anicteric in hepatitis C.
- Hepatitis B and C can progress to chronic phase in 1–2% and 80% cases respectively. However, 90% infants and neonates with hepatitis B infection develop chronicity.
- Mortality in hepatitis E is particularly high (10–20%), if it occurs during pregnancy.

CHRONIC HEPATITIS

Chronic hepatitis is defined as persistent inflammation and necrosis of liver for at least 6 months. Progression is slow in mild forms but severe forms progress rapidly and lead to cirrhosis. The causes of chronic hepatitis are given in **Table 3.16**.

Chronic hepatitis is classified on the basis of its cause, its histological activity and its degree of progression. Various tests required to identify the cause are given in **Table 3.17**.

Table 3.14: High risk individuals who require hepatitis B vaccination.
- Medical, dental and nursing students
- Persons on hemodialysis
- Patients requiring multiple transfusions
- IV drug abusers
- Medical, nursing, other health workers and laboratory staff
- Newborns of HBsAg positive mothers
- Persons with multiple sexual partners

Table 3.15: Post-exposure prophylaxis of Hepatitis B.

	Source patient -HBsAg positive	Source patient-HBsAg negative	Source unknown or not available for testing
Unvaccinated			
Non-immune	HBIG (0.06 mL/kg) single dose and initiate HBV vaccination	Initiate HBV vaccination	Initiate HBV vaccination
Previously vaccinated- anti-HBs titer known/Test for anti-HBs in exposed HCW			
Known responder (Anti-HBs titer ≥ 10 mIU/mL)	No treatment	No treatment	No treatment
Known non-responder (Anti-HBs titer < 10 mIU/mL)	HBIG × 1 dose and boost or initiate revaccination or HBIG × 2 doses (1 month apart)*	No treatment Consider Revaccination	Treat as HBsAg positive if high risk source
If test facility is not available	HBIG and vaccine booster	No treatment	Treat as HBsAg positive if high risk source
If still undergoing vaccination	HBIG × 1 dose; complete vaccination	Complete vaccination	HBIG × 1 dose; complete vaccination

*In persons who have completed two full courses of vaccination and still have anti-HBS antibody titer of <10 MIU/mL, two dosage of HBIG is recommended at interval of one month.
(mIU/mL: milli-international units per milliliter)

Table 3.16: Causes of chronic hepatitis.

- Viral hepatitis
  - Hepatitis B
  - Hepatitis C
  - Hepatitis D
- Alcohol-related liver disease
- Nonalcoholic steatohepatitis (NASH)
- Autoimmune hepatitis
- Drug induced (INH)
- Wilson's disease
  - Hemochromatosis
- Alpha-1 antitrypsin deficiency

Table 3.17: Tests for chronic hepatitis.

HBsAg (Hepatitis B surface antigen)	Hepatitis B
Anti-HCV (Hepatitis C antibody)	Hepatitis C
Autoantibodies (antinuclear antibody, smooth muscle antibody, antimitochondrial antibody)	Autoimmune hepatitis
Immunoglobulins	Autoimmune hepatitis
Ferritin	Hemochromatosis
α1-antitrypsin	α1-antitrypsin deficiency
Ceruloplasmin	Wilson's disease

Chronic Viral Hepatitis

Hepatitis B and C can progress to chronic phase in 1–2% and 80% cases respectively.

Clinical Features

The clinical features of chronic viral hepatitis are fatigue and persistent or intermittent jaundice. Patients may present with features of cirrhosis and its complications. Extrahepatic presentations like arthralgia and arthritis, immune complex glomerulonephritis, polyarteritis nodosa (hepatitis B) and essential cryoglobulinemia (hepatitis C) may occur.

Laboratory Features

High and fluctuating levels of serum aminotransferases are characteristic features. Serum bilirubin is only mildly raised whereas alkaline phosphatase is usually normal. Serum albumin is low. Prothrombin time is increased in severe cases.

Biopsy of the liver is required for assessment of histological activity to grade the chronic hepatitis as mild, moderate or severe.

Serological tests are needed to identify the viral types and their replication patterns.

Treatment

- *Chronic hepatitis B:* The treatment of chronic hepatitis B is needed if there are markers of viral replication and elevated to twice the above level of normal **(Table 3.18)**. Different drugs used are interferon alpha, entecavir, tenofovir, lamivudine, telbivudine and adefovir dipivoxil.

 Pegylated interferon alpha is given subcutaneously once a week for 48 weeks. Interferon is contraindicated in the presence of cirrhosis.

 Entecavir and tenofovir are potent antiviral agents and are more effective than lamuvidine or adefovir. Entecavir or tenofovir is preferred as first line agent as chances of resistance are minimal with these agents. Entecavir is used in the doses of 0.5 mg daily, 1 mg daily is given in lamivudine resistant patients. The dose of tenofovir (TDF) is 300 mg orally daily. Lamivudine is used in daily oral dose of 100 mg. Adefovir is safe and effective and given orally in the dosage of 10 mg daily **(Table 3.19)**.

- *Chronic hepatitis C:* All patients with chronic HCV infection need treatment. The goal of treatment is eradication of HCV. Sustained viral response (SVR) is defined as undetectable HCV RNA 12 weeks after treatment. Treatment reduces complications of HCV infection (cirrhosis, hepatocellular carcinoma), morbidity and mortality in patients who achieve SVR.

 Direct antiviral agents (DAA) are now available for use in chronic hepatitis C and combination of these oral DAAs are the first line treatment for hepatitis C (interferon sparing regimen). Duration of treatment is also shorter when these newer agents are used.

 Combination of subcutaneous weekly pegylated interferon alpha (PEG-IFN) and daily oral ribavirin were used earlier. Triple therapy including PEG-IFN, ribavirin and a direct antiviral agent is sometimes given.

 The DAA are given for 12–24 weeks. The response to treatment varies according to the genotype of the HCV. The best response is observed in genotypes 2 and 3 **(Tables 3.20 and 3.21)**.

 Daclatasvir, sofusbuvir, velpatasvir and ledipasvir are now available in India. Regimen in Chronic hepatitis C depends on viral genotype, viral load (estimated by PCR), presence of cirrhosis and prior treatment failure.

 Genotype 3 is most prevalent in India. Some of the newer regimens recommended for treatment of chronic hepatitis C are given below:
 - Sofusbuvir (400 mg) + Daclatasvir (60 mg) for 12 weeks.
 - Sofusbuvir and velpatasvir (pan-genotypic) for 12 weeks.
 - Sofusbuvir (400 mg) + Daclatasvir (60 mg) ± Ribavarin for 24 weeks in patients with cirrhosis and previous nonresponders.
 - Fixed dose combination of Ledipasvir (90 mg)/Sofusbuvir (400 mg) for 12 weeks.
 - Fixed dose combination of Ledipasvir (90 mg)/Sofusbuvir (400 mg) ± Ribavarin for 24 weeks in patients with cirrhosis and previous non-responders.

 Ledipasvir is currently recommended for treatment of genotypes 1, 4, 5 and 6.

- Treatment of other causes of chronic hepatitis is given in **Table 3.22**.

Table 3.18: Indications for treatment of chronic hepatitis B.

HBeAg POSITIVE

HBV DNA	ALT	Treatment	Follow up	Drugs	Duration	Comments
>20,000 IU/mL	≤2 x ULN	No treatment recommended	Consider treatment if: • ALT becomes elevated >2 x ULN • Liver biopsy shows moderate/severe inflammation or fibrosis • Non-invasive testing suggests moderate/severe fibrosis			Treatment may be considered in: • Patients > 40 years • Those with family history of hepatocellular carcinoma (HCC)
>20,000 IU/mL	>2 x ULN	Treat if no spontaneous HBeAg loss occurs after 3 to 6 months of observation	Monitor for Seroconversion from HBeAg to anti-HBe	Entacavir (ETV), Tenofovir (TAF/TDV), or PegIFN alfa	ETV, TAF, TDV-at least 12 months after seroconversion PegIFN alfa- 48 weeks	

HBeAg NEGATIVE

HBV DNA	ALT	Treatment	Follow up	Drugs	Duration	Comments
>2000 IU/mL	>2 x ULN	Treatment required	Monitor for HBsAg loss	Entacavir (ETV), Tenofovir (TAF/TDV), or PegIFN alfa	ETV, TAF, TDV-for years/indefinite PegIFN alfa- 48 weeks	Endpoint of treatment- Loss of HBSAg
≤2000 IU/mL	≤ULN	No treatment recommended	Monitor HBV DNA and ALT			Treat if HBV DNA and ALT increases

PATIENT WITH CIRRHOSIS (Regardless of HBeAg status)

HBV DNA	ALT	T	Treatment	Follow up		Duration	Comment
Detectable	Any ALT	**Compensated**	Treatment recommended		ETV, TAF, or TDF	Indefinitely	
		Decompensated	Treat immediately	Monitor urea/creatinine if TDF is given	ETV-preferred TDF may be given Refer for liver transplant		Evaluate for liver transplant
Undetectable	Any ALT	**Compensated:**	Observe	HBV DNA			Evaluate for other causes of cirrhosis
		Decompensated		HBV DNA	Refer for liver transplant		Evaluate for other causes of cirrhosis

(ETV: entacavir; TDF: tenofovir disoproxil fumarate; TAF: tenofovir alafenamide; ALT: alanine aminotransferase; Peg IFN alfa: pegylated interferon alfa; ULN: upper limit of normal, >35 IU/mL in males and > 25 IU/mL in females)

Table 3.19: Agents used for treatment of chronic hepatitis B.

Name	Dose	Comments
Injectable		
Peginterferon alfa-2a	180 mg SC once weekly for 48 weeks	Alternative to oral agents
Peginterferon alfa-2b	1.5 mcg/Kg SC once weekly for 48 weeks	Used in chronic hepatitis D infection
Oral		
Entecavir	0.5 mg orally once daily 1 mg orally once daily for patients resistant to lamivudine	**Entacavir and tenofovir are preferred first line agents.** Resistance rare
Tenofovir disoproxil fumarate (TDF)	300 mg orally once daily	Preferred as first line agent, resistance rare. May cause renal and bone toxicity
Tenofovir alafenamide (TAF)	25 mg orally once daily	Preferred as first line agent, resistance rare, less toxic
Lamivudine	100 mg orally once daily	Not used now
Adefovir dipivoxil	10 mg orally once daily	Least potent Not used now
Telbivudine	600 mg orally once daily	Associated with resistance, not preferred now

Table 3.20: Treatment of chronic hepatitis C.

Oral
Direct antiviral agents (**DAA**)

Injectable
PEG interferon alpha 2a 180 mcg weekly
or
PEG interferon alpha 2b 1.5 mcg/kg weekly
plus
Oral ribavirin 800–1200 mg/day

Table 3.21: Direct antiviral agents (DAA) for hepatitis C.

	Drug	Dose (orally)
NS5A inhibitors	**Daclatasvir**	60 mg once daily
	Velpatasvir	100 mg once daily
	Ledipasvir	90 mg once daily
	Elbasvir	50 mg once daily
	Ombitasvir	25 mg once daily
	Pibrentasvir	120 mg once daily
NS5B inhibitors (NPIs)	**Sofosbuvir**	400 mg once daily
NS5B inhibitors (NNPIs)	Dasabuvir	250 mg twice daily
NS3/4A protease inhibitors	Telaprevir	1125 mg twice daily
	Boceprevir	800 mg thrice daily
	Simeprevir	150 mg once daily
	Paritaprevir	150 mg once daily
	Grazoprevir	100 mg once daily
	Voxilaprevir	100 mg once daily
	Glecaprevir	300 mg once daily
Host targeting antiviral drugs	Alisprovir	400 mg twice daily

Table 3.22: Treatment of non-viral chronic hepatitis.

Autoimmune hepatitis
Prednisolone
Azathioprine
Mycophenolate mofetil

Wilson's disease
Zinc
Trientine
Penicillamine

α1-antitrypsin deficiency
Liver transplantation (only effective treatment)

Hemochromatosis
Regular therapeutic phlebotomy

Drug-induced chronic hepatitis
Withdrawal of causative drug

- Liver transplantation is indicated in advanced liver disease.

Prognosis

The course of the chronic hepatitis is variable. The sequelae of chronic hepatitis are cirrhosis, liver failure and hepatocellular carcinoma. Upto 40% patients with chronic hepatitis B and 30% with chronic hepatitis C will eventually develop cirrhosis in 5–30 years. The risk of development of hepatocellular carcinoma is 3–5% per year in patients with cirrhosis.

Non-alcoholic Steatohepatitis (NASH)

Non-alcoholic fatty liver disease (NAFLD) is characterized by fat accumulation in the liver with no history of high alcohol consumption. It is a progressive disease and is associated with overweight/obesity, insulin resistance, type 2 diabetes and hypertension. NAFLD is also associated with obstructive sleep apnea, polycystic ovary syndrome, and bacterial overgrowth in small bowel. Ethnic and racial factors also influence fat accumulation in the liver. If there is inflammation along with fatty infiltration, the condition is known as NASH (Non-alcoholic steatohepatitis) which is seen in around 25% patients with NAFLD. Patients with NAFLD may progress to cirrhosis and liver cancer. The annual risk of developing cirrhosis in NAFLD is 6%.

Diagnosis depends on detection of increased liver fat with or without rise in aminotransferases levels in the absence of excess alcohol consumption (not more than 1 drink daily in women and more than 2 drinks daily in men). However other causes of fat deposition and liver inflammation such as viral hepatitis, drugs, autoimmune hepatitis, metabolic causes (iron or copper excess, α-1 antitrypsin deficiency) must be ruled out.

NAFLD is frequently asymptomatic and detected incidentally when routine tests show abnormal blood aminotransferases levels and fatty liver on imaging. However, it may be associated with fatigue and discomfort in right upper quadrant.

Features of advanced liver disease in NAFLD/NASH:
- Clinical features: Presence of splenomegaly, ascites, encephalopathy, variceal hemorrhage, spider angiomata, palmar erythema.
- Blood tests revealing Hepatic dysfunction: Hyperbilirubinemia, hypoalbuminemia, prothrombin time prolongation.
- Imaging for liver stiffness: Magnetic resonance elastography (MRE), transient elastography (FibroScan).
- Liver biopsy for the evidence of severe liver injury and fibrosis.

Treatment

- Diet and exercise: Lifestyle modification can improve hepatic steatosis and liver dysfunction. Loss of at least 3–5% of body weight improves steatosis, up to 10% weight loss improves steatohepatitis.
- Drugs: No pharmacological agent is currently approved for the treatment of NAFLD/NASH. A new agent Obeticholic acid, an oral farnesoid X receptor (FXR) agonist is being tested for the treatment of liver fibrosis in NASH. Saroglitazar, a dual PPARα/γ agonist, results in a significant decrease in aminotransferase (ALT) levels

in patients with NAFLD. Saroglitazar is approved for treatment diabetic dyslipidemia in India. Pioglitazone has shown to be of some benefit in NAFLD. Vitamin E (800 IU/day) was demonstrated to be beneficial in non-diabetic NASH patients, but its use was also associated with increased risk of all-cause mortality.
- Bariatric surgery may be useful for weight reduction, however it is not indicated in advanced disease (cirrhosis and portal hypertension).
- Treatment of comorbidities: Diabetes, obesity, and dyslipidemia should be appropriately managed.
- Treatment of the complications such as cirrhosis and portal hypertension and primary liver cancer.
- Liver transplantation: Patients with end-stage liver disease should be evaluated for liver transplantation.

CIRRHOSIS OF LIVER

Cirrhosis of liver is the end result of the hepatocellular injury characterized by the presence of extensive fibrosis, regenerative nodules and loss of liver architecture.

Two of the commonest causes of cirrhosis are viral hepatitis (B, D and C) and prolonged excessive use of alcohol. Important causes of cirrhosis are given in **Table 3.23**.

Pathology

- The activation of stellate cells (fat storing cells, Ito cells) is the central event in the development of cirrhosis irrespective of the cause. The activated stellate cells transform into multifunctional cells upon interaction with hepatocytes, Kupffer cells and cytokines. The transformed cells form type I collagen leading to fibrosis.
- The cirrhosis can be micronodular typically in alcoholics where the regenerating nodules are small (<1 mm). The macronodular form is characterized by larger nodules and is seen in posthepatitic or postnecrotic cirrhosis. However, either form can occur at different stages of disease.
- Clinical features of the cirrhosis are derived from the changes in the liver morphology as well as from liver cell dysfunction **(Table 3.24)**.
    - Fibrosis and distorted vasculature may lead to portal hypertension and complications associated with it.
    - Hepatocellular dysfunction leads to jaundice, edema, coagulopathy and metabolic abnormalities.

Table 3.23: Important causes of cirrhosis.
- Viral hepatitis (postnecrotic)
- Alcohol (Laennec's cirrhosis)
- Non alcoholic steatohepatitis (NASH)
- Autoimmune hepatitis
- Drug induced
- Biliary cirrhosis
- Hemochromatosis
- Wilson's disease
- Cardiac cirrhosis (prolonged CHF)
- Alpha-1 antitrypsin deficiency
- Cryptogenic (unknown etiology)

Table 3.24: Clinical features of cirrhosis.

Features due to hepatocellular dysfunction
- Jaundice
- Ascites
- Hepatomegaly (initial phase)
- Spider nevi, palmar erythema
- Gynecomastia, testicular atrophy
- Menstrual abnormalities, breast atrophy
- Bleeding tendency
- Hepatic encephalopathy

Features due to portal hypertension
- Ascites
- Splenomegaly
- Variceal bleeding
- Hepatic encephalopathy

Others
- Parotid and lacrimal gland enlargement
- Clubbing
- Opaque nails (leukonychia)
- Dupuytren's contracture
- Skin pigmentation

- Ascites and hepatic encephalopathy can result from both mechanisms.

Clinical Features

Cirrhotic patients may be asymptomatic and may be diagnosed incidentally.
- Mostly symptoms such as weakness, fatigue, weight loss, anorexia, nausea, vomiting and abdominal discomfort occur insidiously.
- The liver is firm, nontender and nodular and is enlarged initially. The liver size reduces due to fibrosis as the disease progresses.
- Jaundice is generally absent or mild initially. It may become severe at later stages.
- Patient may present with features of *portal hypertension* mainly abdominal distension due to ascites and splenomegaly, hematemesis and melena due to variceal rupture or hepatic encephalopathy **(Table 3.24)**.
- The signs of *chronic hepatic dysfunction* such as spider nevi, palmar erythema, gynecomastia, testicular atrophy and loss of hair may occur due to disturbances in hormonal metabolism. Females may have loss of libido, menstrual abnormalities and breast atrophy. Palmar erythema is redness of thenar and hypothenar eminences which may also be found in normal persons and in hyperdynamic circulation. Spider nevi are dilated central arterioles with radiating small vessels (like spider) found mainly on the upper part of the body. They can also be seen in normal persons and also during pregnancy.
- Patients may have hemorrhagic manifestations such as epistaxis and increased menstrual flow.
- Other features include parotid gland and lacrimal gland enlargement, digital clubbing, Dupuytren's contracture and skin pigmentation. Complications of the cirrhosis are given in **Table 3.25**.

Table 3.25: Complications of cirrhosis.

- Portal hypertension
  - Upper GI bleed
  - Ascites
  - Spontaneous bacterial peritonitis (SBP)
- Hepatic encephalopathy
- Hepatorenal syndrome
- Hepatocellular carcinoma
- Coagulopathy

Laboratory Features

- *Blood examination:*
  - Aminotransferases (ALT, AST) are frequently elevated whereas a rise in the serum bilirubin and ALP may occur later.
  - Serum albumin is low.
  - PT is frequently prolonged.
  - Anemia can occur due to bleeding, folate deficiency, marrow suppression or hypersplenism.
  - Leukopenia and thrombocytopenia suggest hypersplenism.
- *Imaging:* Ultrasonography is helpful in the evaluation of liver size and texture, ascites, portal hypertension and splenomegaly.
- *Endoscopy:* Upper gastrointestinal endoscopy is required to detect esophageal varices and to exclude other causes of upper gastrointestinal bleeding in the stomach and duodenum.
- *Liver biopsy:* Biopsy helps in the assessment of severity of the cirrhotic changes. Typical histological features may suggest the specific cause of the cirrhosis.

Management

Management includes general management, treatment of specific cause, management of the complications and liver transplantation.

- *General management:*
  - The diet should contain an adequate amount of protein and calories. However, protein intake should be reduced in case of hepatic encephalopathy.
  - Vitamin supplementation is helpful.
  - Salt restriction is required in case of ascites.
  - Medications which are hepatotoxic or metabolized in liver should be given with caution.
- *Treatment of specific cause:* Alcohol abstinence is mandatory in alcoholic cirrhosis. Specific therapy is needed in hemochromatosis and Wilson's disease.
- *Management of complications:* (discussed later)
- *Liver transplantation:* The most common indication for liver transplantation is irreversible progressive chronic liver failure due to cirrhosis.

Prognosis

Overall the prognosis of cirrhosis is poor. Child Pugh's classification is used for the grading and the prognosis. The prognosis is favorable if the cause can be corrected. Around 25% of the patients survive for more than 5 years.

PORTAL HYPERTENSION

Portal hypertension is elevation of portal venous pressure above 10–12 mmHg (normal 5–10 mmHg). Portal hypertension results from (a) increased resistance to portal blood flow and (b) high portal blood flow. More commonly, portal hypertension occurs due to increased resistance.

The causes of portal hypertension are classified according to the site of obstruction in relation to hepatic sinusoids— (a) presinusoidal, (b) sinusoidal and (c) post-sinusoidal. Causes of portal hypertension are given in **Table 3.26**. Cirrhosis is the most common cause of portal hypertension. Portal vein obstruction is the next most common cause.

Clinical Features

The clinical features result from portal-systemic collateral formation and portal venous congestion. As there are no valves in the portal vein, retrograde blood flow from portal venous system (high pressure) to systemic venous circulation (low pressure) occurs during portal hypertension.

The main clinical features are:
- Hemorrhage from rupture of varices (hematemesis)
- Ascites
- Splenomegaly
- Hypersplenism
- Hepatic encephalopathy.

Splenomegaly is the cardinal finding of portal hypertension. Hypersplenism may give rise to thrombocytopenia and leukopenia. Anemia is rare.

Collateral formation occurs around the esophagus and stomach (esophageal varices and gastric varices), the rectum (hemorrhoids), retroperitoneal space and periumbilically in anterior abdominal wall. Collateral vessels in the anterior abdominal wall may be visible as tortuous vessels radiating from the umbilicus (caput medusae).

As a result of portal-systemic shunting, various toxic substances enter into systemic circulation without going to

Table 3.26: Common causes of portal hypertension.

Presinusoidal
- Extrahepatic
  - Portal vein obstruction (thrombosis, trauma, malignant diseases of pancreas)
- Intrahepatic
  - Schistosomiasis
  - Sarcoidosis, vinyl chloride

Sinusoidal
- Cirrhosis
- Metastatic liver disease

Postsinusoidal
- Intrahepatic
  - Veno-occlusive disease
- Extrahepatic
  - Budd-Chiari syndrome (hepatic vein thrombosis)

the liver. This is the basis for hepatic encephalopathy. *Musty odor of the breath (fetor hepaticus)* due to the presence of mercaptans can occur in hepatic encephalopathy.

Investigations

- *Endoscopy:* Esophageal varices suggest the presence of portal hypertension. However, it does not detect the cause.
- *Ultrasonography:* It is useful in the evaluation of size and texture of the liver, splenomegaly, diameter and flow pattern of the portal vein, ascites and collateral circulation.
- *CT scan and MRI:* These are usually not needed. However, these are sensitive methods to detect collaterals.
- *Portal venous pressure:* Measurement of portal venous pressure is needed to confirm portal hypertension and to determine the level of obstruction. Portal venography helps in knowing the site and cause of the obstruction.

Management

The management includes—(a) reduction of pressure in the portal vein and (b) treatment of the complications.
a. *Reduction in the portal venous pressure:* Propranolol and nidolol can be used to lower the portal venous pressure. Transjugular intrahepatic portosystemic shunt (TIPSS) and surgical decompression procedures are other options to decrease portal venous pressure.
b. *Treatment of complications:* Complications like upper GI bleed, ascites, spontaneous bacterial peritonitis (SBP), hepatic encephalopathy and hypersplenism are managed as given below.

UPPER GASTROINTESTINAL BLEEDING

Important causes of upper GI bleeding are given in **Table 3.27**. Peptic ulcer is the most common cause of upper GI bleeding. However, the most common cause of upper GI bleeding in the cirrhotic patient is rupture of esophageal varices. Bleeding in cirrhotic patients may also occur due to congestive gastropathy or rupture of gastric varices. The bleeding may be contributed by the presence of coagulopathy, thrombocytopenia, gastric erosions and drugs.

Variceal bleeding presents as painless hematemesis and melena. There may be circulatory shock if the bleeding is massive. GI bleeding can precipitate hepatic encephalopathy.

Upper GI endoscopy is the best method to detect the cause of bleeding. Endoscopy may also be used for therapeutic interventions.

Table 3.27: Causes of upper GI bleeding.

- Peptic ulcer disease
- Variceal rupture
- Erosive gastritis (drugs, alcohol, severe illness/stress)
- Gastric malignancy
- Mallory-Weiss tear (laceration at gastroesophageal junction due to vomiting)

Treatment of Variceal Hemorrhage

- Urgent hospitalization in ICU.
- Restore the intravascular volume by the blood transfusion.
- Fresh frozen plasma is given to correct coagulopathy.
- Reduction of portal venous pressure is achieved by:
    - Somatostatin or its analogue octreotide (50–100 µg bolus followed by 25–50 µg/hour).
    - Terlipressin 1 mg intravenous 6 houly also reduces portal pressure.
    - Vasopressin infusion (0.2–0.4 unit/minute) if both are not available
    - Transjugular intrahepatic portosystemic shunt (TIPS) if bleeding does not respond to drugs and therapeutic endoscopic intervention. A metallic stent is placed between the hepativ vein and portal vein to reduce portal venous pressure and control bleeding.
    - Emergency portosystemic shunt surgery is rarely performed now, it may be considered in patients with good hepatic reserve if bleeding is not controlled by other measures.
- Local measures:
    - *Endoscopic intervention:* It is most widely used as the first line of treatment. Bleeding is stopped in the majority of cases. Ligation of esophageal varices with bands and injection of sclerosing agent (sclerotherapy) are usual procedures **(Figs. 3.4A and B)**.
    Endoscopic injection of glue (cyanoacrylate) is effective in control of bleeding from gastric varices.
    - *Balloon tamponade* (with Sengstaken-Blakemore tube) is used when bleeding is massive and endoscopy is not available.
    - *Esophageal transection* may rarely be needed as a last resort.

Prevention of Variceal Bleeding

- Prevention of first hemorrhage (primary prevention) from varices is accomplished either (a) by the use of non-selective beta-blocker (propranolol) or (b) by prophylactic endoscopic banding.
- *Prevention of recurrent bleeding:*
    - Propranolol and band ligation are useful in reducing recurrent variceal bleeding.
    - TIPSS or portal-systemic shunt surgery may be required in patients not responding to the above measures, however, the risk for hepatic encephalopathy is increased.

HEPATIC ENCEPHALOPATHY

Hepatic encephalopathy is a neuropsychiatric syndrome secondary to acute or chronic hepatic failure or due to portal-systemic shunt.

The toxic substances absorbed from the intestine are either not metabolized by the failing liver or bypass the

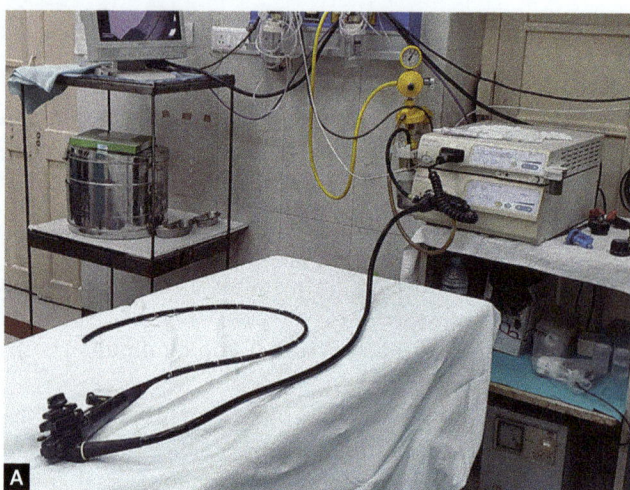 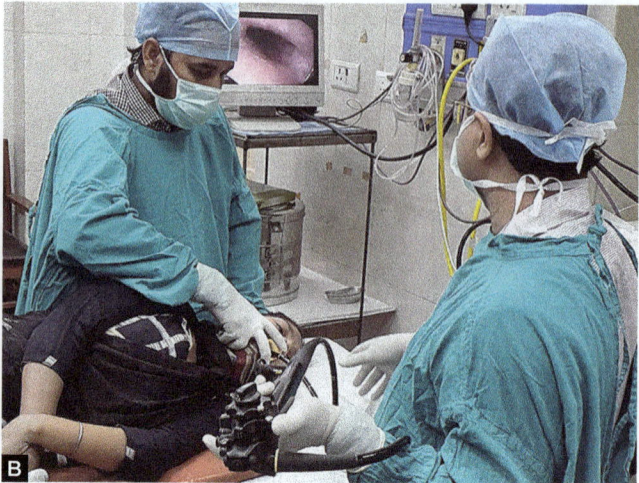

Figs. 3.4A and B: (A) Upper gastrointestinal endoscope; (B) Upper gastrointestinal endoscopy (UGIE).

liver through portal-systemic shunts. Thus, these harmful substances (mainly ammonia, mercaptans, short chain fatty acids and false neurotransmitters) reach the central nervous system and result in alteration in consciousness and other manifestations. The alteration in sensorium may range from mild confusion and disordered sleep patterns to deep coma *(hepatic coma)*. Flapping tremor *(asterixis)* and *fetor hepaticus* are usually present.

Precipitating Factors

Certain factors may precipitate the onset of encephalopathy in otherwise stable cases of cirrhosis. These factors enhance the production of ammonia or other toxic nitrogenous substances or affect the CNS directly. The most common precipitating factor is upper GI bleeding. Other important factors are given in the **Table 3.28**.

Treatment

The treatment of hepatic encephalopathy includes following:
- The precipitating factors should be identified and removed.
- Protein should be withheld from the diet in severe cases or restricted to less than 20 g/day. However, the amount of protein in the diet is increased gradually once the patient improves. Vegetable proteins are preferred over animal proteins. Constipation should be avoided.
- The nonabsorbable disaccharides (lactulose) act as osmotic laxative, favour conversion of ammonia to poorly absorbed ammonium ion and inhibit ammonia production by colonic bacteria. The usual dose is 15–30 mL thrice a day and it is adjusted so as to produce 2–4 soft stools daily.
- Oral neomycin (0.5–1 g 6 hourly) can be used to reduce gut bacteria and ammonia production. Metronidazole (250 mg 8 hourly) can alternatively be used. Recently, nonabsorbable agent *rifaximin* (400 mg orally three times daily) has been found to be effective and safer than neomycin and metronidazole.
- Sedatives and hypnotics should be avoided. However, short acting oxazepam may be given to agitated patients. Flumazenil, a benzodiazepine antagonist may be helpful in some cases.
- Zinc supplementation may sometimes help.
- Liver transplantation may be considered in nonresponding patients.

Management of Hemorrhagic Tendency in Liver Disease

- The administration of vitamin K (10 mg for 3 days subcutaneously) may be helpful in correction of coagulopathy in cases with vitamin K malabsorption.
- Fresh frozen plasma which contains all clotting factors, is indicated in active severe bleeding or prior to surgery.
- Platelet transfusion may be needed in thrombocytopenia with bleeding.

Hepatocellular Carcinoma

Patients with cirrhosis are monitored periodically for the development of hepatocellular carcinoma. This is done by the measurement of serum alpha fetoprotein level and imaging techniques.

Hepatorenal Syndrome

Renal failure occurring in the setting of cirrhosis and ascites without any evidence of specific cause of renal dysfunction is known as hepatorenal syndrome. Kidneys are intrinsically

Table 3.28: Precipitating factors for hepatic encephalopathy.
- Gastrointestinal bleeding
- Increased protein in the diet
- Constipation
- Uremia
- Hypokalemia and alkalosis
- Vigorous paracentesis
- Infections
- Drugs (diuretics, sedatives, hypnotics)
- Portal-systemic shunt (TIPSS or surgery)

normal. The hepatorenal syndrome is believed to be due to altered systemic and renal blood flow. It has a very poor prognosis. Treatment is usually unsuccessful. Liver transplantation may be helpful in appropriate candidates.

ASCITES

Accumulation of excess fluid in the peritoneal cavity is called ascites. Normally there may be a small amount of fluid (<20 mL) in the peritoneal cavity. Ascites can be associated with normal or diseased peritoneum. The most common cause of ascites is cirrhosis with portal hypertension. Tuberculosis and malignancies are the other important causes. **Table 3.29** shows causes of ascites.

Pathogenesis

Increased hydrostatic pressure in portal venous system, dilatation of splanchnic arterial system, hypoalbuminemia and reduced plasma oncotic pressure lead to loss of fluid from vascular compartment into peritoneal cavity. These changes cause reduction in the effective circulatory volume leading to increased activation of renin-angiotensin-aldosterone system, enhanced sympathetic activity, and release of the antidiuretic hormone causing salt and water retention. This further contributes to the development of ascites.

Clinical Features

The main symptoms are distension of abdomen with or without discomfort or pain. Other symptoms may occur according to the cause of ascites. There may be fever in infective pathology while marked weight loss suggests malignancy. Patients should be questioned to ascertain if any risk factors of chronic liver disease such as viral hepatitis, alcohol use, transfusions and IV drug abuse exist.

Inspection: Inspection of abdomen may reveal distension with fullness in the flanks, everted and horizontal umbilicus, abdominal striae, prominent and tortuous veins and hernia.

Palpation: Fluid thrill is present in massive ascites (*see* **Fig. 2.10**).

Percussion: Shifting dullness is demonstrable on percussion in moderate ascites (*see* **Fig. 2.11**).

Other findings will be present depending on the underlying cause of ascites. For example, spider nevi, palmar erythema and gynecomastia suggest chronic liver disease. Splenomegaly is present in portal hypertension.

Investigations

- *Ultrasonography:* Ultrasonography of abdomen can detect presence of minimal amount of fluid and is helpful when clinical signs are not present. It is also used for guiding paracentesis (drainage of fluid). It can also detect features of cirrhosis and portal hypertension and other findings like lymph nodes, masses, metastasis in liver. CT scan can also be done for this purpose. Doppler ultrasound can detect obstruction in portal vein thrombosis and hepatic vein thrombosis.
- *Paracentesis:* Abdominal paracentesis is performed as a routine investigation to determine the cause. It can be performed under ultrasound guidance. 50–100 mL of fluid is drained and examined for the color, total and differential cell count and malignant cells. Biochemical tests include protein and albumin levels, glucose, LDH and amylase. Culture, Gram stain and AFB staining may also be performed.
    - In cirrhosis, the appearance of ascitic fluid is clear, straw colored. The fluid is milky white in chylous ascites while it is cloudy in infections. Hemorrhagic fluid may be seen due to trauma, tumor or tuberculosis.
    - The presence of more than 500 leukocytes/µL suggests inflammatory conditions. Polymorphonuclear count more than 250/µL is characteristic of bacterial peritonitis. Predominantly elevated lymphocytes suggest tuberculosis.
    - Based on the specific gravity and total protein concentration, ascitic fluid has traditionally been classified as transudative and exudative.
        a. Transudative fluid (specific gravity <1.016, protein <25 g/L) is typically found in cirrhosis and CHF.
        b. Exudative fluid (specific gravity >1.016, total protein >25 g/L) is seen in conditions with diseased peritoneum like tuberculosis, malignancy and bacterial peritonitis.
    - Serum-ascites albumin gradient (SAAG) is the best indicator to classify ascites into portal hypertensive and non-portal hypertensive causes. SAAG is the difference between the serum and ascitic fluid albumin levels. Transudative ascites is generally high gradient type and exudative ascites the low gradient type.
        a. High gradient (>1.1 g/dL) suggests that ascites is due to portal hypertension (cirrhosis, CHF).
        b. Low gradient (<1.1 g/dL) is seen in cases without portal hypertension.

    Laparoscopy and peritoneal biopsy may be needed in specific cases.

Table 3.29: Causes of ascites.

Normal peritoneum
- Cirrhosis with portal hypertension
- Congestive heart failure (CHF)
- Hypoproteinemia (nephrotic syndrome, malnutrition)
- Budd-Chiari syndrome
- Pancreatitis
- Biliary ascites
- Chylous ascites (filariasis, trauma, tumor)
- Meig's syndrome

Diseased peritoneum
- Tuberculous peritonitis
- Bacterial peritonitis
- Malignancy (peritoneal, hepatic)

Management

The treatment of ascites in cirrhosis consists of the following steps:
- Salt in the diet is restricted to 2-3 g/day.
- Diuretics are given if there is no response to salt restriction. Spironolactone is initially used in a dosage of 100 mg/day which is increased to 400 mg/day. Frusemide (40-160 mg/day) is added in case the response is inadequate. The goal is to reduce the weight at a rate of not more than 1 kg/day in patients with anasarca and no more than 0.5 kg/day in patients with ascites alone. Vigorous diuresis may precipitate hepatic encephalopathy and renal failure.
- Therapeutic paracentesis is needed in massive ascites with respiratory compromise. A volume of 4-6 liters is removed. Intravenous albumin is given concomitantly to maintain intravascular volume.
- Portacaval shunt surgery or implantation of peritoneovenous shunt (between abdominal cavity to superior vena cava) may be indicated in refractory ascites.
- TIPSS is an alternative to surgical shunting in cases with refractory ascites.

Treatment of underlying cause: Specific treatment is given in patients according to the cause. For example, antitubercular therapy is indicated in tuberculous ascites.

Spontaneous Bacterial Peritonitis

Spontaneous bacterial peritonitis (SBP) or primary bacterial peritonitis (PBP) is a common complication in patients with ascites due to cirrhosis. There is no apparent intra-abdominal source of infection. SBP must be differentiated from secondary bacterial peritonitis characterized by intra-abdominal infections due to appendicitis, perforated peptic ulcer or ruptured gallbladder.

- *Etiology:* The most common organisms responsible for SBP are *E. coli, Klebsiella* and *Streptococcus pneumoniae*.
- *Clinical features:* Clinical features include fever, abdominal pain, worsening or precipitation of hepatic encephalopathy or worsening of renal dysfunction. Abdominal tenderness and decreased bowel sounds are seen in many cases. Some patients may not have any suggestive symptoms or signs.
- *Investigations:* Ascitic fluid is cloudy with high leukocyte counts. Polymorphonuclear (neutrophils) cell count of more than 250/μL strongly suggests SBP. Gram stain may be positive. Culture of ascitic fluid confirms the diagnosis.
- *Treatment:* Treatment of SBP includes commencing of antibiotic therapy. Third generation cephalosporins (cefotaxime 2 g IV 8 hourly or ceftriaxone 1-2 g IV daily) or quinolones (ciprofloxacin 500 mg IV 12 hourly) are given for 5 days.
- *Prevention:* Recurrence of SBP is prevented by using norfloxacin (400 mg daily) or ciprofloxacin (750 mg weekly). Alternatively, a double strength tablet of trimethoprim-sulfamethoxazole may be given daily.

HEPATOMEGALY

Liver is examined when the patient is supine with relaxed abdominal wall. The fingers are placed in the right abdomen and slowly advanced upward as the patient inhales and exhales deeply.

The liver is normally not palpable; however, it may be palpable in thin individuals. It is palpable in the right upper abdomen when enlarged. In emphysema, liver may be palpable without being enlarged as it is pushed downward by the inflated lung. Hence, upper border of the liver should also be ascertained by percussion in order to measure the span of liver, which is normally 12-15 cm in height. Normally the upper liver dullness is at the level of fifth rib in the right mid-clavicular line. Important causes of hepatomegaly are given in **Table 3.30**.

- The size of the liver is usually expressed in centimeters below the right costal margin.
- The consistency of the liver should be noted as soft, firm or hard.
- The surface may be smooth or nodular and edges may be sharp, regular or irregular.
- Liver may be nontender or tender to touch.
- Tender hepatomegaly may occur in CHF, acute hepatitis and liver abscess.
- The liver is soft, smooth and tender in CHF, and firm, regular in cirrhosis.
- Hard, irregular, nontender and nodular liver is detected in metastatic disease.

Table 3.30: Causes of hepatomegaly.

Vascular causes
- CHF
- Hepatic vein thrombosis

Inflammatory causes
- Hepatitis (viral, drugs, alcohol)
- Cirrhosis (early stage)
- Liver abscess (amoebic, pyemic)

Neoplasm
- Hepatoma
- Metastatic
- Lymphoma, leukemia

Granulomatous causes
- Tuberculosis
- Sarcoidosis

Infiltrative causes
- Fatty liver (alcohol, diabetes, toxin)
- Non-alcoholic steatohepatitis (NASH)
- Amyloidosis
- Hemochromatosis
- Storage disorders

Biliary tract obstruction

SPLENOMEGALY

Spleen is normally not palpable. If palpable, it is enlarged. Symptoms due to splenomegaly are abdominal discomfort and pain (for detail, see Chapter 4).

IMPLICATIONS ON DENTAL PRACTICE

- Patients with cirrhosis should be investigated for any hemostatic defects (coagulopathy, thrombocytopenia) before dental procedures. Tests recommended are complete blood count, PT, APTT, bleeding time and platelet count. Fresh frozen plasma and platelet infusion may be needed in patients with marked hemostatic defects.
- Patients with obstructive jaundice may have bleeding tendency due to vitamin K deficiency. Such patients are given injectable vitamin K in order to correct bleeding tendency.
- Neonate with obstructive jaundice may develop green teeth.
- Sedative and tranquillizers should be avoided in patients with cirrhosis as these agents may precipitate encephalopathy.
- Most drugs are metabolized in the liver. Hence, caution should be taken in prescribing medications in patients with liver dysfunction.
- Universal precautions must be taken while doing any procedure or intervention to prevent transmission of infection.
- In case of exposure to hepatitis B positive blood (such as accidental needle prick or by sharp instruments), unvaccinated individuals should take immunoglobulin and vaccine as soon as possible after the exposure. Full course of vaccine should be completed.
- All dentists should get vaccination against hepatitis B.
- Invasive dental or oral surgical procedures may possibly increase the risk of SBP in patients with cirrhosis and ascites. Antibiotic prophylaxis with amoxicillin plus metronidazole may be recommended.

SELF ASSESSMENT

Multiple Choice Questions

1. Following are features of hemolytic jaundice, *except*:
    A. Recurrent jaundice
    B. Mild jaundice
    C. Conjugated hyperbilirubinemia
    D. Increased urobilinogen in urine
2. Most of the bilirubin in normal persons is:
    A. Unconjugated   B. Conjugated
    C. Equal amounts of conjugated and unconjugated
    D. Variable
3. Pruritus (itching) is a symptom of:
    A. Prehepatic jaundice   B. Obstructive jaundice
    C. Both   D. None
4. Causes of hepatocellular jaundice include all, *except*:
    A. Viral hepatitis   B. Drugs
    C. Alcohol   D. Stone in common bile duct
5. Marked elevation of alkaline phosphatase is characteristic of:
    A. Hemolytic jaundice   B. Hepatocellular jaundice
    C. Obstructive jaundice   D. All of the above
6. In obstructive jaundice, urinary examination shows:
    A. No urobilinogen, no bilirubin
    B. Increased urobilinogen, inceased bilirubun
    C. Increased urobilinogen, no bilirubun
    D. No urobilinogen, increased bilirubin
7. In obstructive jaundice all are present, *except*:
    A. Pale stools
    B. Pruritus
    C. Vit K deficiency
    D. Increased urobilinogen in urine
8. Which of the following is transmitted by feco-oral route:
    A. Hepatitis B   B. Hepatitis C
    C. Hepatitis D   D. Hepatitis E
9. Which of the following is not true for hepatitis A:
    A. Feco-oral transmission
    B. Progression to chronic stage
    C. Vaccine against hepatitis A is available
    D. Ig are used for passive immunization
10. Which of the following is not a feature of acute liver disease:
    A. Increased ALT
    B. Prolonged PT
    C. Marked elevation in bilirubin
    D. Low serum albumin
11. Vaccine is available for:
    A. Hepatitis C   B. Hepatitis E
    C. Both   D. None
12. Cirrhosis is a complication of all, *except*:
    A. Hepatitis B   B. Hepatitis C
    C. Hepatitis E   D. Wilson's disease
13. Budd-Chiari syndrome results from the obstruction of:
    A. Portal vein   B. Biliary tract
    C. Hepatic veins   D. Hepatic artery
14. All the following contribute to hepatic encephalopathy, *except*:
    A. GI bleeding
    B. Hypokalemia
    C. Spontaneous bacterial peritonitis
    D. Protein restriction in diet
15. Laennec's cirrhosis is associated with:
    A. Hepatitis B   B. Drugs
    C. Chronic alcoholism   D. Wilson's disease
16. Hepatitis B and C share all the following clinical features, *except*:
    A. Transmission through IV drug abuse
    B. Transmission through sexual contact
    C. Low mortality associated with acute disease
    D. Development of chronic hepatitis in 70–80% patients
17. Patient vaccinated with hepatitis B is positive for:
    A. Hepatitis B surface antigen (HBsAg)
    B. Hepatitis B surface antibody (anti-HBs)
    C. Both HBsAg and anti-HBs
    D. Hepatitis B core antibody (anti-HBc) and anti-HBs

18. Kayser-Fleisher (KF) ring is seen in:
    A. Wilson's disease
    B. Hemochromatosis
    C. Lipid storage disorders
    D. Glycogen storage diseases
19. Jaundice is clinically detectable when serum bilirubin concentration exceeds:
    A. 0.5–1 mg %
    B. 2–3 mg %
    C. 5–8 mg %
    D. 9–12 mg %
20. Tender hepatomegaly is seen in:
    A. Acute viral hepatitis
    B. CHF
    C. Amoebic liver abscess
    D. All
21. Portal hypertension can occur due to:
    A. Portal vein thrombosis
    B. Hepatic vein thrombosis
    C. Cirrhosis
    D. All
22. Gastroesophageal varices is complication of:
    A. Gastric carcinoma
    B. Esophageal carcinoma
    C. Portal hypertension
    D. Varicose vein
23. Immediate treatment of percutaneous exposure (needle prick) in unvaccinated persons to hepatitis B positive blood is:
    A. Interferon and vaccine
    B. Vaccine and lamivudine
    C. Immunoglobulin and vaccine
    D. Immunoglobulin and interferon
24. Following is not used in treatment of chronic hepatitis B:
    A. Interferon
    B. Lamivudine
    C. Adefovir
    D. Ribavirin
25. Prevention of hepatitis C includes:
    A. Administration of vaccine
    B. Administration of immunoglobulin
    C. Both
    D. None
26. Best indicator of acute hepatocellular dysfunction is:
    A. Increased ALT
    B. Increased ALP
    C. Prolonged PT
    D. Decreased albumin
27. All the following can cause ascites with SAAG < 1.1, except:
    A. Tuberculosis
    B. Malignancy
    C. Portal hypertension
    D. Bacterial peritonitis
28. Treatment of choice in bleeding due to hepatocellular dysfunction is:
    A. Whole blood transfusion
    B. Fresh frozen plasma
    C. Vitamin K administration
    D. Packed red blood cell transfusion
29. Which of the following is used for prevention of recurrent variceal bleeding in patients with cirrhosis and portal hypertension:
    A. Amlodipine
    B. Atenolol
    C. Propranolol
    D. Vitamin K
30. Which of the following is now preferred drug for treatment of chronic hepatitis B?
    A. Tenofovir
    B. Lamuvidine
    C. Adefovir
    D. Acyclovir
31. A person who has suffered from hepatitis B infection earlier gets needle prick injury contaminated with blood of hepatitis B patient. Best option will be to:
    A. Give Hepatitis B vaccine
    B. Administer HBIG one dose
    C. Administer HBIG two doses
    D. Do nothing
32. A person has anti-HBs titer of 6 IU/mL after vaccination gets needle prick injury contaminated with blood of hepatitis B patient. Best option will be to:
    A. Give Hepatitis B vaccine and HBIG both
    B. Administer Hepatitis B vaccine only
    C. Administer HBIG only
    D. Do nothing
33. A previously vaccinated person has anti-HBs titer of 24 IU/mL gets needle prick injury contaminated with blood of hepatitis B patient. Best option will be to:
    A. Give Hepatitis B vaccine and HBIG both
    B. Administer Hepatitis B vaccine only
    C. Administer HBIG only
    D. Do nothing
34. A hepatitis B positive patient has compensated cirrhosis with detectable HBV DNA levels of 2000.
    The best therapy for him is:
    A. Pegylated interferon alpha
    B. Entacavir
    C. Administer HBIG only
    D. Sofosbuvir

Fill in the Blanks

1. Normal portal vein pressure is _____ mm Hg.
2. Porto-systemic collaterals around umbilicus may be visible as_____.
3. Normal bilirubin level is _____.
4. Conjugation of bilirubin occurs in _____.
5. Vitamin K dependent coagulation factors are _____.
6. AST : ALT ratio of more than two is suggestive of _____.
7. All coagulation factors except factor VIII are synthesized in _____.
8. Sweet, musty odor present in patient of hepatic encephalopathy is known as_____.
9. Shifting dullness is a sign of _____.
10. Child-Pughs classification is used in assessing the prognosis in patients of _____.

Hematological System

ANEMIA

Anemia is defined as a decrease in the level of hemoglobin below normal for that age and sex. The normal hemoglobin level varies from 13-16 g/dL in the adult male and 12-15 g/dL in the female. The **Table 4.1** shows the values of RBC count, hematocrit and hemoglobin, below which patient is diagnosed to have anemia.

Normal Hematopoiesis

- Hematopoiesis in adult life takes place in the marrow of flat bones such as ribs, vertebrae, pelvic bones, sternum, scapula and the proximal ends of long bones.
- All blood cells arise from a population of cells called hematopoietic stem cells **(Fig. 4.1)**. About 2.5 billion red blood cells (RBCs), 1 billion granulocytes and 2.5 billion platelets per Kg of body weight are produced each day.
- The amount of hemoglobin is maintained by erythropoietin, the hormone secreted by renal peritubular cells.
- The average lifespan of RBCs is 90-120 days and around 1% of RBCs are destroyed in the spleen and replaced by the marrow everyday.

Clinical Presentations

The symptoms and signs of anemia depend on a number of factors. Important factors are:
- Severity of anemia
- Rapidity with which it develops
- Cause of anemia
- Presence of comorbid diseases.

Patients, who develop anemia acutely, such as following massive bleeding, may be highly symptomatic whereas those with gradually developing anemia may have mild symptoms. This is due to the development of various compensatory mechanisms in order to improve tissue oxygenation.

The symptoms and signs of anemia are due to the anemia *per se* or due to conditions which have resulted in anemia.

Table 4.1: Values below which anemia is diagnosed.

	Male	Female
RBC count (million/μL)	<4.5	<4.0
Hemoglobin level (g/dL)	<13	<12
Hematocrit %	<40	<37

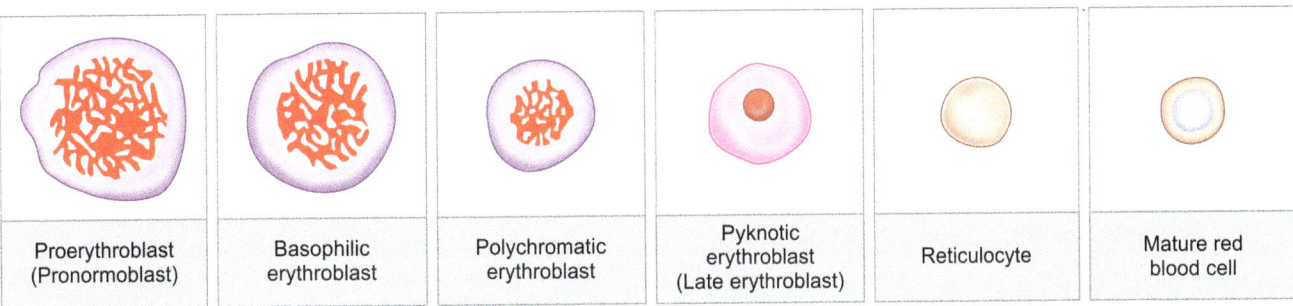

Fig. 4.1: Normal erythropoiesis.

Following are symptoms and signs due to anemia itself:

General: Pallor, weakness, malaise, feverishness, tiredness, vertigo, tinnitus.

Central nervous system: Lack of concentration, decreased memory, syncope, altered sensorium, seizures.

Cardiorespiratory: Palpitation, dyspnea, angina, tachycardia, cardiomegaly, congestive heart failure, flow murmur.

Gastrointestinal: Anorexia, nausea, distaste, stomatitis, cheilosis, glossitis, dysphagia, malabsorption, hepatosplenomegaly.

Others: Loss of libido, impotence, menstrual abnormalities.

Classification

Anemia has been classified in various ways.
- Traditionally it is classified into three groups: (1) Dyshematopoietic, (2) Hemorrhagic and (3) Hemolytic anemia.
- Another classification is based on the morphology of RBC (MCV, MCH, and MCHC) and is grouped into normocytic/microcytic/macrocytic and normochromic/hypochromic types **(Table 4.2)**.
- However, the recent classification is based on reticulocyte index, which is a measure of RBC production. The reticulocyte index is increased (>2.5) due to increase in erythropoiesis as occurs in hemolytic and hemorrhagic anemias. A low reticulocyte index (<2) shows decreased marrow production or maturation defects during erythropoiesis **(Table 4.3)**.

Table 4.2: Red blood cell indices (normal values).

Mean corpuscular volume (MCV)	90 ± 8 fL
Mean corpuscular hemoglobin (MCH)	30 ± 3 pg
Mean corpuscular hemoglobin concentration (MCHC)	33 ± 2%

Table 4.3: Classification of anemia.

- **Hypoproliferative (decreased production of red cells): Normocytic normochromic**
  - Bone marrow failure: Aplastic anemia
  - Bone marrow invasion (myelophthisis): Infiltration, fibrosis
  - Mild to moderate iron deficiency
  - Decreased stimulation by erythropoietin: Renal disease, metabolic defects, inflammation
- **Maturation defect of RBC**
  - Nuclear defect (defect in DNA synthesis): B_{12} deficiency, folic acid deficiency, drug toxicity, and refractory anemia (Macrocytic)
  - Cytoplasm defect (defect in hemoglobin synthesis): Severe iron deficiency, thalassemias, sideroblastic anemia, and lead poisoning (Microcytic)
- **Hemolytic anemia**
  - Intrinsic defects: Hereditary spherocytosis, G6PD deficiency, and sickle cell anemia (HbS)
  - Extrinsic defects: Immune mediated, malaria, microangiopathic anemia, and toxins
- **Hemorrhagic anemia**

Investigations

Tests are needed to assess the type of anemia and also to ascertain its cause. **Table 4.4** shows the tests generally performed in anemic patients.
- Mean corpuscular volume (MCV) of less than 80 fL is called microcytosis and MCV of more than 100 fL is known as macrocytosis.
- The variation in red blood cell size and shape is known as anisocytosis and poikilocytosis respectively.
- *Correction of reticulocyte count:* The reticulocyte count needs to be corrected according to the hematocrit. The corrected reticulocyte count is further adjusted if peripheral blood smear reveals prematurely released cells (polychromasia). This is known as reticulocyte index. Reticulocyte index is the main indicator of RBC production.

Approach to a Case of Anemia

A detailed history and physical examination is required in a case of anemia. In order to know about the cause of anemia, one should ask about;
- Duration of anemia
- Dietary history
- Use of drugs such as NSAIDs, antibiotics, heavy metals, etc.
- Blood loss (piles, excessive menstrual bleed, peptic ulcer)
- Bowel disturbances like diarrhea or dysentery
- Worm infestations
- Tobacco, pan masala, alcohol
- Fever, infections, jaundice
- Family history of anemia
- Blood transfusion
- Liver disease, renal disease
- Joint pain, skin rashes, bone pain, fracture.

Physical examination should mainly include:
- Pallor (conjunctivae, oral mucosa, palm)
- Jaundice
- Skin (rashes, purpura, nodules)
- Oral cavity (ulcers, gingiva, tongue, tonsils)
- Congenital abnormalities
- Lymphadenopathy.

Table 4.4: Investigations in anemic patients.

- Hemoglobin, hematocrit
- RBC indices: MCV, MCH, MCHC, and Red cell distribution width (RDW)
- Reticulocyte count and index
- Total and differential leukocyte count
- Platelet count
- Cell morphology: Size, color, anisocytosis, poikilocytosis, and any abnormal features
- Iron status: Serum iron level, total iron binding capacity (TIBC), ferritin, and marrow iron stain
- Serum vitamin B_{12} and folic acid levels
- Bone marrow aspiration and biopsy
- Liver function, renal function and thyroid function tests

- Hepatosplenomegaly
- Cardiac, respiratory and nervous system examination

IRON DEFICIENCY ANEMIA

Iron deficiency anemia (IDA) is the most common form of anemia prevalent worldwide.

Source and Daily Requirement

Iron is mainly available from a diet rich in meat, liver, beans, jaggery and green vegetables. Milk is poor source of iron. Daily iron requirement is 1 mg in males and 2 mg in females.

Metabolism

- Iron is absorbed in the proximal small intestine in the ferrous form. The absorption of iron is facilitated by the presence of acid in the stomach and vitamin C, while antacids, calcium, phosphates, and phytates decrease it.
- Ferrous iron is transported by metal transporter to enterocytes and stored in the form of ferritin. The iron is transferred out of enterocytes by transporter ferroportin into the circulation.
- Iron released into the circulation binds to transferrin and is transported to sites of uses and storage. Hepatocytes, enterocytes and macrophages serve as storage reservoir of iron.
- Recently a liver hormone, hepcidin has been identified as a principal hormone involved in iron regulation. Hepcidin regulates the iron homeostasis by targeting at villus enterocytes, macrophages and hepatocytes. Thus, liver plays a central role in the regulation of iron absorption from the gut and in influencing the release of iron from the storage sites.

Causes of Iron Deficiency Anemia

The most common cause of IDA is blood loss. The blood loss can be due to hookworm infestation (*Ancylostoma duodenale* and *Necator americanus*), gastritis, peptic ulcer, esophageal varices, intestinal polyp, hemorrhoids, or heavy menstrual bleeding. Iron deficiency can occur during physiological states with high iron demand like adolescence and pregnancy. Decreased absorption due to gastrectomy, achlorhydria or diseases of the small intestine can also lead to IDA **(Table 4.5)**.

Clinical Features

Besides having general symptoms of anemia such as weakness, malaise, tiredness, lack of concentration and anorexia, patients with IDA may specifically have pagophagia, i.e., craving for ice, cheilosis and spoon-shaped nails (koilonychia). On examination, patients are quite pale **(Fig. 4.2)**. Mild splenomegaly can occur in iron deficiency anemia, although it is uncommon. Additionally, patient may complain of dysphagia due to formation of post-cricoid web (Plummer Vinson or Patterson Kelly syndrome). *Plummer Vinson or Patterson Kelly syndrome includes:*

- Iron deficiency anemia
- Angular stomatitis
- Glossitis
- Dysphagia.

Post-cricoid web is a premalignant lesion and there is an increased risk of oral squamous cell cancer and esophageal cancer at post-cricoid tissue web.

Table 4.5: Causes of iron deficiency anemia.

- Blood loss
  - Acute blood loss: Accident and surgery
  - Chronic blood loss: Gastritis, peptic ulcer, hookworm infestation, hemorrhoids, and menstrual loss
2. Increased demand
   Infancy, adolescence, and pregnancy
3. Malabsorption
   Post-gastrectomy, sprue, and Crohn's disease
4. Inadequate diet

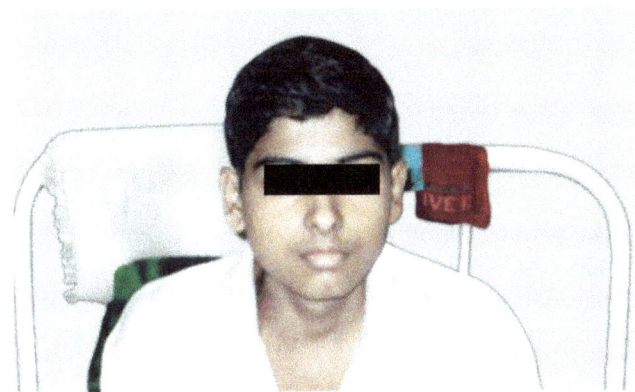

Fig. 4.2: Pallor visible over face.

Investigations

Important investigations are peripheral blood examination, serum iron studies and bone marrow examination **(Fig. 4.3)**.

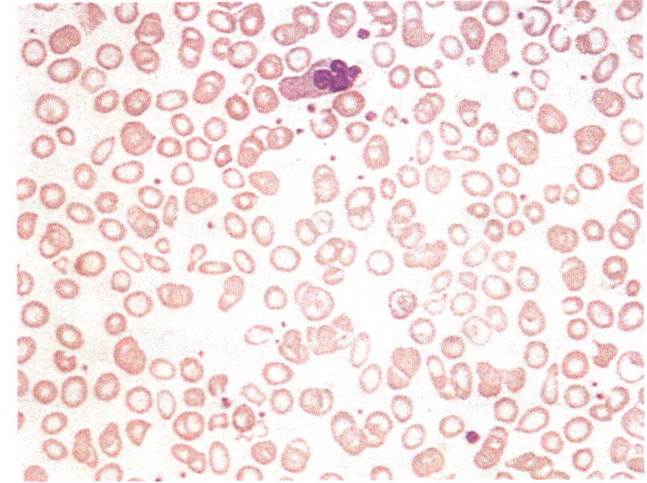

Fig. 4.3: Peripheral blood smear of iron deficiency anemia patient.

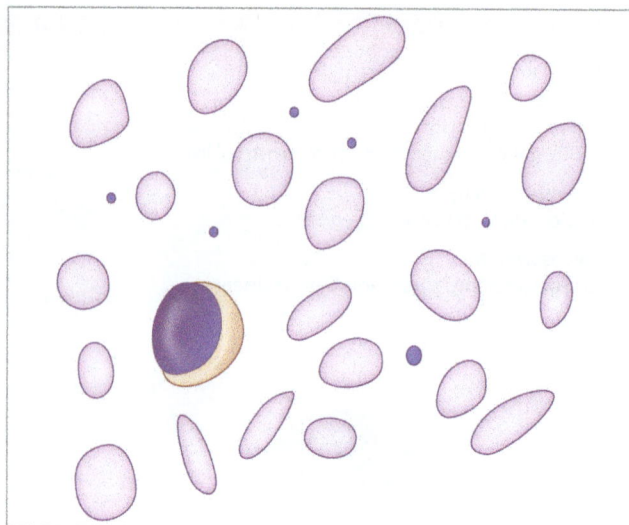

Fig. 4.4: Microcytic hypochromic anemia.

- The general blood picture is microcytic hypochromic (**Fig. 4.4**).
- Serum iron and ferritin are low while total iron-binding capacity (TIBC) is increased. Transferrin saturation is below 16%. Normal level of Transferrin saturation is 30–50%.
- Bone marrow stains for iron reveal decreased or absent iron stores.
- Stool examination for parasites and occult blood is useful for detection of the cause of iron deficiency.
- Endoscopic and radiological examination of gastrointestinal tract is needed to detect the source of bleeding.

Other conditions with microcytic hypochromic anemia should be differentiated from the iron deficiency anemia. These conditions are thalassemia, sideroblastic anemia, chronic inflammation and lead poisoning (**Table 4.6**).

Treatment

Oral Iron Therapy

The drug of choice is ferrous sulfate 200 mg thrice a day (elemental iron 60 mg thrice a day) orally taken in between meals. About 15–20% patients may develop intolerance to oral iron in the form of abdominal pain, nausea, vomiting, diarrhea or constipation. In such cases, the dose may be reduced or the salt is changed to ferrous gluconate, ferrous fumarate, sodium iron edetate or carbonyl iron. The treatment with oral iron is usually given for a long duration and is sustained for 6–12 months even after normalization of hemoglobin. This can be monitored by measuring the level of serum ferritin (normal level 50–200 ug/L).

Parenteral Iron Therapy

Intravenous iron therapy is indicated in following conditions:
- Patient is unable to tolerate oral iron
- Patient has malabsorption
- The needs for iron are relatively acute as in pregnancy or following bleed
- Patients on chronic hemodialysis
- Patient who have undergone gastrectomy
- Achlorhydria.

The total parenteral (intravenous) dose of iron can be calculated by the formula:

$$\text{Body weight (Kg)} \times 2.3 \times (15\text{-Hb level in g/dL}) + 500 \text{ or } 1000 \text{ mg (for stores)}$$

The intravenous iron is generally given at weekly intervals to a total of the calculated dose. Previously used iron compound, iron dextran has been associated with the risk of anaphylaxis which is rarely seen with newer preparations like sodium ferric gluconate, ferric corboxymaltose and iron isomaltoside (ferric derisomaltose) and iron sucrose. Some may develop severe reaction, hence a test dose is preferred before the infusion. One should watch for symptoms like chest pain, wheeze and hypotension and if these occur, the infusion of iron should immediately be stopped and the patient be managed for anaphylactic reaction. Patients may develop minor symptoms like skin rashes, joint pain or fever following intravenous iron; however, these can be managed easily by analgesics and anti-allergic drugs. Occurrence of these minor symptoms does not preclude further dosage.

Red Blood Cell Transfusion

Red cell transfusion is indicated in patients with severe anemia where cardiorespiratory conditions warrant immediate intervention. In these situations, whole blood must be avoided since it may cause volume overload. Whole blood is needed if there is continued and excessive blood loss.

Anemia of Acute or Chronic Inflammation/Infection

Anemia of acute or chronic inflammation is one of the most common types of anemia which forms an important differential diagnosis of iron deficiency anemia because of similar general blood picture and low serum iron. This type of anemia is characterized by mild to moderate anemia associated with inflammatory diseases such as rheumatoid arthritis, serious infections, carcinoma, and liver disease.

Mechanism

There is inadequate delivery of iron to the marrow despite normal or increased iron stores. There is an impaired marrow response to erythropoietin also. These effects are mediated by inflammatory cytokines [interleukin 1 (IL-1), interferon γ (IFN-γ), tumor necrosis factor] and hepcidin. Inflammation causes increased expression of hepcidin by the liver. Hepcidin suppresses iron absorption and inhibits the release of iron from storage sites.

Investigations

Blood tests reveal hemoglobin levels of 8–10 g/dL, low serum iron, low total iron-binding capacity, decreased transferrin saturation, and a normal or increased serum ferritin. Bone marrow stain reveals adequate iron stores.

CHAPTER 4: HEMATOLOGICAL SYSTEM

Table 4.6: Differential diagnosis of microcytic hypochromic anemia.

Test	Iron deficiency	Inflammation	Thalassemia	Sideroblastic anemia
• Serum Iron	Low	Low	Normal/high	Normal/high
• Total iron-binding capacity (TIBC)	Increased	Decreased	Normal	Normal
• Percent saturation	Markedly low	Low	Normal	Normal
• Serum ferritin	Low	Normal/high	High	High
• Hemoglobin pattern	Normal	Normal	Abnormal	Normal

The changes in serum iron profile in different conditions are given in **Table 4.6**.

Treatment

Treatment of underlying inflammatory disease usually corrects anemia. Iron therapy is not indicated. Anemia in inflammatory disorders like rheumatoid arthritis responds to injection erythropoietin. Erythropoietin stimulates production of red blood cells. It is given in doses of 40,000 to 60,000 IU subcutaneously once a week. Erythropoietin is also indicated in anemia of cancers such as in myeloma and chronic lymphocytic leukemia and anemia in chronic renal failure.

MEGALOBLASTIC ANEMIA

Most important causes of megaloblastic anemia are vitamin B_{12} deficiency (cobalamin) and folic acid deficiency. Vitamin B_{12} and folic acid are essential for DNA synthesis and their deficiency may lead to impaired cellular proliferation and maturation. Rapidly dividing cells particularly those of hematopoietic and gastrointestinal tissues are most affected. Because of impaired cellular maturation, a large number of erythroblasts in bone marrow fail to mature and are destroyed. This is called ineffective erythropoiesis. Leukopenia and thrombocytopenia also occur due to impaired proliferation and maturation of respective progenitor cells. Hence, many such patients have pancytopenia.

Cobalamin

- The daily requirement of vitamin B_{12} (cobalamin) is about 2.5 µg.
- Cobalamin is not synthesized in the human body and thus must be supplemented in diet. The only dietary source of cobalamin is animal products like meat and dairy foods.
- It is absorbed in the terminal ileum. The absorption is facilitated by the intrinsic factor produced by the parietal cells of the stomach.
- The cobalamin is largely stored in liver which may last upto 3–6 years.

Folic acid

- Folic acid (pteroylmonoglutamic acid) is found in foodstuff from both animal and plant sources. Dietary folic acid may be destroyed by cooking.
- The body stores are relatively small and may last for only a few months. The average daily requirement is 50–100 µg, although the demand may increase several fold during pregnancy.
- It is mainly absorbed in the jejunum.

Causes of Cobalamin and Folic Acid Deficiency

In tropical countries, megaloblastic anemia occurs mostly due to folic acid deficiency because of malnutrition and during pregnancy. Important causes of cobalamin and folic acid deficiency are given in **Table 4.7**.

Clinical Manifestations

The clinical manifestations are mainly due to the involvement of hematological and gastrointestinal systems. Nervous system is also involved in cobalamin deficiency.

- Patients are anemic and they may also have mild jaundice due to raised plasma unconjugated bilirubin. Purpura may rarely occur due to thrombocytopenia. Spleen may be enlarged. Patients with cobalamin deficiency may have hyperpigmentation of knuckles and oral mucous membrane (**Figs. 4.5 and 4.6**).
- Anorexia, weight loss, diarrhea and smooth and beefy red tongue are important and significant gastrointestinal manifestations.
- Neurological manifestations such as paresthesia, ataxia, sensory-motor paraparesis (subacute combined degeneration), forgetfulness, psychosis are found in cobalamin deficiency and may occur even in the absence of anemia.

Table 4.7: Causes of cobalamin and folic acid deficiency.

Causes of cobalamin deficiency
- Decreased intake: Vegans
- Decreased absorption:
  - Intrinsic factor deficiency: Pernicious anemia and postgastrectomy
  - Diseases of terminal ilium: Sprue, Crohn's disease, and intestinal resection
  - Bacterial proliferation
  - Fish tapeworm (Diphyllobothrium latum) infestation

Causes of folic acid deficiency
- Decreased intake: Unbalanced diet and alcoholism
- Increased demand: Pregnancy, infancy, and hemolysis
- Decreased absorption: Sprue, and celiac disease
- Drugs: Phenytoin, methotrexate, pyremethamine, and trimethoprim

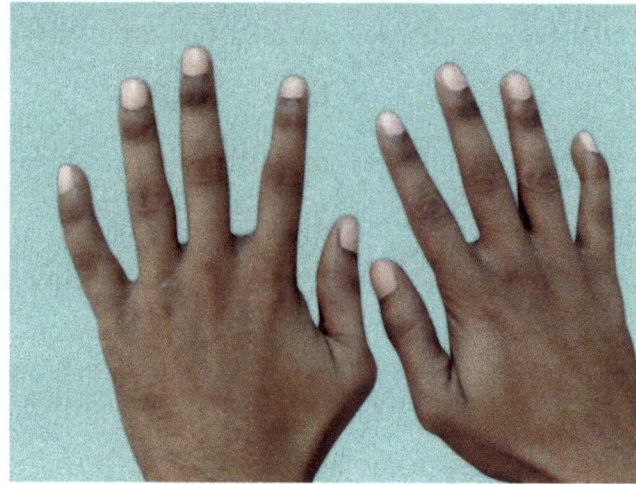

Fig. 4.5: Hyperpigmentaion of knuckles in vitamin B_{12} deficiency.

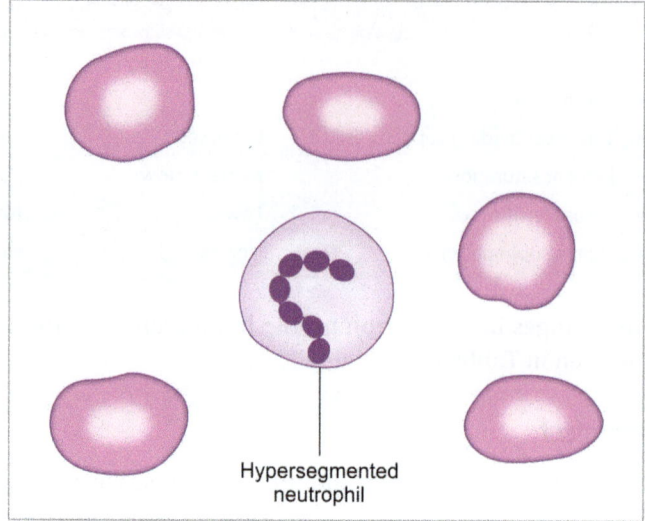

Fig. 4.7: Hypersegmented neutrophil in megaloblastic anemia.

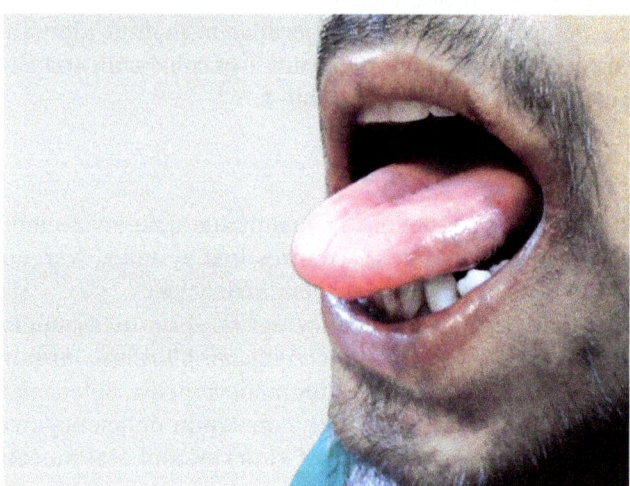

Fig. 4.6: Hyperpigmentaion of oral mucosa in vitamin B_{12} deficiency.

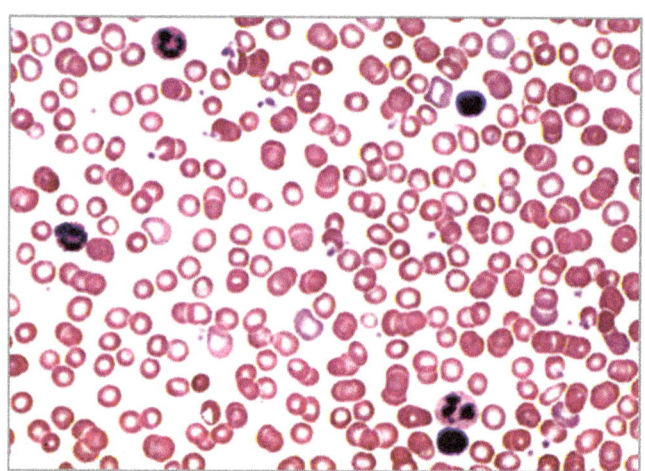

Fig. 4.8: Peripheral blood picture of megaloblastic anemia.

Investigations

- Complete blood count shows decrease in hemoglobin, leukopenia, and thrombocytopenia.
- Peripheral blood smear reveals macrocytosis (MCV >110 fL). Other causes of macrocytosis like hemolysis, liver disease, hypothyroidism and alcoholism must be ruled out. Hypersegmented neutrophils with a nucleus of six or more lobes in a single cell are highly characteristic of megaloblastic anemia **(Figs. 4.7 and 4.8)**.
- Lactate dehydrogenase (LDH 1) and unconjugated bilirubin are raised due to ineffective erythropoiesis.
- Bone marrow is hypercellular and reveals megaloblastic changes. Megaloblasts are abnormally large RBC precursors with nuclei less mature than would be expected from the cytoplasmic development.
- Serum cobalamin and folate levels are determined to detect the specific deficiency.
- Serum levels of both methylmalonic acid and homocysteine are increased in cobalamin deficiency while only homocysteine level is increased in folate deficiency.
- Schilling test is performed to detect the malabsorption of cobalamin. Auto-antibodies against intrinsic factor and parietal cells are found in *pernicious anemia.*

Treatment

Packed red cell transfusion is needed in case of severe anemia with cardiac symptoms. In addition, treatment is directed against the cause of the disease like antibiotics for bacterial overgrowth in the intestine.

Cobalamin deficiency: Parenteral therapy with intramuscular cyanocobalamin or hydroxocobalamin or methylcobalamin is preferred since deficiency is mostly due to malabsorption. The treatment begins with a dose of 1000 μg (1 mg) per week for 8 weeks followed by 1000 μg each month. The treatment is lifelong in case of pernicious anemia.

Folate deficiency: The usual dose of folic acid is 1 mg per day orally. However, higher dosage up to 5 mg daily may be needed in cases of malabsorption. Folinic acid is used in methotrexate-induced anemia.

APLASTIC ANEMIA

Aplastic anemia is characterized by pancytopenia (anemia, leukopenia and thrombocytopenia) and hypocellular bone marrow. In the majority of patients, the cause is not discernible (idiopathic) while the major known causes are drugs, radiation and viral infections **(Table 4.8)**.

Pathogenesis

The pathogenesis of bone marrow aplasia is generally believed to be immune mediated. However, some genetic factors may predispose the individual to develop an abnormal T cell immune response to exogenous stimuli (drugs, viruses) and subsequent marrow failure.

Clinical Features

- The common presentations are bleeding and symptoms of anemia.
- The excessive tendency to bleed is due to thrombocytopenia which may present as easy bruising, epistaxis, gum bleeding, heavy menstrual flow and petechiae (small pinpoint hemorrhage in skin and mucous membrane). Intracranial and retinal hemorrhages may also occur.
- Neutropenia may predispose patients to develop infections.
- Lymphadenopathy and splenomegaly are absent.

Investigations

- Peripheral blood smear shows normocytic or macrocytic anemia, decreased granulocyte and platelet count. Immature cells are absent. Reticulocytes are absent or few **(Fig. 4.9)**.
- The diagnosis is confirmed by the bone marrow aspiration and biopsy **(Fig. 4.10)**.
- Other investigations include viral markers, chromosomal studies, and tests for paroxysmal nocturnal hemoglobinuria (PNH). Chromosomal studies are done in children and younger adults to rule out inherited disorders like Fanconi's anemia.

Table 4.8: Types of aplastic anemia.

- Idiopathic
- Secondary
  - Drugs: Chloramphenicol, sulphonamides, indomethacin, gold, cytotoxic drugs, and anticonvulsants
  - Radiation
  - Chemicals: DDT and benzene
  - Viruses: Hepatitis viruses, parvovirus, HIV-1, Epstein-Barr virus
  - Pregnancy
  - Paroxysmal nocturnal hemoglobinuria (PNH)
- Inherited
  - Fanconi's anemia

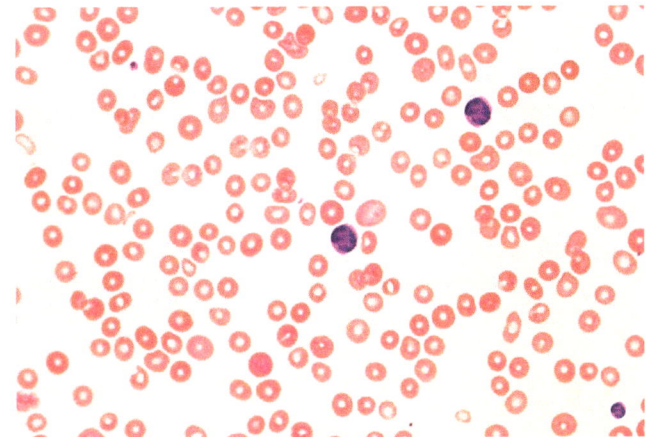

Fig. 4.9: Peripheral blood picture in aplastic anemia.

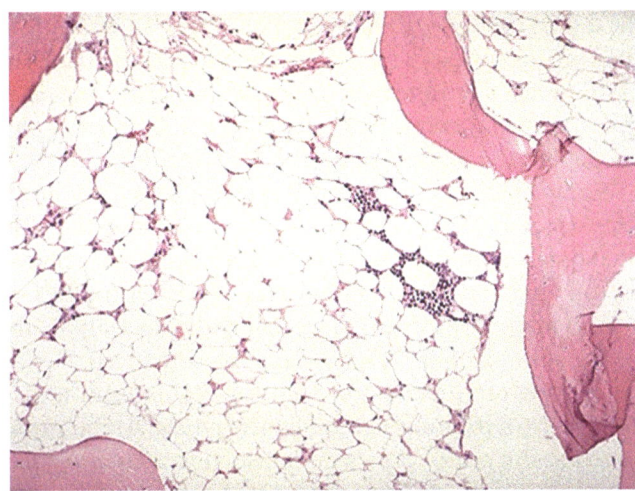

Fig. 4.10: Bone marrow picture in aplastic anemia.

Treatment

- *Bone marrow transplantation:* Allogeneic bone marrow transplantation (BMT) from HLA matched siblings is curative and the preferred mode of therapy in young patients (<40 years). However, this is limited by the high cost, nonavailability of matched donors and the significant morbidity and mortality. Moreover, this facility is available only at a few centers.
- *Immunosuppressive therapy:* Immunosuppressive agents such as anti-thymocyte globulin (ATG) or anti-lymphocyte globulin (ALG) along with cyclosporine is the treatment of choice for patients who cannot be given BMT. Around 60–70% patients respond to this treatment.
- *Other drugs:* The role of anabolic steroids like stanozolol is not clear, though some patients may respond to them. Recently thrombopoietin mimetic agent, eltrombopag is recommended as a front line treatment of aplastic anemia along with cyclosporine. The response is quite encouraging. The use of alemtuzumab, anti CD 52 monoclonal antibody has produced encouraging results in relapsed or refractory cases of aplastic anemia.

d. *Supportive therapy:*
   - Severe anemia is managed with packed red cell transfusion.
   - Platelet concentrates are used to maintain platelet count at or more than 10,000/ μL. Aspirin and NSAIDs which inhibit platelet function should be avoided.
   - Infections should be aggressively dealt with broad-spectrum antibiotics and antifungal agents. Granulocyte transfusion has also been used in overwhelming infections. Aseptic precautions must be observed to prevent infections.

HEMOLYTIC ANEMIA

The average lifespan of RBC is 90–120 days and around 1% of RBCs are destroyed in the spleen and replaced by the bone marrow every day. Hemolytic anemia results due to increased premature destruction of RBCs if the bone marrow is not able to replenish them adequately.

Hemolysis may be extravascular or less commonly intravascular. The hemoglobin, released following RBC breakdown is immediately bound to a plasma protein, haptoglobin. The hemoglobin also binds with albumin to form methemalbumin. In case of severe hemolysis, the haptoglobin binding capacity of plasma is reduced. Hence, free hemoglobin passes through renal glomeruli and is converted to ferritin and hemosiderin in proximal tubules and passed in the urine (hemosiderinuria). Excess hemoglobin that is not absorbed by proximal tubules is passed as such in the urine (hemoglobinuria). Unconjugated bilirubin is raised due to increased hemolysis (prehepatic or hemolytic jaundice).

Hemolytic anemia can be acquired or hereditary. Hemolysis can occur due to defects in the RBC (intracorpuscular or intrinsic defects) or due to causes other than in RBC (extracorpuscular or extrinsic defects). The classification is given in **Table 4.9**.

Hemoglobinopathy

Normal hemoglobin (Hb) consists of heme and tetramer of globin polypeptide chains. Major adult Hb (HbA) has two alpha chains and two beta chains ($\alpha_2\beta_2$) and represents 98% of total Hb. During fetal life, fetal hemoglobin (HbF), containing two alpha chains and two gamma chains ($\alpha_2\gamma_2$), predominates. A small amount of HbA$_2$ ($\alpha_2\delta_2$) is also found in normal adults. The defect in Hb such as in thalassemia and sickle cell disease can result in hemolysis.

Thalassemias: Thalassemias are hereditary disorders characterized by reduced production of globin chains. Reduction in alpha chain synthesis leads to alpha thalassemia and that of beta chain leads to beta thalassemia. Hence in alpha thalassemia, excess beta chains form β_4 tetramer called HbH. In beta thalassemia, there is relative increase in the amount of HbF and HbA$_2$ as beta chains are missing and are substituted by gamma and delta chains respectively. Beta thalassemia major (Cooley's anemia) is a severe disease and manifests in childhood. This condition is transfusion dependent and generally fatal by 30 year of age. Beta thalassemia minor is mild disease, nontransfusion dependent, and patients can live full normal lives. In case of severe thalassemia, the expansion of bone marrow (due to extramedullary hematopoiesis) may cause bony deformities, pathological fractures and osteopenia.

Sickle cell anemia: Sickle cell anemia is caused by mutation in the beta globin gene that replaces the sixth amino acid from glutamic acid to valine (HbS, $\alpha_2\beta_2^{6\ Glu-val}$). Under hypoxic conditions, HbS polymerizes leading to sickling of the RBCs which are more liable to hemolysis.

Clinical Features

- The important clinical manifestations are anemia, recurrent mild jaundice and splenomegaly.
- Patients may have fever with chills during hemolysis.
- Other manifestations are gallstones (pigment stones) and red brown urine (hemoglobinuria).
- The family history may be positive in hereditary disorders like sickle cell disease, thalassemia and hereditary spherocytosis.
- A history of drugs and exposure to chemicals should also be obtained. This is important in patients with G6PD deficiency.
- Characteristic facial features due to marrow expansion and growth retardation may be seen in inherited disorders for example in thalassemia **(Fig. 4.11)**.

Investigations

- Peripheral blood smears reveal features of hemolysis like anisocytosis, poikilocytosis, macrocytosis and target cells. Characteristic RBC morphology is seen in specific causes **(Table 4.10 and Figs. 4.12A and B)**.

Table 4.9: Classification of hemolytic anemias.

Congenital (Intrinsic)
1. Membrane defects: Hereditary spherocytosis and hereditary elliptocytosis
2. Hemoglobinopathies:
   a. Abnormal chain synthesis; thalassemia
   b. Amino acid substitution: Sickle cell disease (HbS), HbC, HbD
3. Enzyme defects: Glucose-6-phosphate dehydrogenase and pyruvate kinase deficiency

Acquired (Extrinsic)
1. Immune: Autoimmune hemolytic anemia (AIHA)
2. Non-immune:
   a. Mechanical: Disseminated intravascular coagulation (DIC), toxemia of pregnancy, and artificial heart valve
   b. Malarial and clostridium infections
   c. PNH (intrinsic)*

*Paroxysmal nocturnal hemoglobinuria (PNH) is characterized by acquired RBC membrane defect (intrinsic).

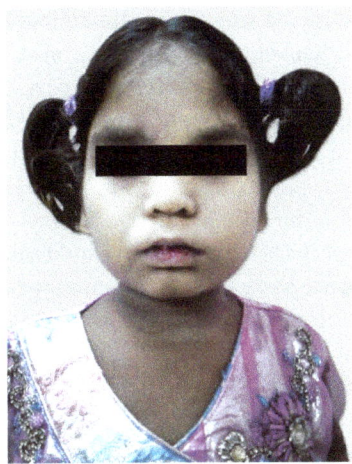

Fig. 4.11: Facial look of a thalassemic child.

Table 4.10: Red cell morphology in hemolytic anemias.	
Spherocytes	Hereditary spherocytosis and AIHA
Target cells	Thalassemia
Microcytes	Thalassemia
Schistocytes	DIC, eclampsia, and artificial heart valve
Sickled cells	Sickle cell syndrome

(AIHA: autoimmune hemolytic anemia)

- Reticulocyte count is increased and is most useful in the diagnosis of hemolytic anemia.
- Bone marrow examination is generally not required.
- Serum unconjugated bilirubin, methemalbumin, and LDH are increased. Serum haptoglobin is decreased or absent **(Table 4.11)**.
- Urine examination may reveal presence of hemosiderin or hemoglobin.
- Serum iron and ferritin levels are normal.
- Tests such as hemoglobin electrophoresis, HPLC (High performance liquid chromatography) for hemoglobin variants, osmotic fragility, Coombs' test, Glucose-6-phosphate dehydrogenase (G6PD) levels, sickling tests, and genetic studies are helpful in the diagnosis of the specific causes.
- Amniocentesis and chorionic villi biopsy are performed for prenatal diagnosis of inherited conditions like thalassemia and sickle cell disease.

Treatment

Supportive treatment in form of packed cell transfusion may be needed. However, repeated transfusion may lead to iron overload which in turn may require treatment with chelating agents, deferoxamine. Folic acid, 5 mg daily is given to meet the increased demand. Following are other modes of treatment in specific situations:
- Bone marrow transplantation is curative in thalassemia and sickle cell disease.
- Splenectomy may be needed in hereditary spherocytosis and AIHA.

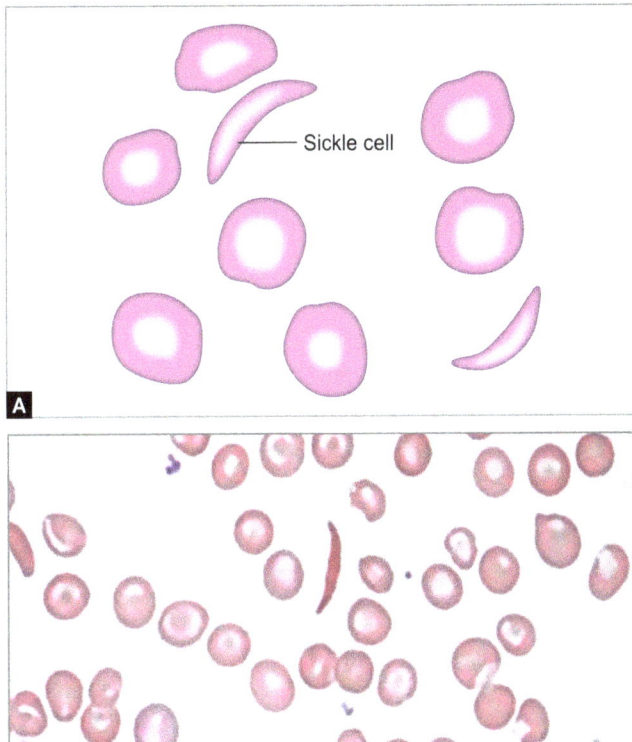

Figs. 4.12A and B: Sickle cell anemia.

Table 4.11: Findings suggestive of hemolysis.
Increased RBC Destruction:
• High serum indirect bilirubin
• Low serum haptoglobin
• High serum LDH
• Hemoglobinuria and hemosiderinuria (in intravascular hemolysis)
• Decreased RBC lifespan
Increased RBC Production:
• High reticulocyte count
• Nucleated RBCs in peripheral smear
• Erythroid hyperplasia in bone marrow

- Steroids and other immune suppressive drugs are given in immune-mediated anemias.
- Factors including infections, dehydration, hypoxia (in sickle cell disease) and drugs (primaquine, sulphonamides) that may precipitate hemolysis in persons with G6PD deficiency should be avoided.

Management of Sickle Cell Disease

General

Proper hydration must be maintained particularly during exercise, infection or exposure to heat.

Prophylactic antibiotics are given before any dental procedures, especially in splenectomized patient.

Pneumococcal and *H. influenzae* vaccines should be given.

Table 4.12: Modalities in the management of sickle cell disease.

- Hydration
- Oxygen
- Analgesics
- Exchange blood transfusion
- Prophylactic vaccines
- Hydroxyurea
- Glutamine
- Anti-P-selectin monoclonal antibody
- Gene therapy
- Bone marrow transplantation

Drugs

Hydroxyurea is the mainstay of treatment in patients with severe symptoms. It increases HbF (fetal hemoglobin) in blood, improves vascular endothelial function, and decreases white blood cells (WBCs) and reticulocytes. Hydroxyurea offers beneficial effects in symptomatic patients and has been shown to offer survival advantage. The dose is generally 15–20 mg/kg/day and is titrated on the basis of WBC count.

Other drugs known to offer beneficial effect are Glutamine and Anti-P-selectin monoclonal antibody (Crizanlizumab).

Bone marrow transplantation is a curative method of treatment but it is effective and safe only in children with sickle cell disaease.

The development of a new technology CRISPR (Clustered regularly interspaced short palindromic repeats) has allowed gene editing. This may prove a promising method of therapy (gene therapy) in future **(Table 4.12)**.

Prophylactic exchange transfusion seems to substantially reduce the chances of stroke.

ANEMIA OF ACUTE BLOOD LOSS

Acute blood loss due to trauma and surgery may lead to anemia. A loss of about 20% of blood volume (1 liter) can be tolerated; however, a loss of more than 40% can lead to shock.

Anemia may be apparent only after volume replacement in patients with acute blood loss.

Other findings include raised total leukocyte count and platelets, and presence of nucleated RBCs and immature leukocytes in the peripheral blood. Maximal rise in reticulocytes occur after 1 week. A rise in serum unconjugated bilirubin and fall in serum haptoglobin may occur in case of bleeding in an internal cavity.

The management includes treatment of the underlying conditions and the blood transfusion. Patient may need iron replacement.

LEUKEMIA

- Leukemia arises from malignant transformation of hematopoietic cells leading to increased number of white blood cells in blood and/or bone marrow.
- Depending on the onset and the course of the disease, leukemia is classified as acute or chronic.
- The course in acute leukemia is aggressive and the lifespan is short if not treated. The course in chronic leukemia is indolent and the survival period is much longer.
- Leukemia is also named as myeloid or lymphoid depending on the type of cell of origin.

In majority of cases the etiology of leukemia is not known. However, some are associated with ionizing radiation, drugs (alkylating agents), toxins (benzene) and viral infections. There may be a genetic predisposition for the development of leukemia.

ACUTE LEUKEMIAS

Acute leukemia is life threatening hematological malignancy characterized by >20% blasts in either peripheral blood or bone marrow. Acute leukemias are broadly classified in two catogories, i.e., acute lymphoblastic leukemia (ALL) and acute myeloblastic leukemia (AML). Eighty percent of pediatric leukemias are acute lymphoblastic leukemia in contrast to preponderance of AML in adults and elderly. Classification of acute leukemia based on morphology is given in **Table 4.13**. Recently AML and ALL have been further subclassified based on WHO 2016 revision.

Types of AML

- AML with recurrent genetic abnormalities
- AML with myelodysplasia related changes
- Therapy-related AML
- AML not otherwise specified
- Myeloid sarcoma
- Myeloid proliferations related to Down syndrome.

Types of ALL

- B lymphoblastic leukemia/lymphoma
- T-lymphoblastic leukemia/lymphoma
- Mature B cell leukemia
- Early T-cell precursor -ALL

Table 4.13: Classification of acute leukemias based on morphology.

Acute myeloid leukemia (AML)
(French-American-British classification)
- M0 Undifferentiated
- M1 Myeloblastic
- M2 Myeloblastic with differentiation
- M3 Promyelocytic
- M4 Myelomonocytic
- M5 Monoblastic
- M6 Erythroleukemia
- M7 Megakaryoblastic

Acute lymphoblastic leukemia (ALL)
- ALL-L1: small uniform cells.
- ALL-L2: large varied cells
- ALL-L3: mature medium size cells.

Pathophysiology: Various cytogenetic and molecular abnormalities lead to uncontrolled proliferation of immature precursors and their defective maturation and differentiation. These immature cells are known as Blasts. These blasts do not function well and also replace the normal hematopoietic system in bone marrow leading to various cytopenias (low blood counts) and bone pains. These cytopenias give rise to various manifestations of disease like anemia, bleeding and infections. Immunocompromised status also adds to the risk of infections.

Acute Myeloid Leukemia

Clinical Features

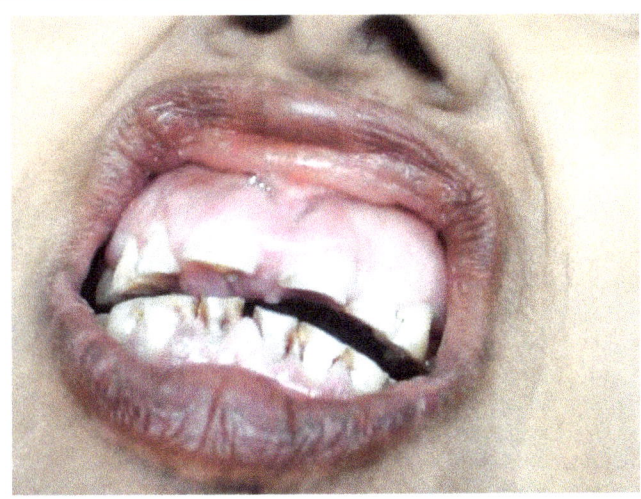

Fig. 4.12: Gum hyperplasia in an AML-M5 patient.

Median age of a patient with AML is 70 years. Most cases have no apparent cause but some may have history of prior irradiation, chemotherapy, chemical exposure or prior myeloproliferative/myelodysplastic disorder. Usually the symptoms are acute onset. Patient can present with a few weeks to few months history of following features
- **Fever:** Fever is very common in acute leukemia. It can be a manifestation of disease as well as the opportunistic infection due to functional neutropenia and compromised immune status. Bacterial and fungal infections are common in AML.
- **Weakness/lethargy:** These are symptoms due to anemia and disease itself. Rapid onset weakness, exertional breathlessness and loss of stamina is very common.
- **Bleeding symptoms:** Usually patients have bleeding due to thrombocytopenia. Severe thrombocytopenia is not rare in AML. Although coagulopathy is less common but some variants of AML, i.e., Acute promyelocytic leukemia (APML) can present with diffuse bleeding due to associated disseminated intravascular coagulopathy.
- **Bone pains:** Bone pain occurs due to expansion of bone marrow because of rapidly proliferative leukemic cells. Rib pain, joint pain and pain in extremities is quite common in acute leukemia.
- **Hyperviscosity:** AML with a blast count of >1,00,000/cmm or a monocytic variant with a count of >50,000 can present with hyperviscosity due to large size and more sticky nature of blasts in AML. They can present with visual symptoms, giddiness, breathlessness and confusion/altered mentation.
- **Other clinical features:** Malignant cells can also infiltrate various organs leading to hepatosplenomegaly and lymphadenopathy. Some times mass lesions and proptosis can be there due to localized blast collection known as Myeloid sarcoma. Gum hyperplasia is a common feature in monocytic leukemias (AML M4 and M5) and occurs due to gum infiltration by monocytic cells **(Fig. 4.12)**.

Diagnosis

Peripheral blood examination and bone marrow is helpful in suspecting the type of leukemia and counting blast %

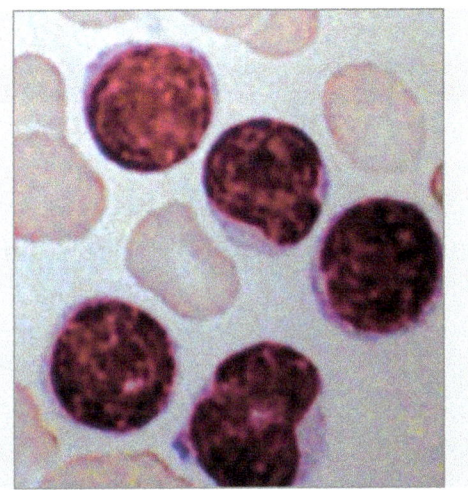

Fig. 4.13: Acute myeloid leukemia.

(Fig. 4.13). A blast which is 3–5 times larger than a mature lymphocyte having scant to moderate eosinophilic cytoplasm and multiple prominent nucleoli are suggestive of myeloid blast. Auer rods if present are characteristic of AML and it is present in almost 45% of AML cases. Flowcytometry using acute leukemia panel is the investigation of choice to confirm AML. **Table 4.14** shows the baseline diagnostic workup of acute leukemia patients.

Risk stratification: Underlying cytogenetic and molecular abnormalities play a major role in risk stratification. **Table 4.15** gives the major abnormalities and their prognostic significance. Overall survival (OS) ranges from 30–40%. Good risk patients have OS of 50–60% compared to poor risk patients having survival of 10–20%. Age, performance status and comorbidities like obesity, diabetes, hypertension, and cardiac disorders also have major impact on treatment related complications.

Treatment

After diagnosis, patient as well as the family members should be counseled regarding the disease, prognosis, treatment-

Table 4.14: Diagnostic work up in acute leukemia.

Diagnostic and prognostic workup
- Complete blood counts and peripheral smear
- Bone marrow aspiration and biopsy
- Flowcytometry (acute leukemia panel)
- Karyotyping
- Molecular studies
- CSF examination

Biochemical parameters
- Serum LDH
- Serum uric acid
- Serum electrolytes; sodium, potassium, calcium and phosphate
- Serum urea/creatinine
- Liver function tests

Coagulation parameters
- Prothrombin time
- Activated partial thromboplastin time
- FDP, D-Dimer

Microbiology: HbsAg, HCV, HIV

Table 4.15: Risk stratification in acute myeloid leukemia.

Cytogentics	Incidence	Prognosis
Cytogenetic Abnormalities		
t(8:21)	8–12%	Good
t(15:17)	6–13%	Very Good
t(16:16)		Good
Inv16	5–12%	Good
-5, del 5q	7–10%	Poor
-7, del 7q	10–12%	Very Poor
Normal cytogenetics	50%	Intermediate Risk
Complex karyotype	10–20%	Very Poor
Molecular Abnormalities		
FLT-3 Mutation	20–30%	Poor
NPM-1 Mutation	20–40%	Good
CEBPA Biallelic	5–10%	Good
C-KIT	3–5%	Poor

related complications, need for blood components, cost of treatment, and family and psychological support to these patients.

Supportive Treatment

Anemia is managed with transfusion of packed red cells with a target Hb of 8 g/dl and above. Severe thrombocytopenia (platelet count<10,000/cmm) or <20,000 with fever or any thrombocytopenia with bleeding manifestations should be managed with platelet transfusions. One unit of single donor platelet (SDP) or 4-6 units of random donor platelets (RDP) should be used. If patient presents with fever, sample for blood cultures should be sent before starting antibiotics. Empirical broad-spectrum antibiotics should be started immediately. Proper investigations should be done to localize and identify these infections.

Specific Treatment

Treatment of AML depends on age, performance status, cytogenetics and molecular abnormalities. Patients who are young with good performance status are treated with induction chemotherapy like 3+7 protocol. This includes Daunorubicin and Cytarabine. Those patients achieving remission should undergo 3–4 cycle of consolidation with high dose cytosine arabinoside. High risk patients should undergo allogeneic stem cell transplant after induction remission. Patients with comorbidities, active infections or elderly patients should be treated with low intensity treatment options like demethylating agents (Azacitidine, Decitabine) or low dose cytarabine. Targated therapies like FLT-3 inhibitors and C-Kit inhibitors also have role in treatment of AML patients having these molecular abnormalities. Commonly used drugs are mentioned in **Table 4.16**.

Acute Lymphoblastic Leukemia

Acute lymphoblastic leukemia (ALL) is the most common pediatric leukemia. Two major types of ALL are B-ALL and T-ALL. B-ALL accounts for 80% of all ALLs and Pre-B ALL is the most common type (80%) in this category. Evolution in management of ALL has lead to >80% overall long-term survival (cure) of pediatric patients. In adults this remains poor in the range of ~40%.

Clinical Presentation

Patients present with weakness, lethargy, fever, bleeding manifestations, swellings in the neck and armpits and bone pains. Bone and joint pain is common in pediatric patients. Clinical examination reveals pallor, lymphadenopathy and variable hepatosplenomegaly. Bone tenderness can also be elicited.

Diagnosis and Risk Stratification

Diagnostic workup is similar to AML including CBC, peripheral smear, bone marrow evaluation, flowcytometry,

Table 4.16: Drugs commonly used to treat acute leukemias.

Acute myeloid leukemia
- Daunorubicin
- Cytosine arabinoside
- Etoposide
- All –trans-retinoic acid*

Acute Lymphoblastic leukemia
- Vincristine
- Prednisolone
- Daunorubicin
- L-asparaginase
- Methotrexate
- Etoposide
- Cytosine arabinoside
- Mercaptopurine

*This is a vitamin A analog, used in the treatment of AMLM3.

Table 4.17: Cytogenetic abnormalities in acute lymphoblastic leukemia.

Cytogenetic abnormality	Molecular transcript	Incidence (Pediatric patients)	Prognosis
t(12:21)	TEL-AML1	20–25%	Good
t(9:22)	BCR-ABL	4%	Very poor
t(4:11)	MLL-AF4	8%	Very poor
t(8:14)	IgH/MYC	2%	Good
Hyperdiploidy		20–25%	Good
Hypodiploidy		6%	Poor

CSF analysis, cytogenetics and molecular studies. Lymphoblasts are 2–3 times larger than mature lymphocyte and have very high N:C ratio, scant basophilic agranular cytoplasm and inconspicuous nucleoli. Flowcytometry helps in diagnosing ALL as well as subtyping it. Baseline evaluation for tumor lysis is very important as ALL patients with high TLC >1,00,000/cmm or having Burkitt leukemia have very high chances of tumor lysis syndrome (TLS). Baseline CSF evaluation is also important as 5% patients can have CNS involvement needing CNS directed therapy. **Table 4.17** shows major cytogenetic abnormalities in pediatric patients and their prognostic significance.

Treatment

Counseling of patients as well as family members regarding prognosis, treatment-related complications, future need for stem cell transplant, cost of treatment, and need for family and psychological support should be done in detail. Supportive care in the form of tumor lysis prophylaxis (hydration and allopurinol/febuxostat/rasburicase), antibiotic prophylaxis and antiviral prophylaxis should be started. Supportive care including tumor lysis prophylaxis, viral and bacterial prophylaxis, blood component support should be started as indicated.

Specific Treatment

Pediatric ALL protocols are well developed. MCP-841, BFM-95, BFM 2002, UKALL are some of the protocols commonly used in clinical practice. Adolescents and young adults are also managed on the similar lines. Treatment includes combination of chemotherapies spaced over phases of induction, consolidation and maintenance. Total duration of treatment is around 2.5 years. Induction usually includes steroids (Dexamethasone/prednisolone), anthracycline (Daunorubicin), vincristine and L-asparaginase. The purpose of induction chemotherapy is to reduce the disease burden to the minimum and achieve complete remission. Consolidation includes high-dose Methotrexate or high-dose Cytarabine-based chemotherapy to further boost the response achieved by induction chemotherapy and eradicate resistant clones. Long-term maintenance with 6-mercaptopurine and oral methotrexate is needed to prevent relapse at sanctuary sites.

High-risk patient needs allogeneic stem cell transplant as consolidation in second complete remission. Philadelphia positive patients benefit from addition of tyrosine kinase inhibitors (TKIs) like Imatinib, Nilotinib or Dasatinib. Elderly patients need different protocols or dose modifications.

CNS-Directed Therapy

Intrathecal therapy is given according to the selected protocol to prevent CNS relapse. Single agent methotrexate or triple agent combination (Methotrexate, cytarabine and hydrocortisone) should be used based on status of CNS involvement. Prophylactic cranial radiotherapy (12–18 Gy) should also be planned according to the protocol to prevent CNS relapse.

Chronic Myeloid Leukemia

Chronic myeloid leukemia (CML) is a type of myelo-proliferative disorder. It is classified as one of the myeloproliferative neoplasms as per WHO classification of myeloid malignancies **(Table 4.18)**.

It occurs as a result of malignant transformation of pluripotent stem cell leading to accumulation of large number of immature leukocytes in the blood. The underlying chromosomal abnormality in CML is the Philadelphia chromosome (short 22) which results due to the reciprocal translocation between chromosomes 9 and 22 **(Figs. 4.14A and B)**. The translocation leads to the formation of hybrid gene *(bcr-abl)* and synthesis of a 210 KD protein. This protein has intrinsic tyrosine kinase activity and is responsible for the initiation and maintenance of the malignant proliferation in CML.

Typically the course of CML consists of three phases if left untreated:
1. The initial phase is the chronic phase which, without treatment, may last for 2–3 years.
2. This evolves into an accelerated phase which finally transforms into a terminal blast phase.
3. The blast phase is like acute leukemia, which is mostly myeloblastic but in about 20% cases, it can be lymphoblastic.

Prior to the advent of specific BCR-ABL tyrosine kinase inhibitors (TKIs), the median survival of CML patients was 3–4 years and 10 years survival was less than 30%. But with TKIs, 10 years survival is around 85%.

Table 4.18: Myeloproliferative neoplasms (MPN).

- Chronic myeloid leukemia *BCR-ABL 1-positive* (CML)
- BCR-ABL 1-negative MPNs
  - Polycythemia vera
  - Primary myelofibrosis
  - Essential thrombocythemia
- Chronic neutrophilic leukemia
- Chronic eosinophilic leukemia not otherwise specified (CEL-NOS)
- Mastocytosis
- Myeloproliferatiev neoplasms unclassified (MPN-U)

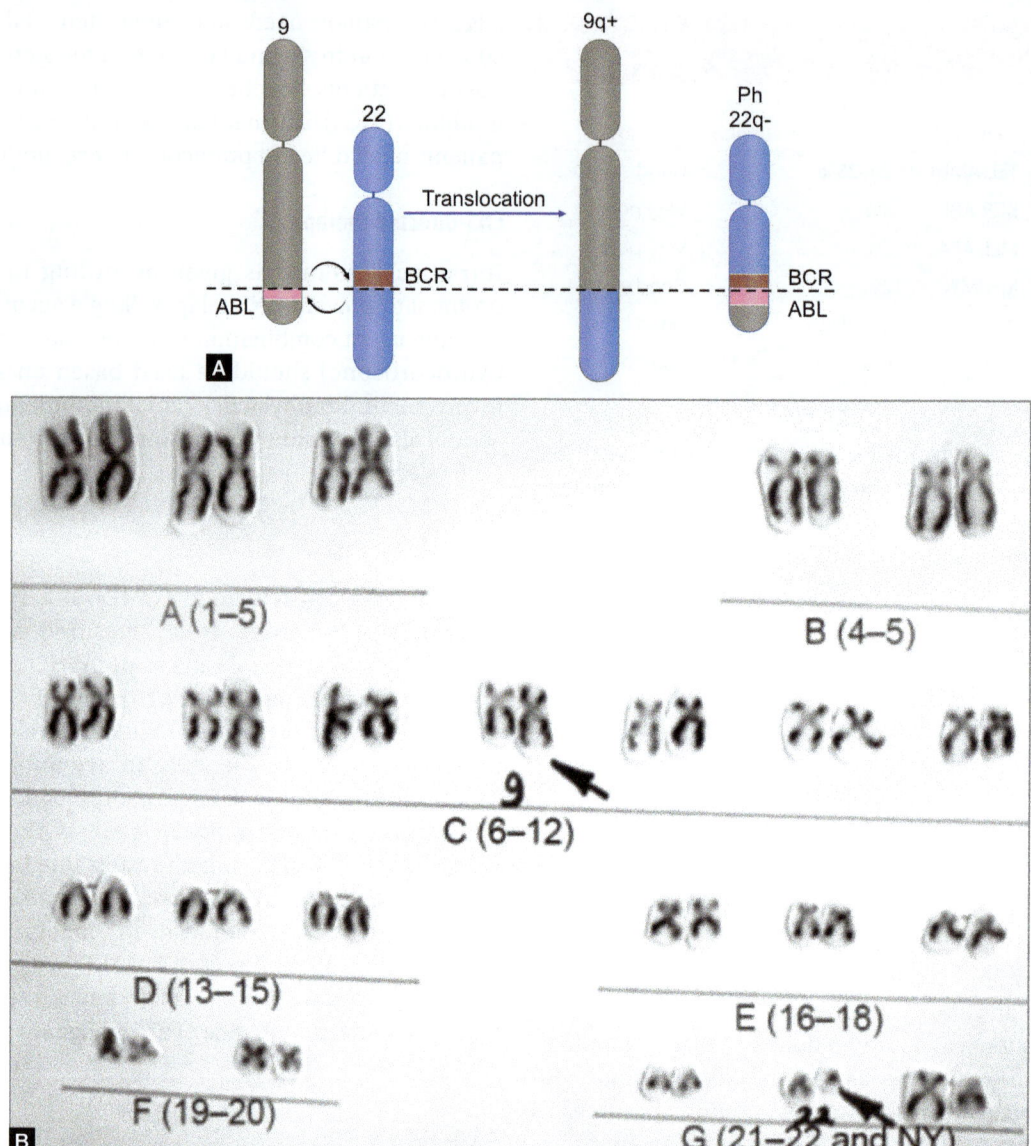

Figs. 4.14A and B: (A) Philadelphia chromosome; (B) Cytogenetic study showing short chromosome 22.

The incidence of CML in India is not well known, however it is the most common type of chronic leukemia in India in contrast to the West where most common type of chronic leukemia is chronic lymphocytic leukemia. There is slight male predominance. The median age of patients is 35-40 years which is lower than that is reported from West (55-60 years). The reason why disease occurs at younger age in India is not known.

No etiological cause is known to be associated with CML. It is not causally related to viruses, toxins, insecticides or pesticides. There is no familial basis of the disease. However exposure to high dose of radiation in atomic bomb survivors in Japan has been associated with occurrence of CML.

Clinical Presentations

The clinical presentations of CML depends upon the duration of disease when patient presents. In developed countries, CML is incidentally detected on routine blood examination when the patient is asymptomatic. However in India, most patients have weakness, weight loss, fatigue, and splenic enlargement at presentation. Other manifestations may be due to thrombotic complications such as priapism, stroke, myocardial infarction, visual disturbances, venous thrombosis, etc. Patients in advanced disease such as in accelerated or blast phase may have fever, lymphadenopathy, bone and joint pain and bleeding.

Investigations

- The peripheral blood examination reveals high total leukocyte count (generally in lacs), normocytic normochromic anemia and high platelet count. Differential count reveals neutrophilic predominance and presence of band cells, metamyelocytes, myelocytes, promyelocytes, and blast cells (generally less than 5% in chronic phase) **(Fig. 4.15)**.

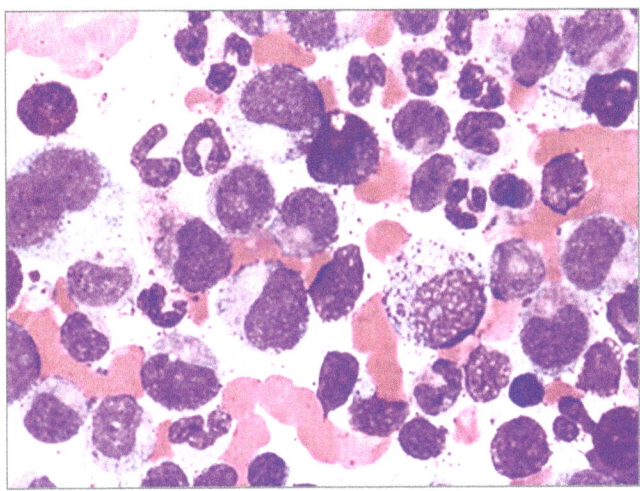

Fig. 4.15: Blood picture in CML patient.

- The presence of low platelet count denotes worsening of the disease. Presence of 20% or more blast cells in bone marrow or peripheral blood is diagnostic of the blast phase of CML.
- The diagnosis of CML is confirmed by the demonstration of Philadelphia chromosome on cytogenetic analysis or the presence of *bcr-abl* fusion gene by molecular techniques.

Treatment

- The drug of choice in CML chronic phase is one of the TKIs. These are new targeted drugs which specifically inhibit the *bcr-abl* tyrosine kinase. The selection of a particular TKI is made based on its cost, availability, comorbidity in the patient, and stage of the disease. Various TKIs are imatinib, dasatinib, nilotinib, bosutinib, and ponatinib **(Table 4.19)**. This can result in molecular remission in around 60–70% patients. The usual dose of imatinib is 400 mg oral daily. In case of suboptimal response, the dose can be increased to 800 mg/day. Those who are non-responder to imatinib or do not tolerate imatinib are given other tyrosine kinase inhibitor, *Dasatinib* or *Nilotinib*. Ponatinib, a newer tyrosine kinase inhibitor is found to be useful in resistant cases who have T315I kinase domain mutation. The duration of treatment is generally lifelong. Trials are underway to find out the possibility of stopping the drug once patients have achieved complete molecular response for more than 2 years.
- At present the only known curative method of treatment of CML is allogeneic bone marrow transplantation (Allo BMT). However, since most patients respond to tyrosine kinase inhibitors and live almost normal lifespan and majority cannot avail Allo BMT due to the high cost, lack of proper donor or the high risk involved in the procedure, this mode of treatment is reserved for those patients who are resistant to drug therapy.
- Other agents like interferon alpha and hydroxyurea are now no longer used in CML due to advent of TKIs. However hydroxyurea is sometimes used to lower the leukocyte count if it is very high in order to reduce the complications of leukostasis.
- The blast phase is managed as acute leukemia. Alternatively imatinib in larger dosage (600 mg daily) or dasatinib can be tried in blast phase of lymphoid lineage.

Chronic Lymphocytic Leukemia

Chronic lymphocytic leukemia (CLL) is a malignancy of mainly B cell origin, although it can be T cell type in some. It has slowly progressive course. The median age at presentation is 65 years.

CLL is characterized by the presence of large number of mature looking small lymphocytes in the blood smear and lymphoid organs like lymph nodes, liver and spleen. The classic features of CLL include absolute clonal B lymphocyte count in the peripheral blood >5000/cmm with varying degree of cytopenias and hepatosplenomegaly. The patients are immunocompromised because B cells are less responsive to antigenic stimuli.

Clinical Manifestation

- The onset is insidious.
- In many, the disease is asymptomatic and is diagnosed during incidental blood examination.
- The usual clinical features are painless lymphadenopathy, splenomegaly and anemia.
- Autoimmune hemolytic anemia and thrombocytopenia may also occur.
- Binet and Rai staging systems are used for the prognostic classification of CLL. Rai staging is commonly used in clinical practice **(Table 4.20)**.

Investigations

- Examination of the blood reveals high lymphocyte count (WBC usually >20,000/µl). Majority of the cells are mature lymphocytes **(Fig. 4.16)**.
- Bone marrow examination reveals infiltration with mature lymphocytes.
- Coombs test is positive in autoimmune hemolytic anemia.
- Thrombocytopenia may occur due to immune destruction or marrow failure.
- Serum immunoglobulin levels may be low which gives an idea about the degree of immunosuppression.
- Newer prognostic markers like CD38, ZAP 70 mutation and VIg mutation are helpful in the management of CLL.

Table 4.19: Tyrosine kinase inhibitors for treatment of CML.

Name	Route	Dose	Indications
Imatinib	Oral	400 mg daily	All phases
Dasatinib	Oral	70–140 mg daily	All phases
Nilotinib	Oral	600–800 mg daily	All phases except blastic phase
Bosutinib	Oral	500 mg daily	All phases except frontline
Ponatinib	Oral	45 mg daily	All phases except front line

Table 4.20: Rai clinical staging for CLL.

Rai staging	Risk	Details	Median overall survival (months)
0	Low	Lymphocytosis in blood (>5000/cmm)	>120
I	Intermediate	Above plus enlarged lymph nodes	95
II	Intermediate	I plus enlarged liver/spleen	72
III	High	Lymphocytosis + enlarged liver/spleen or lymphadenopathy with anemia (<11 gm%)	30
IV	High	Lymphocytosis + enlarged liver/spleen or lymphadenopathy with thrombocytopenia (<100000/cmm)	30

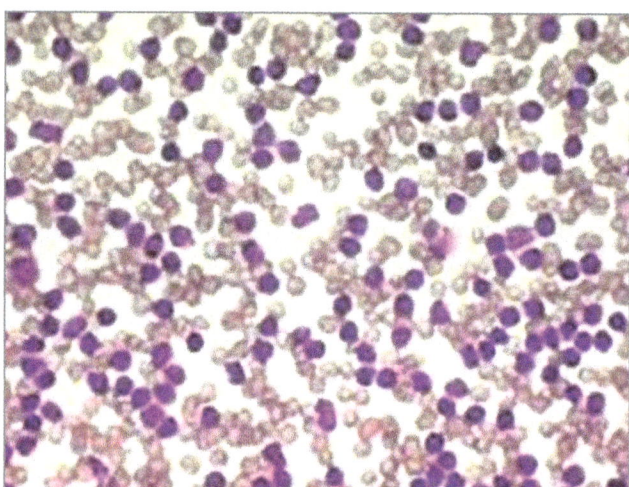

Fig. 4.16: Blood picture in CLL patient.

Treatment

- Most patients do not require treatment in the early stage of the disease.
- Those with features of progressive disease such as symptomatic lymphadenopathy, anemia or thrombocytopenia need chemotherapy.
- The therapy of choice in young and fit patients is fludarabine based chemotherapy (fludarabine alone or in combination with cyclophosphamide and/or anti-CD 20 monoclonal antibody) which provides better response and survival.
- Alternatively oral chlorambucil may be given. Prednisolone is administered in cases of autoimmune hemolytic anemia.
- Recently an oral drug Ibrutinib (Bruten tyrosine kinase inhibitor) has been approved in CLL as front line treatment as well as in relapsed cases. The dose is 420 mg/day. Another agent venetoclax (BCL2 inhibitor) has been shown to be effective in relapsed cases.

LYMPHOMAS

Lymphomas are tumors of lymphoid cells presenting with lymphadenopathy, organomegaly, bone marrow involvement or a combination of these. Broadly lymphomas are classified histologically into two groups, i.e., Hodgkin lymphoma (HL) and Non-Hodgkin lymphoma (NHL). Most of the NHLs are of B cell origin and Hodgkin lymphoma is also proposed to originate from B-cells. A simplified classification of lymphomas is given in **Tables 4.21**.

Staging of Lymphomas

CT scan of neck, thorax, abdomen and pelvis or FDG-PET-CT whole body (Fluorodeoxy glucose-Positron emission tomography) is required for staging of lymphoma. PET-CT is preferred nowadays. It tells about anatomical extension as well as metabolic activity of involved node or tissue. Bone marrow study is required to rule out marrow involvement. Modified Ann Arbor staging system was initially prepared for staging of Hodgkin lymphoma but currently used to stage most lymphomas **(Table 4.22)**. Stage of lymphoma decides the prognosis as early stage lymphomas (stage I, II) have better prognosis compared to advanced stages (III,IV) **(Table 4.23)**.

Hodgkin Lymphoma

Hodgkin lymphoma is a lymphoid malignancy characterized by presence of Reed-Sternberg (RS) cells of B cell origin. The background on histopathological examination is mostly reactive and made of lymphocytes, eosinophils and plasma cells. It is a slowly growing lymphoma which originates at single nodal site usually and then spreads contiguously.

Table 4.21: Classification of lymphoma.

Hodgkin lymphoma	Non-Hodgkin lymphoma
Nodular lymphocytic predominant Hodgkin lymphoma (NLPHL)	**B-Cell Origin (~80%)** **Precursor cell** • B-Lymphoblastic lymphoma **Mature cell** • Diffuse large B cell lymphoma • Follicular lymphoma • Mantle cell lymphoma • Marginal zone lymphomas • Small lymphocytic lymphoma (CLL/SLL) • Lymphoplasmacytic lymphomas • Other rare lymphomas
Classical Hodgkin lymphoma Nodular sclerosis type Mixed cellularity type Lymphocyte rich type Lymphocyte depletion type	**T-Cell origin (~20%)** **Precursor cell** • T-Lymphoblastic lymphoma **Mature cell** • Peripheral T-cell lymphomas NOS • Anaplastic large cell lymphoma • Angioimmunoblastic T-cell lymphoma (AITL) • Gamma-delta T-cell lymphoma • Mycosis fungoides and Sezary syndrome • Other rare lymphomas

Table 4.22: Ann Arbor staging system.	
Stage I	Involvement of single lymph node region or lymphoid structure*
Stage II	Involvement of two or more lymph node regions on same side of the diaphragm
Stage III	Involvement of lymph node regions or lymphoid structures on both sides of the diaphragm
Stage IV	Disseminated disease with liver or bone marrow involvement

A. No systemic symptoms
B. Weight loss >10 percent in 6 months, fever, and night sweats

*The lymphoid structures are defined as spleen, thymus, Waldeyer's ring, appendix and Peyer's patches.

Table 4.23: Staging of lymphoma.	
Stage	Disease involvement
I	Single lymph node region (I) or one extralymphatic site (I_E)
II	Two or more lymph node regions, on the same side of the diaphragm (II) or local extralymphatic extension plus one or more lymph node regions on the same side of diaphragm (II_E)
III	Lymph node regions on both sides of the diaphragm (III), which may be accompanied by local exralymphatic extension (III_E)
IV	Diffuse involvement of one or more extralymphatic organs or sites
A	No B symptoms
B	Presence of at least one of: unexplained weight loss >10% baseline during 6 months prior to staging; recurrent unexplained fever >38°C; recurrent night sweats
X	Bulky tumor: Either a single mass exceeding 10 cm in largest diameter or a mediastinal mass exceeding one third of the maximum transverse transthoracic diameter measured on a standard posterior-anterior chest radiograph

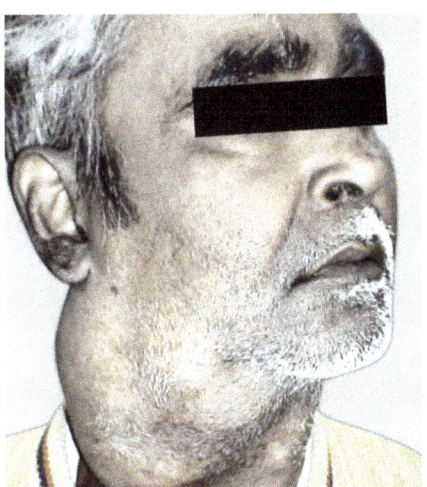

Fig. 4.17: Cervical lymphadenopathy.

Extranodal involvement is not common but may involve any other organ or tissue.

Etiology

Etiology is not known in most of the cases. HIV infection has been found to be associated with Hodgkin lymphoma especially with mixed cellularity and lymphocyte depletion type. Epstein-Barr virus (EBV) is commonly found in Hodgkin lymphoma but etiological association is not clear. Familial association has also been reported in Hodgkin lymphoma.

Clinical Features

- It has a unique bimodal age distribution with peak age between 15–35 years and second peak after 55 years.
- Most common clinical presentation is painless lymphadenopathy in neck, supraclavicular area or axillae. Mediastinal involvement is common in nodular sclerosis type of Hodgkin lymphoma (**Fig. 4.17**).
- B symptoms including fever (>38°C for 3 consecutive days in last 3 months without evidence of any infection), night sweats (drenching night sweats needing change of clothes) and weight loss (unintentional weight loss >10%) is found in one third of the patients at presentation. B-symptoms occur due to underlying inflammatory milieu of lymphoma.
- Some unusual features like generalized pruritus and pain in lymph nodes following alcohol ingestion may also be present in patients with Hodgkin lymphoma.

Classification

Hodgkin lymphoma can be classified into classical Hodgkin lymphoma (cHL) and nodular lymphocytic predominant Hodgkin lymphoma (NLPHL). Classical Hodgkin lymphoma can be further subcategorized into nodular sclerosis, mixed cellularity, lymphocyte rich and lymphocyte depletion type. Nodular sclerosis is the most common variety in USA while mixed cellularity is the most common subtype in India.

Diagnosis and Staging

Complete blood count, ESR, Serum albumin, liver function tests (LFT) and renal function tests (RFT) are useful initial tests before planning chemotherapy. Fine needle aspiration cytology (FNAC) of lymph node is inadequate for diagnosis and biopsy should be preferred. Characteristic histopathological finding with presence of Reed Sternberg cells (Owl's eye appearance, **Fig. 4.18**) and background inflammatory milieu is helpful in diagnosis. On immunohistochemistry, RS cells are CD15, CD30 and PAX-5 positive and CD 45 and EMA negative. Staging should be done as discussed in the staging section.

Nodular Lymphocyte-Predominant Hodgkin Lymphoma

It is a special type of Hodgkin lymphoma characterized by nodular pattern in lymph node and, absence of RS cells and presence of LP cells also known as L and H cells or

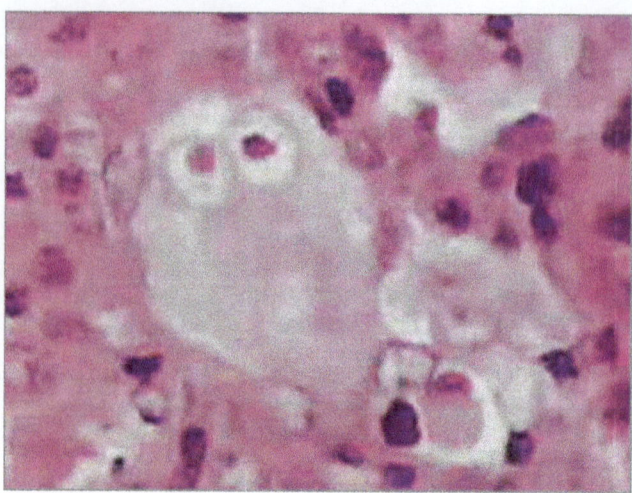

Fig. 4.18: Reed-Sternberg cell in Hodgkin's lymphoma.

popcorn cells. These cells are rosetted by T Cells. It usually presents with single site lymphadenopathy and responds well to chemotherapy but relapses are very common. On Immunohistochemistry (IHC) the tumor cells (LP cells) are positive for CD 20, CD45 and EMA and negative for CD15 and CD30.

Treatment of Hodgkin Lymphoma

Localized early stage nonbulky disease (STAGE IA,2A): should be treated with III - IV cycles of ABVD chemotherapy (Doxorubicin, bleomycin, vinblastine, dacarbazine) alone or II cycles of ABVD chemotherapy followed by involved field radiotherapy.

Advanced stage disease or early disease with bulk: Treated with VI cycle of ABVD chemotherapy followed by radiotherapy (RT) to bulky site/residual site if present.

Availability of anti CD 30 antibody (Brentuximab vedotin) has provided option for management of HL in upfront setting as well as relapsed refractory conditions. This drug has also been used as bridge to transplant. Autologous transplant remains the only curative option for relapsed HL. Early stage patients have a long-term survival of >90% while advanced stage HL has much lower survival in range of 50–70%.

Early stage NLPHL can be treated by involved field radiotherapy and advanced stage can be treated with rituximab (anti-CD 20 antibody) with chemotherapy cycles either R-ABVD or R-CHOP (Rituximab, cyclophosphamide, doxorubicin, vincristine, prednisolone).

Rarely Hodgkin lymphoma can transform into non-Hodgkin lymphoma or chronic lymphocytic leukemia.

Non-Hodgkin Lymphoma

Non-Hodgkin lymphoma classification has been discussed early in this chapter. Clinically it can be subdivided into indolent and aggressive type of lymphoma. Indolent lymphomas usually occur in elderly age group, progress very slowly and are not life threatening but usually incurable. Follicular lymphoma, small lymphocytic lymphoma and marginal zone lymphomas are the common examples. Aggressive lymphomas usually occur in young age and pediatric population. They are generally curable but have very aggressive course and life threatening if not treated well in time. Diffuse large B cell lymphoma and Burkitt lymphoma are classical examples of aggressive lymphomas.

Etiology

- Viruses like Epstein-Barr virus, HIV, Hepatitis C virus and Human herpes virus-8 (HHV-8) have been implicated in causation of various lymphomas. EBV has been associated with Burkitt lymphoma and primary CNS lymphoma, HIV with primary effusion lymphoma and plasmablastic lymphoma, HCV with lymphoplasmacytic lymphoma and HHV-8 with Castleman disease.
- *Helicobacter pylori* has been associated with gastric MALT (Mucosa associated lymphoid tissue) also known as MALTOMA (a type of marginal zone lymphoma). Chlamydia psittaci is a causative agent for conjunctival MALT.
- Congenital and acquired immunodeficiencies and autoimmune disorders predispose for development of lymphomas.
- Chemotherapy and irradiation are well known risk factors for development of non-Hodgkin lymphoma.

Clinical Features

- Patient can present with localized or generalized lymphadenopathy along with hepatomegaly and/or splenomegaly.
- Patients can have B symptoms like fever, night sweats and weight loss in 30–50% cases.
- Extra nodal presentation is not uncommon. Patient can present with involvement of central nervous system (CNS), testis, orbit, thyroid, breast, bone marrow, liver or any other organ.
- Sometimes, superior vena cava obstruction, spinal cord compression, intestinal obstruction or tumor lysis syndrome can be the first manifestation in NHL.
- Symptom duration can vary from one to three months in aggressive lymphomas to 6–12 months or even more in indolent lymphomas.

Investigations

Routine investigations like Complete blood count (CBC), Peripheral blood smear examination, Serum LDH, Serum uric acid, LFT, Serum protein albumin, RFT, Viral markers including HBsAg, HCV, HIV and Pregnancy test for females of child bearing age. High serum LDH is one of the poor prognostic factors.

Diagnostic Investigations

Biopsy of the involved node or organ/tissue is mandatory for diagnosis. Excisional biopsy is preferred but sometimes core needle biopsy is adequate if the site is abdomen or mediastinum or a site difficult to biopsy. Fine needle aspiration cytology (FNAC) is not reliable and gives poor diagnostic yield in lymphoma. Bone marrow examination helps in staging the patient but sometimes it can be helpful in diagnosis too. Histopathological examination (HPE) of lymph node by expert hematopathologist and appropriate immunohistochemistry (IHC) panel test are needed to diagnose and subclassify the type of lymphoma. **Table 4.24** shows different IHC patterns of different B cell NHLs. Fluorescent in situ hybridization (FISH) is used to detect specific cytogenetic abnormalities associate with lymphomas. Common cytogenetic abnormalities are translocation t(8:14) in Burkitt lymphoma, t(14:18) in follicular lymphoma and t(11:14) in mantle cell lymphoma.

Staging and Management

Whole body PET-CT scan or CT scan of neck, thorax, abdomen and pelvis should be done in all patients. Bone marrow examination should be done to rule out marrow involvement. Pre-chemotherapy workup includes 2D-ECHO heart and pulmonary function test. International prognostic index (IPI) is used to risk stratify these patients. Age, performance status, stage of disease, serum LDH and extranodal involvement are the five major risk factors used in IPI to risk stratify these patients.

- DLBCL is the most common type of NHL and accounts for 30–40% of all cases. R-CHOP (Rituximab, Cyclophosphamide, Adriamycin, Vincristine, and Prednisolone) is the standard chemotherapy protocol for DLBCL. Early stage disease can be treated with IV cycles of chemotherapy and advanced stage disease can be treated with VI cycles of R-CHOP chemotherapy.
- Burkitt lymphoma is treated by short duration intensive protocol like Hyper-CVAD protocol and DA-EPOACH protocol.
- Low grade lymphomas can be treated with B+R (Bendamustine+ Rituximab chemotherapy) or R-CVP (Rituximab, Cyclophosphamide, Vincristine, and Prednisolone) chemotherapy. Targeted therapies like Bruton tyrosine kinase inhibitors (BTKi) such as ibrutinib and acalabrutinib are now available for nonchemotherapy treatment options for low grade lymphomas like SLL, Mantle cell lymphoma and Lymphoplasmacytic lymphoma in first/second line treatment.
- Relapsed refractory aggressive non-Hodgkin lymphomas are treated by salvage chemotherapy with either of R-ICE, R-DHAP or R-GDP protocols followed by autologous stem cell transplant.
- T-cell lymphomas like PTCL and ALCL are treated using CHOP or CHOP-E chemotherapy and need autologous transplant in first remission as they have very poor prognosis otherwise.

Prognosis

Early stage DLBCL has long-term survival in range of 80–90% while patients with stage IV disease have only 40–50% long term survival. Low grade lymphomas have good long-term survival but tend to relapse. PTCLs have poor survival of 30–40% in long term. Relapsed refractory lymphomas have very poor prognosis.

MULTIPLE MYELOMA

Multiple myeloma (MM) is a clonal plasma cell disorder characterized by malignant proliferation of plasma cells. Incidence of multiple myeloma increases with age. Median age of disease in western world is 7th decade while median age in India is in 5th decade. Etiology of MM is not well known. Normally plasma cells produce polyclonal immunoglobulin while clonal plasma cells produce monoclonal immunoglobulins composed of a single type of heavy and light chain.

Pathophysiology

Clonal plasma cell proliferation leads to replacement of bone marrow by malignant cells. This results into progressive anemia and other cytopenias. Excessive amount of light chain is produced and subsequently deposited in renal tubules and glomerular apparatus leading to cast nephropathy and renal amyloidosis respectively. Increased osteoclastic activity leads to bone resorption and osteolytic lesions. Bone marrow environment also helps in growth and survival of plasma cells.

Clinical Features

- Most patients with multiple myeloma (60–80%) present with bone pain and symptomatic anemia.

Table 4.24: Immunohistochemistry (IHC) findings in lymphoma.

Type of lymphoma	CD20	CD10	CD5	BCL-2	BCL-6	Others
DLBCL	++	+-	-	+-	+-	
Follicular lymphoma	++	+	–	+	+	
Burkitt lymphoma	++	+	-	–	+	C-Myc +
Marginal zone lymphoma	++	-	-	-	-	
Mantle cell lymphoma	++	-	+	-	-	Cyclin-D1+
SLL	+	-	+	-	-	CD23+

- Renal failure is present in 20–40% of cases.
- Patients have history of pathological fractures in almost 20% of cases.
- Patients can also present with recurrent infections, peripheral neuropathy, cord compression, swellings in body (plasmacytomas), altered sensorium and seizures.
- Combination of bone pain, anemia and renal failure is highly suggestive of multiple myeloma. Acronym **CRAB** (Hyper**C**alcemia, **R**enal failure, **A**nemia, **B**one lesions) is used for diagnosis of multiple myeloma. At least one of these features should be there to call it as symptomatic myeloma.

Diagnosis

- Complete hemogram and peripheral smear examination show anemia, rouleaux formation, and occasionally plasma cells in smear.
- Renal function test, serum calcium, ESR, C-reactive protein, serum LDH, serum alkaline phosphatase and Beta-2 microglobulin are other important investigations.
- Bone marrow shows increase in plasma cells with presence of atypical plasma cells and plasmablasts.
- Serum protein electrophoresis and immunofixation reveal the presence of Myeloma band (M-band) and involved heavy and light chains.
- Skeletal survey is done using whole body PET-CT or low dose whole body CT or X-ray skull, pelvis, both femur, humerus, spine and chest **(Fig. 4.19)**.

Treatment

Combination drug treatment followed by autologous stem cell transplant is treatment of choice. A combination of steroid, proteosome inhibitor and immunomodulatory drug is the preferred combination. Dexamethasone, bortezomib and lenalidomide combination is the most commonly used combination. Thalidomide or cyclophosphamide can also be used in place of lenalidomide. A total of IV-VI cycles is given with response monitoring every month. If patient achieves more than partial response (Complete response, Very good partial response) he should be taken for autologous transplant. Post-transplant single agent maintenance is also preferred. Intravenous bisphosphonate should be given on monthly basis to prevent bone related events. Some patients may develop bisphosphonate-induced osteonecrosis of jaw and need withdrawal of this drug. Newer monoclonal antibody (Daratumumab) proteasome inhibitors (Carfilzomib, ixazomib) and immunomodulators (Pomalidomide) based treatment is coming up.

Prognosis

The survival of myeloma patients has improved from an average of 3 years to 7–10 years. This has been possible due to newer drugs coming up. Hence myeloma is now a chronically manageable condition but still incurable.

NORMAL HEMOSTASIS

The blood remains fluid in the vessels while it clots at the site of breach or injury. The anticoagulant and procoagulant mechanisms are intricately regulated so that no clotting occurs in flowing blood or at unwanted sites whereas there is an immediate platelet plug formation and fibrin deposition at the site of bleeding.

Exposure of blood to the subendothelial connective tissue following surgery, trauma or disease initiates primary and secondary hemostatic processes.

Primary Hemostasis

Within seconds of injury, the constriction of minor vessels like arterioles, capillaries and venules and the formation of platelet plug lead to the arrest of bleeding temporarily and allows time for fibrin deposition.

Platelet Plug Formation

Platelet plug formation requires three critical events, namely: (a) platelet adhesion, (b) granule release, and (c) platelet aggregation.

- Normally platelets do not adhere to the intact endothelium. This is mainly due to endothelial prostacyclin (PGI_2) which inhibits platelet activation. However, following injury, platelets adhere to the subendothelial collagen tissue through GpIa/IIa and Gp VI receptors. The von Willebrand factor (vWF) also helps in adhesion via linking platelet Gp Ib/IX receptor to the subendothelial collagen. **(Fig. 4.20)**.
- Platelets become subsequently activated and release products like thromboxane A_2 (TXA_2), ADP, vWF and fibrinogen that promote platelet aggregation.
- The released ADP changes the conformation of platelet GpIIb/IIIa complex. The fibrinogen binds with the GpIIb/IIIa receptor on the platelets, linking adjacent platelets

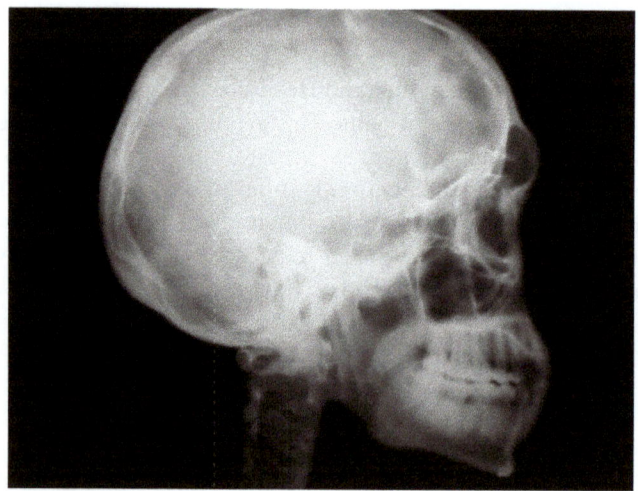

Fig. 4.19: X-ray skull showing multiple osteolytic lesions.

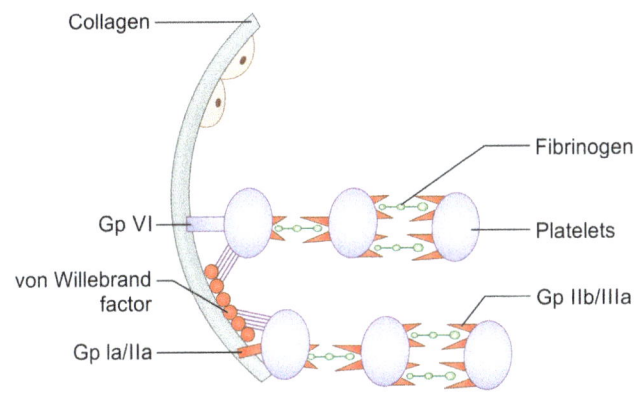

Fig. 4.20: Platelet plug formation.

into a hemostatic plug. The balance between the activity of TXA$_2$ and PGI$_2$ determines the rate and extent of platelet activation.

Secondary Hemostasis

Secondary hemostasis is important for bleed from larger vessels and involves activation of the plasma coagulation system as a result of which the platelet plug is stabilized by the fibrin deposition (clot formation). It requires several minutes and prevents recurrent bleeding hours or days after the initial injury.

Coagulation Mechanism

The process of coagulation involves specific plasma proteins (Coagulation factors) and other substances like phospholipids, calcium and the tissue factor. Most coagulation factors are synthesized in the liver. Factors II (Prothrombin), VII, IX (Christmas factor) and X (Stuart factor) require vitamin K for their synthesis.

There are two pathways which initiate the process of coagulation: intrinsic and extrinsic (**Fig. 4.21**).

a. The intrinsic pathway is activated by negatively charged surfaces and activated platelets. It involves coagulation factors XII (Hageman factor), XI, IX and VIII. The activity of the intrinsic process is assessed by determining the APTT (*activated partial thromboplastin time*).

b. The extrinsic pathway is initiated by the tissue factor released from damaged cells. The tissue factor activates factor VII. This is measured by determining the PT (*Prothrombin time*).

Both pathways converge to activate factor X which converts prothrombin to thrombin in the presence of factor V, calcium and phospholipids. Thrombin changes fibrinogen into fibrin monomer. The conversion of fibrinogen into fibrin can be measured by *thrombin time*. Fibrin monomers are crosslinked by activated factor XIII to form a stable fibrin polymer. An interpretation of different coagulation tests is given in **Table 4.25**.

Clot Lysis

The lysis of clot (fibrinolysis) and repair of vessel starts after the clot formation. Physiological fibrinolysis activators, tissue plasminogen activator (tPA) and urinary plasminogen activator (uPA or urokinase) are released from the endothelial cells and convert plasminogen into plasmin.

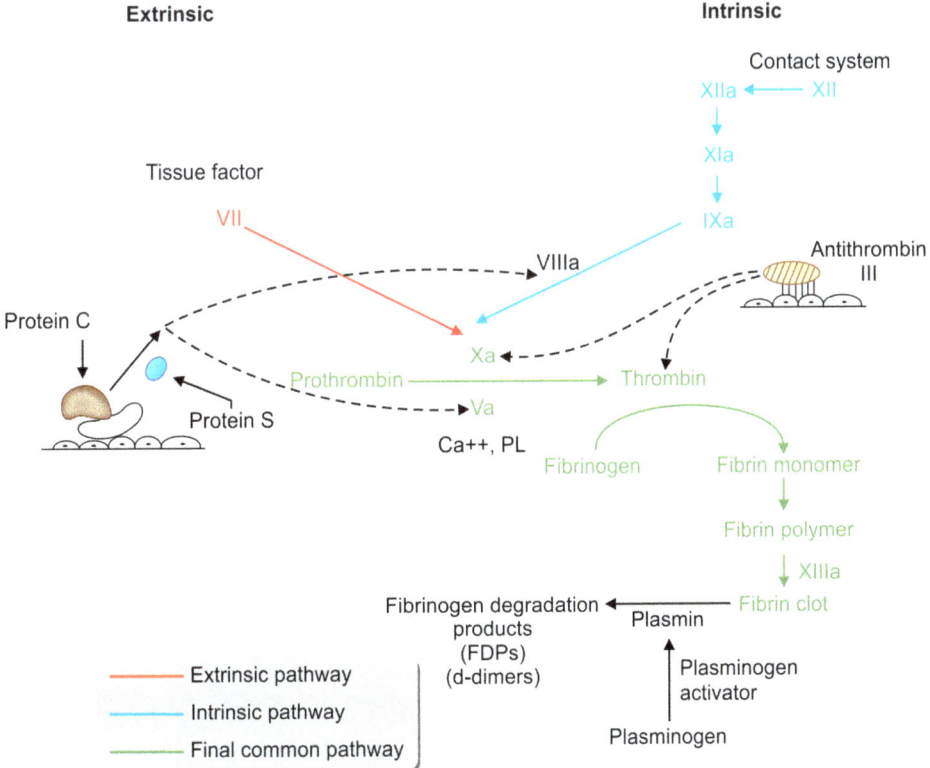

Fig. 4.21: Coagulation pathway.

> **Table 4.25:** Coagulation test abnormalities in various factor deficiencies.
>
> - **Prolonged APTT:** Factors XII*, XI, IX, VIII deficiency von Willebrand disease
> - **Prolonged PT:** Factor VII deficiency, early vitamin K deficiency
> - **Prolonged APTT and PT:** Factors II, V, X, late vitamin K deficiency, warfarin, heparin
> - **Prolonged thrombin time (TT):** Heparin, afibrinogenemia and dysfibrinogenemia
> - **Clot solubility in 5M urea:** Factor XIII deficiency (in this PT, APTT, TT are normal)

*No clinical bleeding occurs in Factor XII deficiency.

Plasmin degrades the fibrin polymer into small fragments, fibrin degradation products (FDPs) which are cleared by the monocyte-macrophage scavenger systems.

Coagulation Inhibitors

The formation of clot is limited to the site of injury only. This is tightly regulated by the coagulation inhibitors such as antithrombin III, protein C and protein S. These collectively maintain the fluidity of blood.

Disorders of Hemostasis

Bleeding due to vessel or platelet disorders is generally localized to superficial sites like the skin and mucous membrane; it occurs immediately after trauma and is controlled by local measures. In contrast, bleeding due to coagulation disorders occurs in deeper tissues (subcutaneous, muscle, joint, and body cavities), hours or even days after the injury and is not affected by local therapy. The disorders of hemostasis can be classified into three types:
- Vessel wall abnormalities
- Platelet disorders
  - Decreased platelet count (Thrombocytopenia)
  - Platelet dysfunction
- Coagulation disorders
  - Congenital: Hemophilia A and hemophilia B
  - Acquired: Liver diseases, vitamin K deficiency, DIC and coagulation inhibitors (warfarin, heparin).

Table 4.26 shows laboratory abnormalities in some common hemostatic disorders.

Vessel Wall Abnormalities

The abnormalities of vessel wall, both congenital and acquired, may result in purpura (Bleeding in the skin and mucous membrane). Platelet count, platelet function and bleeding time are normal. Important causes are senile purpura, Henoch-Schönlein purpura, vasculitis, paraproteinemia, scurvy and Ehlers-Danlos syndrome.

PLATELET DISORDERS

The most common sites to observe bleeding in platelet disorders are skin and mucous membrane.
Collection of blood in skin is called purpura.
- Petechiae are small pinpoint hemorrhages into the dermis due to the leakage of red blood cells through capillaries.
- Ecchymoses are large subcutaneous collection of blood due to leakage from small arterioles or venules (common bruises).
- Deeper and palpable collection of blood is called hematoma.
- The bleeding in mucous membrane may present as gum bleeding, epistaxis, and menorrhagia.

The normal platelet count is 1,50,000 to 4,00,000/μL.
- Patient is usually asymptomatic if platelet count is more than 1,00,000/μL.
- Bleeding occurs only from severe trauma when the platelet count is 50,000 to 1,00,000/μL.
- There is a tendency to easy bruising and purpura after minor trauma at counts between 20,000 to 50,000/μL.
- Patients with counts lower than 20,000/μL bleed spontaneously and may have intracranial or internal bleeding.
- It is to be noted that bleeding does not always correlate with the platelet count; patient may bleed at a higher platelet count and vice versa.

The causes of thrombocytopenia are given in **Table 4.27**.

Idiopathic (Autoimmune) Thrombocytopenic Purpura

Idiopathic (Autoimmune) thrombocytopenic purpura (ITP) is an autoimmune disorder in which antibodies (IgG) are produced against platelet antigens (gpIIb/IIIa). The antibody-coated platelets are destroyed by phagocytic cells in the spleen.

Table 4.26: Laboratory abnormalities in some common hemostatic disorders.

Conditions	Bleeding time	Platelet count	PT	APTT	Others
Hemophilia A	Normal	Normal	Normal	Raised	Low factor VIII level
Hemophilia B	Normal	Normal	Normal	Raised	Low factor IX level
Von Willebrand's disease	Prolonged	Normal	Normal	Raised	Decreased vWF level, abnormal platelet adhesion
Idiopathic thrombocytopenic purpura (ITP)	Prolonged	Low	Normal	Normal	Increased megakaryocytes on bone marrow examination
Disseminated intravascular coagulation (DIC)	Prolonged	Low	Raised	Raised	High FDP, Low fibrinogen

Table 4.27: Causes of thrombocytopenia.

• Marrow disorder (decreased production)
   – Marrow failure – aplasia, hypoplasia
   – Infiltration – tumor, fibrosis
   – Vit B_{12}/Folate deficiency
• Splenic sequestration: Splenic tumor and portal hypertension
• Increased destruction of circulating platelets
   – Immune: ITP, SLE, drug induced, lymphoma, CLL, and HIV
   – Non-immune: DIC, sepsis, prosthetic valve, and TTP

Clinical Features

- In children, the onset is generally sudden (acute ITP). Purpura appears 2–3 weeks after viral infection. In most cases the condition is self-limiting.
- The onset is insidious in adults and the disease may persist for years (chronic ITP). Chronic ITP is more common in females.

The common presentations are skin and mucosal bleeding in the form of petechiae, ecchymosis, gum bleeding, epistaxis, and menorrhagia **(Figs. 4.22 and 4.23)**. Bleeding in gastrointestinal and genitourinary tract may also occur. Spleen is usually not palpable.

Diagnosis

- The peripheral blood examination reveals low platelet count.

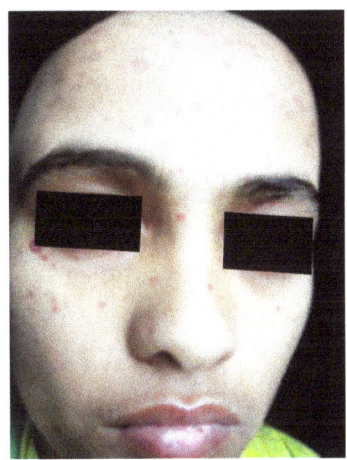

Fig. 4.22: Purpuric rashes on the face.

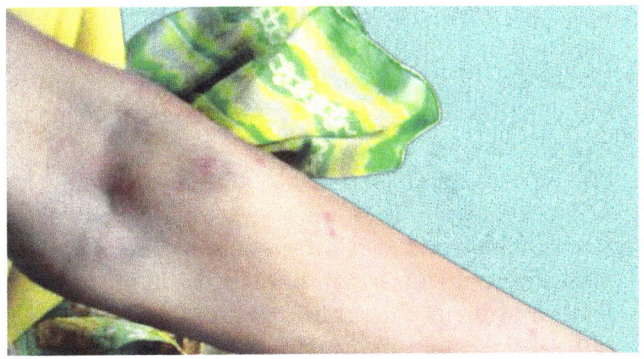

Fig. 4.23: Purpuric rashes on the upper limb.

- Bone marrow examination shows normal morphology with increased megakaryocytes.
- Bleeding time is increased whereas clotting time, prothrombin time and APTT are normal.
- Tests are done to exclude the possibilities of HIV infection, SLE, viral hepatitis and infectious mononucleosis (EBV, CMV) since these conditions may be associated with thrombocytopenia.

Treatment

The treatment of ITP is indicated if platelet count is below 10,000 to 20,000/µL or there is extensive bleeding. The aim is to maintain the platelet count at or more than 20,000/µL.

- The initial treatment is with oral prednisolone 1–2 mg/kg/day. In most patients, platelet count improves within few days. The dose of prednisolone is tapered when the platelet count becomes normal.
- In case of severe and life-threatening bleeding, intravenous immunoglobulin (IV Ig) is given in the dosage of 1g/kg for 1–2 days.
- Splenectomy is indicated when there is no response to medical therapy or an unacceptably large dose of steroid is needed to maintain adequate platelet count. Most patients will respond to splenectomy which is curative in around 70–80% cases. Patient should be given prophylactic pneumococcal and influenza vaccine at least 3 weeks prior to splenectomy.
- Patients who fail to respond to steroid and splenectomy may be given danazol, vincristine, azathioprim, cyclophosphamide or cyclosporine. Monoclonal antibody (Anti-CD20, rituximab) has also been used in some cases with success and the dose is 375 mg/m^2 weekly for 4 weeks given as intravenous drip.
- Recently, thrombopoietin receptor agonists (eltrombopag 50 mg/day oral and romiplostim 250 microgm subcutaneously weeekly) have been shown to be effective in steroid non-responsive ITP patients. These are also indicated as upfront treatment in ITP.
- Platelet transfusion provides only a transient effect and is reserved only for cases with life-threatening bleeding.

Functional Platelet Disorders

Prolonged bleeding time despite normal platelet count indicates functional disorder of platelets. There may be defect in the platelet adhesion, aggregation or granule release. Important causes are given in **Table 4.28**. Commonly used drugs, aspirin and clopidrogel cause inhibition of platelet function. Aspirin irreversibly inhibits platelet cyclooxygenase-I (COX-I) thus blocking synthesis of thromboxane A2. Clopidogrel inhibits ADP-mediated platelet aggregation.

Renal Diseases

The bleeding in renal disorders is generally due to platelet dysfunction caused by low molecular weight products.

Table 4.28: Causes of functional platelet disorders.

Congenital
- Bernard-Soulier syndrome (defect in platelet receptor GpIb/IX)
- Glanzmann's thrombasthenia (defect in platelet receptor GpIIb/IIIa)
- Von Willebrand's disease
- Storage pool disorders

Acquired
- Uremia
- Drug induced (aspirin, NSAIDs, and clopidogrel)
- Myeloproliferative disorders

Mild thrombocytopenia also contributes to bleeding. The treatment consists of platelet and red cell transfusion and dialysis. Desmopressin may also promote hemostasis in renal failure.

VON WILLEBRAND DISEASE

Von Willebrand disease (VWD) is the most common inherited hemostatic disorder. It is mainly inherited in an autosomal dominant manner. von Willebrand factor (vWF) is a multimeric plasma glycoprotein synthesized by megakary-ocytes and endothelial cells. It serves two major functions.

1. It is a carrier protein for factor VIII. Deficiency of the vWF leads to secondary reduction in the factor VIII level.
2. Platelets adhere to subendothelial collagen tissue through GpIa/IIa and Gp VI receptors. von Willebrand factor helps in adhesion via linking platelet GpIb/IX receptor with subendothelial collagen.

There are several subtypes of VWD.
- The most common is type I which is characterized by mild to moderate decrease in the plasma vWF.
- The vWF is qualitatively abnormal in type II VWDs, although its plasma level is normal.
- Type III VWD is the most severe form where vWF is nearly absent.

Clinical Features

In most cases, mild symptoms in form of epistaxis, gum bleeding, menorrhagia and superficial bruises may be present. Gastrointestinal bleeding may also occur. Excessive hemorrhage may be observed after trauma, dental extraction or surgery. Unlike hemophilia, hemarthrosis (bleeding in joints) generally do not occur.

Investigations

- Platelet count is normal.
- Bleeding time and APTT are prolonged.
- The factor VIII activity is low.
- The plasma vWF level is reduced.
- The platelet adhesion activity of vWF as measured by ristocetin cofactor assay is reduced.

Treatment

- Mild bleeding episodes can be managed by giving desmopressin (DDAVP) which increases the vWF level.
- Cases with persistent and severe bleeding are managed with plasma derived factor VIII concentrate that also contains considerable amount of vWF.
- Cryoprecipitate (rich in factor VIII and vWF) can be used alternatively.
- Antifibrinolytic agent (e.g. tranexamic acid) is useful as an adjunctive therapy during dental procedures. The dose of tranexamic acid is 25 mg/kg thrice a day for 5-7 days.

COAGULATION DISORDERS

Inherited Coagulation Disorders

In inherited coagulation disorders, only a single coagulation factor is involved (reduced or defective). The most common inherited coagulation abnormalities are factor VIII deficiency (hemophilia A) and factor IX deficiency (hemophilia B).

Hemophilia

Hemophilia is an X-linked recessive disorder characterized by the deficiency of factor VIII (Hemophilia A) or factor IX (Hemophilia B). The disease manifests in males while females are carriers **(Fig. 4.24)**. Rarely it may also manifest in females in case the father is a hemophilic and mother is carrier or if the patient has Turner's syndrome (45 XO).

Clinical Manifestations

The clinical manifestation of hemophilia depends on the severity of deficiency of the factor VIII or IX.

The bleeding is spontaneous in severe cases (Factor activity <1%) while it may occur after minor trauma or surgery in moderate cases (Level 1-5%).

- People with mild disease (factor activity 5-40%) rarely bleed spontaneously but can bleed following severe trauma or surgery.
- Severe cases generally manifest in early childhood when the child starts crawling or walking whereas mild and moderate cases may clinically manifest later in life.
- The bleeding occurs mainly in joints (hemarthrosis), muscles (hematoma), viscera or in retroperitoneum but it can involve any organ system.
- The most common joint involved is the knee joint **(Fig. 4.25)**. Ankle, elbow and hip joints are also involved. Warmth, pain and swelling are initial presentations of joint involvement. Recurrent bleeding in the joint can lead to synovial thickening, destruction of cartilage, fibrosis and deformity of joints.

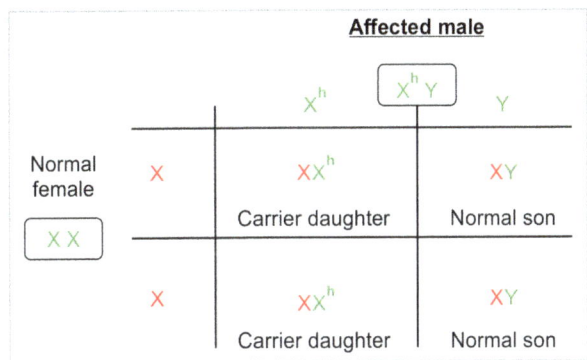
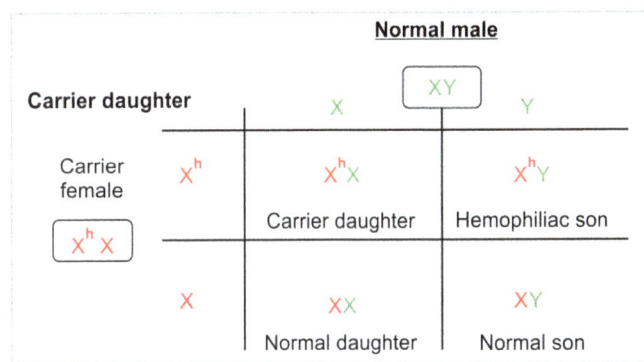

Fig. 4.24: Genetics of haemophilia.

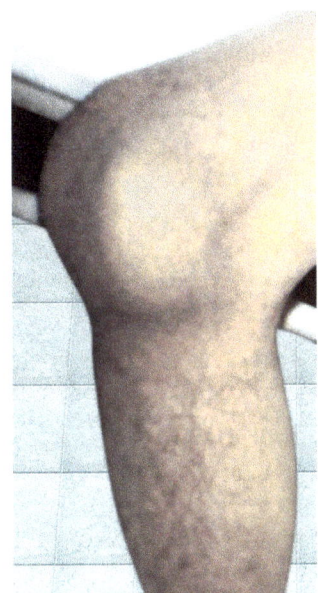

Fig. 4.25: Hemarthrosis of the knee.

- Calf and psoas muscles are most commonly affected with hematoma. Bleeding into iliacus muscle often causes femoral nerve palsy. Patients can also develop large calcified mass of blood with inflammation that may be mistaken as tumor (pseudotumor syndrome).
- Hematuria is also common in hemophilia.
- Intracranial and oropharyngeal bleeding may be fatal.

Investigations

- Activated partial thromboplastin time (APTT) is prolonged.
- Prothrombin time (PT), bleeding time and platelet count are within normal limits.
- Diagnosis is confirmed by the assay of factor VIII or IX.
- *Prenatal diagnosis* can be made by chorionic villi biopsy or amniocentesis.

Management

The management includes supportive and specific therapy.

Supportive Therapy

- The joint is immobilized with splint to reduce pain and bleeding.
- Ice cold packs are applied to the involved joints intermittently for few hours. This helps to arrest the bleeding.
- Physiotherapy is indicated once active bleeding stops to prevent joint deformity.
- Non-steroidal anti-inflammatory drugs and intramuscular injections should be avoided.

Specific Therapy

- Specific therapy of hemophilia A includes intravenous administration of factor VIII. The dose, frequency and duration of factor administration depend on the severity of the bleeding. A dose of 1 unit/kg factor VIII raises the activity of the factor by 2%. An increase to around 20–50% activity is generally needed to control bleeding. The chances of transmission of infections such as hepatitis, Parvovirus and HIV with uses of plasma derived factor can be eliminated by the use of recombinant factor.
- In case the factor is not available, cryoprecipitate which is rich in factor VIII, fibrinogen and vWF may be used.
- Mild hemophilics may benefit from desmopressin (DDAVP) which increases factor level to 2–3 folds.
- Antifibrinolytic agents like ε-amino caproic acid (EACA) and tranaxemic acid can be used in minor dental and oral mucosal bleed. These agents inhibit plasminogen activator in oral tissue and stabilize the clot formation. EACA is given orally or IV in dosage of 100 mg/kg upto 10 g initially followed by 50 mg/kg upto 5 g 6 hourly for 2–7 days. EACA can also be used as a mouthwash. Tranexamic acid can be given in dosage of 0.5–1 g 8 hourly orally. The filling of carious tooth requires single infusion of factor VIII combined with antifibrinolytic agents for 3–4 days after the procedure. In case of major oral and periodontal surgery and extraction of permanent teeth, the patient needs hospitalization and regular infusion of factor VIII along with EACA.

Therapy of Hemophilia B

The specific treatment of hemophilia B is the intravenous administration of factor IX. Desmopressin and cryoprecipitate are not effective.

Acquired Coagulation Disorders

Acquired coagulation disorders are common and generally complex. There is deficiency of multiple coagulation factors. Most common acquired coagulation disorders are DIC, hemorrhagic diathesis due to liver disease, vitamin K deficiency and complications of anticoagulant therapy.

Liver Diseases

- Most of the coagulation factors are synthesized in liver. Hence, there may be deficiency of these factors in liver diseases.
- Vitamin K absorption is reduced in cholestatic liver diseases leading to decreased synthesis of vitamin K dependant factors (II, VII, IX, X).
- The bleeding in liver diseases is compounded by the presence of anatomical lesions like esophageal varices, gastritis and peptic ulcer disease.
- Thrombocytopenia can occur in patients having chronic liver disease with splenomegaly *(hypersplenism)*.

Most patients have prolonged PT and APTT. Prolongation in PT correlates with bleeding risk. Treatment includes parenteral vitamin K and infusion of fresh frozen plasma as it contains all coagulation factors.

Protein C, protein S and antithrombin III are also synthesized in the liver. Deficiency of these coagulation inhibitors favors coagulation and can predispose the patients to develop DIC.

Disseminated Intravascular Coagulation (DIC)

Disseminated intravascular coagulation is characterized by widespread coagulation in the microcirculation leading to consumption of coagulation factors and platelets.

Mechanism: Endothelial damage in septicemia and other situations cause release of the endothelial tissue factors which activate the coagulation process. Thromboplastin released from placenta, damaged tissue and injured brain also activates the coagulation cascade. The formation of fibrin stimulates the fibrinolytic system generating fibrin degradation products (FDP). The deficiency of coagulation factors and platelets leads to hemorrhagic manifestation which is further exacerbated by the activation of the fibrinolytic system. The important causes of DIC are mentioned in **Table 4.29**.

Clinical Features

- Since DIC leads to both thrombosis and bleeding, the manifestations are either in the form of tissue infarction, digital ischemia and gangrene or bleeding at various sites. Spontaneous oozing from venepuncture sites or wounds is an important clue to the diagnosis of DIC.
- DIC can present as recurrent deep or superficial vein thrombosis, particularly in cancer patients.
- Microangiopathic hemolysis can lead to anemia.

Table 4.29: Causes of DIC.

Infections
- Gram-negative bacterial infections
- Gram-positive bacterial infections
- Fungal infections
- Malaria

Obstetric
- Retained dead fetus
- Amniotic fluid embolism
- Abruptio placentae

Malignancies
- Lung, pancreas, prostate cancer
- Acute promyelocytic leukemia

Tissue injury
- Burns
- Head injury

Investigation

The DIC is suspected when there is a suggestive clinical situation (as mentioned in **Table 4.29**) along with following laboratory findings:
- Low platelet count
- Increased PT and APTT
- Low plasma fibrinogen level
- Elevated plasma FDP (d-Dimer assay)
- Schistocytes (fragmented RBC) on peripheral blood smear.

Management

This includes the following steps:
- Prompt management of underlying disorders such as:
  - Antibiotics in septicemia
  - Delivery of fetus in obstetric complications
- Patients with bleeding manifestations should receive fresh frozen plasma (FFP) to replace coagulation factors and platelet transfusion to correct thrombocytopenia.
- Heparin is indicated in patients where the predominant manifestation includes thrombosis and gangrene. Role of heparin in patients with bleeding manifestations is controversial. However, it may be given in such situations where the bleeding is not controlled despite adequate replacement with FFP and platelets.

Agranulocytosis

The mean blood neutrophil count is around 3,600/µl. The important function of neutrophil is to prevent and contain bacterial and fungal infections. The decrease in neutrophil count is called neutropenia (<1,500/mL). The neutrophil count below 500/mL is called severe neutropenia. Agranulocytosis term is used to describe a state of severe neutropenia or absence of circulating neutrophils.

Causes

Neutropenia can occur due to:
a. Decreased production
b. Increased destruction
c. Excessive peripheral pooling of neutrophils.
   Important causes of neutropenia are given in **Table 4.30**.

Manifestations

The manifestations depend on the severity and duration of neutropenia and the type of underlying illness. Oral ulcers are usual in agranulocytosis. The patient develops fever and infections mainly of oropharynx, perirectal area, sinuses, lungs and skin. Common organisms responsible for infections are Gram-negative enteric bacilli, *Pseudomonas* spp., *Staphylococcus* spp., *Candida* and *Aspergillus*.

A careful history of exposure to drugs, toxins and duration of illness should be asked. A careful examination of oropharynx and perirectal area should be done. The presence of lymphadenopathy and hepatosplenomegaly should also be noted.

Investigations

Peripheral blood examination reveals the degree of neutropenia. It can also reveal the presence of hematological malignancies. Bone marrow examination is necessary to diagnose aplasia, infiltration, fibrosis and hematological malignancies. Investigations for the presence of auto-antibodies are conducted as needed.

Management

Patients with neutropenia and fever must be admitted to the hospital. Sample for culture should be obtained and empirical parenteral broad spectrum antibiotics must be started immediately. Antifungal agents are to be given if fever does not respond to antibiotics. Neutrophil transfusion may help in severe refractory infections.

Prevention of infection is very crucial. Handwashing is an effective method for preventing the spread of infections. Growth factors (G-CSF or GM-CSF) are used to reduce the chance and severity of neutropenia after chemotherapy and radiation therapy.

SPLENOMEGALY

Spleen is a reticuloendothelial organ which lies in the left upper quadrant of abdomen. The important functions of spleen are:
- Removal of old and defunct red blood cells from circulation
- Synthesis of antibodies in the white pulp
- Removal of antibody-coated bacteria and blood cells
- Spleen can form blood cells when the bone marrow is unable to meet the demand (extramedullary hematopoiesis).
- It also serves as a reservoir (store) for platelets and neutrophils.

Increase in the normal function can lead to splenomegaly. Causes of splenomegaly are given in **Table 4.31**.

The spleen is normally not palpable. If palpable, it is enlarged (**Fig. 4.26**). The direction of enlargement is towards right iliac fossa. The maximum diameter of spleen on ultrasonographic assessment is around 13 cm. Massive splenomegaly is defined as the spleen palpable more than 8 cm below costal margin. The common causes of massive splenomegaly are mentioned in **Table 4.32**.

Clinical Manifestations

The symptoms due to splenomegaly are abdominal discomfort and pain. Massive splenomegaly may cause early satiety and

Table 4.30: Important causes of neutropenia.

Drug induced
- Anti-cancer drugs, antibiotics (sulphonamides, chloramphenicol), anticonvulsants (carbamazepine), and antithyroid drugs

Hematological diseases
- Aplastic anemia, acute leukemia, myelofibrosis, tumor invasion and megaloblastic anemia

Infections
- Tuberculosis, typhoid, kala azar, malaria, infectious mononucleosis, and HIV

Autoimmune
- Systemic lupus erythematosus, and Felty's syndrome

Congenital
- Cyclic neutropenia

Table 4.31: Causes of splenomegaly.

Hyperplasia in response to infection
- Malaria and kala azar
- Infectious mononucleosis, cytomegalovirus infection, HIV infection, and viral hepatitis
- Endocarditis, tuberculosis, typhoid fever, and septicemia
- Histoplasmosis

Hyperplasia due to excessive function of red cell removal
- Spherocylosis, thalassemia, and early sickle cell disease

Hyperplasia in response to immune disorder
- Felty's syndrome, SLE, and sarcoidosis

Extramedullary hematopoiesis
- Myelofibrosis and marrow infiltration

Congestive splenomegaly
- Portal hypertension (cirrhosis, hepatic vein obstruction, portal vein thrombosis)

Infiltration of spleen
- Leukemias, lymphomas, myeloproliferative disorders, amyloidosis, and storage diseases (Gaucher's disease, Niemann-Pick disease)

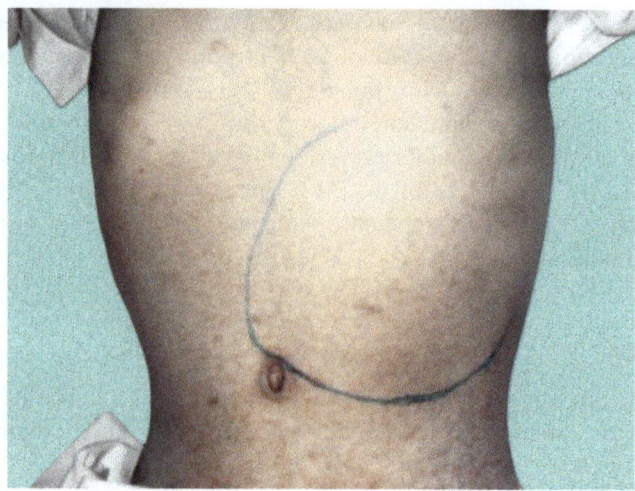

Fig. 4.26: Splenomegaly.

Table 4.32: Causes of massive splenomegaly.
- Chronic myeloid leukemia
- Portal hypertension
- Myelofibrosis
- Malaria
- Kala azar
- Storage disorders (Gaucher's disease)

abdominal bloating due to abdominal compression. Splenic infarction may result in severe pain radiating to the left shoulder. Repeated splenic infarction in sickle cell disease may lead to splenic destruction (autosplenectomy). Rupture of enlarged spleen can occur spontaneously or due to trauma and this may be fatal. Pancytopenia may occur in patients with splenomegaly (hypersplenism).

Diagnosis

A detailed history and clinical examination are helpful in knowing the underlying cause of splenomegaly. One should particularly look for the presence of fever, bleeding, lymphadenopathy and hepatomegaly. The following investigations can be helpful in making a diagnosis:
- Complete blood count
- Bone marrow examination
- Imaging (ultrasonography, CT scan)
- Screening for infections and autoimmune diseases
- Endoscopy of the upper gastrointestinal tract.

LYMPHADENOPATHY

Enlarged lymph nodes may be localized or generalized. The **Table 4.33** shows important causes of lymphadenopathy.

Generalized lymphadenopathy is defined as the enlargement of three or more noncontiguous lymph node areas. Inguinal lymph nodes upto 2 cm size and submandibular lymph nodes upto 1 cm are generally considered normal.
- Lymphadenopathy may be the presenting symptom or it may be noticed incidentally when examined for other reasons.

Table 4.33: Causes of lymphadenopathy.

Infections
- Viral: EBV, CMV, and HIV
- Bacterial: Streptococci, Staphylococci, and tuberculosis
- Spirochaetal: Syphilis
- Fungal: Histoplasmosis, and coccidioidomycosis
- Parasitic: Filariasis, kala azar, and toxoplasmosis

Malignancies
- Primary: Lymphomas, ALL, and CLL
- Metastasis: From various primary sites

Immunological diseases
- Rheumatoid arthritis, SLE, and drugs (phenytoin)

Miscellaneous
- Sarcoidosis and amyloidosis

- In more than two-third of the cases, the cause of lymphadenopathy is nonspecific or reactive.
- The enlargement of supraclavicular and scalene lymph nodes is always abnormal. The left supraclavicular node can be enlarged in metastasis from GI malignancy (Virchow's node, **Fig. 4.27**).
- The most common site of localized lymphadenopathy is the neck (**Fig. 4.28**) which is generally due to upper respiratory infections, oral and dental lesions and viral illnesses (infectious mononucleosis and others). In India, tuberculosis is an important cause of lymphadenopathy.
- Metastasis from cancer of head and neck, lung and thyroid may also lead to cervical lymphadenopathy.
- Generalized lymphadenopathy may be found in viral infections (due to EBV, CMV, HIV), connective tissue disorders (SLE) and malignancies (ALL, CLL, lymphomas). Malignancy should be considered in elderly patients with lymphadenopathy.

Diagnosis

History: A detailed history of the presence of fever, weight loss, cough, sore throat, pain in lymph nodes, occupation, sexual behavior and drug intake is taken.

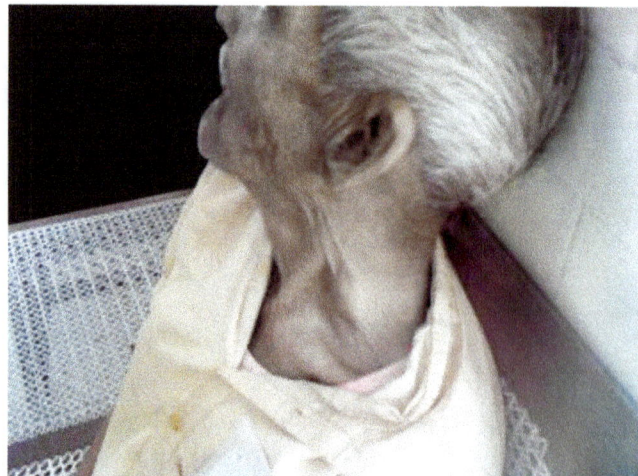

Fig. 4.27: Left supraclavicular lymphadenopathy (Virchow's node).

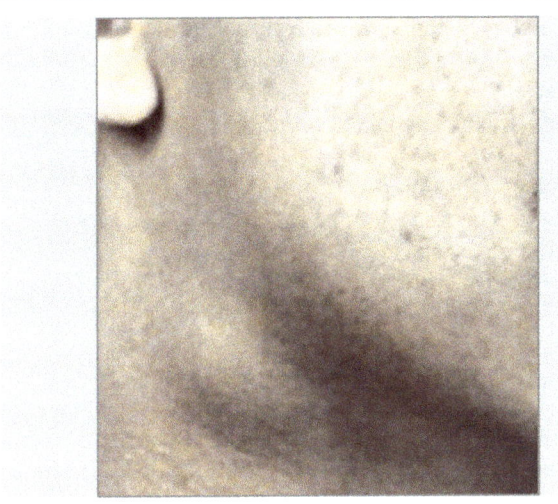

Fig. 4.28: Cervical lymphadenopathy.

Examination:
- The lymph nodes are examined for the size, texture, tenderness, mobility and for the signs of inflammation over the node **(Fig. 4.29)**.
  - Hard, fixed and nontender lymph nodes are metastatic.
  - Rubbery lymph nodes are found in lymphoma.
  - Matted lymph nodes are characteristic of tuberculosis.
- The presence of skin lesions, hepatomegaly and splenomegaly should be noted.
- Careful oral, dental and throat examination is performed in cases with cervical lymphadenopathy.
- Abdominal and mediastinal lymphadenopathy may only be detected by imaging.

Investigations: The following investigations are helpful in making a diagnosis:
- Complete blood count
- Lymph node biopsy/FNAC
- X-ray chest, ultrasonography, CT scan
- Bone marrow examination
- Screening for infections and autoimmune illnesses.

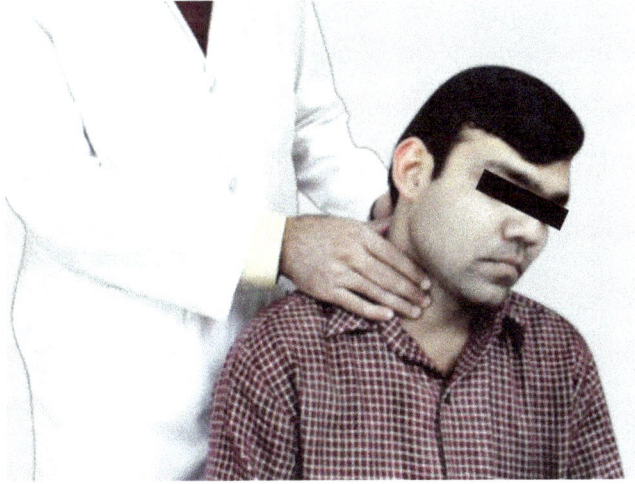

Fig. 4.29: Examination of cervical lymph node.

IMPLICATIONS ON DENTAL PRACTICE

- Elective oral surgical and periodontal procedures should be avoided in patients with severe anemia. Increased bleeding and impaired wound healing may occur in presence of anemia.
- Glossitis, burning mouth, angular stomatitis and aphthous stomatitis can be early manifestations of iron, vitamin B_{12} or folate deficiency. These may occur before the appearance of anemia.
- Iron syrups may lead to staining of teeth. This can be prevented by using sodium ironedetate.
- General anesthesia is not administered if Hb level is <10 g/dL. Hemolytic anemias, particularly sickle cell disease may pose difficult problem during general anesthesia.
- Painful infarcts in the jaws in sickle cell disease may be mistaken for toothache or osteomyelitis.
- Patients with splenectomy are more prone to infections. Hence, dental procedures in such patients should be done under prophylactic antibiotics.
- Infection and bleeding pose major problem in the dental management in patients with aplastic anemia. Gingival bleeding may be controlled by the use of local hemostatic measures and use of systemic antifibrinolytic agents (tranexamic acid, aminocaproic acid). Oral infection can be reduced by use of chlorhexidine oral rinses.
- Cyclosporin (used in patients with aplastic anemia) can result in gingival swelling.
- Intramuscular injections and nerve block anesthesia are avoided in patients with thrombocytopenia. However, intraligamentary anesthesia can be used safely.
- Oral ulcers, advanced periodontal disease, pericoronitis and pulpal infections can lead to life-threatening septicemia in patients with severe neutropenia. The patients should be given appropriate antibiotics and mouth rinses.
- Oral bleeding, oral ulcers, gingival infiltrates, oral infections and cervical lymphadenopathy may be the presenting features of leukemias. Hence, the dentist may be the first clinician to suspect the disease.
- Spontaneous gingival bleeding is common when platelet count is below 20,000/mm³.
- A history of any bleeding manifestations (including family history) must be asked in patients undergoing dental procedures. In case of such history, investigations should be performed to diagnose or exclude hemostatic disorders.
- A history of anticoagulant therapy must be noted. Non-surgical treatment can be carried out provided the PT/INR is not grossly above the therapeutic range and trauma is minimal. Surgical treatment is not recommended for those who have INR >3.5. At an INR <3.5 where bleeding is expected (in procedures like multiple extractions, removal of wisdom teeth, full mouth or arch extraction) local measures should be used along with the reduction

of INR to 2–3. Extensive flap surgery or multiple bony extraction may require an INR of <1.5.
- The transfusion of blood and blood components should be done if absolutely necessary to avoid the risk of transfusion-associated infections such as HIV, hepatitis B, hepatitis C, syphilis, malaria, cytomegalovirus and parvovirus.

SELF ASSESSMENT

Multiple Choice Questions

1. **Raised PT and PTT are seen in:**
   A. Thrombocytopenia B. VWD
   C. DIC D. Hemophilia.
2. **Which of the following manifestations is characteristic of hemophilia?**
   A. Gum bleeding B. Petechiae
   C. Hemarthrosis D. Epistaxis
3. **Gum hypertrophy can be seen in:**
   A. AML B. CLL
   C. CML D. ALL
4. **Gum bleeding can occur in:**
   A. ITP B. Acute leukemia
   C. VWD D. All of the above
5. **Microcytic hypochromic anemia is seen in all, except:**
   A. Thalassemia B. Iron deficiency
   C. Folate deficiency D. Pyridoxine deficiency
6. **In hemolytic anemia the following can occur:**
   A. Indirect hyperbilirubinemia
   B. Splenomegaly
   C. Gallstones
   D. All of the above
7. **Which is true in VWD:**
   A. Normal PT
   B. Normal APTT
   C. Decreased platelet count
   D. Raised plasma FDP
8. **The most preferred way to assess RBC production is to measure:**
   A. Serum ferritin B. Reticulocyte count
   C. RBC half life D. Total RBC count
9. **Following may be seen in megaloblastic anemia:**
   A. Paresthesia B. Macrocytosis
   C. Smooth tongue D. All of the above
10. **Plummer-Vinson syndrome is seen in:**
    A. Iron deficiency B. Esophageal carcinoma
    C. Alcohol withdrawal D. Lead poisoning
11. **Following test is used to examine the intrinsic coagulation pathway:**
    A. PT B. PTT
    C. Both of the above D. None of the above
12. **The bleeding due to oral anticoagulation therapy is managed by:**
    A. Aspirin B. Vitamin K
    C. Factor VIII D. Platelet transfusion
13. **Most of the coagulation factors are synthesized by:**
    A. Kidneys B. Bone marrow
    C. Liver D. Capillary endothelial cells
14. **Most of the bilirubin is formed in:**
    A. Liver B. Spleen
    C. Gallbladder D. Red blood cells
15. **Platelet dysfunction can be found in following, except:**
    A. VWD B. Uremia
    C. Aplastic anemia D. Aspirin therapy
16. **The following can be found in aplastic anemia, except:**
    A. Thrombocytopenia B. Splenomegaly
    C. Low reticulocyte count D. Infections
17. **Which one of the following is seen in ITP:**
    A. Raised bleeding time B. Raised PT
    C. Raised PTT D. High plasma FDP
18. **A 20-year girl develops excessive and prolonged bleeding following tooth extraction. Tests reveal raised PTT, normal PT, normal platelet count. The most probable diagnosis is:**
    A. VWD B. ITP
    C. Hemophilia D. DIC
19. **Following are vit K dependent coagulation factors:**
    A. VIII, IX, and IX B. II, VII, IX, X
    C. II, V, VII, IX D. V, VII, X, XII
20. **The mechanism of action of tranexamic acid is:**
    A. Anticoagulation
    B. Antifibrinolysis
    C. Enhancing platelet aggregation
    D. All of the above
21. **The following are found in DIC:**
    A. Thrombocytopenia B. Excessive bleeding
    C. Thrombosis D. All of the above
22. **Presence of gum bleed, infections, sternal tenderness and low platelet count suggests:**
    A. ITP B. Acute leukemia
    C. Sickle cell disease D. Aplastic anemia
23. **The following may retard iron absorption, except:**
    A. Phytates B. Calcium
    C. Vitamin C D. Achlorhydria
24. **Following can be found in hemolysis, except:**
    A. Low plasma haptoglobin
    B. Raised bilirubin
    C. Hemoglobinuria
    D. Low reticulocyte count
25. **Which of the following is generally given in hemolytic anemia:**
    A. Parenteral iron B. Folic acid
    C. Cobalamin D. Vitamin E
26. **Bleeding time is prolonged in:**
    A. Thrombasthenia B. Thrombocytopenia
    C. Uremia D. All of the above
27. **The following can be found in iron deficiency anemia, except:**
    A. Microcytosis
    B. Koilonychia
    C. Raised reticulocyte count
    D. Low plasma ferritin
28. **The therapy of choice in bleeding secondary to liver dysfunction is:**
    A. Cryoprecipitate B. Fresh frozen plasma
    C. Factor VIII D. Platelet transfusion
29. **All of the following conditions are classified as hypoproliferative anemia, except:**
    A. Aplastic anemia
    B. Anemia due to renal disease

C. Hemolytic anemia
D. Vitamin B₁₂ deficiency anemia
30. **High reticulocyte count is a feature of:**
    A. Aplastic anemia
    B. Iron deficiency anemia
    C. Sideroblastic anemia
    D. Autoimmune hemolytic anemia
31. **The patient has presented with anemia and mean corpuscular volume of 122 fL, most likely cause is:**
    A. Aplastic anemia
    B. Iron deficiency anemia
    C. B₁₂ deficiency anemia
    D. Hemolytic anemia
32. **All of the following are features of hemolysis, *except*:**
    A. High indirect bilirubin
    B. High serum haptoglobin
    C. High serum LDH
    D. High reticulocyte index
33. **Which of the following drug can be used in treatment of Immune thrombocytopenic purpura (ITP):**
    A. Eltrombopag   B. Dasatanib
    C. Abatacept   D. Teriparatide

Fill in the Blanks

1. The most common type of leukemia in children is _____.
2. Philadelphia chromosome is present in patients of_____.
3. Oral anticoagulant therapy is monitored by _____ test.
4. PTT is used to monitor_____therapy.
5. Koilonychia is seen in _____.
6. The plasma level of haptoglobin is_____in hemolytic anemia.
7. Imitanib mesylate is used in the therapy of _____.
8. Spontaneous bleeding can occur in thrombocytopenia if platelet count falls below_____.
9. Reed-Sternberg's cells are seen in_____.
10. Coombs' test is positive in _____anemia.
11. Most common inherited bleeding disorder is _____.
12. Hard, fixed and non-tender lymphadenopathy suggests a diagnosis of _____.
13. Virchow's node is _____.
14. Fish tapeworm can cause_____deficiency anemia.
15. Vegetarians are prone to develop_____deficiency.
16. Massive splenomegaly is defined as _____.
17. Localized lymphadenopathy most commonly occurs in _____region.
18. Matted lymph nodes are seen in_____.
19. The daily dose of oral iron for treatment of iron deficiency anemia is_____.
20. The MCV is_____in pernicious anemia.
21. The most common cause of microcytic hypochromic anemia is_____.
22. Normal absolute eosinophil count is_____.
23. The lifespan of RBC is_____.
24. Hypersegmented neutrophils are characteristically found in_____anemia.
25. Schilling test is useful in the diagnosis of_____.

CHAPTER 5

Cardiovascular System

SYMPTOMS AND SIGNS OF CARDIOVASCULAR DISEASES

Symptoms

Following are important symptoms in patients with cardiac diseases:
- Dyspnea
- Chest pain
- Palpitation
- Edema
- Syncope
- Fatigue
- Cough
- Reduced urine output (circulatory failure)
- Right upper abdomen discomfort.

Dyspnea

Dyspnea is an abnormally uncomfortable awareness of breathing. Main causes of dyspnea are diseases of cardiovascular system and pulmonary system (see also Chapter 6). In cardiovascular system this is mostly due to heart failure.

In heart failure elevated pulmonary venous and capillary pressure leads to pulmonary congestion. Pulmonary congestion leads to decreased lung compliance and increased airway resistance. Hence, an extra effort is needed to ventilate lungs. Other mechanisms of dyspnea are respiratory muscle fatigue and acidosis. Rapid, shallow breathing is characteristic of cardiac dyspnea.

Dyspnea is classified in four grades depending on severity, that is, level of exertion required to provoke its onset **(Table 5.1)**. The breathlessness in cardiac patients may be on exertion, at rest or in the supine position (orthopnea).

Table 5.1: The New York Heart Association (NYHA) grading of dyspnea.

Grade 1	No breathlessness
Grade 2	Breathlessness on severe exertion
Grade 3	Breathlessness on mild exertion
Grade 4	Breathlessness at rest

Orthopnea: Orthopnea, breathlessness on lying flat, is due to redistribution of fluid from abdomen and lower extremities to chest in recumbent position (increased venous return) and elevation of diaphragm.

Paroxysmal nocturnal dyspnea (PND): PND is a condition when patients may wake up in the night (usually after 2-3 hours of sleeping) with complaints of severe breathlessness and wheezing. Patient is relieved by sitting upright or standing. Patient usually opens window or door for fresh air. PND is a variant of orthopnea and is due to same mechanisms. In advanced failure, patient may not be able to lie supine at all.

Palpitation

Palpitation is an unpleasant awareness of the beating of the heart. It may occur due to abnormalities in the rate, rhythm or force of contraction of the heart.
- Important causes of palpitation are atrial, junctional and ventricular tachyarrhythmias.
- Rapid irregular palpitation is due to atrial fibrillation.
- Other causes are extrasystole, high cardiac output states (anemia, thyrotoxicosis) and valvular regurgitation (mitral regurgitation, aortic regurgitation).

Chest Pain

Chest pain is the common presentation in the cardiac disease, although it can also occur in diseases of the lungs, chest wall or in anxiety states **(Table 5.2)**.

Table 5.2: Causes of chest pain.

• **Cardiac causes**
  – Myocardial infarction
  – Pericarditis
  – Dissection of aorta
• **Non-cardiac causes**
  – Functional
  – Disease of thorax
  – Herpes zoster
  – Costochondritis
  – Myalgia
  – Pleurisy
  – Pneumothorax
  – Pulmonary embolism
• **Extrathoracic causes**
  – Esophagitis
  – Peptic ulcer
  – Cholecystitis
  – Pancreatitis

- The chest pain due to ischemic heart disease typically is constricting, heavy or choking in character, occurs in retrosternal area, may radiate to left arm or shoulder and is provoked during exertion. The pain may be accompanied by sweating, nervousness, breathlessness or marked anxiety (see Chapter 1: **Table 1.1**).
- The chest pain may also occur due to aortic dissection, pericarditis, pneumothorax, esophagitis, pleuritis, costochondritis.
- The pain in pericarditis is sharp central or to the left side of the chest which increases on deep inspiration and during coughing or postural changes.

Fatigue

Fatigue is an important symptom of cardiac failure. It is due to decreased oxygen delivery to muscles.

Edema

Edema in heart failure is a manifestation of systemic venous congestion and increased salt and fluid retention which occurs as compensatory mechanism. Edema generally presents first in the dependent parts of the body. This is usually bilateral and presents initially in feet, and is more marked at the end of the day **(Fig. 5.1)**. However, edema may be localized in the sacral area in bed-ridden patients (see also Chapter 1).

Syncope

Syncope is defined as transient loss of sensorium due to decreased cerebral blood flow. There is generally a spontaneous recovery. Important cardiac causes of syncope are arrhythmias, aortic stenosis and massive myocardial infarction. A syncopal attack due to heart blocks is known as *Stokes-Adams attacks* (see page 127).

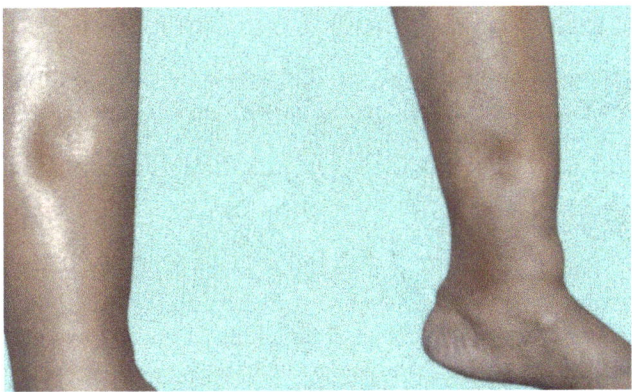

Fig. 5.1: Bilateral pedal edema (pitting type).

Cough

It is usually a symptom of respiratory diseases, but may be found in cardiac diseases as well. Pathophysiology behind cough in cardiac diseases is pulmonary venous congestion. Here it is predominantly nocturnal usually with minimal expectoration, which increases on lying down.

Hemoptysis

It is defined as coughing out blood in sputum. It is also a symptom predominantly of respiratory diseases. Patients with mitral stenosis may have hemoptysis. Pink frothy sputum associated with sudden severe breathlessness and cough signifies pulmonary edema.

Reduced Urine Output

Decreased urine output in cardiac diseases suggests decreased end organ perfusion and it must be given immediate attention. Regular monitoring of urine output is important in guiding therapy in patients with heart failure.

Right Upper Abdomen Discomfort

The patient may also complain of pain in right hypochondrium and decreased appetite due to congestive hepatomegaly in right sided heart failure. Sometimes this may also lead to icterus.

GENERAL EXAMINATION

The clinical examination in a cardiac patient should include a complete general examination together with a systemic cardiac examination. Other relevant systems are also examined for making a complete diagnosis.

A thorough examination is mandatory. One should specifically look for chest deformities, anemia, cyanosis, clubbing of fingers and toes, edema, hepatomegaly, cutaneous signs of infective endocarditis, arterial pulses, jugular venous pulsations and blood pressure.

Anemia

Anemia may be a precipitating factor in ischemic heart disease and heart failure. It can be present in infective endocarditis.

Cyanosis

Cyanosis is a bluish discoloration of the skin and mucous membrane caused by increased concentration of reduced hemoglobin (>4 g %) in superficial blood vessels. Cyanosis is looked for at lips, nail beds, malar area, earlobes and the mucous membrane of the oral cavity.

Cyanosis is classified into central and peripheral types **(Table 1.9)**.
a. The imperfect oxygen saturation or abnormal hemoglobin derivatives lead to *central cyanosis* which is seen in both the mucous membrane (tongue) and skin and also nail beds. The extremities are warm.
b. *Peripheral cyanosis* is due to excessive extraction of oxygen from the capillaries when the flow of blood is slow. The extremities are cyanosed and cold while mucous membrane of the oral cavity and tongue are spared. Warming of the cyanotic extremity may increase blood flow and abolish peripheral (but not central) cyanosis.
c. Cyanosis due to heart failure is of *mixed type*, both central and peripheral.

Cardiac causes of cyanosis are cyanotic congenital heart disease (Fallot's tetralogy, Eisenmenger's syndrome) and pulmonary edema. Central cyanosis is seen in such cases. Cyanosis in congestive heart failure can be both central and peripheral types.

Edema

Edema which pits on digital pressure is a feature of cardiac failure **(Fig. 5.1)**. Later the edema may progress to anasarca.

Clubbing

It is defined as selective bulbous enlargement of the distal segments of fingers and toes due to excessive proliferation of connective tissue.

The enlargement of the distal portion of the fingers and toes, due to proliferation of connective tissues, is known as clubbing (*see* **Fig. 1.11A**). The clubbing is graded as follows:
- Grade I: There is thickening of tissues at the nail base.
- Grade II: In addition to the features of grade I, the angle between nail base and the adjacent skin fold of the finger is obliterated. There is reduction in the space between thumb nails when placed in apposition (*Schamroth's window test*).
- Grade III: In addition to the features of grade I and grade II, the shape of the nail becomes convex in both horizontal and vertical directions. In severe cases there is bulbous enlargement of the distal segment of the fingers (drumstick appearance) (*see* **Fig. 1.11B**).

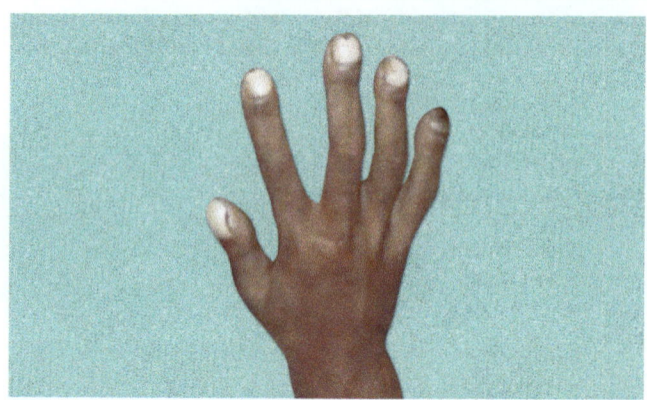

Fig. 5.2: Clubbing in cyanotic heart disease.

- Grade IV: Along with the clubbing, there may be swelling above the wrist and ankles due to periosteitis of long bones *(hypertrophic osteoarthropathy)*.

The exact mechanism of clubbing is clearly not known. However, it is thought to be due to some humoral substances leading to increased vascularity in the nail bed.

Clubbing of fingers and toes is found in cyanotic heart disease and infective endocarditis **(Fig. 5.2)**.

Peripheral Signs of Infective Endocarditis

Petechial hemorrhages, splinter hemorrhages in the nail bed, Osler's nodes (tender erythematous nodules at the finger pulp), Janeway lesions (painless red lesions of the palms) and Roth's spots (erythematous lesion on ocular fundi) should be looked for as an evidence of infective endocarditis.

Arterial Pulse

Arterial pulse should be examined for the rate, rhythm, volume, character and radio-femoral delay. The rate and rhythm are assessed by palpating radial artery **(Fig. 5.3)**. The character of the pulse is better assessed by palpating the carotid artery **(Fig. 5.4)**.

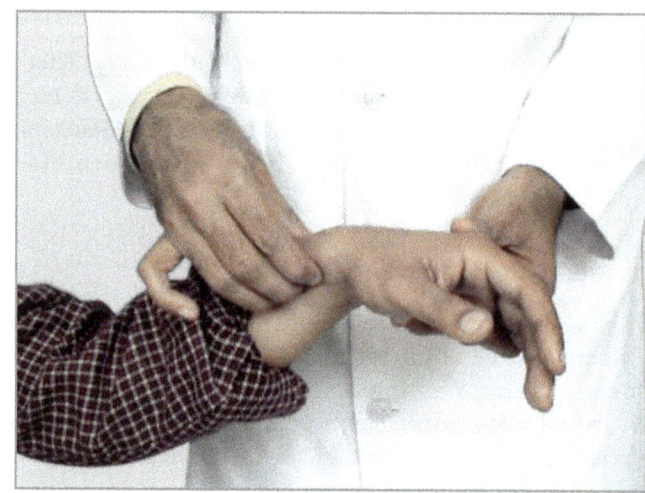

Fig. 5.3: Palpation of the radial artery.

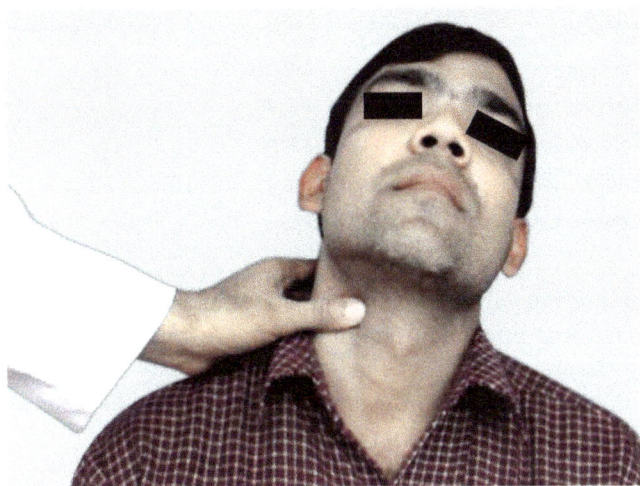

Fig. 5.4: Palpation of the right carotid artery with the left thumb.

Other peripheral arteries like brachial, popliteal, posterior tibial and dorsalis pedis can also be palpated. The pulse may be *absent or weak* in obstruction in the proximal part of the artery due to thromboembolism and atherosclerosis.

Rate: The *pulse rate* is determined by counting it for at least 30 seconds. The normal pulse rate varies from 60–100 per minute (*see* **Table 1.5**).
- Bradycardia is defined as pulse rate <60/min. Important causes are raised intracranial pressure, heart blocks and sinus node disease, cholestatic jaundice, hypothyroidism and drugs (beta blockers, verapamil, digoxin). Bradycardia may also be present in athletes.
- Tachycardia (pulse rate >100/min) occurs due to fever, exercise, anxiety, thyrotoxicosis, anemia, tachyarrhythmias, shock and drugs.
- Pulse is slower than would be expected from the height of fever in typhoid fever *(relative bradycardia).*

Rhythm: Normally the rhythm of the pulse is regular. An *irregular rhythm* is seen in atrial fibrillation (irregularly irregular) and frequent ectopic beats (regularly irregular).

Character:
- A low volume and slow rising pulse *(parvus et tardus)* is found in aortic stenosis (AS).
- A large bounding pulse *(hyperkinetic pulse)* is seen in hyperkinetic states (anemia, fever, anxiety, exercise), patent ductus arteriosus, ventricular septal defect, and aortic regurgitation (AR).
- *Bisferiens pulse* which has two systolic peaks is found in mixed lesions of AS and AR.
- Alternating strong and weak pulse *(pulsus alternans)* is present in severe left ventricular failure.
- Normally there is a fall in systolic arterial pressure of <10 mmHg during inspiration. An accentuation in this phenomenon can lead to weakening or disappearance of pulse during inspiration *(paradoxical pulse).* This is found in cardiac tamponade and obstructive airway disease.

Radio-femoral delay: The femoral pulse is weak and delayed as compared with the radial pulse *(radio-femoral delay)* in coarctation of aorta.

Blood Pressure

Blood pressure is measured in both arms and also in the lower limb. In coarctation of aorta, the arterial pressure in the upper limb is much higher than in lower limbs. The pulse pressure is defined as difference between systolic and diastolic pressures, it is wide in aortic regurgitation (AR), anemia and pregnancy whereas it is narrow in aortic stenosis (AS). Hypotension may occur in cardiac failure (see Chapter 1).

Jugular Venous Pulse

Pulsations and pressure in internal jugular vein in the neck are noted.
- *Venous vs arterial pulsation:* Venous pulsations must be differentiated from carotid artery pulsations. Venous pulsations are better seen while arterial pulsations are better palpable. The upper level of venous pulsation varies with the change in posture and phases of respiration.
- The venous pulse has three positive waves, a, c, and v, and two negative waves or descents, x and y. The a wave is due to atrial contraction. This is followed by x descent (due to descent of tricuspid valve ring) which is interrupted by a small c wave. The v wave is due to passive filling of blood from veins into the right atrium during ventricular systole. This is followed by y descent due to rapid flow of blood from the right atrium to the right ventricle when the tricuspid valve is open.
- Jugular veins are distended and pulsatile in congestive heart failure and pericardial effusion.
- Normally there is fall in the jugular venous pressure (JVP) during inspiration. There may be a paradoxical rise in the JVP during inspiration in constrictive pericarditis and cardiac tamponade *(Kussmaul's sign).*
- A raised jugular venous pressure (JVP) is a sign of right heart failure. "a" wave is absent in atrial fibrillation whereas it is prominent in tricuspid stenosis (TS). Prominent "y" descent is seen in tricuspid regurgitation.

Others

- *Inspiratory* crepitations over the lung bases are present in patients with heart failure. In patients with pulmonary edema, coarse crepitations are heard widely along with wheezing.
- *Tender hepatomegaly* may be present in cases with heart failure.
- *Splenomegaly* can be found in subacute infective endocarditis.
- *Ascites* may occur in severe heart failure.
- *Abdominal bruit* over renal area may be found in hypertension due to renal artery stenosis.

CARDIAC EXAMINATION

Inspection and Palpation

- The lowermost and outermost distinct cardiac pulsation is known as cardiac impulse or apex beat. It is normally situated in the fifth intercostal space just medial to mid-clavicular line. The apex beat may be shifted inferiorly or laterally in cardiac enlargement. The apex beat is insignificant in cases of pericardial effusion and mitral stenosis (MS) whereas prominent in mitral regurgitation (MR), aortic regurgitation (AR) and aortic stenosis (AS). The apex beat is palpated to determine its location and character. It is "tapping" in character in MS while thrusting in AS and AR.
- Pulsations in left parasternal area and epigastrium may be seen in cases of right ventricular enlargement.
- Pulmonary component of second heart sound (P_2) is palpable in second left parasternal area in case of pulmonary hypertension.
- A thrill (palpable murmur) may be palpable in systolic phase (MR, AS, ventricular septal defect) or diastolic phase (MS, AR) in corresponding areas.

Auscultation

- The first heart sound (S_1) corresponds to the closure of mitral and tricuspid valves. It is loud in MS and muffled in MR.
- The second heart sound corresponds to the closure of aortic (A_2) and pulmonary valve (P_2). The pulmonary component of the second heart sound (P_2) is loud in pulmonary hypertension and soft in pulmonary stenosis. Aortic second sound (A_2) is soft in AS. There is a wide and fixed split of second heart sound in atrial septal defect (ASD).
- The presence of third heart sound (S_3) in children may be physiological. However, after the age of 40 years it may signify ventricular failure.
- The fourth heart sound (S_4) occurs due to vigorous atrial contraction with a noncompliant ventricle (as in hypertension, AS).
- Opening snap (OS) is audible due to forceful opening of the mitral valve in diastolic phase preceding the murmur and is heard in cases of noncalcific mitral stenosis.
- Ejection click may be heard due to opening of the stenosed aortic or pulmonary valve.

The murmurs are found because of turbulent flow within the heart and great vessels. An increased flow across

Table 5.4: Types of murmur and their causes.

Pansystolic	MR, TR, VSD
Ejection systolic	AS, PS
Early diastolic	AR, PR
Mid-diastolic	MS, TS, Austin Flint in AR
Continuous	PDA

the normal valve may also generate murmur (innocent or functional murmur). The murmurs are generally defined by characters such as site, loudness, quality, timing and radiation. Different murmurs found in heart diseases are mentioned in **Tables 5.3 and 5.4**.

INVESTIGATIONS

Chest X-ray

Chest X-ray is useful in detecting cardiomegaly **(Fig. 5.5)**. Dilatation of individual chambers can also be recognized on X-ray of the chest. Straight left heart border may suggest mitral stenosis. X-ray may also reveal signs of increased pulmonary blood flow (pulmonary plethora) and pulmonary hypertension.

Electrocardiogram (ECG)

It is one of the basic and most important bedside tests for cardiac evaluation. The electrical activity in the heart can be recorded at the surface with the help of electrodes and is reflected in waveforms (P, Q, R, S, T). The P wave denotes

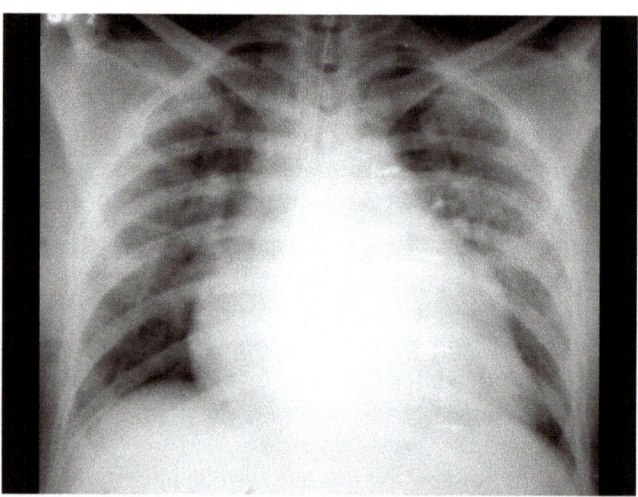

Fig. 5.5: X-ray chest showing cardiomegaly.

Table 5.3: Auscultatory findings in rheumatic valvular heart disease.

Mitral stenosis	Loud S_1, Loud P_2	Opening snap	Mid-diastolic murmur
Mitral regurgitation	Soft S_1, Loud P_2		Pansystolic murmur
Aortic stenosis	Soft A_2	Ejection click	Ejection systolic murmur
Aortic regurgitation	Soft A_2		Early diastolic murmur

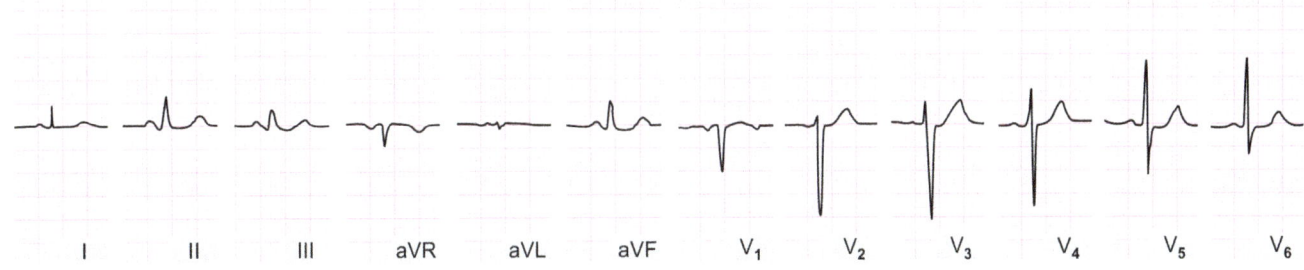

Fig. 5.6: Normal electrocardiogram.

the atrial depolarization while QRS shows the ventricular depolarization. The T wave reflects the ventricular repolarization. A normal ECG pattern is shown in **Figure 5.6**. The ECG is helpful in diagnosing ischemic heart disease. It can also indicate the presence of cardiomegaly and arrhythmias. In stress ECG test, the recording is made while the patient is exercising on a treadmill. This is used to confirm the diagnosis of angina and to evaluate patients with IHD for the purpose of management.

Echocardiography

This very useful noninvasive procedure is employed to diagnose structural and functional abnormalities of the heart and the presence of cardiac vegetations. Doppler echocardiography can detect the abnormal direction of flow as in MR or AR and also the pressure gradient across the stenotic valve.

Transesophageal echocardiography is more sensitive method to detect smaller vegetations, prosthetic valve dysfunction and atrial septal defects.

Cardiac Catheterization

A catheter is passed in the heart via an artery or vein under fluoroscopic monitoring. It is mainly used to assess coronary artery disease, to evaluate valvular heart disease and to measure the chamber pressure. Coronary angiography is done to define coronary anatomy and to determine the extent of coronary artery disease.

Cardiac Biomarkers

Some enzymes are released due to death of cardiac myocytes and these are used in diagnosis of MI (myocardial infarction). These are Troponin I, Troponin T, CPK-MB, LDH.

Pro BNP is a marker suggestive of heart failure.

Others

Myocardial perfusion imaging with radioactive thallium, magnetic resonance imaging (MRI) and positron emission tomography (PET) are other techniques employed in patients with cardiac diseases.

ACUTE RHEUMATIC FEVER

Acute rheumatic fever (ARF) is a multisystem disorder which follows pharyngeal streptococcal infection. This is the commonest cause of acquired heart disease in childhood and adolescence. Acute rheumatic fever is still prevalent in developing countries, although it is less commonly seen in the industrialized world.

Acute rheumatic fever affects children, most commonly between 5 to 15 years of age. It occurs in about 3% individuals who develop pharyngeal infection with certain serotypes of group A β *hemolytic streptococci (serotypes 1,3,5,6)*. Streptococcal antigens have cross reactivity with cardiac tissue; hence, anti-streptococcal antibodies mediate inflammatory reaction in the myocardium, endocardium and pericardium. Joint and skin tissues are also affected due to tissue cross reactivity.

Clinical Features

The manifestations of ARF are fever, malaise, lethargy, anorexia and symptoms caused due to involvement of heart, joints, skin and central nervous system. These manifestations occur generally 2–3 weeks after streptococcal pharyngitis. Its diagnosis is based on updated Jone's Criteria (**Table 5.5**). Presence of two or more major criteria or one major and at least two minor criteria plus evidence of previous streptococcal infection is required for the diagnosis of ARF.

Table 5.5: The WHO criteria (based on Jones criteria) for diagnosis of rheumatic fever.	
Major criteria	**Minor criteria**
Polyarthritis Carditis Chorea Subcutaneous nodules Erythema marginatum	Clinical: Fever, polyarthralgia Laboratory: Elevated ESR or TLC ECG: Prolonged P-R interval
And	
Positive throat culture for streptococci or elevated **or** Increasing streptococcal antibody titer **or** Rapid antigen test for group A streptococcus, **or** Recent scarlet fever	

Polyarthritis (Most Common)

- It is an early feature of ARF and occurs in about 75% of patients.
- There is acute painful inflammatory involvement of the large joints (ankles, knees, elbows) which are red, swollen and tender.
- The pain and swelling in the involved joints subside or disappear as newer joints are affected (migratory polyarthritis).
- The response to salicylates is dramatic.
- The inflammation does not leave any residual joint deformity.

Carditis

- Involvement of pericardium, endocardium and myocardium (pancarditis) occurs in 40 to 60% of patients with ARF.
- The symptoms are chest pain, palpitation and breathlessness.
- Examination may reveal tachycardia, third heart sound, pericardial rub, murmur of mitral regurgitation and cardiomegaly. A mid-diastolic murmur (Carey Coombs' murmur) may be present due to mitral valvulitis.
- Fibrosis and adhesion of the valve may develop following healing of the valvulitis which may lead to stenosis and/ or regurgitation (rheumatic valvular heart disease). The mitral valve is most commonly involved and the aortic valve is next most affected.
- The valvular involvement increases the risk of infective endocarditis.

Chorea

Chorea is a manifestation of central nervous system involvement in ARF. This is also known as Sydenham's chorea or St. Vitus dance. It is characterized by involuntary purposeless movement of hands, feet or face. Chorea is a late manifestation in the course of ARF and is more common in females.

Subcutaneous Nodules

This rare manifestation occurs in less than 10% cases of ARF. These are 0.5 to 2 cm, painless, firm nodules found over extensor surface of joints. The presence of subcutaneous nodules signifies underlying rheumatic heart disease.

Erythema Marginatum

This also occurs in less than 10% patients. These are evanescent red macules with pale center over the trunk and proximal extremities. Erythema marginatum may not be well appreciated in dark skinned people and it is rarely found on face.

Investigations

- The blood examination reveals leukocytosis (with predominantly neutrophils), raised ESR and CRP.
- Throat swab culture may be positive for group A streptococci.
- Anti-streptolysin O (ASO) titer is raised to >200 units in adults or >300 units in children.
- Other antibodies like anti-deoxyribonuclease B and anti-hyaluronidase may also be helpful in the diagnosis.
- Chest radiograph, ECG, and echocardiography are helpful in the diagnosis of carditis.

Treatment

- *Eradication of streptococci:* A 10 days course of erythromycin (250 mg 6 hourly oral) or oral penicillin V (500 mg twice daily) is administered to all patients to eradicate streptococcal infection. Alternatively, a single intramuscular injection of benzathine penicillin G (1.2 million units) may be given.
- *Bed rest:* This is required in patients with severe carditis. This is also helpful in reducing joint pain. The duration of rest is guided by symptoms and markers of inflammation.
- *Salicylates:* Aspirin is given in 6 divided dosages of 60 to 120 mg/kg per day to relieve arthritis. This should be given for 4–6 weeks and then gradually tapered.
- *Steroids:* Prednisolone (1–2 mg/kg/day) may be given to patients with severe carditis with CHF. As the patients improve, steroid should be tapered and salicylates added.

Secondary Prevention

This is used to prevent subsequent pharyngeal infection with group A streptococci. Following drugs may be used for secondary prevention of ARF:
- Oral penicillin V (250 mg twice daily)
- Oral sulphadiazine (1 g daily)
- Erythromycin (250 mg twice daily)
- Intramuscular benzathine penicillin G (1.2 million units) every three weeks

This is given for at least 5 years after the ARF without carditis and for at least 10 years after acute rheumatic fever with carditis. However, in patients with documented rheumatic heart disease or those at high risk of exposure, prophylaxis may be required indefinitely, preferably life long.

RHEUMATIC VALVULAR HEART DISEASE

About half of the patients who have rheumatic carditis will develop valvular disease. The mitral valve is most commonly involved, followed by the aortic valve. Other valves are involved rarely. Valvular defect may be stenotic or regurgitant. The patient may have single or multiple valvular involvements.

Mitral Stenosis (MS)

Mitral stenosis (MS) is more commonly found in females and its commonest cause is rheumatic heart disease. Rarely may it be congenital or degenerative **(Table 5.6)**.

Table 5.6: Causes of mitral stenosis.

1. Rheumatic fever
2. Calcification/degeneration of mitral valve
3. Congenital mitral stenosis

Pathophysiology

The size of the orifice of normal mitral valve is 4–6 cm². The orifice is progressively narrowed by fibrosis and calcification of valve leaflets, fusion of commissures and shortening of chordae tendineae. Mitral valve orifice less than 2 cm² is hemodynamically significant and becomes "critical" at <1 cm². The obstruction to the flow of blood through the stenosed mitral valve during diastole causes a rise in left atrial pressure. This leads to the hypertrophy and dilatation of the left atrium, pulmonary venous congestion and pulmonary arterial hypertension. Right ventricular failure may occur due to pulmonary hypertension. Reduced lung compliance causes breathlessness while decreased left ventricular filling leads to low cardiac output and fatigue. Atrial fibrillation (AF) commonly occurs because of left atrial dilatation. Patients, particularly with AF, are more susceptible to develop left atrial thrombus and systemic thromboembolism.

Table 5.7: Clinical signs of mitral stenosis.

- Malar flush (mitral facies)
- Atrial fibrillation (irregularly irregular pulse)

Cardiac examination
- Tapping apex beat
- Diastolic thrill in mitral area

Auscultation
- Loud first heart sound
- Opening snap
- Mid-diastolic murmur in mitral area (low pitched, rumbling)

Signs of pulmonary hypertension
- Loud P_2
- Right ventricular heave

Signs of raised pulmonary capillary pressure
- Pulmonary crepts

Signs of right heart failure
- Raised JVP
- Tender hepatomegaly
- Bilateral pitting pedal edema
- Ascites and pleural effusion in severe cases

Clinical Manifestations

The early presentations of MS include breathlessness on exertion and fatigue. As the stenosis progresses, patients are dyspneic on rest and even have orthopnea and paroxysmal nocturnal dyspnea (PND). Acute pulmonary edema may also occur. There may be hemoptysis (due to rupture of pulmonary-bronchial venous connections secondary to pulmonary venous hypertension), edema of lower limbs, palpitation and thromboembolic events (stroke, limb ischemia). Signs are given in **Table 5.7**.

Investigations

- ECG may reveal the evidence of left atrial (LA) enlargement, right ventricular (RV) hypertrophy and atrial fibrillation **(Fig. 5.7)**.
- Chest X-ray shows findings suggestive of LA enlargement and pulmonary congestion.
- Echocardiography is the most sensitive and specific of non-invasive methods to diagnose the valvular disease. It may reveal structural abnormalities of the valves, size of cardiac chambers, pulmonary artery pressure, ventricular dysfunction and presence of thrombi. Transesophageal echocardiography provides better information than transthoracic echocardiography.
- Cardiac catheterization is used to assess associated valvular lesions and to detect coronary artery disease.

Treatment

Medical

Medical treatment of mitral stenosis consists of:
- Restriction of physical activity.
- Sodium restriction and diuretics are used in heart failure.
- Digoxin is given to control ventricular rate in patients with AF. Beta blocker and calcium antagonists (verapamil, diltiazem) can also be used.
- Oral anticoagulant (warfarin) is given to patients with a history of thromboembolic events or to those with AF (INR of 2.0–3.0).
- Prophylaxis should be given to all patients to prevent rheumatic fever (see secondary prevention of rheumatic fever).
- Prophylaxis for infective endocarditis should be given prior to procedures (see prophylaxis for endocarditis). *Recent guidelines recommend prophylaxis only if there is a prior history of endocarditis.*

Surgical

Surgical intervention is needed when patient remains symptomatic despite medical treatment or when mitral stenosis is severe.

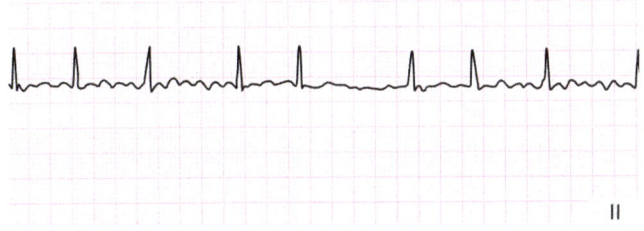

Fig. 5.7: Atrial fibrillation.

- *Mitral valvotomy*
  - Percutaneous balloon valvotomy is indicated when mitral valve is noncalcified and without regurgitation. The procedure involves the passing of catheter across the valve and inflation of the balloon to dilate the orifice.
  - Open valvotomy is carried out in patients where balloon valvotomy is not possible or in cases with restenosis. In this procedure the fusion of the valve is loosened and calcium deposit and thrombi are removed.
- *Mitral valve replacement:* The mitral valve is replaced when there is critical MS (<1 cm^2 orifice size) and/or there is associated significant mitral regurgitation. Replacement is also done when the mitral valve is severely distorted and calcified.

Mitral Regurgitation (MR)

Mitral regurgitation (MR) is the backflow of blood from the left ventricle to the left atrium during systole. Rheumatic heart disease is the principal cause of MR. Other important causes are mitral valve prolapse, ischemic heart disease, dilated cardiomyopathy and connective tissue diseases like Marfan syndrome. Myocardial infarction, infective endocarditis and trauma can lead to *acute MR* **(Table 5.8)**.

Pathophysiology

Mitral regurgitation leads to gradual dilatation of LA with little increase in pressure. However, chronic volume overload leads to left ventricular (LV) dilatation. Eventually the pressure in the LV and LA rises leading to breathlessness and pulmonary congestion. On the contrary, there is sudden elevation of LA pressure in *acute MR* causing severe pulmonary edema.

Clinical Manifestations

The symptoms of chronic MR are similar to that of MS and the main symptoms are fatigue, exertional dyspnea and orthopnea. Thromboembolic events are less common. Patients with acute severe MR commonly present with acute pulmonary edema. Clinical signs are listed in **Table 5.9**.

Table 5.8: Causes of mitral regurgitation (MR).

Chronic MR
- Rheumatic fever
- Mitral valve prolapse
- Infective endocarditis (damage to valve)
- Ischemic
- Dilated cardiomyopathy (dilatation of ventricle/mitral valve ring)

Acute MR
- Infective endocarditis
- Myocardial infarction (papillary muscle rupture)
- Trauma

Table 5.9: Clinical signs of mitral regurgitation.
- Atrial fibrillation (irregularly irregular pulse)

Cardiac examination
- Hyperdynamic and shifted apex beat
- Systolic thrill in mitral area

Auscultation
- Soft first heart sound
- Apical S$_3$ (third heart sound)
- Pan systolic murmur in mitral area

Signs of pulmonary hypertension
- Loud P$_2$
- Right ventricular heave

Signs of raised pulmonary capillary pressure
- Pulmonary crepts

Signs of right heart failure
- Raised JVP
- Tender hepatomegaly
- Bilateral pitting pedal edema
- Ascites and pleural effusion in severe cases

Investigations

- ECG may reveal the evidence of LA and LV enlargement, RV hypertrophy and atrial fibrillation.
- Chest X-ray shows findings suggestive of LA and LV enlargement and pulmonary congestion.
- *Echocardiography is the most sensitive and specific of non-invasive methods* to diagnose valvular disease. It may reveal structural abnormalities of the valves, size of cardiac chambers, pulmonary artery pressure, ventricular dysfunction and presence of thrombi. *Doppler echocardiography* is needed to detect and estimate the MR. Transesophageal echocardiography provides better information than transthoracic echocardiography.
- Cardiac catheterization is used to assess the severity of MR, to detect associated valvular lesions and coronary artery disease.

Treatment

Medical

Medical treatment of mitral regurgitation consists of:
- Restriction of physical activities that cause fatigue and breathlessness.
- Sodium restriction and diuretics are used to reduce pulmonary congestion.
- Digoxin is given to control ventricular rate in patients with AF and to improve the ventricular systolic function.
- Vasodilators like ACE inhibitors are given in chronic MR to reduce regurgitation and improve forward output. Intravenous nitroprusside or nitroglycerine is useful in *acute MR*.
- Oral anticoagulant (warfarin) is given to patients with history of thromboembolic events or to those with AF.
- Prophylaxis should be given to all patients to prevent rheumatic fever.

- Prophylaxis for infective endocarditis should be given prior to procedures. *Recent guidelines recommend prophylaxis only if there is a prior history of endocarditis.*

Surgical

Mitral valve repair/Mitral valve replacement: Patients who are initially on medical therapy are watched for symptomatic worsening and for radiological evidence of progressive cardiac enlargement or deteriorating cardiac function. In this case, surgery is indicated. Surgery includes repair or replacement of the mitral valve.

Acute MR: Acute MR due to endocarditis, myocardial infarction and trauma often requires emergency surgery. Prior to surgery, patients are stabilized by vasodilators or intra-aortic balloon counter pulsation which reduces regurgitation by lowering systemic vascular resistance.

AORTIC STENOSIS (AS)

Aortic stenosis (AS) in *adults* may be due to (a) degeneration and calcification of a normal valve, (b) calcification of a bicuspid valve and (c) rheumatic aortic valve stenosis. Rheumatic AS is always accompanied with mitral valve involvement and presence of AR. Aortic stenosis in *children* is commonly congenital in origin **(Table 5.10)**.

Pathophysiology

The obstruction to the left ventricular outflow causes pressure overload on the LV which subsequently leads to concentric LV hypertrophy. The increase in cardiac output during effort is limited by the valve stenosis. This can cause syncope and hypotension. Left ventricular failure occurs when it is unable to overcome the obstruction.

Ischemic symptoms (angina) may result due to increased oxygen demand by hypertrophied myocardial mass together with decreased coronary supply. Angina may occur even in the absence of coronary artery disease.

Clinical Manifestations

The patients remain asymptomatic for many years. Symptoms occur when AS becomes severe (valve size <1 cm^2). Exertional dyspnea, angina pectoris and syncope are three cardinal symptoms of AS. Sudden death may occur. In the advanced stage, symptoms of LV failure such as orthopnea, PND and pulmonary edema may occur. Clinical signs are given in **Table 5.11**.

Table 5.10: Causes of aortic stenosis (AS).

- Degeneration/calcification of normal valve
- Calcification of bicuspid aortic valve
- Rheumatic fever
- Congenital AS

Table 5.11: Clinical signs of aortic stenosis.

General examination
- Slow rising pulse with delayed peak (pulsus parvus et tardus)
- Carotid thrill
- Narrow pulse pressure

Cardiac findings
Inspection and palpation
- Forceful and sustained apex beat
- Systolic thrill at base of the heart radiating to carotid artery

Auscultation
- Soft or absent A_2
- S_4 at apex (S_3 if LVF)
- Harsh ejection systolic murmur best at aortic area and radiating toward carotid artery

Others
- Basal crackles (crepts) in lungs due to pulmonary congestion
- Signs of RV failure may be present in severe cases

Investigations

- ECG may show the evidence of LV hypertrophy and left bundle branch block.
- Chest X-ray is generally normal. However, it may show post-stenotic dilatation of the ascending aorta and valvular calcification.
- Echocardiography may reveal structural abnormalities of the valves including calcification, size of cardiac chambers, pulmonary artery pressure, ventricular dysfunction and presence of thrombi. Doppler echocardiography is needed to detect associated AR.
- Cardiac catheterization is mainly required to accurately assess the severity of AR, LV dysfunction and to detect the presence of coronary artery disease.

Treatment

Medical

Medical treatment of aortic stenosis consists of:
- Strenuous physical activities should be avoided.
- Sodium restriction is advised in presence of CHF. Diuretics are used with caution to avoid hypotension.
- Digoxin is given to improve the ventricular systolic function in patients with LVF.
- Oral anticoagulant (warfarin) is given if there is AF.
- Prophylaxis for infective endocarditis should be given prior to procedures. *Recent guidelines recommend prophylaxis only if there is a prior history of endocarditis.*
- Statins have been shown to reduce the progression of degenerative calcific AS.

Surgical

- Surgical aortic valve replacement: All symptomatic adult patients with severe AS should be considered for aortic valve replacement.
- Transcatheter aortic valve replacement (TAVR): A stented bioprosthetic valve is placed within the stenotic valve via

a transfemoral, transaortic or subclavian route under fluoroscopic and echocardiographic guidance. It reduces mortality compared to medical treatment in patients with high risk for surgery and has similar results as surgical valve replacement.
- Percutaneous balloon aortic valvuloplasty: It is useful in children with congenital non-calcific AS.

AORTIC REGURGITATION (AR)

- Aortic regurgitation (AR) is the backflow of blood from the aorta through an incompetent aortic valve into the left ventricle during diastole.
- AR may be either due to valvular involvement or dilatation of aortic root or both.
- The important causes of valvular involvement are rheumatic disease, endocarditis, trauma and congenital bicuspid aortic valve. Marfan syndrome and severe hypertension can lead to aortic root dilatation and AR. Syphilis and ankylosing spondylitis can cause AR because of valvular involvement and aortic dilatation **(Table 5.12)**.

Pathophysiology

Regurgitation causes volume overload leading to dilatation and hypertrophy of the LV. The stroke volume is increased to maintain the effective cardiac output. This is the basis for peripheral arterial signs in AR. As the LV function deteriorates, the effective forward output declines even during rest. Myocardial ischemia may occur even in the absence of concomitant coronary artery disease (CAD).

Clinical Manifestations

- The patients remain asymptomatic for years. Palpitations, particularly on lying down are generally an early symptom. Later on, patients present with dyspnea on exertion followed by orthopnea and PND. Angina may also occur frequently in severe AR.
- The presentations in *acute severe AR* are pulmonary edema and/or cardiogenic shock (tachycardia, cold extremities, hypotension, cyanosis). The clinical signs are listed in **Table 5.13**.

Table 5.12: Causes of aortic regurgitation.

Valvular
- Rheumatic fever
- Endocarditis
- Trauma
- Congenital bicuspid aortic valve
- Syphilis
- Ankylosing spondylitis

Aortic root disease
- Aortic dissection
- Marfan syndrome
- Hypertension
- Syphilis
- Ankylosing spondyltis

Table 5.13: Clinical signs of aortic regurgitation.

General examination
Peripheral signs of AR
- Collapsing or water hammer pulse
- Dancing carotids (pulsatile and prominent carotid arteries)
- Quincke's sign (alternate flushing and paling of skin at root of nail on pressure)
- Pistol shot sound over femoral arteries (Traube's sign)
- Duroziez sign (to and fro murmur over femoral artery when it is compressed)
- de Musset's sign (head nodding with the pulse)

Blood pressure
- Increased pulse pressure (low diastolic pressure)
- Hill's sign: Systolic BP in lower limbs is higher (>20 mmHg) than in upper limbs.

Cardiac findings
Inspection and palpation
- Heaving and laterally displaced apex beat
- Diastolic thrill at left sternal border

Auscultation
- Soft or absent A_2
- S_3 (S_4 occasionally)
- High pitched blowing early diastolic murmur best at left sternal border
- Other murmurs include ejection systolic murmur at aortic area radiating to carotid artery and low pitch mid-diastolic murmur over mitral area (Austin Flint murmur).

Others
- Basal crackles (crepts) in lungs due to pulmonary congestion.
- Signs of RV failure (edema and hepatomegaly) may be present in severe cases.

Investigations

- ECG shows the evidence of LV hypertrophy and ST-T changes.
- Chest X-ray reveals cardiomegaly and aortic root dilatation. Features of pulmonary congestion may be present.
- Echocardiography may reveal structural abnormalities of the valves, size of cardiac chambers, pulmonary artery pressure, ventricular dysfunction and presence of thrombi. Doppler echocardiography is needed to assess the severity of AR.
- Cardiac catheterization is mainly required to detect the presence of coronary artery disease.

Treatment

Medical

Medical treatment of aortic regurgitation consists of:
- Strenuous physical activities should be avoided.
- Sodium restriction and diuretics are advised in presence of CHF.
- Digoxin and vasodilators (ACE inhibitors) are given to improve the ventricular systolic function in patients with LVF. Long-acting nifedipine has been found to delay the need for operation.

- Oral anticoagulant (warfarin) is given if there is AF.
- Prophylaxis for infective endocarditis should be given prior to procedures. *Recent guidelines recommend prophylaxis only if there is a prior history of endocarditis.*
- Nitroprusside or ionotrope is given in acute AR to stabilize the patient before surgery.
- Treatment of precipitating or underlying causes (syphilis, endocarditis) should be commenced.

Surgical

Aortic valve replacement and/or aortic root repair: All symptomatic patients with chronic AR should be considered for aortic valve replacement. However, surgery may also be advisable in asymptomatic patients who show evidence of progressive cardiomegaly or deteriorating LV function.

Acute AR: Repair of aortic root abnormalities and aortic valve replacement should urgently be performed in patient with acute AR. Patients may be stabilized by vasodilators or ionotropes before surgery.

INFECTIVE ENDOCARDITIS

Infective endocarditis is microbial infection of endothelium of the heart. The infection most commonly occurs at the site of pre-existing endocardial damage in heart valves (native or prosthesis) and endocardium of the chambers. Similar process involving arterial endothelium in arteriovenous shunts, patent ductus arteriosus and coarctation of aorta is known as infective endarteritis.

Pathology

The endothelium may get damaged due to high pressure jet injury as occurs in valvular or congenital heart disease. The damaged surface of endothelium invites platelet adhesion and aggregation and fibrin deposition (*nonbacterial thrombotic endocarditis*). Organisms which enter into the bloodstream through mucosa, skin or sites of focal infection may colonize the platelets-fibrin deposit and form vegetation. These vegetations can grow in size and cause obstruction or can be dislodged as emboli. Locally, it can lead to abscess formation and damage to the tissues like valves, chordae tendinae and myocardium. Virulent organisms such as *S. aureus* may even colonize normal endothelium.

- Ventricular septal defect (VSD), mitral regurgitation, aortic stenosis, aortic regurgitation are particularly susceptible to endocarditis.
- Whereas conditions with low pressure shunt (atrial septal defect) are at low risk of developing endocarditis.
- Intravenous drug abusers are prone to develop right sided (tricuspid valve) endocarditis.

Endocarditis is classified into acute and subacute types depending on manifestations and their clinical course **(Table 5.14)**.

Table 5.14: Acute and subacute infective endocarditis.

Acute infective endocarditis	Subacute infective endocarditis
Rapid course	Indolent course
Rapid valve destruction and abscess formation	Slow structural damage
Metastatic spread common	Less common
Clubbing, splenomegaly and petechial hemorrhages not found	Clubbing, splenomegaly and petechial hemorrhages are seen
Fatal if not promptly treated	Prolonged course unless complicated by ruptured mycotic aneurysm or embolism
Causative organism: *Staph. aureus*, pneumococci, Beta hemolytic streptococci	*Strep. viridans*, enterococci, HACEK group

- The most common organism causing subacute endocarditis is Viridans group of streptococci. These are commensals in the upper respiratory tract and may enter the blood following brushing, chewing or dental procedures. Other organisms like *Enterococcus faecalis*, *S. bovis* may arise from urinary tract or bowel.
- *Staphylococcus aureus* is the most common cause of acute endocarditis.
- HACEK group of gram-negative bacteria *(Haemophilus, Actinobacillus, Cardiobacterium, Eikenella and Kingella)* can also cause native valve endocarditis.
- Other uncommon organisms which cause endocarditis are fungi (Candida), rickettsia, chlamydia and anaerobes.
- Prosthetic valve endocarditis in the initial 1 year after valve placement is generally due to coagulase negative *Staphy. epidermidis*, a normal skin commensal. After one year even in prosthetic valves, most common cause of endocarditis is *Streptococcus viridans*.
- *Staphylococcus aureus* is the most common cause of endocarditis in intravenous drug abusers.

Clinical Manifestations

Endocarditis is suspected in any patient with cardiac disease who develops persistent fever. The manifestations are listed below:
- *General:* Fever, weight loss, night sweats and weakness
- *Cardiac:* New murmur, heart failure and heart blocks
- *Extracardiac:*
    - Following findings may be present in IE:
        » Anemia
        » Clubbing
        » Splenomegaly
        » Petechial hemorrhages
        » Osler nodes (painful lesions at fingertips)
        » Janeway's lesions (macular lesions over palm and soles)
        » Roth spots on fundus examination
        » Subconjunctival hemorrhages

- Meningitis, embolic infarcts and intracranial bleeding due to rupture of mycotic aneurysms are neurological presentations.
- Septic emboli may disseminate infection to distant organs such as skin, spleen, kidneys, bone and meninges. Embolic events may also be associated with infarction at various sites.
- Immune complex deposition can lead to glomerulonephritis and hematuria.

Investigations

- *Blood culture:* The most important test is blood culture which tells about the organism and guides in antibiotic therapy. Venous blood samples are taken 30 minutes apart from three different sites. Aseptic technique is essential and the sample should be taken prior to antibiotic therapy except in severe cases. Serological tests may be useful if blood culture is negative.
- *Echocardiography:* This can reveal the site and size of the vegetations, abscess formation, evidence of underlying heart disease and heart failure. Transesophageal echocardiography is a more sensitive method as compared to transthoracic echocardiography.
- *Other findings:* These include normocytic normochromic anemia, leukocytosis, high ESR and CRP, microscopic hematuria, and proteinuria. Chest X-ray may show evidence of cardiomegaly and heart failure. Conduction defects may be observed on ECG recording.

Diagnostic criteria: Duke's criteria which are based on clinical, laboratory and echocardiographic findings are used for the diagnosis of endocarditis.

Treatment

The treatment of infective endocarditis should be prompt and adequate. The principles of treatment are:
- The antibiotics should be administered parenterally to achieve high serum concentration since the vegetation is avascular.
- The therapy is generally of prolonged duration. The dose and duration should be meticulously adhered to ensure the proper response.
- The antibiotics should preferably be bactericidal.
- The selection of antibiotics should be based on culture reports and minimum inhibitory concentration (MIC) values. Empirical therapy may be initiated in acute severe cases after drawing blood samples for culture. The antibiotics are later changed, if necessary, based on sensitivity reports.

The list of antibiotics commonly used, their dosage and indications are given in **Tables 5.15 and 5.16**.

Table 5.15: The antibiotics commonly used in infective endocarditis.

Antibiotics	Dose
Penicillin G	2–4 million units IV 4 hrly
Gentamicin	1 mg/kg IV or IM 8 hrly
Ceftriaxone	2 g IV OD
Ampicillin/Amoxycillin	2 g IV 4 hrly
Nafcillin or Oxacillin	2 g IV 4 hrly
Cefazolin	2 g IV 8 hrly
Vancomycin	15 mg/kg IV 12 hrly
Rifampicin	300 mg orally 8 hrly

Table 5.16: Common regimens used in IE.

Organism	Sensitivity	Regimens
Streptococci	Penicillin susceptible (MIC <0.1 µg/mL)	Penicillin G (4 weeks) Penicillin G plus Gentamicin (2 weeks) Ceftriaxone (4 weeks) Vancomycin (4 weeks)
	Relatively penicillin resistant (MIC 0.1–0.5 µg/mL)	Penicillin G (4–6 weeks) plus gentamicin (2 weeks)
	Moderately penicillin resistant (MIC 0.5–0.8 µg/mL)	Penicillin G plus Gentamicin (4–6 weeks)
Enterococci		Penicillin G or Ampicillin or Vancomycin plus Gentamicin (4–6 weeks)
Staphylococci Native valve	Methicillin susceptible	Nafcillin or Oxacillin or Cefazolin (4–6 weeks) plus Gentamicin (3–5 days) Vancomycin (4–6 weeks)
	Methicillin resistant	Vancomycin (4–6 weeks)
Prosthetic valve	Methicillin susceptible	Nafcillin or Oxacillin (6–8 weeks) plus Gentamicin (2 weeks) plus Rifampicin (6–8 weeks)
	Methicillin resistant	Vancomycin (6–8 weeks) plus Gentamicin (2 weeks) plus Rifampicin (6–8 weeks)
HACEK group		Ceftriaxone (4 weeks) Ampicillin plus Gentamicin (4 weeks)
Fungal		Amphotericin B plus flucytosine

Empirical Therapy

Empirical therapy is given when the culture is negative or before culture and sensitivity reports are available. Ceftriaxone plus gentamicin is given in subacute native valve endocarditis. Vancomycin is added to the above regime in case of prosthetic valve endocarditis.

Surgery

Surgery is often needed in patients with prosthetic valve endocarditis and fungal endocarditis who have (a) heart failure due to valve damage, (b) no response to antibiotics, (c) large vegetations and (d) abscess formation.

Prophylaxis

- Antibiotic prophylaxis prevents only a small number of cases of infective endocarditis. Bacteremia associated with routine daily activities like chewing, brushing, and flossing is similar as with dental procedures like tooth extraction. It has been seen that cardiac tissue is exposed to bacteremia causing oral cavity organisms many times greater with routine daily activities than from dental procedures. As per American Heart Association recent guidelines antibiotic prophylaxis is now recommended only for patients at highest risk **(Table 5.17)**.
- Patients with valvular and congenital heart disease who are at high risk of endocarditis should receive prophylactic antibiotics **(Table 5.18)** before undergoing any procedure which may cause bacteremia. Antibiotic prophylaxis is not advised for other cardiac lesions.
- The patients must be advised to maintain good dental and oral health. In patients with poor oral hygiene, routine chewing and brushing of teeth may cause bacteremia. Hence, daily personal care and annual professional dental care is advised.
- Tooth extraction, periodontal surgery, root canal therapy, scaling, removal of tartar and tooth implantation are procedures that require antimicrobial prophylaxis **(Tables 5.19 and 5.20)**. In addition, respiratory, gastrointestinal and genitourinary procedures also require prophylaxis.
- Patients with atrial septal defect, surgically repaired VSD and PDA, prior coronary artery bypass surgery and

Table 5.17: Cardiac lesions (high risk) for which antibiotic prophylaxis is recommended before dental procedures.

- Previous episode of endocarditis
- Patients with prosthetic heart valves
- Cyanotic congenital heart diseases (unrepaired)
- Unrepaired congenital heart defects (VSD, PDA, Coarctation of aorta) or during first 6 months after repair
- Valvulopathy in post-cardiac transplant patients
- Patients with residual defects in incompletely repaired congenital heart disease

Table 5.19: Dental procedures for which endocarditis prophylaxis is advised in patients at high or moderate risk for endocarditis.

- Extractions
- Periodontal procedures, cleaning causing gingival bleeding
- Implant placement, reimplantation of avulsed teeth
- Endodontic instrumentation (root canal) or surgery beyond the apex
- Subgingival placement of antibiotic fibers or strips
- Placement of orthodontic bands but not brackets
- Intraligamentary injections (anesthetic)

Table 5.20: Oral procedures not requiring prophylaxis for infective endocarditis.

- Local anesthetic agent (non-intraligamentary)
- Intracanal endodontic procedure
- Operative and prosthodontic procedures with or without retraction cord
- Adjustment of orthodontic appliance
- Placement of removable prosthodontic or orthodontic appliances
- Impression taking
- Exfoliation of primary teeth
- Oral radiography
- Placement of rubber dams
- Suture removal
- Fluoride treatment

Table 5.18: Antibiotic regimens for high risk cardiac lesions.

Drug	Dose	Route	Timing
Standard regimen			
Amoxicillin	2.0 g	Oral	1 hour before procedure
Penicillin allergy			
Clarithromycin or Azithromycin	500 mg	Oral	1 hour before procedure
Cephalexin	2.0 g	Oral	1 hour before procedure
Clindamycin	600 mg	Oral	1 hour before procedure
Patients unable to take orally			
Ampicillin	2.0 g	IV or IM	1 hour before procedure
Patients with penicillin allergy and unable to take orally			
Cefazolin or Ceftriaxone	1.0 g	IV or IM	30 min before procedure
Clindamycin	600 mg	IV or IM	1 hour before procedure

Cephalosporins should not be used in patients with Type 1 immediate hypersensitivity (anaphylaxis, urticaria, angioedema) to penicillin

Table 5.21: Cardiac conditions where endocarditis prophylaxis is not recommended.

- Atrial septal defect (ostium secondum)
- Mitral valve prolapse without regurgitation and/or thickening
- After surgical repair of ASD, VSD, or PDA
- Coronary artery bypass surgery (CABG) performed more than 6 weeks prior to treatment
- Physiological, functional heart murmurs
- Cardiac pacemakers
- Implanted defibrillators, previous rheumatic fever or Kawasaki disease without valvular dysfunction

implanted pacemakers and defibrillators do not require prophylaxis **(Table 5.21)**.

HYPERTENSION

Elevated arterial pressure (hypertension) is one of the most important public health problems worldwide. A sizable proportion of such patients remain undiagnosed and around half of hypertensive patients are not adequately treated.

There is no definite dividing line between normal and elevated arterial blood pressure. However, hypertension is defined as a level of blood pressure at which there is increased risk for target organ damage and the benefits of treatment outweighs the cost and hazards. An evaluation of additional risk factors should be part of the diagnostic workup in hypertensive patients.

The classification of blood pressure is given in **Tables 5.22 and 5.23**. As per 2020 International Society of Hypertension Global Hypertension Practice Guidelines normal systolic blood pressure is < 130 mmHg and normal diastolic blood pressure is <85 mmHg.

- Isolated systolic hypertension is defined as systolic blood pressure of 140 mmHg or more together with diastolic pressure <90 mmHg. It is common in the elderly due to stiffening of the large arteries with an increase in difference between SBP and DBP (pulse pressure).
- *Labile hypertensives* are those patients who some times have blood pressure in the hypertensive range.

Table 5.22: Classification of blood pressure for adults (>18 years) based on office blood pressure measurement.

Category	Systolic blood pressure (mmHg)	Diastolic blood pressure (mmHg)
Normal	<130	<85
High-normal BP	130–139	85–89
Hypertension	>140	>90
Stage 1	140–159	90–99
Stage 2	>160	>100

Note: Blood pressure values are based on the average of two or more readings taken at each of two or more visits after an initial screening. When systolic and diastolic values fall into different categories, the higher category should be selected for classification.

Table 5.23: Criteria for hypertension based on office-, ambulatory (ABPM)-, and home blood pressure (HBPM) measurement.

Category	Systolic BP (mmHg)		Diastolic BP (mmHg)
Office BP	≥ 140	and/or	≥ 90
Ambulatory BP (ABPM)			
24 hours mean	≥ 130	and/or	≥ 80
Daytime (or awake) mean	≥ 135	and/or	≥ 85
Night time (or asleep) mean	≥ 120	and/or	≥ 70
HBPM	≥ 135	and/or	≥ 85

- *Accelerated hypertension* is defined as significant recent increase in blood pressure over previous hypertensive level associated with rapidly progressive end organ damage.
- Presence of papilledema (swelling of optic disk) along with other features of accelerated hypertension signifies *malignant hypertension*.

Essential Hypertension

Patients with elevated arterial blood pressure without any identifiable cause are said to have essential or primary or idiopathic hypertension. More than 90% patients with hypertension belong to this category. Pathogenesis of essential hypertension is not clearly understood. However, this is thought to be multifactorial. Important environmental factors include high salt intake, heavy alcohol use, obesity and sedentary lifestyle. Genetic factors may also be responsible in some ethnic groups.

Secondary Hypertension

In secondary hypertension, a specific cause is identified. Important causes are given in **Table 5.24**. The most common

Table 5.24: Important causes of secondary hypertension.

Renal disorders
- Renovascular stenosis
- Parenchymal renal disease, particularly glomerulonephritis
- Polycystic kidney disease

Obstructive sleep apnea

Endocrinal disorders
- Pheochromocytoma
- Cushing's syndrome
- Primary hyperaldosteronism
- Acromegaly
- Hypo- and hyperthyroidism

Drugs
- Oral contraceptives
- Corticosteroids
- Sympathomimetic drugs
- Cyclosporine

Miscellaneous
- Toxemia of pregnancy
- Coarctation of aorta
- Raised intracranial pressure

cause of secondary hypertension is renal disease. Secondary hypertension should be suspected if onset of hypertension is at <35 years or >55 years of age, there is abrupt onset of severe hypertension at any age, diastolic hypertension in older adults and drug-resistant hypertension.

Office Blood Pressure Measurement

Blood pressure is measured with the help of a calibrated aneroid or hybrid auscultatory device as mercury sphygmomanometers are banned in most countries.
- BP should be measured in both arms and also in the lower limb. In coarctation of aorta, the arterial pressure in the upper limb is much higher than in the lower limbs.
- Patient should be sitting at ease.
- Cuff should be applied closely to the upper arm; it should not be loose or tight. The lower border of the cuff must be one inch (2.5 cm) above the cubital fossa.
  Neither patient nor staff should talk before, during and between measurements.
- The instrument should be placed at the same level as the cuff on the patient's arm and the observer's eye.
- The standard cuff width for adults is 12.5 cm. The size of cuff is also important since a small cuff may record false high blood pressure.
- The blood pressure must be recorded when the patient is resting quietly as anxiety, exertion, excitement, smoking and intake of coffee and tea within last half an hour will give rise to false readings.
- In elderly and patients on drugs (for hypertension) BP should be recorded in standing and lying down position to detect the occurrence of postural hypotension.

Initially the assessment of systolic BP is made by palpatory method. The radial or brachial artery is palpated while the cuff is inflated to raise pressure about 30 mmHg above the level at which radial/brachial pulse disappears. The stethoscope is placed over the brachial artery and cuff is deflated slowly. The level at which Korotkoff sounds appear (phase 1) is the systolic pressure and the level at which they disappear completely (phase 5) is the diastolic pressure. When the *pulse pressure* (the difference between systolic and diastolic blood pressure) is increased as in cases with hyperdynamic circulation (aortic regurgitation, pregnancy, thyrotoxicosis, anemia, arteriovenous fistula) the sounds may not disappear completely even at 0 level. In such cases the level at which sounds become suddenly muffled (phase 4) is taken as diastolic blood pressure.

The patient is said to be hypertensive if the systolic BP is >140 mmHg and/or diastolic BP is >90 mmHg **(Table 5.22)**. Sometimes the blood pressure recorded by the clinician at clinic or hospital is high while normal readings are obtained at home or when BP is measured under casual circumstances. This is known as *white coat hypertension* and is the result of the anxiety upon visiting a physician or a hospital.

Out-of-Office Blood Pressure Measurement (HBPM and ABPM)

Measurement of blood pressure by patients at home (HBPM) or with 24-hour ambulatory blood pressure monitoring (ABPM) are more closely associated with hypertension-induced organ damage and the risk of cardiovascular events. ABPM and HBPM more reproducible than office measurements, and identify the white coat and masked hypertension.

Out-of-office BP measurement is often necessary for the correct diagnosis of hypertension and for treatment decisions.

In patients having high-normal BP or grade 1 hypertension (systolic 130–159 mmHg and/or diastolic 85–99 mmHg) with office BP measurements, home or ambulatory BP monitoring is advised to confirm BP levels.

Home Blood Pressure Monitoring (HBPM)

It is done with validated electronic upper-arm cuff device (oscillometric) in the sitting position.

3–7-day monitoring in the morning (before drug intake if treated) and the evening is recommended before each visit to the hospital/health professional.

On each occasion after a 5 minutes rest two measurements should be taken at an interval of 1 minute between measurements.

Average home blood pressure ≥135 or 85 mmHg indicates hypertension **(Table 5.23)**.

In patients on treatment 1–2 measurements per week or month is recommended for long-term follow-up.

Ambulatory Blood Pressure Monitoring (ABPM)

ABPM is used to evaluate blood pressure variable using oscillometric methods over 24 hours periods with large number of measurements along with sleep measurement in patients own environment, representing a 'true' reflection of their BP. Modern ABPM devices are small, convenient, non-invasive and automated. It consists of an arm cuff, small monitor with a tube connecting cuff and monitor. At every 15–30 minutes BP is recorded over a period of at least 24 hours and reading are then analyzed using a computer **(Figs. 5.8 and 5.9)**. Multiple readings recorded by ABPM demonstrates the circadian pattern of BP (diurnal rhythmic changes including nocturnal dipping and morning surge) and BP variation with different environmental and emotional changes.

Ambulatory blood pressure monitoring (ABPM) provides superior and more precise assessment of the true BP than clinic BP. Currently clinical practice guidelines in Europe, North America, Australia and Asia recommends the use of ABPM for confirming the diagnosis of hypertension.

Thresholds for hypertension diagnosis based on ABPM: According to European Society of Hypertension (ESH) practice guidelines 24 hour mean SBP/DBP ≥130/80 mmHg, day time mean SBP/DBP ≥135/85 mmHg and night time

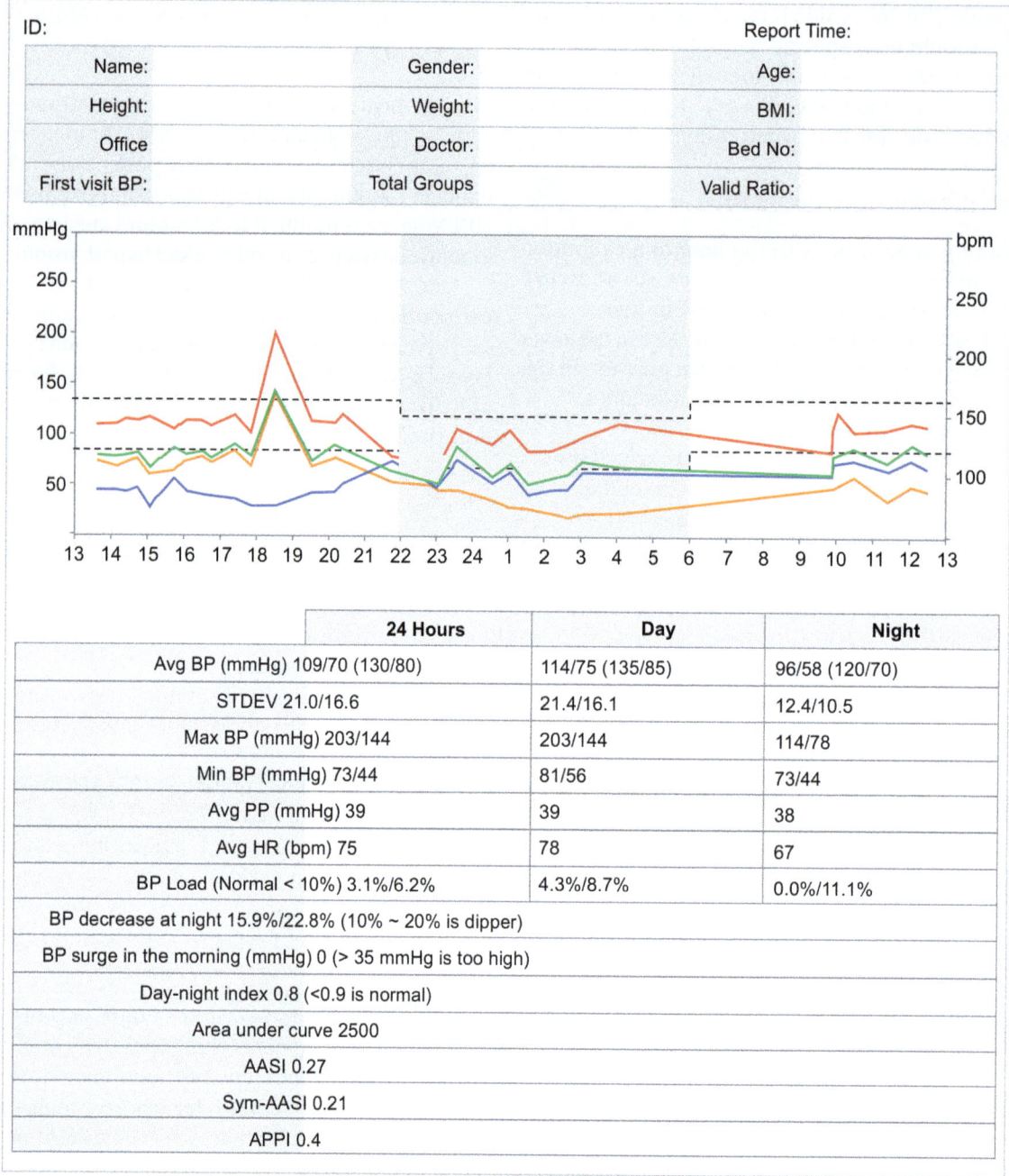

Fig. 5.8: ABPM recording.

mean SBP/DBP ≥120/70 mmHg is defined as hypertension (Table 5.23).

Patients with office BP <140/90 mmHg, 24 hours ABP <130/80 mmHg, Awake ABP <135/85 mmHg but sleep ABP ≥120/70 mmHg defined as 'Isolated nocturnal hypertension'. Night time BP elevation in patient on antihypertensive medications have a poor prognostic outcome in regards to cardiovascular complications.

Indications of ABPM:
- To confirm white coat hypertension
- To confirm masked hypertension
- To look for 24 hour BP patterns
- To assess the response of antihypertensive treatment.

Other situations where it may be useful:
- To measure BP variability
- Information regarding morning BP surge
- Obstructive sleep apnea
- Hypertension in children and adolescents, pregnancy, elderly and endocrine hypertension.
- To identify orthostatic or ambulatory hypotension.

ABPM in clinical practice: ABPM has a diagnostic, therapeutic and prognostic utility in clinical practice. It remains the gold standard test to diagnose hypertension including white coat, masked and nocturnal hypertension (Table 5.25). It also helps in starting antihypertensive treatment in patient with differential cardiovascular risks.

		ID:							Report time:	
		Name:			Gender:				Age:	
		Start time:			End time:				Duration	

	Date	Time	Sys	Dia	HR	MAP	PP	Posture*	Comment
1	12–10	13:35	110	74	78	80	36	S/S	Manual
3	12–10	14:06	112	69	78	79	43	S/M	
4	12–10	14:20	116	73	77	80	43	S/S	
5	12–10	14:41	115	77	80	83	38	S/S	
6	12–10	15:01	119	62	64	68	57	S/S	
9	12–10	15:41	107	66	88	88	41	S/M	
10	12–10	16:01	115	75	78	82	40	S/S	
12	12–10	16:27	115	80	75	85	35	S/S	
13	12–10	16:41	111	74	74	78	37	S/M	
16	12–10	17:20	121	86*	72	92	35	S/S	
18	12–10	17:47	104	71	66	80	33	S/M	
28	12–10	19:28	116	71	77	77	45	S/M	
32	12–10	20:07	114	79	78	92	35	S/S	
33	12–10	20:21	123	77	85	88	46	S/M	
40	12–10	21:42	81	56	104	67	25	S/M	
45	12–10	23:01	73	52	80	54	21	S/M	
46	12–10	23:32	109	78	80	91	31	S/M	
49	12–11	00:30	94	55	72	62	39	L/S	
50	12–11	01:00	108	66	66	74	42	L/M	
51	12–11	01:30	86	44	65	54	42	L/M	
53	12–11	02:06	87	48	61	59	39	L/M	
55	12–11	02:36	94	49	57	64	45	L/M	
56	12–11	03:00	101	66	60	76	35	L/S	
58	12–11	04:00	114	64	61	71	50	S/M	
67	12–11	09:51	84	61	81	63	23	S/M	Manual
68	12–11	09:52	105	73	80	81	32	S/S	Manual
69	12–11	10:00	124	73	83	83	51	S/M	
71	12–11	10:26	105	76	90	88	29	S/M	
76	12–11	11:21	107	66	70	74	41	S/M	
79	12–11	12:01	113	76	82	91	37	S/M	
81	12–11	12:26	110	68	78	83	42	S/M	

Fig. 5.9: ABPM recording.

Patterns of diurnal BP variation (identified by ABPM):
- **Diurnal index/ Dipping**: Dipping of BP during sleep is a common normal phenomenon. Nocturnal BP is 10–20% lower than awake BP or night/day systolic and diastolic BP ratio <0.9 and >0.8
- **Reduced dipping**: Nocturnal systolic or/and diastolic BP fall between 1–10% of daytime values or night/day systolic or/and diastolic BP ratio <1 and >0.9. It is associated with increase cardiovascular risk.
- **Non-dipping and rising**: No reduction in nocturnal BP or there is rise in nocturnal systolic and/or diastolic BP or night/day systolic or/and diastolic BP ratio ≥ 1. It is associated with increase in the cardiovascular risk.
- **Extreme dipping**: Marked nocturnal systolic or/and diastolic BP fall >20% of daytime systolic or/and diastolic values or night/day systolic or/and diastolic BP ratio <0.8. It has a debatable association with the cardiovascular risk.

White coat hypertension: An untreated individual with office BP >140/90 mmHg and 24 hours ABP <130/80 mmHg and Awake ABP <135/85 mmHg and Sleep ABP <120/70 mmHg or Home BP <135/85 mmHg. The term white coat hypertension should be restricted to individuals not on antihypertensive drugs.

Masked hypertension: An untreated individual with Office BP <140/90 mmHg and 24 hours ABP >130/80 mmHg

Table 5.25: Definition of clinical conditions.

Condition	Individuals' status	Office BP (mmHg)	24-hour ABP (mmHg)	Awake ABP (mmHg)	Sleep ABP (mmHg)	Home BP (mmHg)
White coat hypertension	Untreated	>140/90	<130/80	<135/80	<120/70	<135/85
Masked hypertension	Untreated	<140/90	>130/80	>135/80	>120/70	>135/85
Masked uncontrolled hypertension	Treated	<140/90	≥130/80	≥135/85	≥120/70	≥135/85
Isolated nocturnal hypertension	Untreated	<140/90	<130/80	<135/85	≥120/70	<135/85

and/or Awake ABP >135/85 mmHg and/or Sleep ABP >120/70 mmHg or Home BP >135/85 mmHg considered as masked hypertension. Based on ABP readings, more than 30% population with normal BP is diagnosed as masked hypertension. Masked hypertension is a strong predictor of cardiovascular morbidity and mortality and is associated with increased carotid intima-media thickness, LVM index and impaired large artery distensibility.

Patients who are on antihypertensive treatment, the term *Masked uncontrolled hypertension* is used which is defined as treated individuals with Office BP <140/90 mmHg and 24 hours ABP ≥130/80 mmHg and/or Awake ABP ≥135/85 mmHg and/or Sleep ABP ≥120/70 mmHg or Home BP ≥135/85 mmHg.

Effects of Hypertension on Target Organs

There is an increased chance of damage to the vascular bed of several organs mainly retina, heart, brain, kidneys and large arteries.
- *Retinal:* Retinal changes depend on the severity of hypertension. These are classified into four grades (grade I-IV) based on the presence of arteriolar thickening, nicking, hemorrhages, exudates and papilledema.
- *Cardiac:* These include left ventricular hypertrophy, pulmonary edema and high incidence of coronary artery disease.
- *Central nervous system* (CNS): Stroke (infarction and hemorrhage), transient ischemic attacks (TIA), hypertensive encephalopathy (coma, seizures) are important effects on CNS.
- *Renal:* Effect on kidneys consists of proteinuria and renal failure.
- *Large vessels:* Hypertension leads to accelerated atherosclerosis and aneurysmal dilatation.

Risk Factors

An evaluation of additional cardiovascular risk factors should be done in all hypertensive patients **(Table 5.26)**.

Assessment of overall cardiovascular risk should be done according to local guidelines/recommendations based on BP levels and additional risk factors.

Clinical Features
- The majority of patients asymptomatic and is diagnosed on routine clinical examination. However, symptoms due

Table 5.26: Cardiovascular risk factors.

Modifiable risk factors	Relatively fixed risk factors
Current cigarette smoking, second hand smoking	Family history
Diabetes mellitus	Increased age
Dyslipidemia	Male sex
Overweight/obesity	CKD
Physical inactivity/low fitness	Low socioeconomic status
Unhealthy diet	Obstructive sleep apnea
	Psychosocial stress

to raised blood pressure are occipital headache, dizziness, palpitation and fatigue.
- Patient may also present with symptoms related to target organ damage like epistaxis, hematuria, blurred vision, TIA, angina and breathlessness.
- Symptoms pertaining to underlying cause may be present; for example, weight gain (Cushing's syndrome), weight loss (thyrotoxicosis), episodic headache, palpitation and sweating (pheochromocytoma).

History: History must include age, sex, occupation, lifestyle of patient along with history of smoking, diabetes mellitus, hyperlipidemia, alcohol and drug intake and presence of hypertension in family members.

Physical examination: Presence of truncal obesity (Cushing's disease), palpable kidneys (polycystic kidneys), radio-femoral delay (coarctation of aorta), abdominal bruit (renovascular) may help in identifying the secondary cause of hypertension. The signs of complications of hypertension such as heaving apex, fourth heart sound, loud aortic second heart sound, pulmonary crackles and retinal changes may be present.

Investigations

There are some investigations which should be done in all patients with hypertension. Tests are performed to know the cause of hypertension, target organ damage and to detect cardiovascular risk factors. Special tests are performed in others as indicated **(Table 5.27)**.

Management

Hypertension is diagnosed when a systolic blood pressure in office or clinic is equal to or more than 140 mmHg and/or diastolic blood pressure is ≥90 mmHg on repeated

> **Table 5.27:** Investigations in patients with hypertension.
>
> **Basic investigations in all patients**
> - Urine analysis for protein, blood and glucose
> - Fasting blood sugar
> - Serum creatinine and blood urea nitrogen
> - Serum sodium and potassium
> - Serum lipid profile
> - Electrocardiography
>
> **Investigations in special group of patients**
> - Chest X-ray and echocardiography
> - Renal ultrasonography and angiography
> - Serum calcium and phosphate
> - Thyroid stimulating hormone (TSH)
> - Urinary cortisol and catecholamine
> - Plasma renin activity and aldosterone

examination. If on first visit BP is ≥180/110 mmHg and there is evidence of cardiovascular disease the diagnosis can be made on single visit and treatment can be started after the first set of readings.

The treatment of hypertension depends on:
- The level of blood pressure
- The presence of target organ damage
- The presence of cardiovascular risk factors (*see* **Table 5.26**)
- Presence of other disease [Coronary artery disease (CAD), stroke, CKD, HF, and COPD].

The management of hypertension includes general measures **(Table 5.28)** and drug therapy to control blood pressure to target levels and treatment of the other risk factors to reduce cardiovascular risk.

Office BP treatment targets: BP should be lowered to <140/90 mmHg in all patients but should be <130/80 mmHg in most patients. For patients >65 years, SBP goal 130–140 mmHg.

General measures (lifestyle modification):
- *Relief of stress:* Patients are advised to avoid unnecessary tension. Relaxation techniques may also be practised.
- *Salt restriction:* Dietary restriction of sodium chloride upto 6 gm per day reduces blood pressure in some hypertensive patients. Salt restriction also potentiates the effect of almost all antihypertensive agents. Diet rich in potassium and calcium may also be useful in hypertensive patients.
- *Weight reduction:* Caloric restriction in obese patients and weight reduction leads to decline in blood pressure.
- *Control of risk factors:* Restriction of cholesterol and saturated fat in diet reduces the atherosclerotic complications in hypertensive patients. Alcohol intake should be reduced whereas smoking should be stopped. The blood sugar level should be tightly controlled in diabetics.
- *Regular exercise:* Isotonic exercises like jogging and swimming lead to reduction in arterial pressure. Isometric exercises such as weight lifting should be avoided as these can increase arterial pressure. However, exercise should be planned under expert guidance.

Drug Therapy

Various classes of drugs used are given below. Commonly used drugs in each class are given in **Table 5.29**. Mechanism of action and side effects of antihypertensive drugs are given in **Table 5.30**.

- *Diuretics:* Thiazides are the most frequently used diuretics to treat hypertension. The side effects of thiazides such as hyperuricemia, hypertriglyceridemia and hypokalemia can be minimized by restricting the dose of hydrochlorothiazide to 25 mg per day. Recent guidelines recommend use of chlorthalidone. A combination of thiazide and potassium sparing agents (spironolactone, amiloride) may also be used. Loop diuretics (furosemide, torsamide) are used hypertensive crisis and renal failure.
- *ACE inhibitors and angiotensin receptor blockers (ARB):* Angiotensin converting enzyme inhibitors (enalapril, lisinopril, ramipril, perindopril) and ARB (losartan, telmisartan, valsartan) have good antihypertensive effect and cause significant reduction in death, acute MI and stroke. These agents also reduce the progression

Table 5.28: Lifestyle modifications for managing hypertension.

Modification	Recommendation	Approximate systolic blood pressure reduction (Range)
Weight reduction	Maintain normal body weight (body mass index, 18.5–24.9 kg/m²).	5–20 mmHg/10 kg (expect about 1 mmHg for every 1 kg reduction in body weight)
Adoption of DASH eating plan	Consume a diet rich in fruits, vegetables, low-fat dairy products, with reduced content of saturated and total fat.	8–14 mmHg
Dietary sodium reduction	Reduce dietary intake of sodium chloride to no more than 6 g (2.4 g sodium).	5–6 mmHg
Physical activity	Engage in regular aerobic physical activity such as brisk walking, jogging, cycling, swimming (at least 30 min/day, most days of the week). Resistance/strength exercises are also beneficial in reducing blood pressure and are recommended for 2–3 days in a week.	4–9 mmHg
Moderation of alcohol consumption	Limit daily consumption to no more than two drinks for most men and to no more than one drink for women and lighter weight persons.	2.5–4 mmHg
Tobacco	Total abstinence	-

(DASH: dietary approaches to stop hypertension)

Table 5.29: Commonly used antihypertensive agents.

Drug	Total daily dose (mg)	Frequency
Angiotensin-Converting Enzyme Inhibitors		
Ramipril	1.25–20	Once daily
Enalapril	2.5–40	Once daily
Captopril	50–450	Twice/thrice daily
Lisinopril	5–40	Once daily
Quinapril	5–80	Once daily
Perindopril	2–16	Once daily
Angiotensin II Receptor Blockers		
Losartan	25–100	Once daily
Telmisartan	20–80	Once daily
Olmesartan	20–40	Once daily
Valsartan	80–320	Once daily
Azilsartan	40–80	Once daily
Candesartan	8–32	Once daily
Irbesartan	150–300	Once daily
Direct Renin Inhibitor		
Aliskiren	150–300	Once daily
Calcium Channel Antagonists		
Non-dihydropyridine		
Amlodipine	2.5–10	Once daily
Nifedipine	30–120	Thrice a day
Nifedipine XL	30–90	Once daily
Dihydropyridine		
Diltiazem	90–360	Thrice a day
Diltiazem CD	120–480	Once daily
Verapamil	80–480	Thrice a day
Verapamil SR	120–480	Once daily
Diuretics		
Thiazides		
Hydrochlorothiazide	12.5–50	Once daily
Chlorthalidone	12.5–50	Once daily
Indapamide	1.25–5	Once daily
Metolazone	1.25–5	Once daily
Loop diuretics		
Furosemide	20–320	Once daily
Torsemide	5–20	Once daily
Bumetanide	0.5–5	Once daily
Potassium sparing diuretics		
Amiloride	5–10	Once daily
Triamterene	50–200	Twice daily
Spironolactone (Aldosterone antagonist)	25–100	Once daily
Eplerenone (Aldosterone antagonist)	25–100	Once daily
β-Adrenergic Antagonists		
Metoprolol	50–450	Twice daily
Metoprolol XL	50–400	Once daily
Bisoprolol	2.5–20	Once daily
Nebivolol	5–40	Once daily
Propranolol	40–240	Twice daily
Propranolol LA	60–240	Once daily
Labetalol*	200–1200	Twice daily
Carvedilol*	12.5–50	Twice daily
Carvedilol CR	10–80	Once daily
Atenolol	25–100	Once daily
α-Adrenergic Antagonists		
Prazosin	1–20	Twice/Thrice a day
Doxazosin	1–16	Once daily
Terazosin	1–20	Once daily bedtime
Centrally Acting Adrenergic Agents		
Methyldopa	250–2000	Twice/Thrice a day
Clonidine	0.1–1.2	Twice/Thrice a day
Direct-Acting Vasodilators		
Hydralazine	50–300	qid
Minoxidil	2.5–100	Once daily

*α- and β-antagonist properties
(qid: four times a day)

of nephropathy in type II diabetes. The main side effect of ACE inhibitors is cough and angioedema. ARBs have lesser side effects like cough and angioedema than ACE inhibitors. These drugs are contraindicated in bilateral renal artery stenosis and hyperkalemia.
- *Long acting calcium channel antagonist* (amlodipine) is particularly useful in elderly patients with isolated systolic hypertension. Other agents are less commonly used. These groups of drugs can cause pedal edema. Gum hyperplasia has also been reported with use of calcium channel blockers.
- *Beta adrenergic antagonists:* These agents lower heart rate and cardiac output. The cardioselective agents which are preferred include carvedilol, bisoprolol, nebivilol, and metaprolol. They are used with caution in patients with congestive heart failure, heart blocks and asthma, erectile dysfunction.
- *Other groups* of drug occasionally used in hypertension are:
  - Alpha adrenergic receptor blockers: Prazosin, doxazosin
  - Centrally acting agents: Clonidine, methyldopa
  - Vasodilators: Hydralazine, minoxidil
  - Agents with mixed alpha and beta adrenergic antagonist action: Labetalol, carvedilol.

Treatment Guidelines

- *High-normal BP:* Lifestyle modification should be advised **(Table 5.28)**. Drug therapy may be needed in case of presence of other cardiac risk factors or end organ damage.

Table 5.30: Mechanism of action and side effects of antihypertensive drugs.		
Drugs	Mechanism of action	Side effects
Beta adrenergic antagonists	Blockage of sympathetic effects on heart, decreased heart rate and cardiac output	Heart failure, heart blocks, bradycardia, Raynaud's phenomenon, impotence, may precipitate bronchospasm
Calcium channel blockers	Arterial vasodilatation	Pedal edema, flushing, headache, rash, tachycardia (nifedipine), gum hyperplasia
ACE inhibitors	Inhibits ACE and blocks the production of angiotensin II leading to arterial and venous dilatation	Dry cough, angioneurotic edema, hypotension, taste disturbance, hyperkalemia
ARBs	Block angiotensin receptors and cause vasodilatation	Angioedema, rash, hyperkalemia
Diuretics	Cause natriuresis and decrease intravascular volume, may result in mild vasodilatation	*Thiazide;* hyperglycemia, hypercalcemia, hyperlipidemia, hypokalemia and hyponatremia *Loop diuretics;* hypocalcemia, hypokalemia and deafness *K sparing;* gynecomastia, hyperkalemia

- *Hypertension:* In addition to lifestyle modification, drug therapy is indicated. BP should be lowered to <140/90 mmHg in all patients but should be <130/80 mm Hg in most patients (<140/80 in elderly patients). Recent guidelines recommend an ACE inhibitor or angiotensin-receptor blocker (ARB) or calcium-channel blocker (CCB) or thiazide-type diuretic as initial reasonable choices. Combination treatment is recommended for most hypertensive patients, as initial therapy.

It is recommended to initiate an antihypertensive treatment with a two drug combination, preferably in a single pill combination (SPC).

If BP is not controlled with a two-drug combination, treatment should be increased to a three-drug combination, usually a renin-angiotensin system (RAS) blocker + calcium channel blockers (CCB) + thiazide/thiazide-like diuretics, preferably as a SPC

The choice of drug also depends on the presence of co-existing conditions **(Table 5.31)**.

Surgery

Surgical intervention may be required in cases of pheochromocytoma and renal artery stenosis.

Resistant Hypertension

Resistant hypertension is defined as the failure to control blood pressure in patients with maximum doses of three drugs in combination (including a diuretic). In such a case identifiable causes of hypertension must be excluded (chronic kidney disease, aldosterone excess, sleep apnea, renal artery stenosis or coarctation of aorta).

Spironolactone (aldosterone receptor blocker) 25 mg/day is useful in resistant hypertension when added to current therapy as aldosterone may play an important role in resistant hypertension. Renal denervation therapy (radiofrequency ablation of renal sympathetic nerves) may also be effective in resistant hypertension. Stimulation of carotid baroreceptors has also been found to be effective in resistant hypertension.

Hypertensive Crisis

Hypertensive crisis includes hypertensive urgencies and emergencies.

Hypertensive urgencies is defined as substantial increases in blood pressure usually with systolic >220 mmHg or diastolic >120–130 mmHg. It also includes hypertension with disk edema, progressive end organ complications rather

Table 5.31: Choice of antihypertensive drugs and BP goal in various co-existing conditions.			
HTN associated condition	Target BP	Preferred drug	Special comments
Diabetes mellitus (DM)	<130/80 mmHg (<140/80 in elderly patients)	RAAS inhibitor (ACEi/ARBs), CCBs	Monitor for hyperkalemia with RAAS inhibitors
Coronary artery disease (CAD)	<130/80 mmHg (<140/80 in elderly patients)	RAAS blockers (ACEi/ARBs), β-blockers (irrespective of BP)	
Heart failure (HF)	<130/80 mmHg (<140/80 in elderly patients)	RAAS blockers (ACEi/ARBs) or ARNI (sacubitril-valsartan), β-blockers, Diuretics	CCBs are indicated in case of poor BP control
Chronic obstructive pulmonary disease (COPD)	<130/80 mmHg (<140/80 in elderly patients)	CCBs, ARBs	β-blockers should be avoided but β1 selective β-blockers may be used in selected patients (e.g. with CAD, HF)
Pregnancy (Eclampsia and severe preeclampsia)	Immediate reduce SBP <160 mmHg and/or DBP <105 mmHg	IV Labetalol or IV Nicardipine, Methyldopa, CCBs	
Prostatism	<130/80 mmHg (<140/80 in elderly patients)	Alpha blockers	Watch for postural hypotension

(RAAS: renin angiotensin aldosterone inhibitors; ACEi: angiotensinogen converting enzyme inhibitors; ARBs: angiotensin receptor blockers; CCBs: calcium channel blockers)

than damage and severe perioperative hypertension. In this situation, BP must be reduced in several hours. Parenteral therapy is usually not needed.

Hypertensive emergencies include hypertensive encephalopathy, hypertensive nephropathy, intracranial hemorrhage, unstable angina, myocardial infarction, acute left ventricular failure with pulmonary edema, aortic dissection and eclampsia. Malignant hypertension is characterized by nephropathy or encephalopathy with accompanying papilledema.

Control of blood pressure is vital for preventing ongoing end organ damage. Rapidly acting parenteral agents are used. Excessive and rapid decline in the BP should be avoided as it may lead to cerebral hypoperfusion and coronary insufficiency. The goal is to attain a decline of 20-25% in the mean arterial pressure or a diastolic pressure of 110 mmHg. Thereafter, the reduction in blood pressure is attained gradually over several days. The parenteral drugs used are nitroprusside, nitroglycerine, dizoxide, esmolol, labetalol, enalaprilat and hydralazine **(Table 5.32)**. Intravenous frusemide is given as an adjunct. *Sublingual nifedipine should be avoided* in the acute management because it is associated with adverse cardiac events.

ISCHEMIC HEART DISEASE/ CORONARY ARTERY DISEASE

Ischemic heart disease (IHD)/Coronary artery disease (CAD) is the most common cause of premature death.

Table 5.32: Recommended doses of common parenteral agents used for treatment of HT.

Agent	Dose	Comments
Labetalol	IV bolus, 20–80 mg every 5–10 min, upto 300 mg	IV infusion 0.5–2/min until desired BP is obtained
Nicardipine	5 mg/h IV by slow infusion	Titrate up by 2.5 mg/h every 5–15 min (maximum 15 mg/h)
Clevidipine	IV infusion, 1–2 mg/h IV	Titrate by doubling the dose every 2–5 min (maximum 21 mg/h)
Hydralazine	IV bolus, 10–20 mg IV/IM	Repeat after 20 min (maximum 40 mg)
Enalaprilat	1 mg IV bolus over 5 min	Repeat every 6 hours
Sodium Nitroprusside	IV infusion, 0.3–10 mcg/kg/minute	Not to exceed 10 mcg/kg/min
Esmolol	IV bolus, 0.25 – 0.5 mg/kg over 1 minute	Followed by 0.05–0.1 mg/kg/min IV for 4 minutes (maximum dose 300 mcg/kg/min)
Nitroglycerine	IV infusion, 5–250 mcg/minute	Tolerance develops with prolonged use
Methyldopa (for treatment of eclampsia)	IV bolus, 250–500 mg	May lead to hypotension

Table 5.33: Clinical presentations of coronary artery disease/ischemic heart disease.

- Stable angina
- Acute coronary syndromes (ACS)
  - Unstable angina
  - Non-ST segment elevation myocardial infarction (NSTEMI)
  - ST segment elevation myocardial infarction (STEMI)
- Heart failure
- Arrhythmias
- Sudden cardiac death
- Asymptomatic

Table 5.34: Causes of ischemic heart disease.

- Atherosclerosis of coronary arteries
- Spasm of coronary artery
- Vasculitis involving coronary artery
- Emboli
- Congenital anomalies of coronary arteries

The incidence of IHD is increasing worldwide. Ischemia is defined as the lack of oxygen due to reduced perfusion. IHD occurs when there is an imbalance between oxygen supply and oxygen demand. Its spectrum ranges from angina (chronic stable and unstable) to myocardial infarction (Non-ST elevation myocardial infarction/ST elevation myocardial infarction). Clinical presentations of IHD are given in **Table 5.33**.

Causes

The most common cause of IHD is atherosclerosis of coronary arteries. Other less common causes of reduced coronary blood flow are spasm of coronary artery, vasculitis, emboli and congenital abnormalities of coronary artery **(Table 5.34)**.

Pathogenesis of Coronary Atherosclerosis

Atherosclerosis starts in second or third decade of life. The collection of lipoproteins within intimal layer of the coronary artery is the initial event. These lipoproteins undergo modification into oxidized LDL and subsequently are taken up by migrated monocytes in the intima (foam cells). Most foam cells die and result in formation of a lipid rich center. This necrotic area is surrounded by smooth muscle cells which lay down extracellular matrix that forms the bulk of the advance atheromatous lesion (atheromatous plaque or atheroma). Monocyte-mediated cytokines also play an important role in the evolution of the atheromatous plaque. The risk factors for atherosclerosis/cardiovascular disease are given in **Table 5.35**.

The ischemic heart disease can clinically manifest as:
- Angina pectoris (stable or unstable)
- Myocardial infarction
- Arrhythmias
- Heart failure
- Sudden death.

Table 5.35: Important risk factors for atherosclerosis.

- Smoking
- Hypertension
- Lipid disorders (High LDL cholesterol, low HDL cholesterol)
- Diabetes mellitus
- Family history of IHD
- Age (men >45 years, women >55 years)
- Male sex
- Sedentary lifestyle
- Obesity
- Atherogenic diet

Newer risk factors
- Homocysteine
- Lipoprotein (a)

Table 5.36: Characteristics of chest pain in stable angina.

Site of the pain	Retrosternal or precordial
Character of the pain	Squeezing, constricting, piercing, feeling of heaviness or pressure
Precipitating factors	Physical exertion, cold exposure, heavy meals, emotional stress, anemia, thyroid disease, vivid dreams (nocturnal angina)
Associated features	Feeling of impending death, breathlessness, apprehension, nausea, vomiting
Relieving factors	Rest, sublingual nitroglycerine
Radiation	Left shoulder, both arms, jaw, neck
Duration	Typically 2–10 minutes (>30 minutes suggests infarction)

STABLE ANGINA

Stable angina results from transient myocardial ischemia arising because of imbalance between myocardial oxygen supply and demand. The reduced perfusion results from fixed 'stable' obstruction due to atheroma of the coronary arteries **(Fig. 5.10)**.

Clinical Features

- The term angina, derived from Greek language means choking or strangulation.
- Stable angina is characterized by central chest pain or discomfort or heaviness classically precipitated by exertion or stress and relieved by rest. The detailed characteristics of pain are given in **Table 5.36**.
- The diabetics and elderly may present with breathlessness, fatigue and faintness rather than chest pain. Symptoms other than chest pain are known as *anginal equivalents*.
- The physical signs are generally normal. The patient may have signs of cardiomegaly, mitral regurgitation, pulmonary edema and third (S3) or fourth (S4) heart sound (gallop rhythm).
- Evidences of risk factors like hypertension, diabetes mellitus and atherosclerosis (carotid bruit, diminished arterial pulse) may be present. Anemia and thyrotoxicosis may precipitate anginal pain in patients with IHD.

Typical angina: When all the three features are present:
1. Substernal chest discomfort with a characteristic quality and duration.
2. Provoked by stress or exertion.
3. Relieved by rest or nitroglycerine.

Atypical angina: When two of these three features are present.
Noncardiac chest pain: When only one or none of these features is present.

Investigations

Electrocardiogram (ECG)

The ECG changes are present only in around half of the cases. Reversible ST segment depression or elevation with or without T wave inversion during chest pain is specific finding in stable angina.

- *Stress Testing*
  - Exercise ECG: This is used to diagnose IHD and to estimate the prognosis. The ECG is done on a treadmill protocol wherein the recording is made during and after exercise. The symptoms like chest pain, fatigue, breathlessness and changes in ST segment and blood pressure are noted.
  - Myocardial perfusion scanning: The uptake of radioactive thallium 201 or technetium 99m by myocardium is measured during and after exercise or pharmacological stress. This is used in patients who cannot exercise or the results of exercise ECG are inconclusive.
  - Stress echocardiography: This can be used alternatively to diagnose IHD in place of perfusion scanning. Exercise or pharmacological stress may cause the changes in myocardial contraction. The advantage is greater convenience, easily availability and the lower cost.

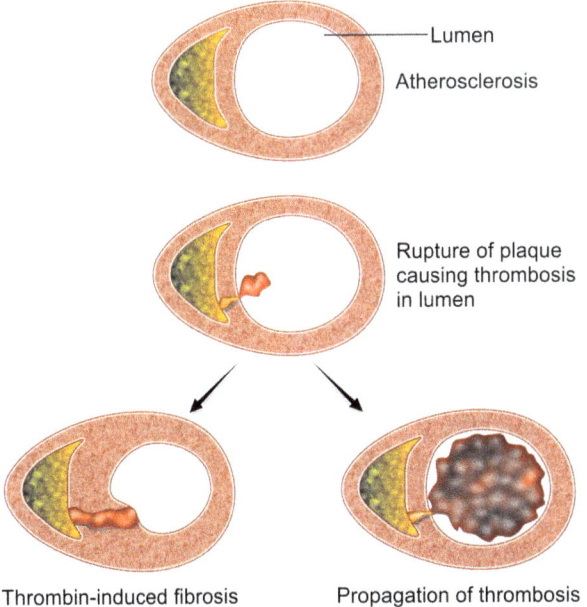

Fig. 5.10: Atheromatous plaque.

- *Coronary arteriography:* It provides information about the severity and extent of coronary artery disease and is useful when other tests have failed to diagnose IHD. This is also indicated in patients who despite medical therapy are symptomatic and may need revascularization.
- Serum lipid profile and plasma glucose are done to diagnose risk factors.

Treatment

The treatment of stable angina includes:
- Medical treatment
- Coronary revascularization
- Identification and control of risk factors
- Education and reassurance.

Medical Treatment

- *Antiplatelet agents*: Low dose aspirin (75–325 mg daily) reduces coronary events in patients of IHD. Aspirin inhibits platelet cyclo-oxygenase irreversibly. Clopidogrel 75 mg daily can be used in place of aspirin if patients develop GI bleeding, allergy, or dyspepsia due to aspirin.
- *Nitrates*: Nitrates cause coronary vasodilatation, thus increasing the myocardial oxygen supply. They also reduce the myocardial oxygen demand by decreasing the preload and afterload on the heart. Nitroglycerine 0.4 to 0.6 mg is given sublingually for acute relief of the anginal pain. For long-term therapy, isosorbide dinitrate (10–20 mg 8 hrly) or isosorbide mononitrate (20–60 mg once or twice daily) is given orally. Nitroglycerine ointment or transdermal patches are also available. It causes headache, light-headedness, black-outs (postural hypotension) and is contraindicated in patients with low blood pressure.
- *Beta blockers*: These reduce myocardial oxygen demand by decreasing heart rate, blood pressure and myocardial contractility. Atenolol (upto 100 mg daily), metoprolol (upto 200 mg daily) and Bisprolol (5–10 mg daily) are commonly used beta blockers. These should be avoided in presence of bradycardia, severe bronchospasm, significant atrioventricular block and uncompensated heart failure.
- *Calcium antagonists*: They reduce arterial pressure and myocardial contractility and cause coronary vasodilatation. These are useful in situations where beta blockers are contraindicated, ineffective or poorly tolerated. Commonly used agents are verapamil, diltiazem, sustained release nifedipine and amlodipine.
- *Ranolazine:* This drug has been recently approved by FDA for use in chronic angina patients. This can be used as first line agent or in patients who are symptomatic despite adequate antianginal therapy. Increase in intracellular sodium concentration in ischemic cardiac monocytes cause calcium overload via the Na+-Ca++ exchanger leading to contractile dysfunction and cellular injury. Ranolazine is piperazine derivative and it acts by inhibiting pathologically enhanced lateral inward sodium current thus preventing sodium overload of ischemic monocytes. This leads to decrease calcium overload via the Na+-Ca++ exchanger and attenuates the accompanying deleterious consequences. It thus minimizes diastolic tension and increases coronary nutrient flow as compression of intramyocardial arterioles is decreased. This drug can be classified as cytoprotective. This is given in the doses of 500–1000 mg per day in two divided doses.
- *Nicorandil:* This is potassium channel opener and given 20 mg BD. It leads reduction of free intracellular Ca++ ions through opening of potassium channels.

Coronary Revascularization

Percutaneous transluminal coronary angioplasty (PTCA): A wire is passed across coronary narrowing under radiographic control and the stenosed part is dilated with the balloon. A metallic stent is placed to maintain maximum dilatation and prevent restenosis. PTCA offers better control of symptoms than medical therapy in patients with chronic stable angina. However, there is no evidence that PTCA improves survival. The most common indication of PTCA in chronic stable angina is the presence of evidence of ischemia during stress test despite medical therapy.

Coronary artery bypass grating (CABG): Internal mammary artery, radial artery or saphenous vein is used as a graft to bypass the obstructive lesion in the coronary artery. The indications for CABG are left main coronary stenosis, two-vessel or three-vessel disease with left ventricular dysfunction, and patients with diabetes mellitus.

Identification and Control of Risk Factors

- Cessation of smoking
- Control of blood pressure
- Control of blood sugar
- Treatment of hyperlipidemia
- Control of weight
- Regular exercise (20 to 30 minutes daily).

UNSTABLE ANGINA

Presently, unstable angina (UA), non-ST segment elevation myocardial infarction (NSTEMI) and myocardial infarction with ST segment elevation (STEMI) are included in a group called *acute coronary syndromes (ACS)*.

UA is defined as angina pectoris or equivalent ischemic discomfort with at least one of three features:
1. It occurs at rest (or with minimal exertion), usually lasting >10 minutes.
2. It is severe and of new onset (i.e., within the prior 4–6 weeks), and/or
3. It occurs with a crescendo pattern (i.e., distinctly more severe, prolonged, or frequent than previously).

The diagnosis of NSTEMI is established if a patient with the clinical features of UA develops evidence of myocardial necrosis, as reflected in elevated cardiac biomarkers [Troponin T and I, Creatine kinase (CK), CK-MB].

Pathophysiology of Unstable Angina

There is rupture or fissuring of coronary artery atheromatous plaque leading to formation of thrombus and acute reduction in the coronary blood flow. This may also be accompanied with coronary artery spasm. The angina due to vasospasm not associated with atheroma is termed as *Prinzmetal's angina*.

The obstruction in the coronary blood flow may progress, hence UA or NSTEMI may evolve into STEMI.

Investigations

- *ECG*: The ECG in patients with UA shows ST segment depression and T wave inversion without a rise in cardiac isoenzymes like creatine kinase MB (CK-MB) or troponin. Prinzmetal's angina is characterized by ST segment elevation.
- *Cardiac markers of necrosis*: NSTEMI is diagnosed when the features of UA are also associated with increased cardiac isoenzymes, i.e., markers of cardiac necrosis.
- *C-reactive protein (CRP)*: CRP levels may aid in initial risk assessment in ACS patients. Increased levels of CRP in ACS are associated with poor prognosis and recurrent cardiac events.

Treatment

The mainstay of treatment of UA/NSTEMI includes following points. Various drugs used in ACS are given in **Table 5.37**.
- Bed rest and supplemental oxygen
- Antiplatelet therapy **(Table 5.38)**
- Anti-ischemic therapy **(Table 5.39)**
- Anticoagulant therapy **(Table 5.40)**
- Risk stratification and revascularization
- Control of risk factors.

- *Bed rest:* The patient should be hospitalized and put on bed rest. Continuous ECG monitoring is done. Supplemental oxygen is given, when oxygen saturation is <90%. Morphine can be used for pain relief.
- *Antiplatelet therapy*: Aspirin and/or clopidogrel are given in the dosage as mentioned in the case of stable angina. Intravenous GpIIb/IIIa inhibitors (Abciximab, Eptifibatide, Tirofiban) are indicated in high risk patients.
- *Anti-ischemic therapy*: It provides pain relief and prevents recurrence of chest pain.
  - *Nitrates* should be given sublingually or by buccal spray. If pain persists, intravenous nitroglycerine is initiated.
  - Initially beta blocker (metoprolol) is given intravenously. Later oral preparations of beta blocker (metoprolol, atenolol) are continued.
  - *Calcium channel blockers* (verapamil, diltiazem) are added when there is inadequate response to

Table 5.37: Drugs used in acute coronary syndromes.

- Antiplatelet therapy
  - Oral
    » Aspirin
    » Clopidogrel
    » Ticagrelor
    » Prasugrel
  - Intravenous
    » Glycoprotein IIB/IIIA inhibitors
    » Abciximab
    » Eptifibatide
    » Tirofiban
    » Cangrelor
- Anti-ischemic therapy/analgesia
  - Nitrates
    » Nitroglycerine
    » Isosorbide dinitrate
    » Isosorbide monotrate
  - Beta blockers
    » Atenolol
    » Metoprolol
    » Esmolol
    » Bisoprolol
    » Nebivolol
    » Carvedilol
  - Calcium channel blockers
    » Amlodipine
    » Diltiazem
    » Verapamil
  - Morphine sulphate
- Heparins (antithrombotics)
  - Unfractionated heparin
  - Low molecular weight heparin, e.g. enoxaparin
  - Fondaparinux
  - Bivalirudin
- Thrombolytic therapy (STEMI only)
  - Streptokinase
  - Alteplase (Recombinant tissue-plasminogen activator, rt-PA)
  - Tenecteplase (TNK-tPA)
  - Reteplase (r-PA)
- Prevention of ventricular remodelling
  - Ramipril
  - Captopril
  - Enalapril
- Plaque stabilization therapy : HMG–CoA reductase inhibitors
  - Atorvastatin
  - Simvastatin
  - Rosuvastatin

Table 5.38: Doses of antiplatelet agents.

Antiplatelet therapy
Oral

Aspirin	162–325 mg initial, then 75–100 mg daily
Clopidogrel	300–600 mg loading dose, 75 mg daily
Ticagrelor	180 mg loading dose then 90 mg bid
Prasugrel	60 mg loading dose, 10 mg daily

Intravenous

Glycoprotein IIB/IIIA inhibitors

Abciximab	0.25 mg/kg bolus, 10 µg/min
Eptifibatide	180 µg /kg bolus, 2 µg/kg/min
Tirofiban	0.4 µg /kg bolus, 0.1 µg/kg/min
Cangrelor	30 µg /kg bolus, 4 µg/kg/min

Table 5.39: Anti-ischemic therapy/analgesia.

Nitrates
• Nitroglycerine	0.4 mg sublingual, 10–200 µg/min IV
• Isosorbide dinitrate	5–40 mg tid
• Isosorbide mononitrate	10–20 mg bid
• Transdermal nitroglycerine patch	5–15 mg daily
• Nitroglycerine daily	0.5–2.0 inch tid

Beta blockers
• Atenolol	50–200 mg daily
• Metoprolol	25–100 mg orally bd
• Esmolol	50–300 µg/kg per minute IV
• Bisoprolol	10–20 mg daily
• Nebivolol	5–40 mg daily
• Carvedilol	3.125–25 mg bid

Calcium channel blockers
• Amlodipine	5–10 mg daily
• Nifedipine	30–180 mg daily
• Diltiazem	Immediate release 30–90 mg daily, Slow release 120–360 mg daily
• Verapamil	Immediate release 80–160 mg daily, Slow release 120–480 mg daily
Morphine sulphate	2–4 mg IV

Table 5.40: Anticoagulants.

Unfractionated heparin	60 units/kg bolus (Max. 4000 U), 12–14 units/kg per hour
Low molecular weight heparin, e.g., enoxaparin	1 mg/kg SC bid
Fondaparinux	2.5 mg SC daily
Bivalirudin	0.75 mg/kg bolus, 1.75 mg/kg per hour

beta blockers and nitrates. Calcium antagonists are also useful in cases where beta blockers are contraindicated.

– *Statins (atorvastatin) and angiotensin converting enzyme (ACE) inhibitors* are given for long-term secondary prevention.

- *Anticoagulant therapy*: Heparin should be given either as intravenous unfractionated heparin (UFH) or subcutaneous low molecular weight heparin (LMWH). Treatment with UFH requires monitoring of PTT (partial thromboplastin time) for adjustment of the dose.
- *Risk stratification*: Based on clinical features, ECG findings and changes in cardiac enzymes, patients are stratified into low and high risk groups. High risk patients are subjected to coronary arteriography and subsequent PTCA or CABG. Low risk patients should undergo early stress test to ascertain the need for angiography.

ACUTE MYOCARDIAL INFARCTION OR STEMI

Acute MI results due to formation of occlusive coronary thrombus on ruptured atheromatous plaque. The prolonged ischemia leads to myocardial necrosis. As opposed to NSTEMI (where there is subendocardial ischemia), there is transmural ischemia in STEMI. The ischemic chest pain is the most common presenting symptom, which is generally:
- Severe, longer lasting (>30 minutes) and may not respond to sublingual nitroglycerine.
- Pain may be absent in diabetics, hypertensive, postoperative and elderly individuals (*silent MI*).
- Other clinical features include marked sweating, breathlessness, nausea, vomiting, syncope and collapse.
- Sudden death may occur due to ventricular arrhythmias or asystole.

General examination may reveal pallor, sweating, tachycardia or bradycardia, breathlessness, mild fever, hypotension, cold peripheries, raised jugular venous pressure and restlessness. Third or fourth heart sounds, murmur of mitral regurgitation, pericardial friction rub may be found on cardiac examination. The presence of crackles (crepts) in lungs suggests left ventricular failure.

Investigations

- *Electrocardiography:* Initially ST segment is elevated and T wave may be tall. Later on, size of R wave diminishes and Q wave develops **(Figs. 5.11 to 5.13)**. Subsequently, T wave become inverted. Finally ST-T wave normalizes while Q wave persists. Arrhythmia may also be present. Right sided leads are required in diagnosis of right ventricular infarction.
- *Cardiac markers*: Intracellular cardiac enzymes and proteins are released into plasma due to myocardial necrosis. Serial estimation to detect the change in the levels of plasma CPK-MB and troponin T and troponin I are most useful for the diagnosis of MI. Troponin T and troponin I increase 3–12 hours after the onset of MI, peak at 24–48 hours, and return to baseline over 5–14 days. Serum CK-MB levels increase 3–12 hours after onset of MI, peak in 24 hours and return to baseline in 48–72 hours.

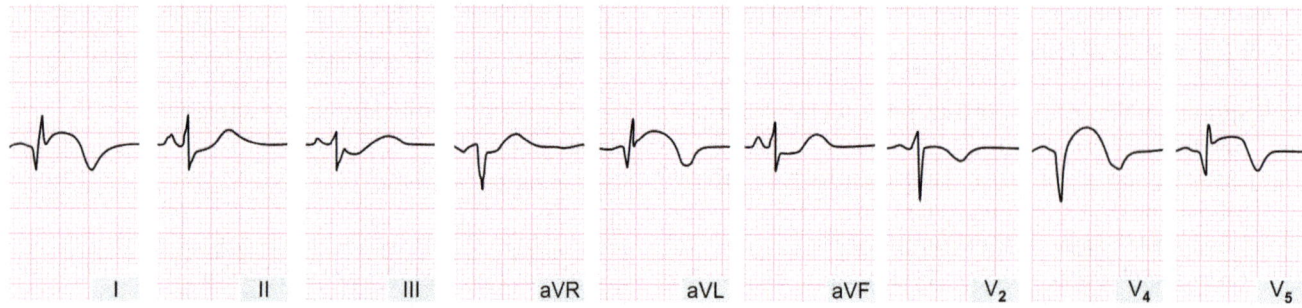

Fig. 5.11: ECG of lateral wall myocardial infarction (early or hyperacute) showing ST segment elevation in leads I, aVL, V4 and V6.

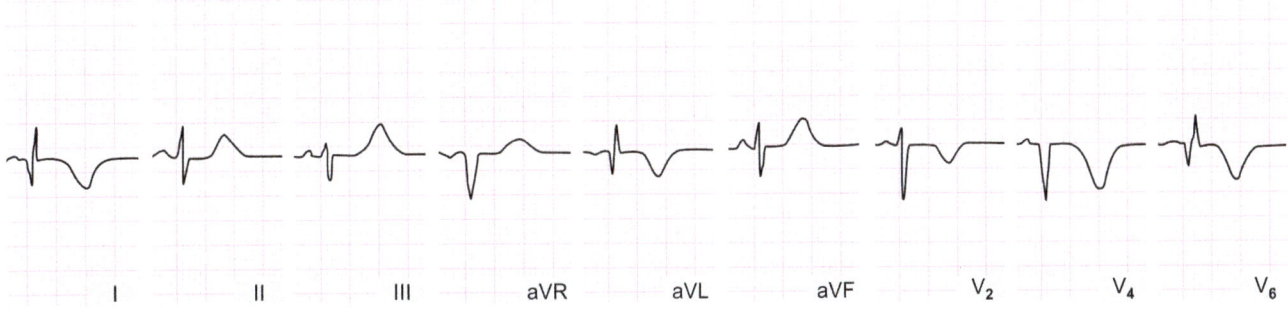

Fig. 5.12: ECG of lateral wall myocardial infarction (recent) showing Q waves and prominent T wave inversion in leads I, aVL, V4 and V6.

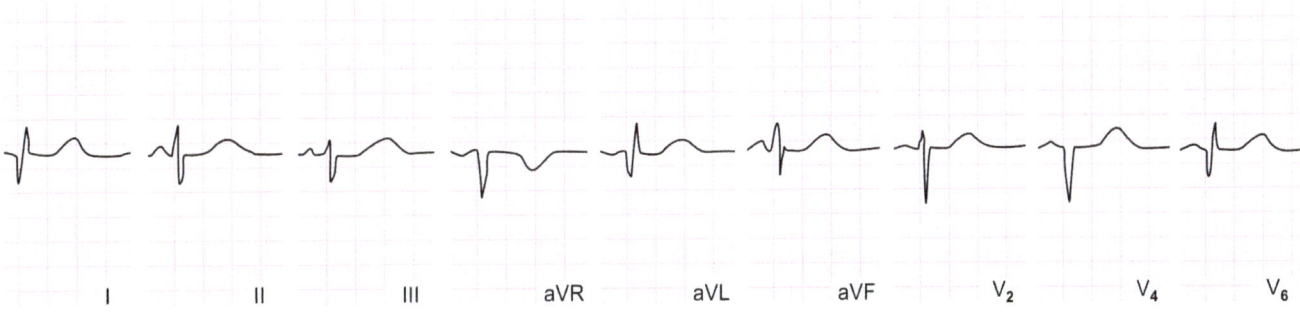

Fig. 5.13: ECG of lateral wall myocardial infarction (old) showing Q waves in leads I, aVL, V4 and V6.

- *Echocardiography*: This is helpful in the detection of wall motion abnormalities, left ventricular dysfunction and other complications such as pericardial effusion, mitral regurgitation, ventricular septal defect and left ventricular thrombus.
- *Other tests*: Chest X-ray may reveal pulmonary edema. Leukocytosis, raised ESR and CRP can also be present. Lipid profile, serum electrolytes, urea and creatinine are also measured.

Management

- *Hospitalization*: Patient should be hospitalized in coronary care unit (CCU) with facilities of continuous ECG monitoring and defibrillator as promptly as possible since many patients die within the first 24 hours of onset of symptoms of MI and over half occur within first hour due to ventricular fibrillation. Patient should be confined to bedrest.
- *Oxygen therapy*: Oxygen is administered, if hypoxemia is present (Oxygen saturation <90%).
- *Antiplatelet agents*: Aspirin (nonenteric coated) in the dosage of 160–325 mg should be given to the patient to chew. Later aspirin is continued in the dosage of 75–162 mg orally daily. Clopidogrel (300 mg loading dose followed by 75 mg/day) can be used if there is allergy or intolerance to aspirin.
- *Relief of pain*:
  – Sublingual nitroglycerine (0.4 mg) is given for pain relief. This may be given at interval of 5 minutes. Intravenous nitroglycerine is started if pain reoccurs or there is associated hypertension.
  – *Morphine* also can be used for pain relief (2–4 mg IV).
  – Intravenous beta blockers such as metoprolol are also helpful for pain relief followed by daily oral therapy.
- *Reperfusion therapy*: This is the mainstay of treatment in STEMI, given to restore the flow in the infarct related artery and to limit the infarct size **(Table 5.41)**.
  – Fibrinolytic agent like streptokinase or tPA (tissue plasminogen activator) is given through intravenous infusion. Alternatively, reteplase or tenecteplase can be administered as bolus (Bolus fibrinolytics). It should be administered as soon as possible. However, it can be useful if given within 6 hours of presentation. The contraindications are history of cerebrovascular accident, severe hypertension and evidence of active internal bleeding. Bleeding is the most frequent side effect of fibrinolytic therapy. Streptokinase can result in hypersensitivity reaction.
  – Primary percutaneous intervention (PCI): Primary percutaneous intervention (Angioplasty, stenting) is expensive and available at select centers. It can be done upto 12 hours or maximum upto 24 hours of symptom onset. When performed by experienced operators it appears to be more effective than fibrinolysis. This can also be performed in case of

Table 5.41: Thrombolytic therapy (STEMI only).	
Streptokinase	1.5 million units IV over 60 min
Alteplase (Recombinant tissue-plasminogen activator, rt-PA)	0.75 mg/kg over 30 min (Max 50 mg), 0.50 mg/kg over 60 min (Max 35 mg)
Tenecteplase (TNK-tPA)	0.5 mg/kg IV bolus (Total dose 30–50 mg)
Reteplase (r-PA)	10 units IV bolus stat and after 30 min

contraindication or failure of fibrinolytic therapy (rescue PCI).
- *Anticoagulant therapy*: Unfractionated heparin as intravenous infusion or low molecular weight heparin as subcutaneous inj. is given to maintain the patency of infarct related artery.
- *3-Hydroxy-3-methylglutaryl-coenzyme A (HMG-CoA) reductase inhibitors (statins)*: Patients with ACS should be given statins (high intensity) within 24 hours of presentation **(Table 5.42)**. Statins are powerful lipid-lowering agents. They also have anti-inflammatory and atherosclerotic plaque-stabilizing effects (pleotropic effects) and have been shown to reduce recurrent ischemia, myocardial infarction and death in patients of atherosclerotic ischemic heart disease.

  A lipid profile should be done in all patients. Statin therapy is given to reduce LDL <70 mg/dL. If LDL remains >70 mg % with use of statins, ezetimibe or PCSK9 inhibitor is given.
- *PCSK9-inhibitors*: Proprotein convertase subtilisin/kexin type 9 enzyme binds to low-density lipoprotein receptors and stops LDL being removed from the blood, leading to an increase in LDL in blood. PCSK9 inhibitors (alirocumab and evolocumab) bind to PCSK9 and inactivate PCSK9 in the liver. It increases the availability of LDL receptors on liver cell surface. LDL receptors transport LDL inside the liver for metabolism. They are given as injections.
- *ACE inhibitors are given to prevent ventricular remodeling*. This is continued indefinitely in patients with hypertension or heart failure **(Table 5.43)**. These are contraindicated in patients with hyperkalemia.
- *Diuretics*: Important part of management in patients, who develop heart failure. Spironolactone is particularly useful (if no contraindication like hyperkalemia) in patients with left ventricular ejection fraction less than 40%.
- *Other measures*: Patients are on bed rest for at least 12 hours. Gradually, the activity is increased depending on the tolerance. Liquid diet is started when chest pain subsides. Later on, low fat, high fiber diet is prescribed. Laxatives are given to relieve constipation. Sedative (diazepam, lorazepam) is generally given for proper sleep.
- *Risk stratification*: Patients are stratified into low and high risk groups depending on presence of persistent ischemia, heart failure and symptomatic ventricular arrhythmias. High risk patients are subjected to coronary angiography and subsequent PTCA or CABG. Low risk patients should undergo early stress test to ascertain the need for angiography.

Secondary prevention: The secondary prevention of MI includes long-term administration of dual anti-platelet therapy (aspirin and clopidogrel), beta blockers, ACE inhibitors, control of risk factors like cessation of smoking, statin therapy for hyperlipidemia, control of blood pressure and blood sugar, weight reduction in obese and regular exercise. Oral anticoagulants may be required in some cases.

Complications of MI

The complications include:
- Arrhythmia: Ventricular fibrillation is the major cause of early death in MI. Other common arrhythmias are atrial fibrillation and heart blocks.
- Pump failure or cardiogenic shock where more than 40% myocardium is damaged. This is an important cause of in-hospital mortality.
- Recurrent ischemia or chest pain
- Pericarditis, Dressler's syndrome
- Thromboembolism
- Ventricular remodeling
- Left ventricular aneurysm
- Mechanical complications like ventricular rupture and cardiac tamponade, mitral regurgitation and rupture of interventricular septum.

HEART FAILURE

Heart failure (HF) is a clinical syndrome in which the heart is unable to pump adequate amount of blood to meet the metabolic demands of the body. Abnormality in cardiac structure or function may be responsible for the inability of heart to pump blood adequately.

HF may be due to abnormalities in myocardial contraction (systolic dysfunction), relaxation and filling (diastolic dysfunction), or both.

Left ventricular (LV) ejection fraction (EF) is used to subdivide HF patients into groups for therapeutic and prognostic purposes. These groups are:
- EF <40%: HF with reduced EF (HFrEF)
- EF 40%–50%: HF with borderline EF
- EF >50%: HF with preserved EF (HFpEF)

Table 5.42: Doses of HMG–COA reductase inhibitors (Statins).

High intensity	Moderate intensity	Low intensity
Reduce LDL cholesterol by ≥50%	Reduce LDL cholesterol by 30% to 50%	Reduce LDL cholesterol by <30%
Atorvastatin 40–80 mg Rosuvastatin 20–40 mg	Atorvastatin 10–20 mg Rosuvastatin 5–10 mg Simvastatin 20–40 mg Pravastatin 40–80 mg Lovastatin 40 mg Fluvastatin XL 80 mg Fluvastatin 40 mg twice daily Pitavastatin 2–4 mg	Simvastatin 10 mg Pravastatin 10–20 mg Lovastatin 20 mg Fluvastatin 20–40 mg Pitavastatin 1 mg

Table 5.43: Drugs for prevention of ventricular remodeling.

Ramipril	5–20 mg
Enalapril	2.5–20 mg

Causes

Heart failure generally occurs due to defect in the myocardial contractility. Ischemic heart disease and cardiomyopathy are the most common causes of HF. Causes of HF are listed in detail in **Tables 5.44 and 5.45**.

Precipitating Factors

In certain situations, the load over an already burdened myocardium is suddenly increased leading to HF. Important precipitating causes are infection, arrhythmias, myocardial ischemia, anemia, excessive physical exertion, drugs like beta blockers and NSAIDs, emotional stress and fluid over load. Pregnancy thyrotoxicosis and accelerated hypertension may also precipitate HF.

Pathophysiology

The pump failure leads to low cardiac output, which activates counter-regulatory neurohormonal mechanisms such as:
- Activation of renin angiotensin aldosterone system (RAAS)
- Stimulation of sympathetic system
- Increased vasopressin secretion.

The net effects of these mechanisms are sodium and fluid retention and vasoconstriction. These tend to improve cardiac output; however, these are also responsible for various manifestations of heart failure due to systemic and pulmonary congestion. Natriuretic peptides are released from the stretched myocytes and mediate vasodilatation, diuresis and sodium loss.

Table 5.44: Important causes of heart failure.
- Ischemic heart disease
- Cardiomyopathy
- Myocarditis
- Valvular heart disease
- Hypertensive heart disease
- Congenital heart disease
- Infective endocarditis
- Pulmonary embolism
- Constrictive pericarditis
- High output states (chronic anemia, thyrotoxicosis, beri beri, arteriovenous fistula)
- Cor pulmonale
- Chronic bradyarrhythmia, chronic tachyarrhythmias

Table 5.45: Causes of heart failure with preserved ejection fraction >40–50%.
- Ischemic heart disease
- Hypertrophic cardiomyopathy
- Hypertension
- Restrictive cardiomyopathy (sarcoidosis, amyloidosis)
- Hemochromatosis
- Fibrosis
- Aging
- Endomyocardial diseases

Symptoms and Signs

Symptoms and signs in CHF are due to:
- Heart failure *per se*
- Underlying causes of heart failure
- Precipitating factor.

Clinical features of heart failure are given in **Tables 5.46 and 5.47**. Mechanisms underlying clinical features are given in **Table 5.48**.

Symptoms of HF mainly arise due to increased pulmonary and systemic venous and capillary pressure and reduced cardiac output. The important symptoms are dyspnea, orthopnea, paroxysmal nocturnal dyspnea, weakness and fatigue, edema and abdominal pain.

Dyspnea is the most important symptom and is multifactorial in origin. The most important mechanism of dyspnea is accumulation of interstitial and alveolar fluid due to increased pulmonary capillary pressure. Initially, the dyspnea occurs only during exertion. Later on, as the disease progresses, the patient is dyspneic even on rest.

- Patients may feel dyspneic in the recumbent position (orthopnea) due to increased venous return to heart and elevation of the diaphragm. The dyspnea is usually relieved by sitting upright.
- There may be episodic severe breathlessness and cough which awaken the patient from sleep (*paroxysmal nocturnal dyspnea*).

Table 5.46: Symptoms of heart failure.
- Dyspnea (breathlessness)
- Orthopnea
- Paroxysmal nocturnal dyspnea
- Fatigue and weakness
- Pink frothy sputum (Acute pulmonary edema)
- Right upper quadrant abdominal pain (Congestion of liver)
- Anorexia, nausea, early satiety (due to edema of intestine)
- Confusion, memory impairment, disorientation (reduced cerebral perfusion)

Table 5.47: Signs of heart failure.

General physical examination
- Tachycardia, Pulsus alternans
- Elevated jugular venous pressure (JVP)
- Bilateral, pitting pedal edema/sacral edema
- Cyanosis of nail bed and lips
- Cold extremities
- Weight loss (cardiac cachexia)

Abdomen
- Tender hepatomegaly
- Ascites

Pulmonary
- Pulmonary rales (crackles, crepitations)
- Wheezing (cardiac asthma)
- Pleural effusion

Cardiac
- Cardiomegaly
- Third heart sounds (S_3)
- Murmurs of mitral and tricuspid regurgitation

Table 5.48: Clinical features of heart failure.

Due to increased preload
Increased systemic venous pressure (right heart failure)
- Raised JVP
- Tender hepatomegaly
- Edema
- Ascites, pleural effusion*

Increased pulmonary venous pressure (left heart failure)
- Dyspnea, orthopnea, PND
- Hemoptysis (pink frothy sputum)
- Central cyanosis
- Crackles on auscultation
- Pleural effusion*

Due to decreased cardiac output and increased afterload
- Cold clammy skin
- Peripheral cyanosis
- Fatigue
- Cardiac cachexia

Due to decreased cardiac contractility
- Ventricular dilatation (cardiomegaly)
- Third heart sound (S_3)
- Pulsus alternans

Arrhythmias
- Sinus tachycardia

*Pleural effusion occurs when both pulmonary and systemic venous pressure are raised

- In its severe form, there is intense bronchospasm and wheeze, a condition known as *cardiac asthma*.
- *Acute pulmonary edema* is a severe form of cardiac asthma wherein the patient has alveolar edema and expectoration of blood-tinged sputum.

Low cardiac output leads to poor effort tolerance, fatigue and weakness. Confusion, lack of concentration, memory impairment, headache and insomnia may occur particularly in elderly patients. There may also be a reduced urine output.

Patients may also have dependent edema in the lower limbs. Edema in the sacral region occurs in bedridden patients. Congestion of liver and portal venous system leads to pain in the abdomen, nausea, anorexia and malabsorption. There may be marked weight loss in severe chronic HF *(cardiac cachexia)*.

The findings on general physical examination in patients with HF include cold extremities, tachycardia, pulsus alternans, hypotension, cyanosis of lips and nail beds, increased jugular venous pressure, pitting edema and tender hepatomegaly. *Pulsus alternans* is regular pulse with regular alteration in pulse amplitude (alternate low and large volume pulse), and is a sign of severe heart failure.

Lung examination reveals inspiratory rales (crepitations) over the bases. In severe cases with pulmonary edema, coarse rales and wheezes all over lung fields are found (cardiac asthma). Third and fourth heart sounds are often heard. Sometimes, patients may exhibit signs of pleural effusion and/or ascites.

Types of Heart Failure

Heart failure has been classified in several ways:
- *Acute or chronic heart failure*: Acute HF occurs suddenly as in massive MI and acute infective endocarditis. Chronic HF presents slowly in conditions like valvular heart disease and cardiomyopathy. Chronic HF may be of the compensated or uncompensated type.
- *Right or left or biventricular heart failure*:
  - Left heart failure: Dysfunction of left ventricles (left ventricular failure) may lead to pulmonary congestion (increased pulmonary venous pressure) that may present as dyspnea, orthopnea, paroxysmal nocturnal dyspnea and crackles in lungs **(Table 5.49)**. The important causes of LVF are rheumatic valvular heart disease (AR, MR, AS), myocardial infarction, cardiomyopathy and hypertension.
  - Right heart failure: Right ventricular failure (RVF) presents in the form of systemic congestion presenting as tender hepatomegaly, raised JVP, pedal edema **(Table 5.50)**. RVF can occur secondary to LVF due to its effects on pulmonary circulation (raised pulmonary arterial pressure). Other important causes of RVF are cor pulmonale (right ventricular enlargement secondary to lung diseases), pulmonary embolism and pulmonary stenosis. Pulmonary congestion is uncommon. Subsequently both ventricular chambers may be affected (biventricular heart failure).
- *Forward or backward heart failure*: The cardiac output is primarily inadequate in forward failure whereas backward failure is characterized by marked salt and water retention causing systemic and pulmonary venous congestion.
- *Systolic or diastolic heart failure*: Heart failure due to impaired myocardial contraction is called systolic HF while failure of ventricle to relax and fill normally is called diastolic HF. The causes of diastolic HF are constrictive pericarditis, restrictive cardiomyopathy and ischemic heart disease.
- *High output or low output heart failure*: High output heart failure occurs in patients with hyperthyroidism, anemia, pregnancy, AV fistula and beri beri. Low cardiac output failure occurs in Ischemic heart disease, hypertension, cardiomyopathy, valvular and pericardial disease.

Table 5.49: Clinical features of left heart failure.

Symptoms
- Dyspnea
- Orthopnea
- Paroxysmal nocturnal dyspnea (PND)
- Acute pulmonary edema

Signs
- Pulmonary rales (crackles, crepitations)
- Third heart sound
- Pulsus alternans
- Pleural effusion

Table 5.50: Clinical features of right heart failure.

- Raised jugular venous pressure (JVP)
- Tender hepatomegaly
- Bilateral pitting pedal edema
- Ascites
- Pleural effusion

Investigations

Investigations are carried out to detect the cause, nature and severity of the HF.
- **Blood tests:** The blood tests generally include hemoglobin, blood urea, electrolytes and thyroid function tests. X-ray chest may reveal cardiomegaly and pulmonary congestion.
- **ECG:** Electrocardiography may show arrhythmia and signs of chamber enlargement.
- **Echocardiography:** Echocardiography is very helpful in knowing about the cause of HF, the type of cardiac dysfunction (systolic or diastolic) and the presence of valvular abnormalities.
- **Brain natriuretic peptide (BNP):** Recently measurement of *brain natriuretic peptide (BNP)* has been shown to be a highly sensitive and specific test for the diagnosis, prognosis and monitoring of the HF. High BNP level can differentiate cardiac asthma from the dyspnea of pulmonary origin.

Treatment

The treatment of HF includes:
- Correction of the underlying cause
- Removal of the precipitating factors
- Control of congestive heart failure.

The treatment of heart failure with preserved ejection fraction (HFpEF) is to control fluid overload with diuretics and correction of reversible factors (hypertension, tachycardias, pericardial diseases). None of the drug has been shown to improve survival in patients with HFpEF.

The treatment of patients with heart failure with reduced ejection fraction (HFrEF) reduces death and hospitalization and prevents sudden cardiac death.

Correction of Precipitating Factors

Precipitating factors in patients with underlying heart disease should be searched and corrected. Some important factors are:
- Excessive salt and fluid intake
- Excessive activity
- Arrhythmias
- Infections
- Anemia
- Pulmonary embolism
- Noncompliance in therapy
- Myocardial ischemia
- Drugs (beta blockers, NSAIDs).

Control of Heart Failure

Control of HF can be achieved by general measures and drug therapy.
- *General measures:*
  - Reduced physical exertion lowers myocardial oxygen demand and thus controls failure. Absolute bed rest may be needed in severe heart failure. In stable patients, regular isotonic exercises are advised.
  - The salt intake is reduced to half of the normal or even less than 2 g per day in some cases.
  - Weight loss in obese patients is also helpful in controlling heart failure.
- *Drug therapy:* Drugs may help in HF by reducing preload and afterload and improving myocardial contractility. This can be achieved generally with the help of more than one class of drugs **(Tables 5.51 and 5.52)**.
  - *Diuretics:* Diuretics lead to increased urinary sodium excretion and reduction in plasma volume. This lowers the preload to the heart.
    » Thiazide diuretics can be used alone in mild HF and in combination with other class of diuretics in severe HF.
    » Loop diuretics are given in severe HF and in cases with renal impairment. Intravenous frusemide causes venodilatation and is useful in acute pulmonary edema.
    » Potassium sparing agents are often used in combination with other diuretics to minimize hypokalemia. Spironolactone in low dosage (25 mg daily) and eplerenone have been shown to improve morbidity and mortality in advanced HF.

    Mineralocorticoid receptor antagonists (MRAs) prevents aldosterone mediated sodium retention. MRAs also reduce vascular reactivity, oxidant stress, inflammation, and fibrosis. Spironolactone is nonselective aldosterone receptor antagonist. Eplerenone is a selective aldosterone receptor antagonist and has no estrogenic side effects of spironolactone.

    MRAs are recommended for use in patients with NYHA class II–IV HF.

Table 5.51: Drugs used in heart failure.

Diuretics
- Thiazide: Chlorthiazide, metolazone
- Loop diuretics: Frusemide, bumetanide, torsemide
- Potassium sparing: Spironolactone, eplerenone, amiloride, triamterene

Vasodilators
Oral:
- ACE inhibitors: Ramipril, enalapril, lisinopril
- ARBs: Losartan, valsartan
- Angiotensin receptor- Neprilysin inhibitor: Sacubitril/Valsartan
- Isosorbide dinitrate
- Hydralazine

Parenteral:
- Sodium nitroprusside
- Nitroglycerine
- Nesiritide (recombinant natriuretic peptide, rBNP)

Inotropic agents
- Digitalis
- Sympathomimetic amines: Dopamine, dobutamine
- Phosphodiesterase inhibitors: Amrinone, milrinone

Beta blockers
- Metoprolol, carvedilol, bisoprolol

Table 5.52: Doses of drugs used in heart failure (HFrEF).

Drug	Usual Initial Dose	Maximum Dose
Angiotensin-Converting Enzyme (ACE) Inhibitors		
Captopril	6.25 tid	50 mg tid
Enalapril	2.5 mg bid	10 mg bid
Fosinopril	5–10 mg od/bid	20 mg daily
Lisinopril	2.5–5.0 mg od	20–30 mg
Quinapril	2.5–5.0 mg bid	10 mg bid
Ramipril	1.25–2.5 mg bid	5 mg bid
Trandolapril	0.5–1.0 mg daily	4 mg daily
Angiotensin Receptor Blockers (ARB)		
Valsartan	40 mg bid	160 mg bid
Losartan	25 mg od/bid	150 mg daily
Irbesartan	75–150 mg daily	300 mg daily
Candesartan	4 mg daily	32 mg daily
Olmesartan	20 mg daily	40 mg daily
Angiotensin Receptor-Neprilysin Inhibitor		
Sacubitril/Valsartan	24/26 mg bid	97/103 mg bid
I_f Channel Inhibitor		
Ivabradine	5 mg bid	7.5 mg bid
Diuretics		
Thiazide Diuretics		
HCTZ	25–50 mg daily	25–50 mg daily
Metolazone	2.5–5.0 mg od or bid	10–20 mg
Loop Diuretics		
Furosemide	20–40 mg od or bid	400 mg
Torsemide	10–20 mg od or bid	200 mg
Bumetanide	0.5–1.0 mg od or bid	10 mg total
Aldosterone Antagonists		
Spironolactone	12.5–25.0 mg daily	25 mg daily
Eplerenone	25 mg daily	50 mg daily
β-Blockers		
Metoprolol succinate	12.5–25.0 mg daily	200 mg daily
Bisoprolol	1.25 mg daily	10 mg daily
Carvedilol	3.125 mg bid	25 mg bid
Digoxin	0.125–0.25 mg daily	0.125–0.25 mg

MRAs (Spironolactone and Eplerenone) have been shown to improve survival and decrease hospitalizations in patients with severe heart failure with low EF and following acute myocardial infarction (MI).

Monitoring of serum potassium is required as life-threatening hyperkalemia may occur with the use of these agents particularly when used with ACE inhibitors. Spironolactone use may cause gynecomastia 10–20% in men (10–20%).

– *Vasodilators:* Activation of renin-angiotensin-aldosterone system (RAAS), adrenergic nervous system and increased secretion of vasopressin cause vasoconstriction and salt and fluid retention. Vasodilators help in HF as they reduce preload and afterload through venodilatation and arterial dilatation respectively.
  » ACE inhibitors improve exercise tolerance and reduce morbidity and mortality in patients with HF. They also prevent the onset of failure in patients with left ventricular dysfunction.
  » Angiotensin II receptor blockers (ARB) are equally effective as ACE inhibitors and have less incidence of cough.
  » Nitrates and hydralazine are also useful for chronic oral administration.
  » Intravenous nitroglycerine, sodium nitroprusside or nesiritide (recombinant BNP) is indicated in acute severe HF.

Sacubitril/valsartan: Sacubitril is neurolysin inhibitor is a neutral endopeptidase is responsible for breakdown of vasoactive peptides (natriuretic peptides, bradykinin, and adrenomedullin). Sacubitril increases the availability of these peptides, which exert favourable effects in HF.

This combination has been shown to improve symptoms and reduce mortality in patients of heart failure. This combination is approved for use in patients with reduced ejection fraction (HFrEF) and NYHA class II–IV symptoms who are already tolerant to ACE inhibitors or ARBs. It causes more angioedema as compared with ACE inhibitors.

– *Ionotropic agents:* They improve myocardial contractility. Various types of ionotropic agents include:
  » Digitalis: Digitalis relieves symptoms of HF and is particularly indicated in patients of HF with atrial flutter or fibrillation.
  » Sympathomimetic amines (Dopamine, dobutamine): Sympathomimetic amines like intravenous infusion of dopamine or dobutamine are useful in acute severe HF.
  » Phosphodiesterase inhibitors (amrinone, milrinone): Amrinone and milrinone (phosphodiesterase inhibitors) also have vasodilator properties and are used alone or together with sympathomimetic amines in severe refractory HF.

d. *Beta blockers:* Metoprolol, carvedilol and bisoprolol are shown to improve symptoms of HF and survival in patients with moderate to severe HF if added to other group of drugs. They also prevent arrhythmias. These agents act by counteracting the adverse effects of enhanced adrenergic stimulation. Beta blockers are started in low dosage initially and the dose is increased gradually with care.

e. *Ivabradine* is an inhibitor of the I_f channel and reduces sinus rate. Use of ivabradine in patients with reduced ejection fraction (EF) has been shown to reduce hospitalization and death in patients with heart failure. It is indicated in patients with EF < 35%

and heart rate ≥70 bpm and taking β-blockers at the highest tolerated dose. It is given to patients with sinus rhythm and not indicated in patients with atrial fibrillation.

3. *Other measures:*
   - *Anticoagulant therapy*: Anticoagulant therapy is given to patients with heart failure and atrial fibrillation or to patients with severe heart failure to prevent thromboembolism.
   - *Antiarrhythmic therapy*: Amiadarone is given to control ventricular arrhythmias.
   - *Pacing*: Biventricular pacing resynchronizes the cardiac contraction and improves the performance in severe heart failure with conduction abnormalities.
   - *Circulatory support*: Mechanical circulatory support like intra-aortic balloon pump is helpful in intractable cases.
   - *Cardiac transplantation*: Cardiac transplantation is considered in patients with refractory severe end stage heart failure.

ACUTE PULMONARY EDEMA (CARDIOGENIC)

Acute pulmonary edema is characterized by the accumulation of fluid in the pulmonary interstitium and alveoli due to increase in the pulmonary venous and capillary hydrostatic pressure. The lungs become less compliant, airways resistance increases and the capillary-alveolar gas exchange is compromised.

Non-cardiac pulmonary edema is characterized by high venous and capillary permeability with low hydrostatic pressure.

Causes

Pulmonary edema can primarily be due to cardiac cause or of noncardiac etiology. The important cardiac causes of acute pulmonary edema are left ventricular failure (acute MI, acute MR and acute AR) and mitral stenosis. The noncardiac causes of pulmonary edema are listed in **Table 5.53**.

Clinical Presentations

There is rapid onset of dyspnea, cough, anxiety and restlessness. The dyspnea is more on lying down and sitting upright may provide some relief. Additionally, patients may have excessive sweating and cyanosis. The sputum may be profuse, pink, frothy or blood stained. The examination may reveal cold extremities, tachycardia and tachypnea with prominent use of accessory muscles of respiration, hypotension. There are extensive rales (crackles, crepitations) and wheezes on lung auscultation. Cardiac examination will reveal findings of underlying heart disease.

Investigations

- The chest X-ray may reveal cardiomegaly and signs of pulmonary edema (prominent interstitial and hilar shadows, Kerley B lines, pleural effusion).
- Echocardiography may help in differentiating cardiac from noncardiac causes by identifying systolic and diastolic ventricular dysfunction and valvular lesions.
- A rise in serum brain natriuretic peptide (BNP) level favors acute left ventricular failure as a cause of pulmonary edema.

Management of Cardiogenic Pulmonary Edema

Acute pulmonary edema is a life-threatening condition and needs prompt management.

Initial Supports

- Oxygen is administered to improve hypoxia. In severe cases, positive pressure ventilation may be needed.
- Patient is placed in sitting posture.

Drug Therapy

- *Intravenous morphine* (2–4 mg) is given to relieve anxiety. It also reduces preload through venodilation and thus reduces dyspnea. This can be repeated if needed.
- *Frusemide* (20–80 mg IV) offers rapid improvement in dyspnea by decreasing pulmonary congestion through its venodilator effect prior to causing diuresis. Hence, it is the diuretic of choice in acute pulmonary edema.
3. *Intravenous nitroglycerine* is also helpful, particularly in cases of ischemic heart disease. Nitroglycerine decreases preload to heart as it is a venodilator. It is contraindicated if there is hypotension. Nitroprusside infusion is indicated in cases of acute pulmonary edema associated with hypertension.
4. *Ionotropic agents* (dopamine, dobutamine) and phosphodiesterase inhibitors (amrinone, milrinone) stimulate myocardial contractility and are useful in patients with hypotension or shock.
5. Intravenous recombinant *BNP* is a potent vasodilator with diuretic properties. It is also effective in acute pulmonary edema.
6. *Hemodialysis* may be needed in patients with severe renal failure.

Table 5.53: Noncardiogenic pulmonary edema.

- Acute respiratory distress syndrome (ARDS)
  - Infections
  - Inhaled toxins
  - Aspiration of gastric contents
  - Disseminated intravascular coagulation
  - Acute pancreatitis
  - Multiple trauma
  - Anaphylaxis
- High altitude
- Narcotic overdose

Correction of Precipitating Factors

The precipitating factors of acute pulmonary edema such as severe hypertension, IHD, arrhythmias, volume overload should be adequately managed.

CONGENITAL HEART DISEASE

Congenital heart disease (CHD) may present in early childhood or may remain asymptomatic till adult life. Its incidence is around 1% of live birth. Congenital abnormalities are due to multifactorial environmental and genetic causes. Rubella infection in mother is associated with patent ductus arteriosus (PDA) and pulmonary artery stenosis. Maternal lupus erythematosus is linked with congenital complete heart block. Use of drugs or toxins (alcohol) during pregnancy can also lead to CHD. Chromosomal abnormalities such as Turner's syndrome and Down's syndrome are associated with coarctation of aorta and septal defects respectively.

Classification

CHD may present with cyanosis or without cyanosis. Overall the most common CHD is ventricular septal defect (VSD) whereas the most common cyanotic heart disease is tetralogy of Fallot. This anomaly can occur in isolation or in combination. The classification of CHD is given in **Table 5.54**.

Ventricular Septal Defect

Ventricular septal defect (VSD) is the most common type of CHD. There is incomplete septation of the ventricles. The defect is most commonly present at the junction of membranous and muscular portion of the interventricular septum. VSD can occur alone or can be accompanied by other defects like aortic regurgitation.

The septal defect allows blood to shunt from left ventricle (high pressure) to right ventricle (low pressure). The right ventricular volume is increased as it receives blood from right atrium (RA) as well as from left ventricle (LV). Hence, the pulmonary flow is increased which in turn leads to an increase in the volume of left atrium (LA) and LV. The increased blood flow and obstructive structural changes in the pulmonary vascular bed result in the increase in pulmonary arterial pressure (pulmonary hypertension).

Pulmonary hypertension can in turn lead to elevated right ventricle (RV) pressure and reversal of shunt (right to left) as the pressure in RV exceeds that of LV. This condition is known as *Eisenmenger syndrome*. Central cyanosis and digital clubbing may also develop.

Clinical Features

The small VSD is generally asymptomatic whereas symptoms of heart failure (fatigue and dyspnea) occur in large VSD. There is an increased incidence of respiratory infection. In advanced cases, cyanosis and digital clubbing appear due to reversal of shunt. There is a pansystolic murmur best heard at left sternal border in smaller VSD (*Maladie de Roger's* murmur). However, the murmur is softer in large VSD as the RV pressure is elevated.

Investigations

Echocardiography is used to detect the location and size of the VSD. The ECG may show biventricular hypertrophy and chest X-ray reveals pulmonary plethora (prominent pulmonary vascular markings).

Treatment

- Small defects should be watched as they may close spontaneously. Surgery is indicated in larger defects.
- Eisenmenger syndrome is a contraindication for surgery where the only option is heart-lung transplantation.
- In VSD, there is a moderate risk of developing infective endocarditis. Hence, endocarditis prophylaxis is mandatory before any procedure.

Atrial Septal Defect

Atrial septal defect (ASD) occurs more commonly in females. The commonest type of ASD is *ostium secundum*. Other types are *ostium primum* and *sinus venosus*. Atrial septal defect may be accompanied by mitral stenosis (*Lutembacher's syndrome*).

A large amount of blood shunts from LA to RA. The right ventricular volume and pulmonary flow are increased which may lead to pulmonary hypertension. The pulmonary hypertension can in turn lead to elevated RV pressure and reversal of shunt (right to left) as pressure in RV exceeds that of LV. This condition is known as *Eisenmenger syndrome*.

Table 5.54: The classification of congenital heart disease.

- **Acyanotic**
  - Left to right shunt
    » Ventricular septal defect (VSD)
    » Atrial septal defect (ASD)
    » Patent ductus arteriosus (PDA)
  - Without shunt
    » Bicuspid aortic valve
    » Coarctation of aorta
    » Congenital aortic stenosis
    » Pulmonary stenosis
    » Congenital mitral stenosis
- **Cyanotic**
  - Increased pulmonary blood flow
    » Complete transposition of great arteries
    » Total anomalous pulmonary venous connection
  - Normal or decreased blood flow
    » Tetralogy of Fallot
    » Tricuspid atresia
    » Pulmonary atresia
- **Others**
  - Dextrocardia
  - Congenital complete heart block

Clinical Manifestations

ASD is generally asymptomatic in early life. However, there is an increased tendency for recurrent respiratory infection. Later during the fourth or fifth decade, it may present as atrial fibrillation, heart failure and Eisenmenger syndrome. Important clinical signs include wide and fixed splitting of second heart sound and a systolic flow murmur over the pulmonary area.

Investigations

Echocardiography is used to detect the location and size of the ASD. The ECG may show incomplete right bundle branch block. Chest X-ray reveals pulmonary plethora and enlargement of the heart.

Treatment

- Large ASD is closed surgically. Eisenmenger syndrome is a contraindication for surgery.
- Isolated secundum lesion has a low risk of developing infective endocarditis, hence prophylaxis is generally not needed.

Patent Ductus Arteriosus (PDA)

In fetal life, the blood from the pulmonary artery does not go to lungs but flows into the aorta through a communication, ductus arteriosus. However, the ductus closes soon after the birth as the blood from pulmonary artery goes to lungs. In some, the ductus fails to close, a condition known as PDA. This is more common in females and is sometimes associated with other congenital abnormalities.

In PDA, the blood flows from high pressure (aorta) to low pressure (pulmonary artery) side, resulting in left to right shunt. Pulmonary artery pressure rises with the rise in pulmonary vascular resistance. As the pressure in pulmonary artery exceeds that of aorta, right to left shunting occurs, the blood flow reverses *(Eisenmenger syndrome)*. This leads to cyanosis, more in the feet than in upper part of the body, also called *differential cyanosis*.

Clinical Manifestations

Patients with small shunt are generally asymptomatic for years. However, there may be retarded growth and development in children with large shunt. With the onset of cardiac failure, the patients develop dyspnea. The arterial pulse is generally high volume. Cardiac finding includes a *continuous 'machinery' murmur* in the left second intercostal space often with a thrill. In advanced cases, P_2 becomes loud and the murmur is shortened. Patients develop cyanosis and features of right heart failure *(Eisenmenger syndrome)*.

Investigations

The echocardiography is used to detect the location and size of the PDA. The ECG may show evidence of RV hypertrophy. Chest X-ray reveals pulmonary plethora and enlargement of heart.

Management

The large PDA is occluded with an implantable device in infancy before pulmonary hypertension develops. However, surgery in small PDA is indicated to reduce the chance of endocarditis but may be delayed until later childhood.

A prostaglandin synthetase inhibitor (ibuprofen or indomethacin) may induce closure in the first week of life if there is no intrinsic abnormality of ductus.

Coarctation of Aorta

Congenital narrowing of aorta (coarctation) occurs most commonly just below the origin of left subclavian artery. "Acquired" coarctation of aorta may result due to trauma or arteritis (Takayasu's disease). This is more common in males and may be associated with other congenital anomalies like bicuspid aortic valve and "berry aneurysms" of cerebral arteries.

Clinical Features

- If severe, it may cause heart failure in the newborn.
- In adults, headache may occur because of hypertension. Blood pressure is raised in upper extremities (in vessels above narrowing) but is normal or low in lower limbs.
- Lower extremities are less developed due to decreased blood supply. Weakness and cramps may occur in lower limbs. On examination, lower limbs are cold and arterial pulsations are weak. Femoral pulsations are delayed in comparison to radial pulse (radiofemoral delay).
- Systolic murmur may be present over the area of narrowing and beat is heard posteriorly.
- Bicuspid valve may cause systolic murmur in aortic area.
- Collateral vessels are well developed on chest and back (involving periscapular, intercostals and internal mammary arteries). Bruit may be heard over collaterals.
- Rupture of "berry aneurysm" may cause cerebral hemorrhage.
- Dissection of aorta and infective endocarditis are other complications.

Investigations

ECG may show LVH. Chest X-ray reveals dilated ascending aorta and indentation at the site of coarctation (the "3" sign). Notching of ribs due to collaterals may be seen. Echocardiography, CT and MRI are helpful in the diagnosis and evaluation of the severity of coarctation.

Management

Surgical correction of the coarctation is indicated in all except very mild cases. Balloon dilatation is used to correct postsurgical restenosis.

Tetralogy of Fallot

The tetralogy consists of following four components;
1. Ventricular septal defect
2. Pulmonary stenosis
3. Overriding of VSD by aorta
4. Right ventricular hypertrophy.

This is the most common cause of cyanotic CHD. The pulmonary flow is reduced due to RV outflow obstruction. This results in shunting of desaturated blood from RV to LV across the VSD leading to cyanosis, clubbing and polycythemia. The cyanosis increases during feeding or crying while it may reduce in squatting posture. There is ejection systolic murmur in the pulmonary area. The complications include infective endocarditis, cerebral infarction or abscess and polycythemia.

Investigations

Electrocardiography shows RV hypertrophy. Chest X-ray reveals 'boot shaped' heart and small pulmonary artery. Echocardiography is diagnostic.

Management

- The treatment is corrective operation which is necessary in almost all cases. This includes correction of pulmonary stenosis and closure of VSD. In case of hypoplastic pulmonary artery, an initial palliative shunt between pulmonary artery and subclavian artery is created to facilitate definitive correction.
- Prophylaxis for infective endocarditis is indicated even after surgical correction.

SYNCOPE

Syncope is defined as a transient loss of consciousness due to diminished cerebral perfusion. Syncope is characterized by loss of postural control and spontaneous recovery.

It may be preceded by symptoms of 'presyncope' such as lightheadedness, visual blurring, dizziness, sweating and nausea.

Causes of Syncope

The causes of syncope can be classified into (Fig. 5.14):
1. Neurally mediated syncope (vasovagal syncope, situational reflex syncope)
2. Orthostatic hypotension
3. Cardiac syncope.

There are some situations which may resemble syncope (Table 5.55).

Neurally mediated syncope is the most common cause of syncope. Cardiac syncope is the next most common cause, particularly in emergency room settings and in older patients. Orthostatic hypotension increases in prevalence with age. The prognosis after a single event is generally benign. Cardiac syncope is associated with an increased risk of sudden cardiac death and mortality. Syncope due to orthostatic hypotension is associated with increased mortality related to age and the associated comorbid conditions.

The normal baroreflex pathway is given in **Figure 5.15**.

Cardiac Syncope

Arrhythmia is the most common cause of syncope due to cardiac cause. The syncope can occur in profound bradycardia or tachyarrhythmia. Under these conditions, the decreased stroke volume can lead to cerebral hypoperfusion. The syncope due to atrioventricular block is known as *Stokes-Adams attack*.

Neurally mediated syncope	Cardiac syncope	Orthostatic hypotension
• Most common (F>M) • Transient change in autonomic efferent activity with increased parasympathetic outflow and sympathoinhibition • Due to multiple triggers	• Decreased cardiac output resulting from arrhythmias and structural heart disease • More common in emergency room settings and in older patients	• Due to failure of the autonomic nervous system, volume depletion or due to drugs • Increases in prevalence with age

Fig. 5.14: Causes of syncope.

Table 5.55: Causes of syncope.

1. **Neurally mediated syncope**
   - Vasovagal syncope
   - Situational reflex syncope
     » Cough syncope, sneeze syncope, airway instrumentation
     » Postmicturition syncope
     » Swallow syncope, gastrointestinal tract instrumentation, rectal examination, defecation syncope
     » Carotid sinus sensitivity, carotid sinus massage
2. **Orthostatic hypotension**
   - Volume depletion
   - Iatrogenic (drug-induced)
   - Primary autonomic failure due to idiopathic central and peripheral neurodegenerative diseases
     » Parkinson's disease, multiple system atrophy (Shy-Drager syndrome)
   - Secondary autonomic failure due to autonomic peripheral neuropathies
     » Diabetes, amyloidosis, autonomic neuropathies
3. **Cardiac syncope**
   - Arrhythmias
     » Sinus node dysfunction, sinus bradycardia
     » Heart blocks
     » Ventricular and supraventricular tachycardia
   - Cardiac structural disease
     » Aortic stenosis
     » Hypertrophic obstructive cardiomyopathy
     » Left ventricular dysfunction
     » Pericardial effusion and tamponade

Conditions which resemble syncope
- Hysterical fainting
- Anxiety
- Hypoglycemia
- Seizures

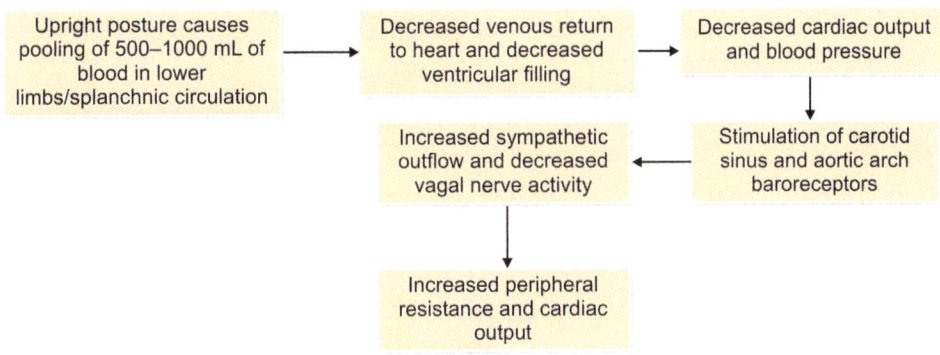

Fig. 5.15: Normal baroreflex pathway.

Vasovagal Syncope

- This is the most common cause of "common faint" in normal persons.
- The precipitating factors are hot or crowded environment, severe pain, extreme fatigue, prolonged standing, hunger and emotional situations.
- The vasovagal syncope occurs generally in the sitting and standing posture. Hence, it is essential that the patient is immediately made to lie down (recumbent position) at the earliest.
- Venous pooling which may occur during prolonged standing or sitting posture reduces the filling of the ventricle. The underfilled ventricle vigorously contracts due to increased sympathetic activation which in turn stimulate myocardial mechanoreceptors and vagal afferent fibers. This causes vasodilation (due to sympathetic inhibition) and bradycardia (increased parasympathetic activity). Vasodilatation and bradycardia produce hypotension and syncope.

Postural Hypotension (Postural Syncope)

- Postural hypotension [orthostatic hypotension (OH)] is a fall in systemic arterial pressure on assumption of upright posture. It is defined as a sustained drop in systolic (>20 mmHg) or diastolic (>10 mmHg) blood pressure within 3 minutes of standing (see also Chapter 11).
- The common causes of postural (orthostatic) hypotension are defective postural reflexes and drugs. There is fall in the systemic arterial pressure on assumption of an upright posture.
- These defective postural reflexes are generally due to autonomic peripheral neuropathy such as in diabetes, parkinsonism and aging.
- Hypovolemia because of diuretic therapy, excessive sweating, diarrhea, or hemorrhage may also lead to postural syncope.
- Drugs that cause postural syncope mainly include vasodilators, diuretics and antidepressants.

Seizures and Syncope

The seizures may easily be confused with syncope. However, careful history and examination may reliably differentiate these situations. The important differences are listed in **Table 5.56**.

Table 5.56: Differences between syncope and seizures.

	Seizure	Syncope
Premonitory symptoms	None or aura	Lightheadedness, nausea, blurring of vision, sweating, palpitation
Precipitating factors	Usually none	Emotional stress, postural hypotension, prolonged standing
Posture	Any posture	Usually erect
Rapidity of onset	Immediate	Gradual
Period of unconsciousness	Prolonged (minutes)	Transient (seconds)
Facial appearance	Cyanosis and frothing	Pallor
Associated findings	Motor seizures, tongue biting, urinary incontinence	Motor movement uncommon and transient
Recovery	Prolonged headache, confusion, focal neurological signs	Rapid and uneventful

Investigations

- Tests like ECG, echocardiography, Holter ECG and electrophysiological studies may be needed to diagnose the cause of syncope.
- Upright tilt test is used to confirm the diagnosis of vasovagal syncope.
- Other tests like EEG, CT, MRI scan may be needed to diagnose any neurological cause.

Treatment

- The treatment depends upon the underlying cause.
- Plasma volume expansion with fluid and salt, avoidance of precipitating factor, reassurance are helpful in management of neurally mediated syncope.
- Treatment of orthostatic hypotension includes patient education regarding staged movement (supine to upright

posture), raising the head of the bed, increased dietary fluid and salts, and administration of fludrocortisone acetate and vasoconstricting agents (midodrine, pseudoephedrine).
- Treatment of cardiac syncope depends upon underlying cause. Various therapies for arrhythmia include:
  – Anti-arrhythmic drugs
  – Cardiac pacing for AV block and sinus node disease
  – Radiofrequency ablation
  – Cardioverter-defibrillator implantation for atrial and ventricular arrhythmia.

However, certain precautions are to be taken regardless of the cause.

Immediate Actions to be Taken During Syncope

- The patient should be placed in supine position with head tilted to the side to maximize cerebral blood flow and to avoid aspiration.
- Peripheral stimulation like sprinkling cold water over the face may help.
- Clothing should be loosened.
- The patient should not be allowed to rise again till weakness persists.

Instructions to the Patients

- Patients are advised to avoid situations that have caused the syncope.
- Patients should try to assume a recumbent position as soon as they feel premonitory symptoms.
- Patients who have recurrent syncope should avoid climbing ladders, swimming alone, driving or operating machines.

ARRHYTHMIA

Abnormalities in the rhythm of heart rate are known as arrhythmias. Cardiac arrhythmias result from abnormalities of impulse generation, conduction or both.

Arrhythmias may present with palpitations, dyspnea, syncope, fatigue, lightheadedness, angina, exercise intolerance and skipped beat. Palpitations are suggestive of tachyarrhythmia. Bradyarrhythmias may present as fatigue, lightheadedness, syncope and exercise intolerance. A classification of arrhythmia is given in **Table 5.57**.

Diagnostic tools for detecting arrhythmia are following:
- 12 lead ECG: An ECG during baseline and at the time of arrhythmia is initial investigation.
- Continuous ambulatory ECG monitoring: Continuous ambulatory monitoring of ECG for 24–48 hours is useful for diagnosis of transient arrhythmias that occur with sufficient frequency. Correlation between symptoms and heart rate recordings aids in diagnosis of arrhythmia.
- Exercise ECG is helpful in diagnosis of exercise-induced arrhythmia or to assess response to exercise.

Table 5.57: Classification of arrhythmias.

- **Sinus rhythms**
  – Sinus arrhythmia
  – Sinus bradycardia
  – Sinus tachycardia
- **Tachyarrhythmias**
  – Atrial tachyarrhythmias
    » Atrial ectopic beats (extrasystoles, premature beats)
    » Atrial tachycardia
    » Atrial flutter
    » Atrial fibrillation (AF)
    » Supraventricular tachycardia (SVT)
      - AV nodal re-entry tachycardia (AVNRT)
      - Atrioventricular re-entrant tachycardia (AVRT)
      - Junctional tachycardia
      - Atrial tachycardia.
  – Ventricular tachyarrhythmias
    » Ventricular ectopic beats (extrasystoles, premature beats)
    » Ventricular tachycardia (VT)
    » Ventricular fibrillation (VF)
    » Torsades de pointes
- **Bradyarrhythmias**
  – Sick sinus syndrome (SSS)
  – Atrioventricular (AV) block
    » First-degree block
    » Second-degree block
      - Mobitz type I (Wenckebach) block
      - Mobitz type II block
    » Third-degree (complete) heart block
  – Bundle branch block
    » Right bundle branch block (RBBB)
    » Left bundle branch block (LBBB)

- Event recorder: They record ECG on activation by the patients when they feel symptoms. This can be kept by the patients for a month or more. These can also be implanted subcutaneously for up to 1–2 years and are useful for patients with infrequent arrhythmia or symptoms.
- Electrophysiological studies (EPS): EPS is an invasive procedure to induce arrhythmia to know their origin. It is particularly useful in supraventricular arrhythmias (SVT) and ventricular arrhythmias (VT).

Anti-arrhythmic Drugs

Anti-arrhythmic drugs are classified into four classes based on their actions **(Tables 5.58 and 5.59)**.

BRADYARRHYTHMIAS

Bradyarrhythmia is a rhythm when heart rate is less than 60 beats per minute.

Sinus Bradycardia

Sinus bradycardia is defined as sinus rate of 60 beats/min with a normal P wave in ECG. In healthy individuals particularly in athletes, heart rate may normally be less than 60/min **(Fig. 5.16)**.

Table 5.58: Classification of anti-arrhythmic drugs.

Class I drugs that block sodium channels (Membrane stabilizing effects)
Ia Prolong action potential:
- Quinidine
- Procainamide
- Disopyramide

Ib shorten action potential:
- Lidocaine
- Mexiletine
- Phenytoin

Ic no effect on action potential:
- Flecainide
- Propafenone

Class II beta-blockers, slow AV conduction:
- Atenolol
- Metoprolol
- Esmolol
- l-sotalol

Class III drugs which prolong action potential:
- Amiodarone
- d-Sotalol
- Ibutilide
- Dofetilide
- Bretylium

Class IV slow calcium channel blockers:
- Verapamil
- Diltiazem

Miscellaneous:
- Adenosine
- Digoxin
- Atropine sulphate

Table 5.59: Intravenous dosage of some commonly used anti-arrhythmic drugs.

- Adenosine: 6 mg IV as a rapid bolus followed by 12 mg after 1–2 min if needed
- Digoxin: 0.5 mg IV over 20 min followed by 0.25 or 0.125 mg increments to 1.5 mg in 24 hours
- Diltiazem: IV bolus of 0.25 mg/kg mg over 2 min, repeat bolus of 0.35 mg/kg if required
- Verapamil: 5–10 mg over 2–3 min, can be repeated after 15–30 min
- Amiodarone: 150 mg IV over 10 min, maintain at 1 mg/min infusion for 6 hours
- Lidocaine: 1–2 mg/kg at 50 mg/min, maintain at 1–4 mg/min
- Ibutilide: 1 mg over 10 min, followed by second infusion of 1 mg
- Flecainide: 50 mg every 12 hours
- Propafenone: 150 mg over every 12 hours
- Metoprolol: 2.5–5 mg IV bolus over 2 min
- Esmolol: 0.5 mg/kg over 1 min

Symptoms: It may cause fatigue, confusion and syncope due to reduced cerebral perfusion. It may also cause breathlessness and angina on exertion.

Causes: Causes of sinus bradycardia are hypothyroidism, hypothermia, myocardial ischemia, primary sinus node disease, drugs (digoxin, beta blockers, calcium channel blockers like diltiazem and verapamil, amiodarone).

Diagnosis: ECG reveals rate of <60/min with normal P wave. PR interval, QRS complexes, ST-T wave pattern are normal.

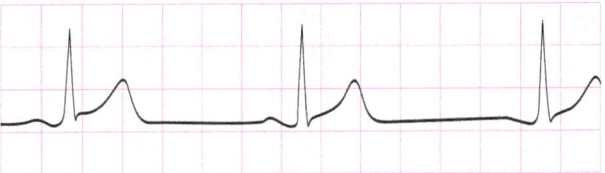

Fig. 5.16: ECG of sinus bradycardia.

Treatment: In symptomatic patients, the treatment is directed towards the underlying cause. Atropine (0.5 to 2.0 mg) intravenously can be given in acute symptomatic patients. Cardiac pacing (transcutaneous or transvenous) may be required.

Sick Sinus Syndrome

Sick sinus syndrome (SSS) is a group of rhythm disturbances that result due to sinus node dysfunction. It includes patients with sinus pause or sinus arrest, tachybrady syndrome and sinoatrial exit block.

Symptoms: Patients with SSS may present with palpitation, dizziness, confusion, syncope because of pauses with sinoatrial or ventricular activity, intermittent tachycardia and bradycardia.

Causes: Sick sinus syndrome occurs most commonly in elderly patients and arises from intrinsic disease (fibrosis, degenerative) of sinus node or cardiac conduction system. Sinus arrest is a condition when sinus node fails to generate an impulse intermittently.

Treatment: Sinus pauses that result in ventricular asystole for 3 sec are indications for permanent pacing.

Atrioventricular Block

Atrioventricular (AV) block is condition when atrial impulse is not conducted or conduction is delayed to ventricles.
- *First-degree heart block* is due to delay of impulse conduction in AV node. ECG reveals prolonged PR interval (> 0.2 seconds). Important causes are increased vagal tone, antiarrhythmic drugs, ischemia, electrolytes disturbances and conduction system disease. It is usually asymptomatic and no treatment is required. However it may worsen heart failure in patients with pre-existing heart disease. In symptomatic patients, dual chamber pacemaker therapy may be considered.
b. *Second-degree heart block* is a condition when some atrial impulses are not conducted to the ventricles. It is of two types:
  1. Mobitz type 1 (Wenckebach) block: Progressive delay in AV conduction occurs prior to blocked beat. ECG reveals progressive prolonged PR interval prior to blocked beat. It is benign and does not progress to complete heart block. Symptomatic patients are managed with IV atropine (0.5 mg). Permanent pacemaker therapy is indicated when cause is untreatable **(Fig. 5.17)**

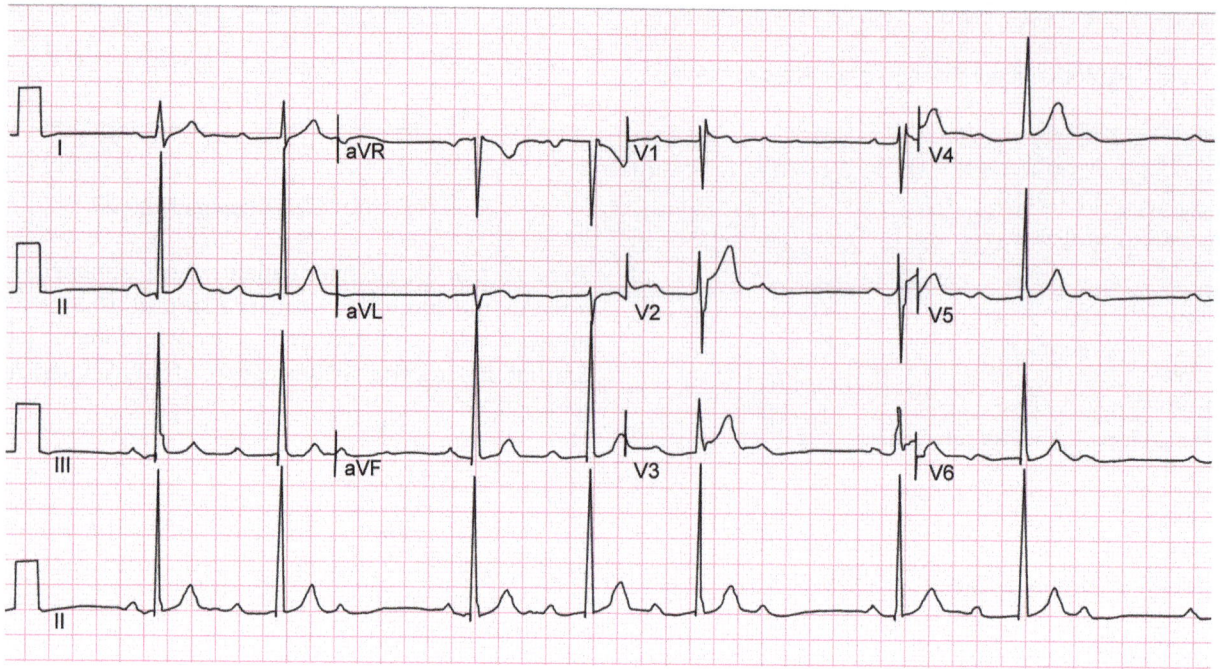

Fig. 5.17: Second degree heart block – Mobitz type 1 (Wenckebach) block.

2. **Mobitz type II AV block** is characterized by abrupt AV conduction block without evidence of progressive conduction delay. ECG reveals no change in PR interval prior to block or non-conducted P wave. Type II block may progress into complete heart block. Permanent pacemaker is indicated.

c. *Complete (third-degree) heart block:* Complete (third-degree) heart block is a more advanced form in which transmission of atrial impulses to ventricles through AV node is completely blocked. Ventricle escape rhythm maintains a regular, slow ventricular rate of <45 beats/min. No increase in heart rate occurs with exercise **(Fig. 5.18)**.

Symptoms: Patient may be asymptomatic or may present with dyspnea and fatigue. Syncope may occur during transition partial heart block to complete heart block due to ventricular asystole, which may last for few seconds to minutes.

Causes: Causes may be congenital or acquired. Acquired causes of complete block are myocardial ischemia/infarction, drugs (digoxin, beta blockers), degeneration of conduction tissue, infiltrative diseases (amyloidosis, sarcoidosis), infectious diseases (Chaga's disease, Lyme disease) and rheumatological diseases.

Diagnosis: Examination of patient reveals "cannon" a waves in jugular veins, varying intensity of first heart sound, changing systolic blood pressure level, slow and regular pulse rate of <45/min.

Treatment: Permanent pacing is indicated if cause is not reversible.

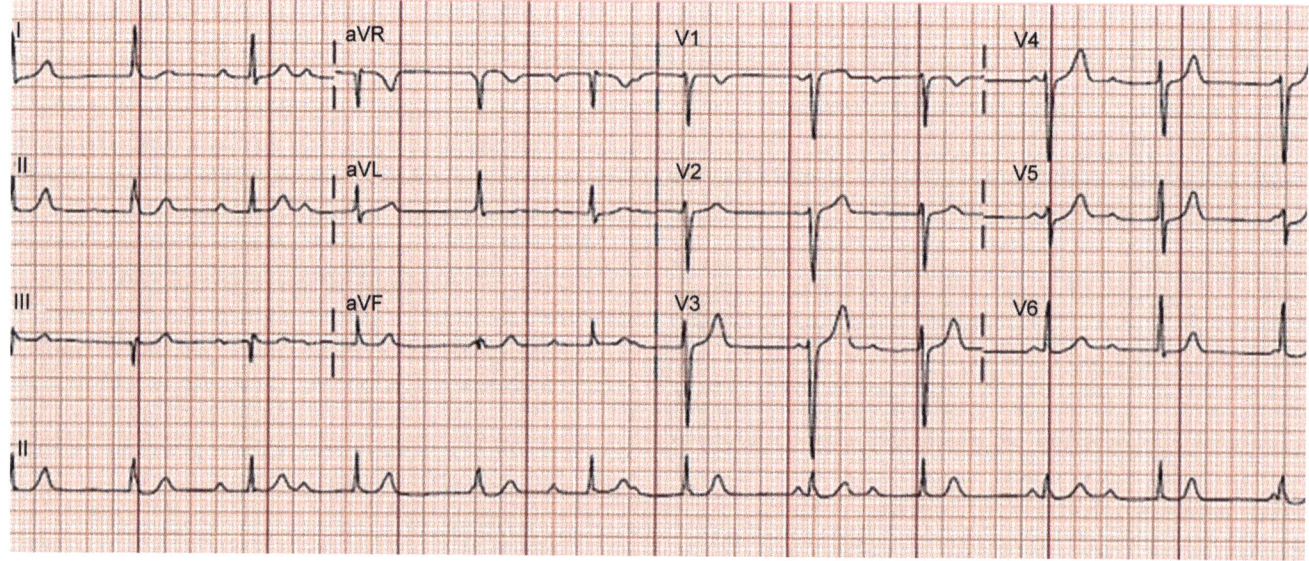

Fig. 5.18: Complete (third degree) heart block.

Stokes-Adams Attacks

Patients with ventricular asystole may present with recurrent syncope due to reduced cerebral perfusion, this is known as Stokes-Adams attack. This occurs in patients with complete heart block, Mobitz type II second degree block and sino-atrial disease.

TACHYARRHYTHMIAS

Tachycardia is defined as a heart rate of more than 100/min. Tachycardias are classified as supraventricular (SVT) and ventricular (VT) depending on site of origin. They are also classified as narrow complex (QRS duration <120 ms) and wide complex (QRS duration >120 ms).

Narrow Complex Tachycardias are of Supraventricular Origin

- *Sinus tachycardia* is defined as sinus rate of >100/min. Increased sympathetic activity due to exercise, anxiety, pregnancy and fever may cause tachycardia. Other cause are myocardial ischemia/infarction, anemia, heart failure, thyrotoxicosis, phaeochromocytoma and drugs which increase sympathetic activity, e.g., beta adrenoceptor antagonists like salbutamol, terbutaline. The ECG reveals rate of 100/min with normal P waves, PR interval and QRS complexes. Treatment is directed at the underlying process. Beta blockers may be useful in reducing rate particularly in the setting of myocardial ischemia.
- *Atrial tachycardia* is defined as rate of more than 100/min with origin of electrical activity within the atrium, not in SA node. It is mostly seen in pulmonary diseases. Other causes are coronary artery disease, digitalis intoxication and acute alcohol ingestion. It produces a narrow complex tachycardia (rate 100–200/min) with abnormal P wave morphology. Paroxysmal atrial tachycardia with atrioventricular block (PAT with block) is associated with digitalis intoxication. Multifocal atrial tachycardia (MAT) is seen in chronic obstructive pulmonary disease and heart failure. Treatment with beta blockers, calcium channel antagonists or digitalis is given to slow the ventricular rate. In digitalis intoxication, the digitalis is stopped and normal potassium levels are maintained. Digoxin antibodies with phenytoin and propranolol are used in refractory condition. Recurrent tachycardia or tachycardia not responding to drugs is treated by radiofrequency catheter ablation or surgical ablation.
- *Atrial flutter* is characterized by single large re-entry circuit within the atrium. ECG reveals flutter waves (saw-toothed appearance) with atrial rate of around 300 beats/min. It is commonly associated with 2:1, 3:1, 4:1 block so heart rate is usually less than the atrial rate (75–150/min). Block is increased by carotid sinus massage or intravenous adenosine and is helpful in diagnosis. Therapy includes: (a) Restoration of sinus rhythm by direct current (DC) cardioversion, (b) digoxin, beta blockers or diltiazem may be used to control ventricular rate, (c) amiodarone, propafenone or fleclainade are also helpful, (d) radiofrequency catheter ablation can be used for cure of atrial flutter in refractory or recurrent cases **(Fig. 5.19)**.
- *Atrial fibrillation (AF)* is the most common sustained arrhythmia. Its prevalence increases with age (affecting 10% of those above 75 years). Conditions which increase atrial size or alter atrial conduction or disrupt atrial refractoriness nonuniformly are particularly

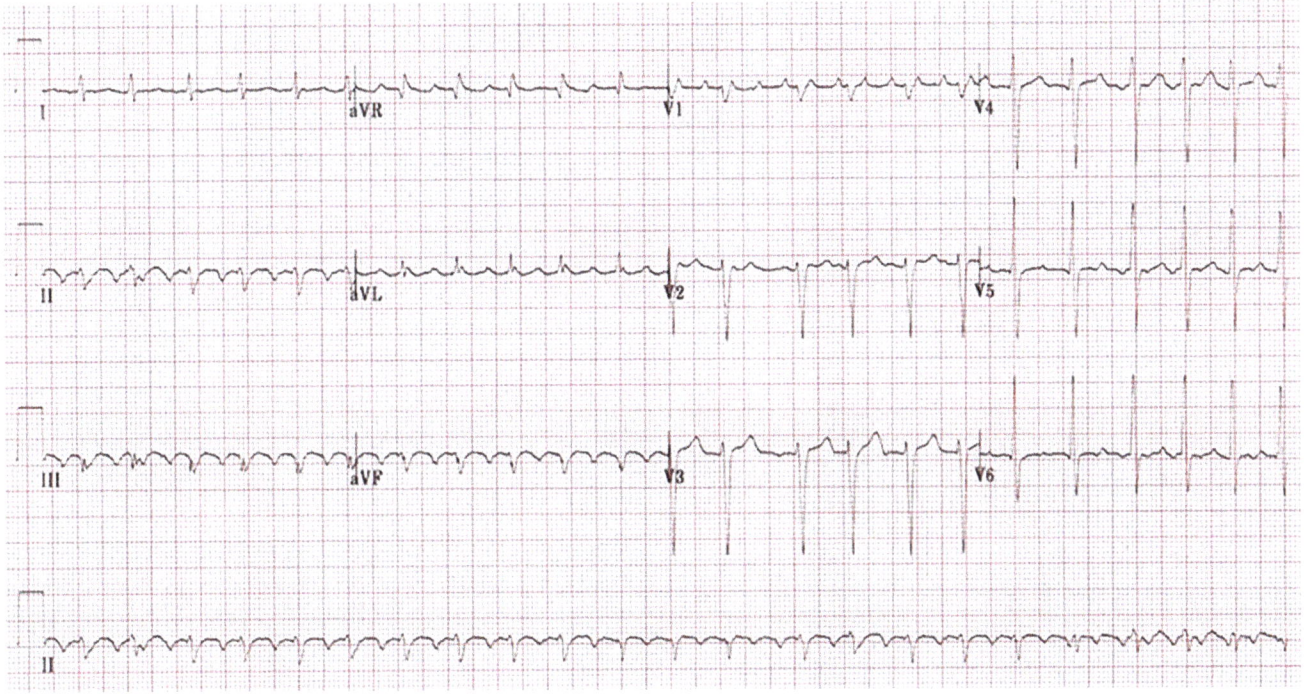

Fig. 5.19: Atrial flutter.

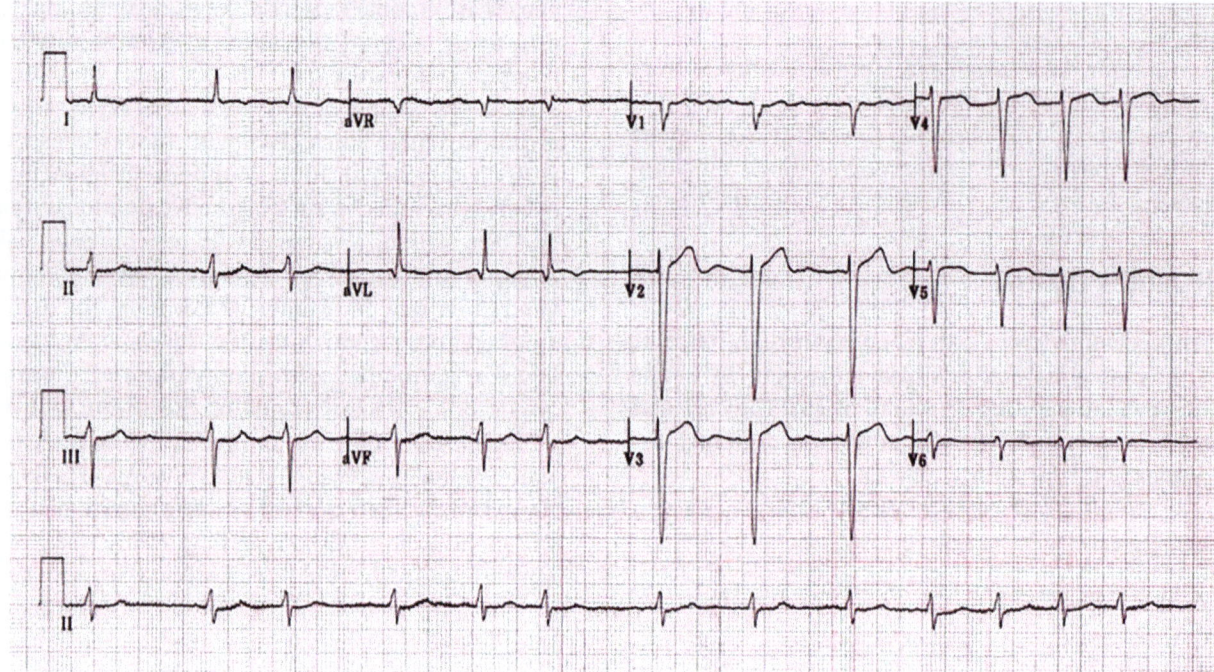

Fig. 5.20: Atrial fibrillation.

susceptible to AF. The most common correctable cause is hyperthyroidism. Atrial fibrillation is due to multiple reentry circuits around the atria. During AF the atria beat rapidly in uncoordinated manner. Ventricles beat irregularly at a rate determined by conduction through AV node producing irregularly irregular pulse **(Fig. 5.20)**.

ECG reveals irregularly irregular rhythm (normal but irregular QRS complexes) with no well defined P waves; ventricular rate is >100/min in untreated cases.

Symptoms of AF are palpitations, breathlessness, angina, syncope and lightheadedness. It may precipitate or worsen heart failure in patients with ventricular dysfunction or structural heart disease. It may be asymptomatic and discovered on routine examination or ECG. Causes of atrial fibrillation are given in **Table 5.60**.

Management of AF: Paroxysmal AF attacks are well tolerated and do not require treatment. In symptomatic patients beta-blockers are used especially if it is associated with coronary artery disease, hypertension or heart failure. Class Ic drugs like flecainide or propafenone are also useful. Radiofrequency ablation and overdrive atrial pacing are other modes of treatment in refractory cases. Management of persistent AF includes:
- Rate control
- Prevention of thromboembolism
- Rhythm control.

Rate Control

Rate control of AF is done by agents which prolong conduction through AV node like beta-blockers, calcium channel blockers (diltiazem, verapamil) and digoxin.

Prevention of Thromboembolism

Loss of atrial contraction and atrial dilatation produces stasis of blood and may precipitate thrombus formation in left atrium. Chronic warfarin ingestion in patients at risk for embolic stroke (cerebrovascular accident) is the most effective therapy for preventing stroke associated with AF. The INR is maintained between 2.0–3.0.

In patients who have AF for >48 hours, anticoagulation with warfarin is recommended for at least 3 weeks before cardioversion.

Rhythm Control

Restoration of sinus rhythm can be achieved with electrical direct current (DC) cardioversion or chemical cardioversion (using antiarrhythmic drugs). If AF is present for <48 hours immediate DC cardioversion or chemical cardioversion (with intravenous ibutilide or flecainide or propafenone) can be done.

Table 5.60: Common causes of atrial fibrillation.
- Valvular heart disease (especially mitral valve disease)
- Ischemic heart disease
- Hypertension
- Hyperthyroidism
- Congenital heart disease
- Acute alcohol ingestion
- Pericardial disease
- Pulmonary diseases
- Drugs (theophylline, etc.)
- Idiopathic (Lone AF)

Supraventricular Tachycardia

Supraventricular tachycardia (SVT) is a generic term for paroxysmal, regular supraventricular tachyarrhythmia. The tachycardia may be due to AV nodal reentrant tachycardia (AVNRT), atrioventricular reentrant tachycardia (AVRT), junctional tachycardia and atrial tachycardia. The term is not generally used for atrial fibrillation (AF) and atrial flutter.

Supraventricular tachycardias (SVT) arise from the atria or the atrioventricular junction and are associated with a narrow QRS complex usually. They are due to re-entry circuit or automatic focus, the AV node is essential component of re-entry circuit.

AV nodal reentrant tachycardia (AVNRT): It is a regular tachycardia and may occur suddenly. Alcohol, tea, coffee or exertion may precipitate or induce arrhythmia. It is due to re-entry in the right atrium and AV node.

ECG reveals normal regular QRS complexes at a rate of 140–240/min.

Symptoms are awareness of fast heart beat (palpitations), breathlessness or syncope. It may present with angina or heart failure if there is structural heart diseases. Polyuria may also occur because of release of atrial natriuretic peptide (ANP) due to increased atrial pressures.

Management

- Carotid sinus massage and other methods which increase vagal tone (Valsalva maneuver, facial immersion in cold water) may terminate the attack. If physical methods are not effective, intravenous adenosine, verapamil, diltiazem, flecainide or beta-blockers may terminate the attack.
- SVTs presenting with hemodynamic instability (hypotension, pulmonary edema) require emergency DC cardioversion.
- For recurrent attacks, prophylactic oral therapy with a verapamil, diltiazem, beta blockers or digoxin may be given. It can also be cured by catheter ablation techniques.

Atrioventricular re-entrant tachycardia (AVRT) and Wolf-Parkinson-White (WPW) Syndrome

This is due to long circuit involving atria, His bundle and ventricles. There is an abnormal connection which connects atria and ventricles (accessory pathway or bypass tract). In some cases this pathway conducts in the retrograde direction, i.e., from the ventricles to atria resulting into normal ECG appearance. In some cases conduction takes place partly through AV node and partly through rapidly conducting accessory pathway during sinus rhythm. If the accessory pathway conducts from the atria to ventricles, the electrical impulses are conducted quickly and depolarize the part of ventricles abnormally (pre-excitation). Premature activation of ventricles produces a short PR interval, and a wide QRS complex with an initial slurred part called as 'delta wave'. Because AV nodes and bypass tracts have different conduction speeds and refractory periods, a re-entry circuit can develop, causing tachycardia. When these patients (with per-excitation ECG) develop symptoms due to tachycardia, this condition is known as Wolff-Parkinson-White (WPW) syndrome.

The ECG appearance may be indistinguishable from AVNRT.

Management

- Carotid sinus massage or intravenous adenosine may terminate the attack.
- If atrial fibrillation occurs, it is treated by DC cardioversion.
- In symptomatic patients, prophylactic therapy is indicated. Flecainide, propafenone or amiodarone is used for prophylaxis.
- Digoxin and verapamil are never used in atrial fibrillation associated with WPW syndrome because they shorten the refractory period of the accessory pathway and may allow a higher rate of conduction and may precipitate ventricular fibrillation.
- In symptomatic patients, catheter ablation of accessory pathway is curative.

Ventricular Tachyarrhythmias

Ventricular Premature Beats

Ventricular premature beats (VPBs) or ventricular extrasystole or ventricular ectopic beats (VEBs) is characterized by wide, bizarre QRS complexes that differ from normal beats in morphology and there is no preceding P wave.
- Every second or third beat if immature, the condition is known as ventricular bigeminy or trigeminy.
- VPC may disappear with exercise and rhythm may become normal if there is no cardiac disease.
- Patient may complain of skipped beat or may be asymptomatic.
- VPC occurring in patients with heart disease are associated with increased chances of sudden cardiac death due to ventricular fibrillation.

Treatment: In asymptomatic patients with no cardiac disease, no treatment is required. If frequent, the underlying cause (hypokalemia, hyperkalemia, hypomagnesemia, hyperth- yroidism and heart diseases) should be treated. Beta-blockers are agents of first choice in symptomatic patients with VPC.

Ventricular Tachycardia (VT)

It is defined as three or more consecutive VPCs. It has to be differentiated from SVT with aberrant conduction.
- The usual mechanism is re-entry or abnormal automaticity or triggered activity in ischemic tissue.
- It may be sustained (>30 sec) or non sustained (<30 sec). Patient may be asymptomatic or presents with syncope or

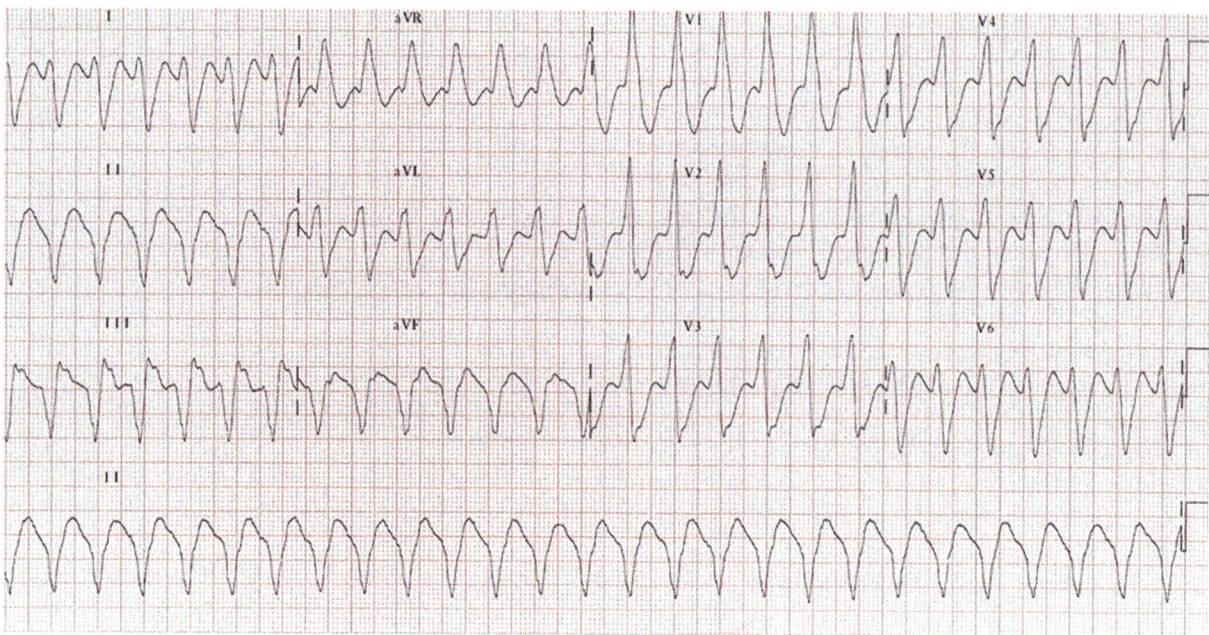

Fig. 5.21: Ventricular tachycardia.

symptoms due to reduced cerebral perfusion (dizziness) or dyspnea.
- VT is a frequent complication of acute myocardial infarction or cardiomyopathy. It may also occur in coronary artery disease, mitral valve prolapse, and myocarditis.
- VT is unfavorable sign in patients with heart disease and may cause hemodynamic compromise or degenerate into ventricular fibrillation.
- ECG shows tachycardia with a rate of >120/min with broad, bizarre QRS complexes **(Fig. 5.21)**.

Ventricular Fibrillation (VF)

It is characterized by rapid and irregular ventricular activation resulting into disorganized contraction of ventricle leading to hemodynamic collapse, cardiac arrest and sudden death.
- The patient is pulseless and becomes unconscious and respiration ceases.
- The ECG reveals irregular, rapid oscillations (250–400/min). The QRS complexes and T waves are not identifiable **(Fig. 5.22)**.

Treatment of VT and VF:
- Immediate DC cardioversion is the primary therapy for pulseless VT or VF.
- Intravenous antiarrhythmic agents may also be required if patient is resistant to defibrillation. In well tolerated VT, intravenous amiodarone or lidocaine is indicated. Electrolyte imbalance, hypoxemia, acidosis should be corrected because these can worsen the situation.

- Treatment of recurrent symptomatic ventricular arrhythmia includes administration of chronic antiarrhythmic agents (beta blockers, amiodarone).
- Nonpharmacologic treatment of VT/VF includes implantable cardiac defibrillator (ICD) and radiofrequency catheter ablation to interrupt the arrhythmia focus or circuit.
- Torsades de pointes is a form of VT in which QRS morphology twists around the baseline. It may occur in hypokalemia, hypomagnesemia or after any drug that prolongs QT interval. It has poor prognosis.

IMPLICATIONS ON DENTAL PRACTICE

- Patients with cardiac disease should receive dental treatment in minimal stressful environment. Anxiety, exertion and pain should be minimized.
- The blood pressure may preferably be measured before any dental procedure to ensure that this is normal or controlled. A high blood pressure may result into precipitation of other related problems such as angina or heart failure.
- Besides general examination, precordium should be auscultated to rule out any lesion in the heart.
- Irregular pulse, engorged jugular veins and tachypnea may indicate the presence of cardiac disease.
- Angina may present as pain in the mandible, teeth and other oral tissues.
- A history of hypertension, ischemic heart disease or any other cardiac problem particularly congenital heart disease and drug intake (anticoagulant, antiplatelet agents) should be sought.
- Epinephrine in the local anesthesia may raise the blood pressure and precipitate dysarrhythmias.

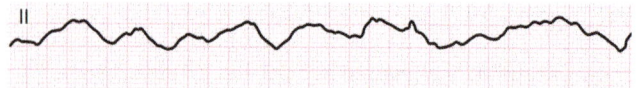

Fig. 5.22: Ventricular fibrillation.

- In patients with IHD, facilities for medical help, oxygen and nitroglycerine should be available.
- General anesthesia should be avoided for at least three months in patients with recent onset angina.
- Elective dental surgery should be deferred for 6 months following acute MI.
- Prophylaxis for infective endocarditis is mandatory in cases where there is a risk.
- Cardiac patients on anticoagulant drugs or aspirin are at increased risk of bleeding following dental procedures. Hence, these drugs should preferably be stopped a week before the procedure.
- Calcium channel blockers may cause gingival swelling and lichenoid lesions in the oral cavity. ACE inhibitors can cause loss of taste, burning sensation in oral cavity, and angioedema. Dry mouth can result due to antihypertensive drugs such as diuretics, beta-blockers and clonidine.
- Sudden change in the posture from supine to standing following dental procedures may cause postural hypotension and syncope, particularly in patients using diuretics and calcium channel blockers.
- Oral abnormalities such as enamel hypoplasia, delayed eruption of both dentitions, positional anomalies, bluish white "skimmed milk" appearance of teeth and vasodilatation in the pulps may be associated with cyanotic congenital heart disease.
- Patient with left ventricular failure should be managed in partially reclining or erect position. Supine position may worsen dyspnea.

SELF ASSESSMENT

Multiple Choice Questions

1. **Differential cyanosis can be seen in:**
   A. Bronchiectasis B. PDA
   C. ASD D. Methemoglobinemia
2. **"a" wave in JVP is absent in:**
   A. Complete heart block B. Severe HF
   C. AF D. All the above
3. **Major criteria for acute rheumatic fever include all, *except*:**
   A. Pancarditis B. Fever
   C. Sydenham's chorea D. Polyarthritis
4. **Following are features of right ventricular failure, *except*:**
   A. Hepatomegaly B. S_3
   C. Pulmonary congestion D. Pedal edema
5. **Most common congenital heart disease is:**
   A. ASD B. VSD
   C. Fallot's tetralogy D. Pulmonary stenosis
6. **Most common congenital cyanotic heart disease is:**
   A. Fallot's tetralogy B. Eisenmenger syndrome
   C. Tricuspid atresia D. Pulmonary atresia
7. **Clubbing may be found in all, *except*:**
   A. Acute infective endocarditis
   B. Fallot's tetralogy
   C. Bronchiectasis
   D. Bronchogenic carcinoma
8. **Following features can be present in SABE, *except*:**
   A. Splinter hemorrhages B. Anemia
   C. Erythema nodosum D. Splenomegaly
9. **Most common organism causing SABE is:**
   A. *S. aureus* B. HACEK group
   C. *Strep. viridans* D. Enterococci
10. **Following may be found in rheumatic AS, *except*:**
    A. Water hammer pulse B. Forceful apex beat
    C. Syncope D. Angina
11. **Prophylaxis for infective endocarditis is not indicated in:**
    A. Implanted pacemaker B. Secondum ASD
    C. CABG D. All the above
12. **Following is the feature of ASD:**
    A. Continuous murmur
    B. High chance of SABE
    C. Wide and fixed second heart sound
    D. Commonest type of congenital heart disease
13. **Following can be found in mitral stenosis, *except*:**
    A. Loud S_1 B. Mid-diastolic murmur at apex
    C. Opening snap D. Aortic ejection click
14. **"T" wave in ECG is due to:**
    A. Atrial depolarization
    B. Atrial repolarization
    C. Ventricular depolarization
    D. Ventricular repolarization
15. **All are features of LVF, *except*:**
    A. Orthopnea B. Hepatomegaly
    C. Pulmonary edema D. S_3
16. **Which antihypertensive drug is contraindicated in bradycardia:**
    A. Amlodipine B. Atenolol
    C. Thiazide D. None
17. **The most common form of hypertension is:**
    A. Renovascular B. Essential hypertension
    C. Endocrinal D. Drug induced
18. **Stokes-Adams attack is due to:**
    A. AF B. Complete heart block
    C. Atrial extrasystole D. Severe hypertension
19. **The preferred antihypertensive agent in diabetics is:**
    A. Beta-blocker B. ACE inhibitor
    C. Diuretics D. Centrally acting drugs
20. **Most common cause of secondary hypertension is:**
    A. Pheochromocytoma B. Eclampsia
    C. Renal D. Primary hyperaldosteronism
21. **The diuretic preferred in acute pulmonary edema is:**
    A. Loop diuretics B. Potassium sparing
    C. Thiazides D. All
22. **Which of the following is most common cause of syncope:**
    A. Neurally mediated syncope (vasovagal syncope)
    B. Volume depletion
    C. Obstructive cardiomyopathy
    D. Heart block (atrioventricular block)
23. **All of the following are common features of aortic stenosis, *except*:**
    A. Exertional dyspnea B. Angina
    C. Syncope D. Pedal edema

24. **Hill's sign in aortic regurgitation refers to:**
    A. Pulsatile carotid arteries
    B. To and fro murmur over femoral artery
    C. Blood pressure in lower limbs higher (> 20 mmHg) than in upper limbs
    D. Pulsatile liver

25. **Empirical therapy of subacute infective endocarditis (SABE) include:**
    A. Ceftriaxone plus gentamycin +/- Vancomycin
    B. Doxycycline plus gentamycin +/- Vancomycin
    C. Azithromycin plus gentamycin +/- Vancomycin
    D. Ampicillin plus gentamycin +/- Vancomycin

Fill in the Blanks

1. Differential cyanosis is seen in _____.
2. Austin flint murmur is found in_____.
3. Carey-Coombs murmur is present in_____.
4. Reversal of shunt in VSD is known as_____.
5. Graham-Steel murmur is found in_____.
6. Maladie de Roger's murmur is found in_____.
7. Continuous machinery murmur is a feature of _____.
8. Most common type of ASD is_____.
9. Antihypertensive drug that can cause gum swelling is_____.
10. Brain natriuretic peptide (BNP) measurement is helpful in the diagnosis of_____.
11. Prehypertension is defined as systolic BP_____ and diastolic_____.
12. Patients with coronary artery bypass surgery require prophylaxis for infective endocarditis (Yes/No)
13. Janeway's lesions are seen in_____.
14. Berry's aneurysm is a feature of_____.
15. Mycotic aneurysm is found in_____.
16. Hill sign is present in_____.
17. Wide fixed splitting of second heart sound is found in_____.
18. First heart sound is_____ in mitral stenosis.
19. Crackles are feature of_____ ventricular failure (right or left).
20. Drugs used for the prophylaxis of rheumatic fever are 1_____, 2_____ and 3_____.

CHAPTER 6

Respiratory Diseases

Diseases of respiratory system are not uncommon. The respiratory tract may be primarily involved or it may be affected secondary to diseases of other systems. A thorough history and detailed clinical examination are mandatory in order to make a proper diagnosis.

The respiratory system is customarily divided into the upper and lower respiratory tract.
- The upper respiratory tract includes the nose, nasopharynx and the larynx
- The lower respiratory tract includes trachea, bronchi and further structures.

The right lung is divided into three lobes: upper, middle, and lower, while the left lung has two lobes: upper and lower. Each lobe is further divided into bronchopulmonary segments. Upper and middle lobe on the right side and upper lobe on the left side occupy most of the area of the chest anteriorly **(Fig. 6.1)**.

SYMPTOMS

The important respiratory symptoms are:
- Dyspnea
- Cough
- Sputum
- Hemoptysis
- Chest pain

Dyspnea

Dyspnea is defined as an abnormally uncomfortable awareness of breathing. The pathophysiology of dyspnea is multifactorial and mainly includes:
a. Hypoxia
b. Hypercapnia
c. Altered lung and chest wall compliance

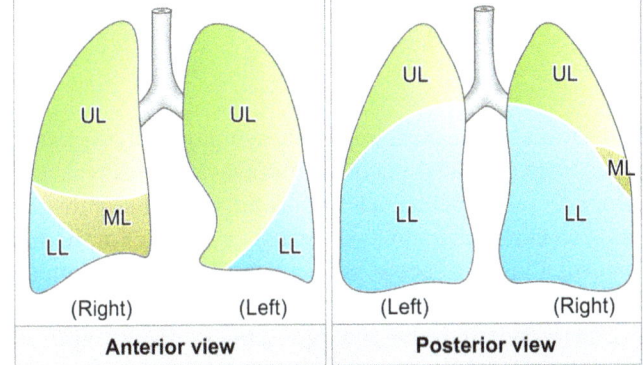

Fig. 6.1: Anterior and posterior aspects of the lung.
(UL: upper lobe; ML: middle lobe; LL: lower lobe)

d. Increased respiratory effort and respiratory muscle weakness

The dyspnea can be acute or chronic: The respiratory causes of acute dyspnea are:
- Severe asthma
- Acute exacerbation of chronic obstructive pulmonary disease (COPD)
- Pneumonia
- Pneumothorax
- Pulmonary embolism (PE)
- Foreign body inhalation
- Laryngeal edema
- Acute respiratory distress syndrome (ARDS)

Important respiratory causes of chronic dyspnea are COPD and interstitial lung disease (ILD). Other causes of dyspnea are given in **Table 6.1**.

Dyspnea can occur only during exertion or it may be present even at rest, depending on the severity of disease. The dyspnea which occurs mainly at the night *(noctural dyspnea)* may be due to asthma, sleep apnea, gastroesophageal reflux

Table 6.1: Important causes of dyspnea.

Acute dyspnea	Chronic dyspnea
a. Respiratory causes 　– Asthma 　– Acute exacerbation of COPD 　– Pneumonia 　– Pneumothorax 　– Pulmonary embolism 　– ARDS 　– Foreign body inhalation 　– Laryngeal edema	a. Respiratory causes 　– COPD 　– Interstitial lung disease 　– Pleural effusion
b. Cardiac causes 　– Acute pulmonary edema	b. Cardiac causes 　– Chronic heart failure
c. Other causes 　– Metabolic acidosis (uremia, diabetic ketoacidosis) 　– Psychogenic	c. Other causes 　– Anemia 　– Obesity

(ARDS: acute respiratory distress syndrome; COPD: chronic obstructive pulmonary disease)

or left ventricular dysfunction. Episodic dyspnea typically occurs in asthma.

Cough

Cough is one of the most important symptoms in respiratory diseases. It may also occur in diseases of cardiovascular system. Duration of cough is important, it may be acute (less than 3 weeks), subacute (3–8 weeks) or chronic (more than 8 weeks). Causes of acute, subacute and chronic cough are given in **Table 6.2**.

The cough may be *dry* or associated with sputum *(productive cough)*.

Table 6.2: Causes of cough.

Acute	Subacute	Chronic
Upper respiratory tract infection	Post infectious	Chronic bronchitis
Pneumonia	Sinusitis	Postnasal drip
Aspiration	Asthma	Asthma
Pulmonary edema		Gastroesophageal reflux
Pulmonary embolism		Drugs (ACE inhibitors)

(ACE: angiotensin converting enzyme)

- Dry cough can occur in bronchial asthma, early phase of pneumonia and ILD. Episodic dry cough particularly in the night may be an early symptom of asthma
- Common causes of productive cough are bronchiectasis, chronic bronchitis, pneumonia, lung abscess and tuberculosis.

The cough may have different characteristics based on the sites involved. These are given in **Table 6.3**.

Sputum

Sputum production is a common symptom in respiratory diseases. Its characteristics such as amount, color and consistency are helpful in making the diagnosis.
- Large amount of sputum is produced in bronchiectasis and lung abscess while scanty thick sputum is found in asthma
- Sputum is mucoid, scanty and thick in chronic bronchitis
- Purulent yellow or green sputum signifies infection
- Foul smelling sputum is present in anaerobic infection
- Pink frothy sputum suggests pulmonary edema
- Patients with bronchiectasis or lung abscess may bring out large amount of sputum in a particular posture which forms the basis of *"postural drainage"* in the management.

Hemoptysis

The coughing of blood in the sputum is called hemoptysis. The blood may be coughed up alone (frank hemoptysis) or there may be streaking of sputum with blood. Expectoration of 200–600 mL blood in 24 hours is defined as massive hemoptysis. Hemoptysis should be differentiated from bleeding from other sites such as gums, nose and stomach. The differentiating features between hemoptysis and hematemesis (bleeding from gastrointestinal tract) are given in **Table 6.4**.

Common causes of hemoptysis are chronic bronchitis, pulmonary tuberculosis and bronchogenic carcinoma. Other causes are given in **Table 6.5**.

Wheezing

Wheeze is a high-pitched continuous musical sound heard due to narrowing of airways. This may be noticed by the patient or relatives or others as in case of asthma.

Table 6.3: Characteristics of cough.

Site of origin	Character of cough	Common causes
Pharynx	Persistent, throat pain	Pharyngitis, postnasal drip
Larynx	Harsh, painful, persistent. May have stridor	Laryngitis, tumor, whooping cough, vocal cord palsy (bovine cough)
Trachea	Persistent, painful, stridor	Tracheitis, tumor
Bronchi	• Dry or productive, wheeze • May have hemoptysis	• Bronchitis, bronchial asthma • Bronchogenic carcinoma
Lung parenchyma	• Dry initially followed by productive cough, rusty sputum • Dry, distressing • Often nocturnal, pink frothy sputum	• Pneumonia • Interstitial fibrosis • Pulmonary edema

Table 6.4: Differences between hemoptysis and hematemesis.

Hemoptysis	Hematemesis
Bright red appearance	Coffee ground or dark red
Presence of cough or other respiratory symptoms	Presence of vomiting or other abdominal symptoms
Alkaline pH	Acidic pH
Melena generally not found	Associated with black tarry stool (melena)

Table 6.5: Causes of hemoptysis.

Respiratory
- Chronic bronchitis
- Tuberculosis
- Bronchogenic carcinoma
- Bronchiectasis
- Pulmonary infarction
- Pneumonia

Cardiac
- Mitral stenosis
- Left ventricular failure

Others
- Goodpasture's syndrome
- Wegener's granulomatosis
- Hemorrhagic disorders
- Anticoagulant therapy

A low-pitched inspiratory sound heard in the obstruction of larynx or trachea is known as "stridor".

Chest Pain

Chest pain in respiratory diseases is mainly due to the involvement of parietal pleura. The pain is sharp "stabbing" which increases on deep inspiration and coughing (pleuritic chest pain). The causes of pleuritic pain are conditions with pleural inflammation and malignancies involving pleura. The pain due to pleural inflammation may occur in pneumonia and pulmonary infarction if parietal pleura is involved. Chest pain due to cardiac diseases should be differentiated from that of pleural origin. Important differentiating points are given in **Table 6.6**.

Table 6.6: Differences between pain of pleural and cardiac origin.

Pleural origin	Cardiac origin
Site is usually lateral, axilla or back	Central, retrosternal
Character of pain is stabbing, cutting or tearing	Heaviness or constriction type
Referred to abdomen or back	Referred to neck or left upper limb
Aggravated by respiratory movement or cough	Aggravated by exertion, emotions
Relieved by rest or decreased movement of chest	Relieved by rest or nitroglycerine
Examination reveals pleural rub localized to the site of pain	Pericardial rub may be present

Inflammation of trachea and large bronchi may cause pain in upper sternal region or on either side of the sternum.

EXAMINATION

General

The general examination in the patients with respiratory disease is of great importance. Particularly one should look for the
- Physique
- Cyanosis
- Digital clubbing
- Elevation of jugular venous pressure (JVP)
- Edema
- Lymph node enlargement.

Physique: Weight loss may be apparent in cases of tuberculosis, chronic suppurative lung diseases and malignancies of the lung or pleura.

Cyanosis: Patients with respiratory failure may have central cyanosis. This may occur acutely in extensive pneumonia, pulmonary edema and massive PE. Chronically, cyanosis is present in COPD. The presence of polycythemia in COPD may lead to cyanosis even in mild hypoxemia.

Clubbing: Digital clubbing may be found in patients with chronic suppurative lung diseases (bronchiectasis, lung abscess, empyema), primary and metastatic lung cancers, mesothelioma, chronic ILD and advanced pulmonary tuberculosis. The presence of digital clubbing along with swelling above the wrist and ankle due to periostitis of long bones (*hypertrophic pulmonary osteoarthropathy*) is particularly associated with bronchogenic carcinoma. Clubbing develops rapidly in patients with lung abscess and bronchogenic carcinoma *(see* **Table 1.8**).

Edema: Pedal edema can be found in patients with respiratory disease and it indicates the presence of cor pulmonale (right ventricular enlargement secondary to pulmonary disease) and right ventricular failure.

Swelling over the face and neck may also occur in superior vena cava obstruction due to enlarged lymph nodes or malignant mass.

Lymph node enlargement: The enlargement of lymph nodes, mainly axillary and cervical may indicate tuberculosis or carcinoma lung. Other groups of lymph nodes like mediastinal, hilar and paratracheal can only be detected by imaging.

Respiratory System Examination

The respiratory system, like other systems, should be examined under four headings: Inspection, palpation, percussion and auscultation **(Table 6.7)**.

Table 6.7: Inspection of chest.
• Shape and symmetry • Movements • Use of accessory muscles • Rate, rhythm and depth of respiration • Trail sign • *Others*: Venous prominence, scar, sinuses

Inspection

Shape and symmetry of chest:
- The shape of the chest is normally bilaterally symmetrical and transverse diameter is more than anteroposterior diameter (elliptical). Over-inflated *barrel-shaped* chest (AP diameter is equal or more than transverse diameter) can be present in COPD. Other deformities of the chest like *kyphosis* (forward bending) or *scoliosis* (lateral bending) should be noted. Deformities such as *pigeon chest* (marked bulging of sternum) and *Harrison's sulcus* (a horizontal groove at the lower part of chest) can rarely be seen
- Tracheal shift can be assessed by looking for the prominence of clavicular end of sternocleidomastoid muscle which becomes more prominent on the side of shift *(Trail sign)*
- Localized bulging in the chest may occur in aneurysm, empyema or cardiac hypertrophy whereas localized recession (flattening) can be seen in pleural or lung fibrosis.

Movements: The movement of the chest is normally equal on both sides. The movement is decreased on the side of disease. Drawing of intercostal spaces with inspiration indicates severe upper airway obstruction. Use of accessory muscles of respiration (intercostals, sternocleidomastoid, etc.) denotes significant pulmonary impairment.

Rate, rhythm and depth of respiration:
- The rate, rhythm and depth of the respiration should also be noted. The normal respiratory rate is around 12–16 per minute. An increase in the respiratory rate is known as tachypnea
- Rapid and deep respiration *(Kussmaul's breathing)* is present in metabolic acidosis whereas rapid shallow breathing is a feature of restrictive lung disease
- *Cheyne-Stokes* respiration is characterized by cyclical waxing and waning of the rate and depth of the respiration intervened with a short period of apnea **(Fig. 6.2)**. It is observed in narcotic overdose and severe left ventricular failure.

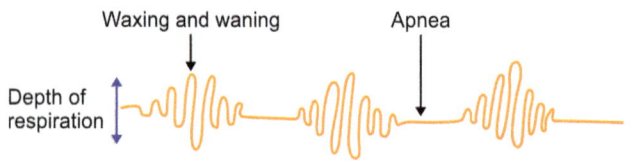

Fig. 6.2: Cheyne–Stokes respiration.

Palpation

- The *trachea and the apex beat* are palpated to find out the shift of the mediastinum. The shift of the mediastinum to the side of the disease occurs in fibrosis and collapse. Mediastinum is pushed to the opposite side in cases of pleural effusion and pneumothorax
- The *expansion of the chest* is measured and compared on both sides
- *Tactile vocal fremitus* is detected with the flat of the hand placed on the chest wall. This occurs due to the transmission of sound waves produced in the larynx and proximal airways to the chest wall. The vocal fremitus is diminished in pleural effusion and pneumothorax and increased in consolidation (pneumonia)
- Palpation can also detect tenderness which may occur in rib fracture and costochondritis.

Percussion

Normally, the percussion note over the chest is resonant.
- It is *impaired* or *dull* in fibrosis, collapse, consolidation and pleural thickening
- The note is "*stony dull*" in pleural effusion
- A *hyperresonant* note is found in pneumothorax and emphysema
- Normal liver dullness is masked in emphysema.

Auscultation

Type of breath sound: Normal breath sounds heard over the chest wall are called *vesicular*. This is a rustling sound heard throughout the phase of inspiration and during initial phase of expiration. There is no pause in-between. The intensity of the vesicular breath sounds is reduced in cases with emphysema, pleural effusion or thick chest wall. Individuals with very thin chest wall may have vesicular breath sounds with increased intensity. Vesicular breath sounds with prolonged expiration are heard in asthma and COPD.

The *bronchial* breath sounds are higher pitched hissing sounds typically heard over trachea in normal individuals. The presence of bronchial breath sounds over other areas of the chest is abnormal. These are classically heard over areas of consolidation and cavity. These sounds are hollow in character, louder during expiration and last for most of the expiratory phase. There is a gap between inspiratory and expiratory phases **(Fig. 6.3)**.

Added sounds: Added sounds include wheezes (rhonchi), crackles (crepitations or rales) and pleural rub.
- *Wheezes* are high-pitched continuous musical sounds associated with narrowing of airways. Diffuse wheezes (polyphonic) are heard in cases of bronchial asthma and COPD whereas localized wheezes (monophonic) are generated at narrowed bronchus due to tumor or foreign body
- *Crackles* are bubbling or clicking brief interrupted sounds produced by the explosive opening of small

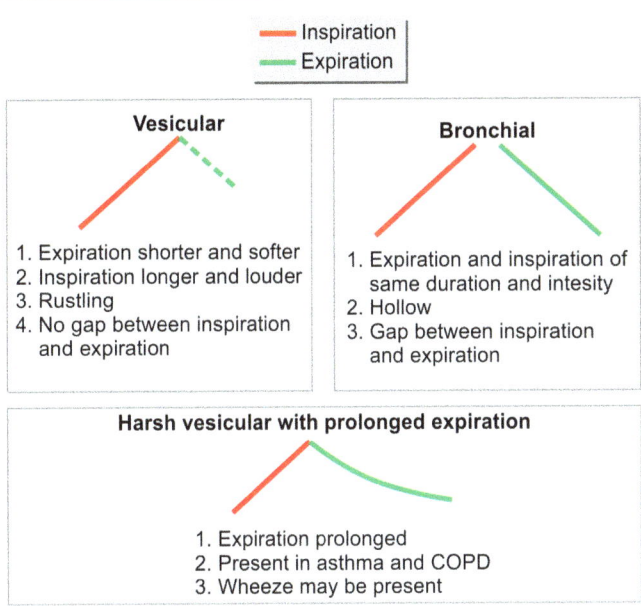

Fig. 6.3: Breath sounds.
(COPD: chronic obstructive pulmonary disease)

airways due to sudden changes in gas pressure. Fine crackles are heard in interstitial fibrosis and early pulmonary edema while coarse crackles are heard in pneumonia, bronchiectasis, chronic bronchitis and late pulmonary edema.
- *Pleural rub* is a leathery rubbing sound found in cases with pleural inflammation.

Vocal resonance: In consolidation, spoken or whispered sounds are auscultated louder and more clearly over the chest wall. These are called *bronchophony* and *whispering pectoriloquy*, respectively. The voice may sound nasal or bleating over the level of pleural effusion (*egophony*).

The chest examination findings in common respiratory diseases are given in **Table 6.8**.

INVESTIGATIONS

Chest X-ray: Chest radiograph is an important initial investigation in patients with respiratory diseases. Consolidation, pleural effusion, pneumothorax, cavity and infiltrates can be reliably diagnosed.

Posteroanterior (PA) view is the standard view. Lateral view provides additional information in certain conditions like minimal pleural effusion (lateral decubitus view) and mediastinal lesions. Comparison with old films is sometimes helpful to detect new lesions or any change in size.

Sputum examination: Examination of the sputum provides useful information. Gram staining, acid fast bacilli (AFB) smear and culture/sensitivity of the sputum are needed to diagnose pulmonary infections. Malignant cells can be seen in sputum in cases of bronchogenic carcinoma. Nebulization with hypertonic saline can be used to obtain sputum samples. Sample can also be obtained by bronchoscopy or transtracheal aspiration.

Computed tomography: This is useful in the diagnosis and staging of lung and pleural malignancies. High resolution CT is particularly helpful in the diagnosis of bronchiectasis, interstitial fibrosis and PE.

Radioisotope imaging: Combined ventilation-perfusion scanning is useful in the diagnosis of pulmonary thromboembolism.

Pulmonary angiography is the definitive method of diagnosing pulmonary emboli.

Arterial blood gas (ABG) analysis: Partial pressures of oxygen (PaO_2), carbon dioxide ($PaCO_2$) and pH can be measured in arterial blood sample. This is helpful in the assessment of the degree and type of respiratory failure.

Table 6.8: Chest examination findings in common conditions.

Condition	Inspection/Palpation	Percussion	Auscultation
Consolidation (Pneumonia)	• Reduced chest wall movement over the affected area • No mediastinal shift • Increased vocal fremitus	Dull note	• Bronchial breath sounds • Crackles • Increased vocal resonance • Whispering pectoriloquy present
Pleural effusion	• Reduced movements over affected side • Mediastinal shift to opposite side • Decreased vocal fremitus	Stony dull note	• Diminished or absent breath sounds • Pleural rub rarely (above effusion) • Egophony
Pneumothorax	• Reduced movements over affected side • Mediastinal shift to opposite side • Decreased vocal fremitus	Hyper-resonant	Diminished or absent breath sounds
Emphysema	• Reduced movements bilaterally • Barrel-shaped chest • No mediastinal shift • Decreased vocal fremitus	• Normal or hyper-resonant • Liver dullness masked	• Diminished vesicular breath sounds with prolonged expiration • Wheezes (rhonchi)
Chronic bronchitis	• Movement normal or symmetrically reduced • No mediastinal shift • Normal vocal fremitus	Normal note	• Vesicular breath sounds with prolonged expiration • Wheezes (rhonchi) • Coarse crackles

Bronchoscopy: Trachea or bronchi are directly visualized by flexible or rigid bronchoscope. Samples from airways can also be obtained by bronchial washings, aspiration or biopsy. Foreign body can be removed by bronchoscopy (Therapeutic bronchoscopy).

Pleural biopsy and aspiration: These are helpful in the detection of the cause of pleural effusion.

Spirometry: Lung volumes are measured by spirometry **(Fig. 6.4)**. This is most useful in differentiating obstructive from restrictive lung diseases.
- Forced expiratory volume (FEV_1) is the amount of gas exhaled in the first second of this maneuver which is around 80% of the forced vital capacity (FVC) in normal subjects FVC in normal subjects **(Fig. 6.5A)**.
- Forced vital capacity is the total amount of gas which can be forcefully exhaled following a maximal inhalation
- In obstructive lung diseases such as COPD, asthma, and bronchiectasis, the FEV_1/ FVC ratio is reduced **(Fig. 6.5B)**.
- The ratio is normal or raised in restrictive lung diseases such as pulmonary fibrosis

- *Peak expiratory flow rate* (PEFR) can be measured by a portable meter and is helpful in the diagnosis and management of patients with asthma.

PNEUMONIA

Pneumonia is defined as the infection of the lung parenchyma (alveoli and distal airways) and interstitium of the lung.

Etiology

Pneumonia is more common at extremes of age and in winter months.
- The risk factors for developing pneumonia are smoking, alcohol use, immunocompromised states (HIV disease, end stage renal disease), diabetes mellitus, congestive heart failure, COPD and malignancies
- Pneumonia is broadly divided into two types, community acquired pneumonia (CAP) and nosocomial pneumonia
- Nosocomial pneumonia: It consists of two entities
    - Hospital acquired pneumonia (HAP): Pneumonia developed after 48 hours after hospital admission

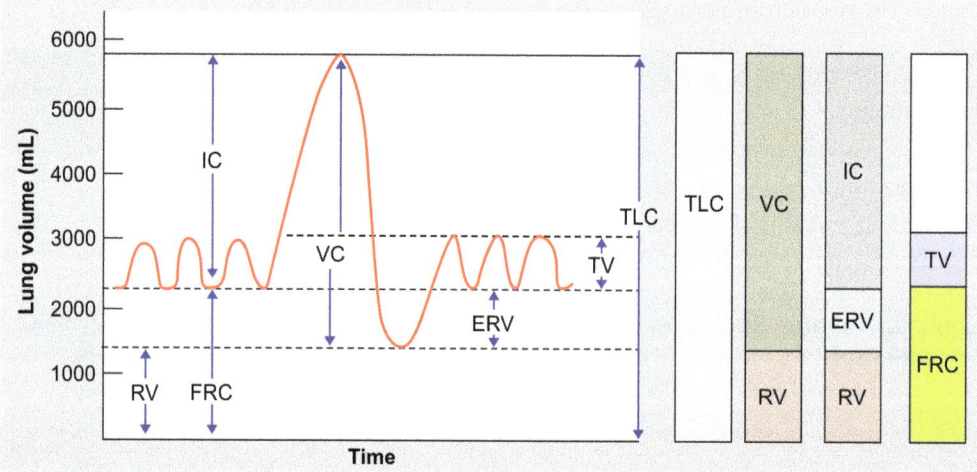

Fig. 6.4: Lung volumes.
(RV: residual volume; FRC: functional residual capacity; ERV: expiratory reserve volume; IC: inspiratory capacity; TLC: total lung capacity; TV: tidal volume; FRC: Functional residual capacity)

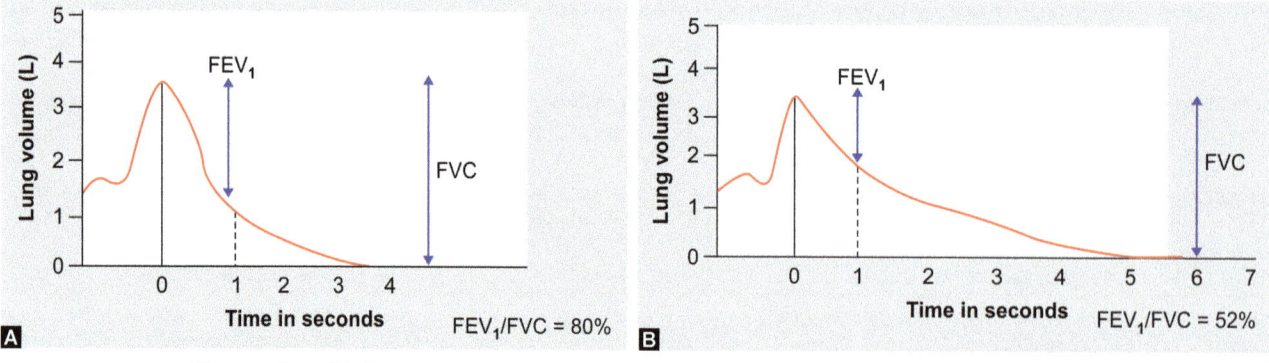

Figs. 6.5A and B: Spirometry in (A) Normal person; (B) Patient with obstructive lung disease.
(FEV_1: forced expiratory volume; FVC: forced vital capacity)

- Ventilator associated pneumonia (VAP): Pneumonia diagnosed 48 hours or more after endotracheal intubation and ventilator support.

Route of Infection

The most common route of infection is microaspiration of oropharyngeal secretions colonized with pathogenic microorganisms. Other routes are gross aspiration, aerosolization, hematogenous spread from a distant site and spread from adjacent tissues.

Organisms

More than 100 organisms including viruses, bacteria, fungi and parasites are reported to cause pneumonia. Common organisms responsible for CAP and healthcare-associated pneumonia (HCAP) are listed in **Tables 6.9 and 6.10**, respectively.

By far the most common organism causing CAP is *S. pneumoniae* (>50%). The etiological organism may vary according to the age of the patient and the specific clinical situations. *P. carinii* occurs in HIV infection while anaerobic and gram-negative bacilli (mixed etiology) can cause pneumonia due to aspiration in patients with stroke, epilepsy, and dental caries. Pseudomonas infection is common in case of bronchiectasis.

Pathology

Pathologically, pneumonia is classified into four types:
1. *Lobar pneumonia:* This type is typically seen in pneumococcal pneumonia. Generally, entire lobe of the lung is involved.

Table 6.9: Common pathogens causing community acquired pneumonia.

Bacteria
- *Streptococcus pneumoniae*
- *Mycoplasma pneumoniae*
- *Haemophilus influenzae*
- *Chlamydia pneumoniae*
- *Staphylococcus aureus*
- *Legionella spp.*

Viruses
- Influenza
- Adenoviruses
- Respiratory syncytial viruses

Table 6.10: Common pathogens causing healthcare-associated pneumonia.

Non-MDR pathogens	MDR pathogens
Streptococcus pneumoniae	Pseudomonas aeruginosa
Haemophilus influenzae	Methicillin resistant S. aureus
Methicillin sensitive S. aureus	Acinetobacter spp.
Enterobacteriacae (E. coli, Klebsiella)	Enterobacteriaceae (antibiotic resistant)

- The first stage is known as *congestion*, which occurs within 24 hours. The lung parenchyma is highly vascular and edematous with plenty of bacteria and scanty neutrophils
- Second stage (*red hepatization*) is characterized by the presence of numerous erythrocytes, neutrophils, desquamated epithelial cells and fibrin in alveoli resulting in a red and airless lung, and a consistency similar to that of liver
- In the third stage (*gray hepatization*), lung parenchyma becomes gray, dry and friable
- Finally, in the *stage of resolution*, the exudates are digested and removed by scavenger cells or coughed out.

2. *Bronchopneumonia:* This type is most commonly seen in HCAP. There is neutrophilic exudate in bronchi and bronchioles with peripheral spread of infection to alveoli. One or several lobes of the lung may be involved. Generally, lower and posterior segments of lobes are affected.
3. *Interstitial pneumonia:* This is seen in viral and pneumocystis jiroveci pneumonia. There is predominant involvement of the interstitium, alveolar wall and connective tissue around the bronchovascular tree. The pattern may be patchy or diffuse.
4. *Miliary pneumonia:* Hematogenous spread of pathogens to the lung may result into diffuse and discrete 2–3 mm lesions resembling millet seeds.

Clinical Manifestations

The onset may be sudden or insidious, and the disease may be mild or severe. Fever with chills or rigors, cough (dry or productive), pleuritic chest pain, breathlessness are typical manifestations of pneumonia. Other symptoms are headache, nausea, vomiting, diarrhea, altered sensorium, myalgia and arthralgia. The signs of lobar pneumonia are depicted in **Table 6.11**.

The severity of pneumonia is indicated by respiratory rate >30 per minute, pulse rate >125 per minute and blood pressure less than 90 mm Hg. Other markers of severity are altered mentation, hypoxia (PaO_2 < 60 mm Hg),

Table 6.11: Respiratory signs in lobar pneumonia.

Inspection and palpation
- Tachypnea
- Decreased movement of the chest on the side of disease
- No shift of trachea or apex beat (no mediastinal shift)
- Increased vocal fremitus

Percussion
Impaired or dull note

Auscultation
- Bronchial breath sounds
- Whispering pectoriloquy
- Increased vocal resonance
- Egophony
- Crackles (crepts)
- Pleural rub

Table 6.12: CURB-65 criteria.

C	Confusion
U	Blood urea nitrogen >20 mg/dL
R	Respiratory rate >30 minutes
B	Blood pressure systolic <90 mm Hg or diastolic <60 mm Hg
65	Age >65 years

hyponatremia, acidosis and azotemia. Pneumonia due to certain organisms like *P. aeruginosa, Klebsiella spp, E. coli, S. aureus* are associated with high mortality rate. The CURB-65 criteria **(Table 6.12)** are helpful in deciding whether patient should be treated on out patient basis or hospitalized. Patients with two or more criteria need hospitalization.

Complications

The complications of pneumonia are given in **Table 6.13**.

Investigations

- *Radiological:* Chest X-ray shows homogeneous opacity localized to the lobe or segment (lobar consolidation) or diffuse infiltrates in bronchopneumonia **(Figs. 6.6 to 6.9)**. Other findings may include pleural effusion, lung abscess

Table 6.13: Complications of pneumonia.

Pulmonary
- Parapneumonic pleural effusion
- Empyema
- Suppurative pneumonia/lung abscess
- ARDS
- Pneumothorax (in *S. aureus* pneumonia)

Extrapulmonary
- Hepatitis, pericarditis, meningoencephalitis
- Multiorgan failure
- Ectopic abscess formation

(ARDS: acute respiratory distress syndrome)

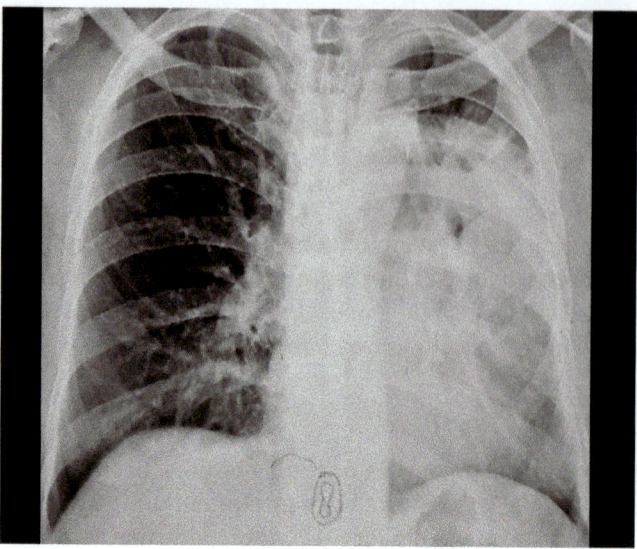

Fig. 6.7: X-ray chest showing left lower pneumonia.

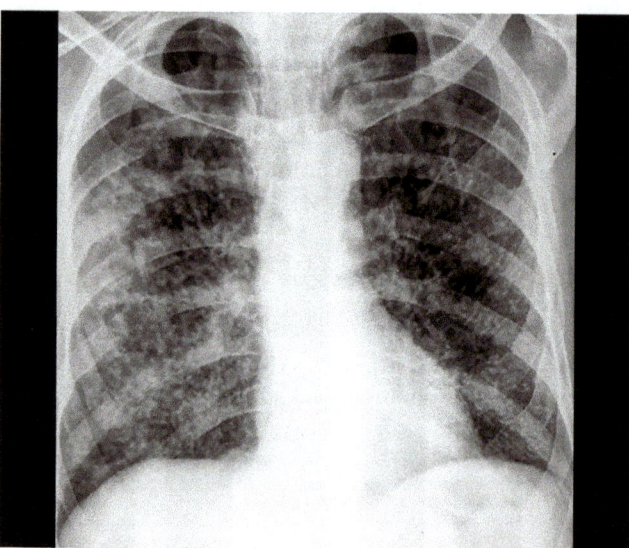

Fig. 6.8: X-ray chest showing bilateral interstitial pneumonia.

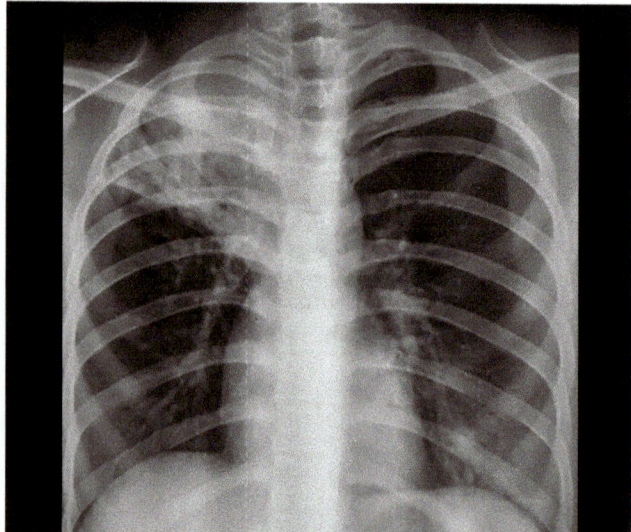

Fig. 6.6: X-ray chest showing right upper lobe consolidation with air bronchogram

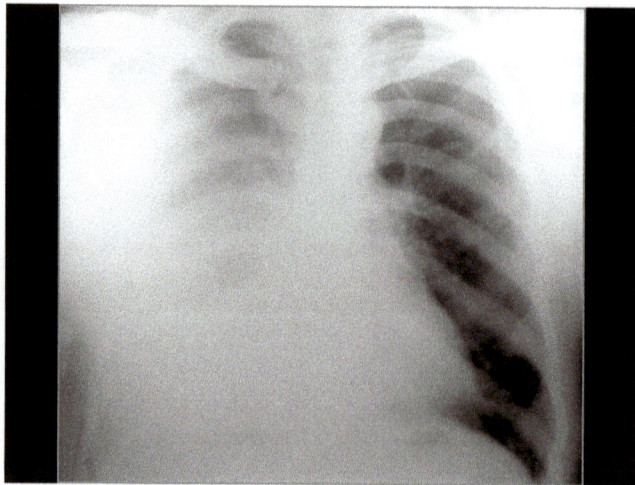

Fig. 6.9: X-ray chest showing consolidation in the right lung.

and hilar lymphadenopathy. Pneumatoceles may be seen in *S. aureus* pneumonia.
- *Sputum or pulmonary secretion examination:* Gram staining and culture are helpful in identifying the causative organisms and finding out the sensitivity pattern.
- *Blood tests:* These include blood culture, ABG analysis, and total and differential leukocyte counts. Neutrophilic leukocytosis is commonly found in bacterial pneumonia while leukopenia may indicate viral etiology.
- *Serological tests:* The detection of antibodies may be helpful in the diagnosis of *Chlamydia*, *Mycoplasma* and *Legionella pneumonia.*
- *Other tests:* Polymerase chain reaction (PCR) based tests and specialized culture tests may be needed in some cases.

Treatment

- *General principles:* The patients are managed as outpatient or inpatient (hospitalized) depending upon the severity of the disease. The severity is generally assessed using CURB-65 criteria. Other criteria used are PORT (Pneumonia Patient Outcomes Research Team) and CPIS (Clinical Pulmonary Infection Score).
- *Supportive therapy:* Oxygen therapy is given to all hypoxemic patients. Those who do not respond may need mechanical ventilation. Intravenous fluids may also be required in hospitalized patients.
- *Antibiotic therapy:* The antibiotics should be started as early as possible. If possible, the specimen should be sent for culture and sensitivity before starting antibiotics. The etiology is commonly unknown; hence, the initial choice of antibiotics is empirical. However, this may be modified once culture reports are available.
    - In outpatients with CAP with no recent antibiotic exposure and comorbidities, the preferred empirical antibiotic options are macrolide or doxycycline or fluoroquinolones (with activity against *S. pneumoniae*) **(Table 6.14)**. A 10–14 days therapy is generally required.

Table 6.14: Empirical antibiotic options in out patients with CAP.

1.	Macrolides	
	a. Clarithromycin	500 mg orally twice a day
	b. Azithromycin	500 mg orally on day 1 then 250 mg daily × 4 days
2.	Doxycycline	100 mg orally twice a day
3.	Fluoroquinolones	
	a. Gatifloxacin	400 mg orally once a day
	b. Levofloxacin	500 mg orally once a day
	c. Moxifloxacin	400 mg orally once a day
4.	Alternative regimens	
	a. Erythromycin	500 mg orally 4 times a day
	b. Amoxicillin-clavulanate	625 mg orally thrice a day
	c. Amoxicillin	500–1,000 mg orally thrice a day
	d. Cefpodoxime	200 mg orally twice a day
	e. Cefuroxime axetil	500 mg orally twice a day

Outpatients with recent antibiotic exposure (within the past 90 days), comorbidities, age < 65 years and immunosuppression should receive respiratory fluoroquinolone or macrolide plus a beta lactam (high dose amoxicillin or amoxicillin-clavulanate).
- Empirical antibiotic options for hospitalized patients with CAP are following. These are given intravenously. The duration of treatment is 10-14 days.
    » Beta lactum (cefatrixone 1–2 g/day or cefotaxime 2 g 6 hourly) plus a macrolide or fluoroquinolones
    » Beta lactam/beta lactamase inhibitor (ampicillin/sulbactam or piperacillin/tazobactam) plus macrolide or fluoroquinolones
    » Patients with aspiration pneumonia should receive fluoroquinolones plus clindamycin or metronidazole
    » In pseudomonas infection (as in patients with underlying bronchiectasis), a combination of fluoroquinolones with carbapenem or cefepime.

LUNG ABSCESS

Suppurative pneumonia is characterized by destruction of lung parenchyma by the inflammatory process generally leading to microabscess formation. When a large collection of pus occurs within the lung parenchyma lined by chronic inflammatory tissue, the condition is known as lung abscess.

The most commonly involved areas are dependent segments of the lungs, *posterior segments of the upper lobes and superior segments of the lower lobes* in supine position.

Risk Factors

Aspiration of oropharyngeal secretion is the most important cause of lung abscess. Predisposing factors for aspiration include:
- Altered consciousness due to any cause (alcohol, drugs, seizures, stroke and general anesthesia)
- Impaired swallowing due to esophageal disorders (achalasia, gastroesophageal reflux)
- Vocal cord palsy
- *Poor oral hygiene and gross oral sepsis is also associated with greater risk of pulmonary infection* due to aspiration.

Causative Organisms

Mostly the lung abscess is caused by mixed bacterial flora, both aerobic and anaerobic.
- Common aerobic pathogens responsible for lung abscess are *S. pneumoniae, S. aureus, S. pyogenes, H. influenzae, E. coli* and *Pseudomonas*
- Anaerobic bacteria such as bacteroides, *Prevotella, Fusobacterium* and *Peptostreptococcus* species are generally responsible in cases with poor dental hygiene or oral sepsis.

Clinical Features

The presentation is generally insidious in anaerobic infection while more acute presentation is typical of aerobic infection. Important symptoms are high remittent fever, weight loss, malaise, night sweats, cough with large amount of purulent sputum. The foul smelling sputum suggests anaerobic infection. Chest pain may occur due to pleural involvement.

General examination may reveal clubbing. Respiratory examination shows signs of consolidation or cavity such as bronchial breath sound and coarse crackles.

Diagnosis

- The chest X-ray may show, in early stages, a homogenous opacity due to consolidation. This may cavitate and present as large cavity with air-fluid level (**Fig. 6.10**). Other causes of cavitatory lung disease should be excluded (**Table 6.15**)
- Sputum or pulmonary secretion obtained by bronchoscopy is cultured for both aerobic and anaerobic organisms
- CT thorax can be helpful to exclude the presence of tumor or other underlying causes in patients not responding to treatment.

Treatment

Medical

- The antibiotic therapy should be chosen according to the organism isolated
- The therapy is generally given for prolonged period (6–8 weeks) until the radiographic resolution of the cavity
- Commonly, a combination of penicillin (amoxicillin) and metronidazole is effective. However, with the emergence of beta lactamase producing organisms, clindamycin (150–300 mg 6 hourly) is now considered standard therapy. Beta lactam/beta lactamase inhibitors may also be used
- Postural drainage is also helpful in the management of lung abscess.

Surgical

Surgical intervention like percutaneous drainage or lobectomy is needed in case there is no response to medical treatment or there is a large abscess.

BRONCHIECTASIS

Abnormal and permanent dilatation of bronchi is called bronchiectasis. There is inflammation of the medium sized airways leading to the destruction of the wall. The inflammatory cells, chiefly neutrophils are primary mediators and they release proteolytic enzymes leading to destruction and fibrosis of bronchial structures. Repeated obstruction and infections are important factors. Common causes of bronchiectasis are suppurative pneumonia and tuberculosis. Other important causes of bronchiectasis are given in **Table 6.16**.

Clinical Manifestations

Chronic persistent or intermittent cough with large amount of purulent sputum is the main symptom. Patient may also have fever, weight loss and hemoptysis. Recurrent lung infection may lead to pneumonia and pleurisy.

Clinical examination reveals digital clubbing and anemia. Lung signs are nonspecific and include basal coarse crackles and wheezes. There may be signs of right heart failure (cor pulmonale).

Investigations

- Chest X-ray may be normal or it may show small cystic spaces (**Figs. 6.11 and 6.12**)

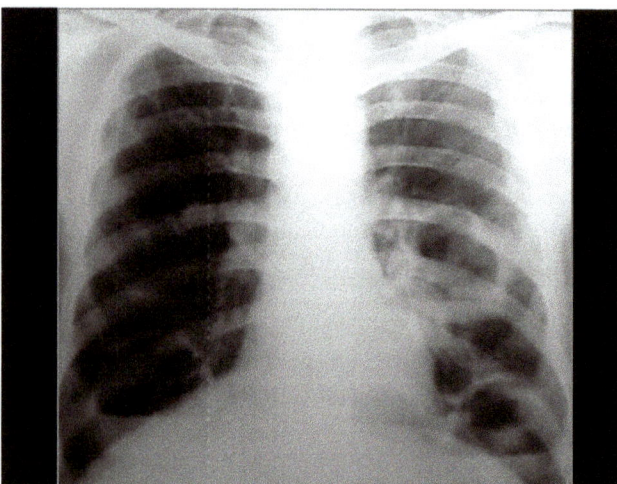

Fig. 6.10: X-ray chest showing lung abscesses with horizontal air-fluid level.

Table 6.15: Causes of cavitary lung disease.
• Lung abscess
• Tuberculosis
• Fungal infections
• Cavitating carcinoma
• Pulmonary infarction
• Wegener's granulomatosis

Table 6.16: Important causes of bronchiectasis.
Congenital
• Kartagener's syndrome*
• Cystic fibrosis
Acquired
• Suppurative pneumonia
• Tuberculosis
• Post-viral infection (in children, adenovirus, influenza virus)
• Foreign body
• Bronchial tumor
• Allergic bronchopulmonary aspergillosis

*Sinusitis and transposition of the viscera

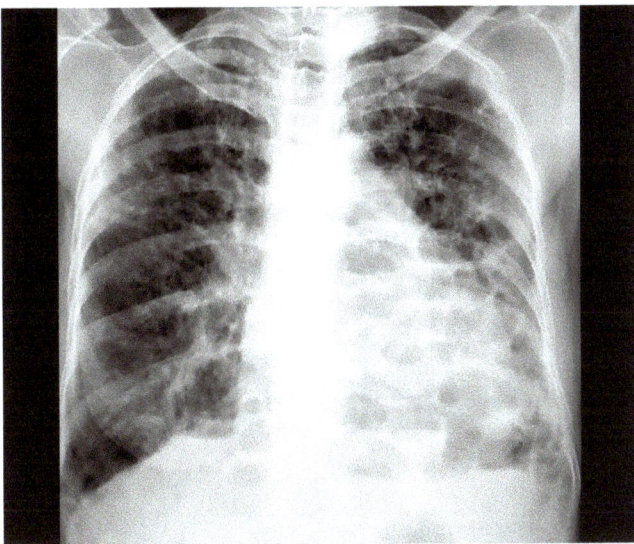

Fig. 6.11: X-ray chest showing diffuse cystic bronchiectasis in left lung.

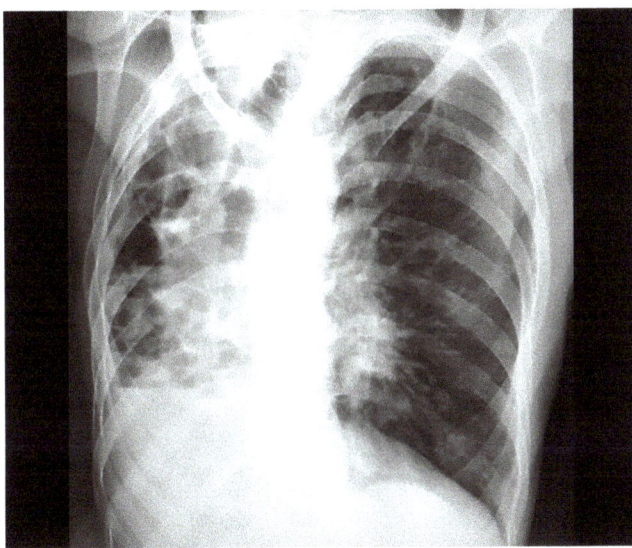

Fig. 6.12: X-ray chest showing post-tubercular fibrobronchiectasis.

- High resolution CT scan (HRCT scan) is the test of choice to make the diagnosis **(Fig. 6.13)**
- Sputum examination and culture guide in choosing the antibiotics.

Treatment

- The main steps in the management of bronchiectasis are antibiotics, postural drainage and inhaled bronchodilators
- Surgery is indicated in cases of massive hemoptysis and localized bronchiectasis which fail to respond to adequate medical therapy.

Complications

The complications of bronchiectasis are amyloidosis, cor pulmonale and abscess at distant site.

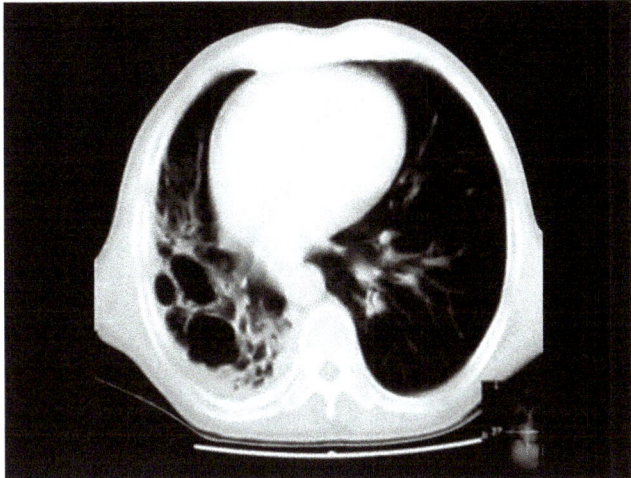

Fig. 6.13: CT scan showing bronchiectasis.

BRONCHIAL ASTHMA

Asthma is a disease of the airways in which there is a chronic inflammation and increased responsiveness to a wide variety of stimuli, leading to reversible airway obstruction. Patients generally have paroxysms of cough, wheeze, chest tightness and dyspnea, interspersed with symptom-free periods.

Pathophysiology

Genetic and environmental factors play a role in the pathogenesis of bronchial asthma.
- Early onset (extrinsic) asthma begins in childhood and a family history of atopy and other allergic disorders such as allergic rhinitis and eczema is usually present. Skin test to antigens is positive and serum levels of IgE are raised. The symptoms resolve in about 80% of children as they grow
- Late onset (intrinsic) asthma starts in adulthood in nonatopic individuals with no family history of allergic disorders. Skin test is negative and serum levels of IgE are normal. This type of presentation is found in minority of asthmatic patients (10%).

Atopic individuals are sensitized after an exposure to allergen and develop IgE antibodies. Subsequent exposure to the allergen causes a two-phase bronchoconstrictor response. Early reaction (type I) occurs because of rapid interaction of allergen with mast cells via IgE-dependent mechanism. It results in the release of preformed mediators like histamine and leukotrienes which cause broncho-constriction (*see* **Table 6.17**). Late reaction (type II) is characterized by T-cell mediated influx of inflammatory cells, chiefly eosinophils. It leads to chronic inflammatory reaction in the bronchial wall.

The pathological changes are:
- Bronchial smooth muscle hypertrophy and hyperplasia
- Hyperplasia of mucous glands
- Mucosal edema with infiltration of granulocytes
- Hyperplasia of mucosal and submucosal vessels

Table 6.17: Key mediators of asthma.

Mediators	Source cells	Mechanism
Chemokines like Eotaxin	Epithelial cells	These are important in recruitment of inflammatory cells in to the airways and are mainly expressed in airway epithelial cells
Cysteinyl leukotrienes	Mast cells and eosinophils	Potent bronchoconstrictors and proinflammatory mediators
Cytokines, e.g., IL-4, 5, 9, 13	Th2 helper cells	It causes inflammatory response in asthma and determine its severity
Histamine	Mast cells	Causes bronchoconstriction
Nitric oxide	Airway epithelial cells	It is potent vasodilator
Prostaglandin D2	Mast cells	Bronchoconstrictor

- Thickening of basement membrane
- Infiltration with eosinophils, lymphocytes, mast cells, neutrophils.

A wide variety of stimuli can provoke bronchospasm in an asthmatic. Stimuli can be allergic or nonallergic **(Table 6.18)**.

Clinical Features

The symptoms of bronchial asthma may be episodic or persistent.

- *Episodic asthma* is characterized by paroxysm of dyspnea, cough, chest tightness and wheezing which occurs more commonly in children and young adults. The attacks may be mild or severe and may last for hours, days or rarely weeks. Between episodes, the patients are usually asymptomatic
- In older nonatopic patients, the asthma is chronic and persistent. Symptoms are worse in the early morning. This can be confused with the COPD.

Examination

- The examination may reveal tachypnea, tachycardia and involvement of accessory respiratory muscles

Table 6.18: Stimuli that can provoke asthma.

Allergic
- Inhaled allergens: Pollen, house-dust, feathers, animal danders, fungal spores
- Ingested allergens: Fish, eggs, milk, nuts, strawberries, yeast, wheat
- Additives in food: Monosodium glutamate (ajinomoto), metabisulfite preservative used in beers, wine and preserved food
- Occupational: Grain-dust, wood-dust
- Environmental: Cold air
- Physiochemical agents: Gases, fumes and smoke
- Drugs: Aspirin, NSAIDS, beta-blockers

Nonallergic
- Infections: Respiratory viral infections
- Exercise
- Emotional outburst

- The breath sound is harsh vesicular with prolonged expiration
- Prominent wheeze is audible in both phases of respiration. Depending on the symptoms, signs, frequency of exacerbations and PEF rate, the asthma is classified as mild, moderate or severe.

Acute severe asthma: This is a severe life-threatening attack of asthma, previously known as *status asthmaticus*. The patient may additionally have tachycardia, pulsus paradoxus, cyanosis and active accessory respiratory muscles. The air entry is drastically reduced (silent chest on auscultation). The patient may become confused or drowsy.

Investigations

Pulmonary function tests:
- Spirometry:
  - Demonstration of reversible air flow obstruction is the hallmark of the diagnosis
  - In bronchial asthma, FEV_1, FEV_1/VC ratio and PEFR are reduced
  - *Demonstration of reversibility*: In adults there is increase in FEV_1 >12% and >200 mL and in children there is increase >12% predicted following administration of bronchodilator [(salbutamol 400 mcg metered dose inhaler (MDI) with spacer or 2.5 mg by nebulizer)] is diagnostic of bronchial asthma
- *Peak flow meter*: It is easily available, inexpensive and handy and easy to use, patient should measure PEFR twice daily for 1–2 week. Normally diurnal variability of PEFR is 10%. There is significant bronchodilator reversibility if PEFR improve by >20% on >3 days/week.

Peak expiratory flow rate is generally used for long-term home monitoring **(Fig. 6.14)**.

- *Bronchial provocation tests*: It is done when there is high index of suspicion of asthma and spirometry/PEFR is normal. It measure airway hyper responsiveness to various stimuli like methacholine (most common), histamine, mannitol, exercise, cold air exposure, etc.

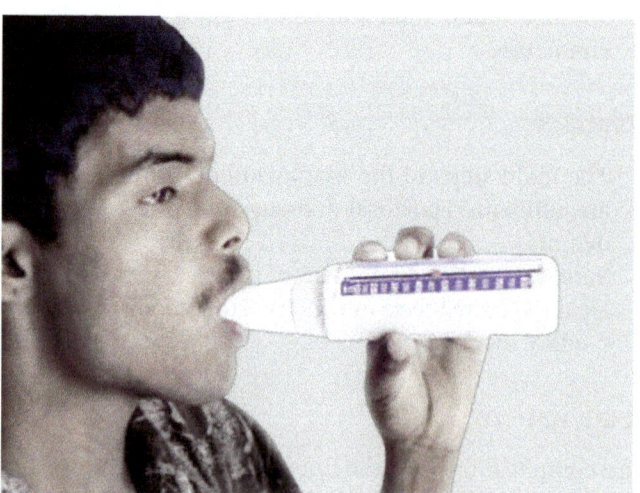

Fig. 6.14: Peak expiratory flowmeter.

Concentration of these agents which causes significant bronchoconstriction ($FEV_1 > 20\%$) is measured and leveled as PC20 or PD20.

These tests can cause life-threatening bronchoconstriction so should be done in tertiary care center in emergency settings only.

- An objective measurement of airflow obstruction is essential to the evaluation of exacerbation. The severity of exacerbation is classified as:
  » Mild (PEF or FEV_1 > 70% of predicted or personal best)
  » Moderate (PEF or FEV_1 > 40% to 69%)
  » Severe (PEF or FEV_1 < 40%)
  » Life-threatening/impending respiratory arrest (PEF or FEV_1 < 40%).

Chest X-ray: This is usually normal. However, it may appear hyperinflated. This is also helpful in ruling out other conditions.

Arterial blood gas analysis: Initially $PaCO_2$ is low. A normal or high $PaCO_2$ is a sign of impending respiratory failure. PaO_2 < 60 mm Hg signifies severe bronchoconstriction and respiratory failure.

Allergy tests: Atopic status can be identified by skin prick testing or by measuring the level of specific immunoglobulin E (SIgE) in serum (not reliable). These can be done when there is suspected allergy to 2–3 substance only.

Others: Peripheral blood may show eosinophilia. Sputum may also contain an increased number of eosinophils.

Management

The overall aim of management as per Global Strategy for Asthma Management and Prevention, Global Initiative for Asthma 2021 should be:
- To abolish or minimize symptoms.
- To attain the best possible PEF
- To prevent exacerbation.
- To normalize exercise capacity.

Non-pharmacological Management

Avoidance of factors: The identification of allergens is possible only in a few cases. Wherever possible, the exposure to such agents must be avoided **(Table 6.19)**.

Desensitization: Desensitization by repeated administration of allergen has not been proven effective in most studies.

Pharmacological Management

Drug therapy: The drugs used in asthma can be grouped as:
- Medications are used to control symptoms, reduce airway inflammation and decrease exacerbations and related decline in lung functions (Controller medications).

Table 6.19: Non-pharmacological management.
- Avoidance of tobacco smoke exposure
- *Physical activity:* Encouraged because of its general health benefits. Provide advice about exercise-induced bronchoconstriction.
- *Weight reduction:* Prevent obesity-induced asthma.
- *Avoid occupational irritants:* Remove sensitizers as soon as possible.
- Avoid medications that may worsen asthma like Aspirin and other NSAIDs in Aspirin-induced asthma
- Remediation of dampness or mold in homes
- Avoid Pet animals in sensitized individual's home
- *Avoidance of indoor pollution:* Wash bed-sheet, carpet, blankets regularly to avoid house dust mites.
- Avoidance of outdoor allergens like pollen, molds, etc.
- *Healthy diet:* Consume a healthy diet high in fruits and vegetables.
- *Avoidance of foods and food chemicals:* If allergy or food chemical sensitivity.
- *Vaccination:* Yearly influenza vaccine in age >50 years.

b. Medications are used for relief of breakthrough symptoms such as exacerbations of asthma or during worsening of symptoms (Reliever medications).

Assessment of asthma symptoms control is important and helps in stepping treatment up or down. Poor control of symptoms is associated with increased exacerbations risk. Patient is asked about following in the past four weeks: Frequency of symptoms, any night waking, limitation of activity and frequency of use of reliever medication (short-acting beta-2 agonist) for relief of symptoms **(Table 6.20)**.

Medications used for asthma are given in **Tables 6.21 and 6.22**.

Chronic Persistent Asthma

A stepwise approach is chosen according to the severity of disease. Once the disease is controlled, a step down therapy is attempted.

Recommended Asthma Treatment for Adults and Adolescents

Preferred (option **a**) and alternative (option **b**) treatment based on initial symptoms is given below. In option **a** patient uses low dose ICS-formoterol (single inhaler) for relief of symptoms (reliever therapy) and takes ICS-formoterol as daily controller therapy. Low dose ICS-formoterol (inhaled

Table 6.20: Asthma control with medication.

In past 1 month, do you have following asthma related symptoms?	
Daytime symptoms: >twice/week?	Yes/No
Extra dose of inhaler: >twice/week?	Yes/No
Any night time waking?	Yes/No
Any physical activity limitation?	Yes/No

Interpretation and action:
Count yes
None = Controlled: Reduce the dose (step down)
Any 1–2 = Partly Controlled: Continue
Many 3–4 = Uncontrolled: Review, optimise and step up

TABLE 6.21: Bronchodilator drugs used in asthma.

Group	Route of administration	Major side effects
Adrenergic (Beta-2 receptor agonist) • Epinephrine • Salbutamol, albuterol, terbutaline • Salmeterol, formoterol, indacaterol, vilanterol (long acting)	• Subcut. injection • Oral and inhaled • Inhaled	Tremor, tachycardia
Methylxanthines • Theophylline • Aminophylline	• Oral and IM/IV • IV	• Nausea, vomiting • Arrhythmia, seizures
Anticholinergics • Ipratropium bromide • Tiotropium • Glycopyrronium • Umeclidinium	Inhaled	No major side effects

TABLE 6.22: Anti-inflammatory drugs used in asthma.

	Route of administration	Major side effects
Steroids *Systemic* • Methyl prednisolone • Prednisolone	• Oral and IV • Oral	Long-term side effects: Adrenal suppression, cataract, growth retardation, osteoporosis, hyperglycemia, hypertension
Inhaled • Beclomethasone • Budesonide • Fluticasone • Ciclesonide • Mometasone	Inhaled	Dysphonia, thrush, long-term use may cause systemic side effects as above
Mast cell stabilizers • Cromolyn sodium • Nedocromil	Inhaled	
Leukotriene modifiers • Montelukast • Zafirlukast • Zileuton	Oral	Hepatic toxicity, drug interaction
Biologics *Anti-IgE* • Omalizumab *Anti-IL5/5R* • Mepolizumab • Benralizumab • Reslizumab *Anti-IL4R* • Dupilumab	Subcutaneous Subcutaneous Subcutaneous Intravenous Subcutaneous	

Note: Long acting inhaled adrenergic agents (salmeterol, formoterol) and theophylline also have anti-inflammatory properties.

corticosteroids plus formoterol) as initial treatment reduces risk of exacerbations. In option **b** patient uses low dose SABA and low dose inhaled corticosteroids (ICS) together for relief of symptoms (reliever therapy) and takes ICS-containing medication as daily controller therapy.

Educate and always check inhalation technique and adherence to therapy.

Step down once symptoms have been controlled for 3 months.

1. Asthma symptoms < 2 in a month without risk factors for exacerbation
   a. Low dose ICS-formoterol as needed (single inhaler).
   b. Low dose inhaled corticosteroids (ICS) whenever low dose short-acting beta-2 agonist (SABA) taken (separate inhalers or in combination inhaler).
2. Asthma symptoms or need for reliever > 2 in a month
   a. Low dose ICS-formoterol as needed.
   b. Low dose maintenance ICS with as needed low dose SABA. Check adherence to daily ICS.
3. Asthma symptoms on most days/waking due to symptoms ≥ 1/week, presence of any risk factor for exacerbation
   a. Low dose ICS-formoterol maintenance and reliever therapy.
   b. Low dose ICS-LABA (inhaled corticosteroids- long-acting beta-2 agonist) with as needed SABA. Check adherence to daily controller therapy.
4. Daily symptoms, severe uncontrolled asthma/acute exacerbation, low lung function:
   a. Medium dose ICS-formoterol maintenance and reliever therapy. Oral corticosteroids may be required (short course).
   b. High dose ICS or medium dose ICS-LABA with as needed SABA. Oral corticosteroids may be required (short course). Check adherence to daily controller therapy.
5. In addition to above treatment consider addition of long-acting muscurinic agents (LAMA), anti-IgE (omalizumab), Anti-IL5/5R (subcutaneous mepolizumab, subcutaneous benralizumab, intravenous reslizumab), anti-IL4R (subcutaneous dupilumab), high dose ICS-LABA. Bronchial thermoplasty with localized radiofrequency pulse may be considered in some patients with severe asthma.

Acute Severe Asthma

- *Hospitalization and oxygen therapy:* The patient should be hospitalized for urgent management. ABG analysis, chest X-ray and ECG should be done to assess severity and to rule out other causes. A high concentration oxygen inhalation is given to maintain PaO_2 > 60 mm Hg.
- Repeated dosage of short-acting adrenergic drugs (salbutamol 2.5–5 mg or terbutaline 5–10 mg) is given through a nebulizer at an interval of 20–30 minutes. The PEFR should be recorded frequently to assess the response. MDI with a spacer device can alternatively be used. Ipratropium bromide can be added to get additional bronchodilator effect.

- *Systemic steroids:* This is essentially needed in all cases of severe asthma. Prednisolone (30–60 mg daily) or methylprednisolone is given orally or intravenously. The dose of inhaled corticosteroids (ICS, ICS-formoterol) increased.
- *Others:*
  - Mechanical ventilation is needed in patients with coma, respiratory arrest, exhaustion and deteriorating blood gases despite adequate treatment.
  - IV fluid is administered to prevent dehydration.
  - Antibiotics are not used routinely. These are only given if infection is present.
  - Opiates, sedatives or tranquillizers are contraindicated.
  - Intravenous magnesium may be considered for severe exacerbations not responding to initial treatment.

Patient Education and Monitoring of Therapy

- The patients are educated about the nature of disease and its treatment
- They should also be trained to recognize the severity of their disease and monitor the response to therapy with the use of peak flow meter
- Patients should also be demonstrated the proper use of inhalation devices such as MDIs (pressurized aerosol system), rotahaler (dry powder system) and nebulizers **(Figs. 6.15A to C)**
- Use of inhaler therapy should be encouraged as it is effective in lower dosage together with a rapid onset of action and has fewer side effects.

Complications

The main complications of bronchial asthma include pneumothorax, respiratory failure and cor pulmonale.

CHRONIC OBSTRUCTIVE PULMONARY DISEASE

Definition

Chronic obstructive pulmonary disease is a common, preventable and treatable disease that is characterized by persistent respiratory symptoms and airflow limitation that is due to airway and/or alveolar abnormalities usually caused by significant exposure to noxious particles or gases and also influenced by host factors including abnormal lung development. Associated co-morbidities have an impact on mortality and morbidity [GOLD (Global Strategy for the Diagnosis, Management, and Prevention of Chronic Obstructive Pulmonary Disease) 2021].

It includes chronic bronchitis and emphysema. Other causes of pulmonary obstruction (asthma, bronchiectasis, cystic fibrosis, bronchiolitis) are not classified as COPD.

- *Chronic bronchitis* is defined as a condition with a history of cough and sputum on most days for at least 3 consecutive months for more than 2 successive years (provided other causes of chronic productive cough are excluded). Recently, chronic bronchitis has been described as clinically defined condition with chronic cough and sputum.
- *Emphysema* is defined as irreversible destruction and enlargement of air spaces distal to terminal bronchioles. Pure forms of these two conditions are rare and in the majority of cases they coexist.

Etiological Factors

- *Cigarette smoking* is the most important etiological factor for COPD. There is a positive correlation between the intensity of smoking (number of cigarettes and duration of smoking) and the development of COPD. However, individual susceptibility varies since only 15% smokers develop clinically significant COPD
- *Biomass fuel smoke exposure:* This is most common nonsmoking risk factor for development of COPD in developing countries like India. Burning of fuel like cow dung, wood, coal, kerosene, etc. emits various noxious particles in its smoke which causes COPD especially in female population
- *Air pollution* in the environment may also be associated with the development of COPD
- *Infections:* Childhood lung infection like whooping cough can lead to COPD in adult life
- *Post tubercular COPD:* Tuberculosis damages lung parenchyma including small airway and alveoli which

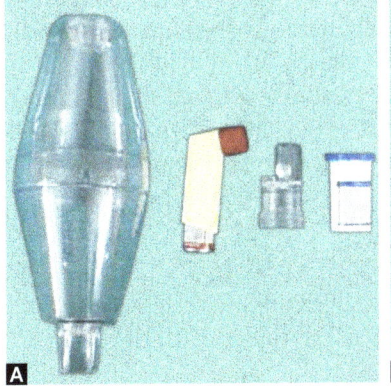
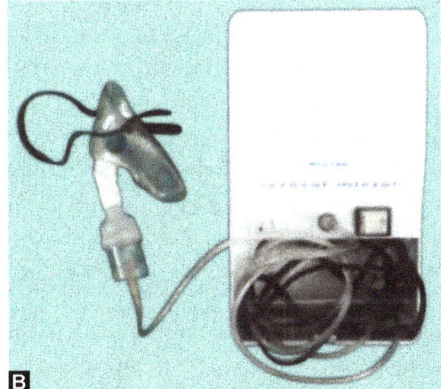
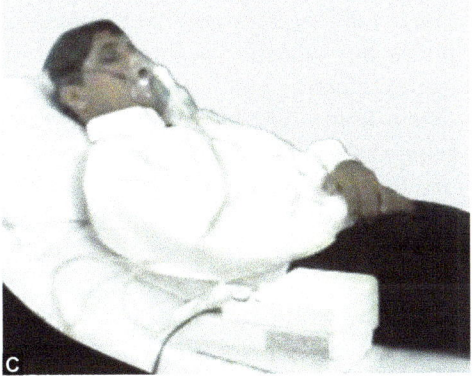

Figs. 6.15A to C: Inhalation devices, nebulizer and patient on nebulizer therapy.

may lead to airway obstruction. This entity called tuberculosis obstructive pulmonary diseases (TOPD)
- Other factors are occupational exposure to dusts, bronchial hyper-responsiveness, chronic asthma, poverty and low birth weight
- Severe alpha-1 antitrypsin deficiency is a proven genetic risk factor for the development of emphysema.

Pathophysiology

The important pathological changes in the airways are inflammation, hypertrophy of the mucous secreting glands and increase in the number of goblet cells. This leads to decreased mucociliary clearance. The mechanical obstruction in the airflow and loss of elastic recoil of lungs result in air flow limitation.

The emphysema in smokers is generally centriacinar which involves mostly the upper lobes of the lung (centriacinar emphysema). In alpha-1 antitrypsin deficiency, the lower lobes of lung are predominantly affected (panacinar emphysema).

The persistent hypoxia and pulmonary vascular changes cause pulmonary hypertension, right ventricular hypertrophy (cor pulmonale) and failure.

Clinical Features

The important symptoms are cough, sputum production and exertional dyspnea. Initially, the cough and expectoration are more marked in winters but later these may occur throughout the year. Sputum is mucoid, scanty and thick. There may be streaking of sputum with blood; massive hemoptysis is rare. Increased production of purulent sputum and fever indicates bacterial infection. As the disease advances, dyspnea becomes more severe and occurs even during rest.

In mild cases, the physical examination may be normal
- Chest examination reveals vesicular breath sound with prolonged expiratory phase and generalized wheeze. The crackles (crepitations) may be heard mainly in the lower zones
- The patient with predominant emphysema shows barrel-shaped chest (increased AP diameter) **(Fig. 6.16)**, loss of cardiac and liver dullness and diminished vesicular breath sound
- The use of accessory respiratory muscles, breathing with pursed lips and lack of cyanosis characterize emphysema (pink puffers)
- Cyanosis and right heart failure are more common and seen earlier in the course of disease in patients with predominant chronic bronchitis (blue bloaters).

The signs are also depicted in **Table 6.23**. Clubbing is not a feature of COPD. If clubbing is present, evaluation for other conditions especially lung cancer should be done.

Many comorbid conditions may influence mortality and hospitalization in COPD patients. These include cardiovascular diseases, depression, skeletal muscle dysfunction, metabolic syndrome and lung cancer. These comorbidities should be looked and treated in COPD patients.

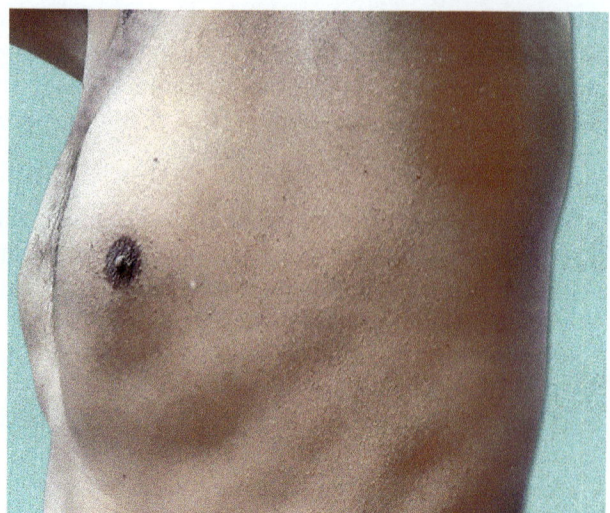

Fig. 6.16: Emphysematous chest: AP diameter is more than lateral diameter.

Table 6.23: Clinical signs in COPD.

General
- Cyanosis
- Signs of right heart failure
  - Pedal edema, raised JVP, hepatomegaly, ascites
- Signs of CO_2 retention
  - Flapping tremor (asterixis), bounding pulse obtundation
- Pursed lip breathing
- Wasting and weight loss

Respiratory
- Use of accessory muscles of respiration (scalene, sternocleidomastoid)
- Indrawing of intercostal muscles during inspiration (Hoover's sign)
- Increased AP diameter of the chest
- Loss of cardiac dullness and liver dullness
- Diminished vesicular breath sounds
- Prolonged expiratory phase
- Generalized wheeze
- Crackles mostly at bases

(COPD: chronic obstructive pulmonary disease; JVP: jugular venous pressure; AP: anteroposterior)

Investigations

- *Pulmonary function tests*: Spirometric demonstration of airway obstruction without significant reversal is the hallmark of the diagnosis of COPD. Significant reversibility of the obstruction (as seen in asthma) is defined as more than 12% or 200 mL increase in FEV_1 after two puffs of short-acting beta adrenergic agonist like salbutamol. An abnormal FEV_1 (< 80% predicted) with an FEV_1/VC ratio of < 70% strongly suggests COPD. Lung volumes (total lung capacity and residual volume) are increased due to air trapping.

COPD is classified according to GOLD 2020 guidelines as:
- Mild: When FEV_1 is >80% predicted

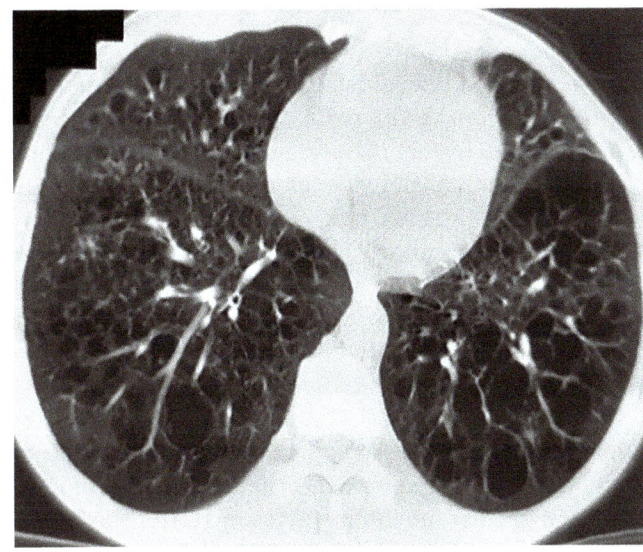

Fig. 6.17: HRCT thorax showing diffuse emphysema.

- Moderate: When FEV_1 is 50–79% predicted
- Severe: When FEV_1 is 30–49% predicted
- Very severe: When FEV_1 is <30% predicted (FEV_1 value following inhaled bronchodilator)
- *Diffusion study:* Diffusing capacity of the lung for carbon monoxide (DLCO) is markedly low in emphysema.
- *Chest X-ray* may demonstrate bullae, hypertranslucent lung fields, flattened diaphragms and prominent pulmonary arterial shadows. The X-ray is also helpful in excluding other conditions presenting with chronic cough and dyspnea. CT is used to diagnose emphysema and to detect its severity **(Fig. 6.17)**.
- *Arterial blood gas analysis* reveals hypoxemia (low PaO_2) and hypercarbia (high $PaCO_2$).
- *Serum alpha-1 antitrypsin* level should be measured in young patients with family history of COPD.
- Polycythemia reflects a physiologic response to chronic hypoxemia. It may also indicate inadequate supplemental oxygen use.

Assessment

According to recent COPD guidelines (GOLD-2021), the management of COPD includes assessment of symptoms, risk of exacerbations and comorbidities.
- *Symptoms:* Patient's symptoms are assessed by modified British Medical Research Council Scale (score 0 to 4) or by COPD assessment test (CAT) which has 8 questions and each question has score 0 to 5 (Total max score 40). Based on these scores, patients are grouped into less symptomatic (mMRC 0-1, CAT < 10) and more symptomatic group (mMRC >2, CAT > 10).
- *Risk of future exacerbations:* Patients are grouped into low risk (0–1/year or not leading to hospital admission) or high risk (≥ 2/year or any history of hospital admission due to exacerbation).

Based on above assessment, they are divided into four groups for purpose of treatment.

≥ 2 exacerbation/year	C	D
0–1 exacerbation/Year	A	B
	mMRC 0–1. CAT < 10	mMRC ≥ 2 CAT > 10

- Group A: Low risk, low symptoms
- Group B: Low risk, more symptoms
- Group C: High risk, less symptoms
- Group D: High risk, more symptoms.

Treatment

Treatment of COPD can be described as of (a) stable COPD, and (b) acute exacerbation. Management of COPD is given in **Tables 6.24 and 6.25**.

Stable COPD

Most forms of therapy are directed to relieve the symptoms and to decrease the frequency and severity of acute exacerbations. These measures do not alter the natural course of the disease. However, interventions **(Table 6.24)** like cessation of smoking, oxygen therapy in chronically hypoxic patients and lung volume reduction surgery (LVRS) in selected patients are known to influence the natural history of COPD.
- *Smoking cessation:* All patients with COPD should be encouraged to stop smoking since it improves the rate of decline in the pulmonary function. The patients should be educated and adequately counseled. Bupropion or nicotine replacement therapy may be employed to enhance the chance of smoking cessation.
- *Oxygen therapy:* Long-term oxygen therapy at home is required in patients with PaO_2 < 55 mm Hg or in patients with PaO_2 55–60 mm Hg who have pulmonary hypertension, heart failure or polycythemia. Oxygen is given in low concentration (2 liter/minute) for at least 15 hours a day.
- *Bronchodilators:* Inhaled bronchodilators are mainstay treatment of COPD and are given on regular basis to

Table 6.24: Non-pharmacological treatment of COPD.

- **Smoking cessation:** Prolong survival
- **Pulmonary rehabilitation:** Improves symptoms, quality of life, and physical and emotional participation in everyday activities
- **Nutrition:** Nutrition supplementation in malnourished patient with emphysema
- **Phlebotomy:** Repeated blood removal to reduce polycythemia
- **Long-term oxygen therapy:** In patients with severe resting chronic hypoxemia
- **Long-term noninvasive ventilation:** In patients with severe chronic hypercapnia
- **Surgical or bronchoscopic interventional treatments:** Advanced emphysema refractory to optimized medical management
- **Lung transplant**
- **Vaccines:** Influenza vaccine yearly and pneumococcal vaccination. Tdap vaccination in adults (if not vaccinated in adolescence)
- **End of life and palliative care**

Table 6.25: Pharmacologic therapies for stable COPD.

Group	Therapy
Group A: (Mild symptoms, low risk of exacerbation)	Inhaled short-acting or long-acting bronchodilator
Group B: (More symptoms, low risk of exacerbation)	• Long-acting bronchodilator (LABA or LAMA) • If no improvement: Combine both bronchodilator (LAMA/LABA)
Group C: (Less symptoms and high risk of exacerbation)	• Long-acting anticholinergic drug (LAMA) • If no improvement in symptoms: Combine both bronchodilator (LAMA+LABA) • If exacerbation occurs then give LAMA+LABA or LABA+ICS/LABA+LAMA+ICS (ICS to be added only if serum Eosinophil count >300)
Group D: (More symptoms and high risk of exacerbation)	• First give LAMA Or LAMA+ LABA if CAT score > 20 Or LAMA + ICS or LABA +LAMA + ICS if blood eosinophil count > 300 or further exacerbation • Add roflumilast if there is further exacerbation and FEV_1 < 50% and have predominant chronic bronchitis • Add azithromycin if there is further exacerbation and patient is not current smoker

(ICS: inhaled corticosteroid)

reduce or prevent symptoms. Anticholinergic agents (ipratropium bromide, tiotropium, glycopyrronium) are used as inhalational therapy. Short-acting beta-2 agonists (salbutamol), long-acting beta-2 agonists (salmeterol, formoterol) and ultra-long-acting beta-2 agonists (indacaterol and vilanterol) are also useful **(Table 6.26)**. The addition of beta agonists with anticholinergic agents provides incremental response. Oral theophylline may result in improved exercise tolerance and quality of life in moderate-to-severe COPD.

d. *Corticosteroids:* ICS have been shown to decrease the frequency of acute exacerbations of COPD. Low dose inhaled steroids(ICS) in combination with bronchodilators (LABA or LAMA/LABA) are indicated in patients with history of hospitalization for exacerbation, ≥ 2 exacerbations per year, blood eosinophils > 300/μL or history of asthma/concomitant asthma. However, chronic use of oral corticosteroid is not recommended in view of side effects.

e. *Combination therapy:* A combination of medications may yield superior efficacy and reduced potential for side effects. The combination of ICS and a long-acting bronchodilator agent (LABA and/or LAMA) is effective in reducing the frequency of exacerbations with an increased risk of pneumonia. The combination of LABA and long-acting anticholinergic agent (LABA plus LAMA) sustains improved lung function compared to either agent alone. Combining short-acting beta-agonist with a short-acting anticholinergic agent (SABA plus SAMA) results in greater increase in FEV_1 in acute exacerbation phase of COPD. Triple combinations of LABA/LAMA/ICS improve symptoms, lung function and reduces exacerbations.

f. *Antibiotics:* Respiratory infections must be treated promptly as they may precipitate acute exacerbation. The most common bacteria responsible for infection are *S. pneumoniae* and *H. influenzae*. The antibiotics of choice are amoxicillin, amoxicillin-clavulanate combination or clarithromycin given for at least 5–10 days. Influenza vaccine is recommended annually.

g. *Phosphodiesterase 4 (PDE4) inhibitors*: Roflumilast (500 mcg q day) appears to be safe when used as an additional therapy to chronic bronchodilators. It is indicated in severe COPD (FEV_1 < 50%) and chronic bronchitis with

Table 6.26: Inhalational therapy for stable COPD.

Group name	Name	Dose	Common side effects
Short-acting beta-agonists (SABA)	Salbutamol MDI/DPI/Nebulization	100–200 mcg/puff, 2–4 puffs q4–6h Nebulizer: 2.5 mg q 6–8h	Palpitations, tremor, tachycardia, throat irritation
	Levosalbutamol MDI/Nebulization	50–100 mcg/puff, 2–4 puffs q4–6h Nebulizer: 1.25 mg q 6–8h	
Long-acting beta-agonists (LABA)	Salmeterol	DPI: 50 mcg, MDI: 25 mcg/puff	Palpitations, headache, upper respiratory tract infections
	Formoterol	DPI: 6–12 mcg, MDI: 6–12 mcg/puff	
	Indacaterol	DPI 150 μg o.d.	
Short-acting anticholinergics OR Short-acting muscarinic antagonist (SAMA)	Ipratropium	MDI: 20 mcg/puff, 2 puffs q 4–6h DPI: 40 mcg q 6–8h	Xerostomia, cough, nausea/vomiting
Long-acting anticholinergics (OR) Long-acting muscarinic antagonist (LAMA)	Tiotropium	MDI: 9 mcg/puff, 2 puffs OD DPI: 18 mcg qd	
	Glycopyrronium Bromide	DPI: 25 mcg OD or 12.5 mcg BD Nebulization: 25 mcg BD	
Inhaled corticosteroid (ICS)	Budesonide	MDI/DPI: 100, 200, 400 OD or BD	Oral candidiasis, aphthous ulcer, etc.
	Fluticasone	MDI/DPI: 50, 100, 125, 250 mcg OD or BD	
	Ciclesonide	DPI 80/160 mcg OD or BD	
	Beclomethasone	MDI/DPI: 100, 200, 400 OD or BD	

(MDI: metered dose inhaler; DPI: dry powder inhaler)

frequent exacerbations. Side effects include weight loss and increased psychiatric symptoms.
h. *Mucolytics and antioxidants*: Regular treatment with these agents (N-acetylcysteine, Carbocysteine, Erdosteine) may reduce the exacerbations.
i. *Pulmonary rehabilitation*: Exercise and pulmonary rehabilitation programs improve dyspnea and quality of life. It also reduces frequency of exacerbations in patients of COPD.
j. *Vaccinations:* Annual influenza vaccine is recommended. It reduces the incidence of influenza related acute respiratory illness in COPD patients. It is reasonable to give pneumococcal vaccination. Tdap vaccination to protect whooping cough (pertussis) is recommended in adults if they have not received it in adolescence.
k. *Surgery*:
   – Lung volume reduction surgery (LVRS) may be indicated in patients with emphysema. It improves pulmonary functions and symptoms and also provides mortality benefit
   – Bronchoscopic lung volume reduction can also be achieved especially in heterogeneous emphysema by using one way endobronchial valves (allow air to come out while expiration but doesn't allow air to come inside in lung while inspiration), lung coils and vapor ablation.
   – Surgical resection is also required in patients with large bullae (bullectomy).
   – Severe COPD is an important indication for lung transplantation. Lung transplantation for severe COPD improves quality of life and functional capacity.

Acute Exacerbation

The acute exacerbation of COPD is defined by GOLD 2021 as "an acute worsening of respiratory symptoms that results in additional therapy". Common cause of exacerbation is viral infection (influenza, RSV, adeno virus, etc.), bacterial infections (*S. pneumoniae, Moraxella, H. influenzae*). It usually causes increased breathlessness and cough, production of increased volume of purulent sputum and sometimes as right heart failure. The patients may have cyanosis and impaired sensorium.

Acute exacerbation of COPD should be differentiated from other conditions presenting as acute onset dyspnea (**Table 6.27**).

Chest X-ray, ABG analysis, ECG, blood counts, urea and electrolytes and sputum culture are generally performed to assess severity of the exacerbation and to exclude other causes.

Most patients require hospitalization. The main steps in the treatment include:
- Oxygen therapy. Controlled oxygen therapy should be given to maintain oxygen saturation between 88–90%. Excessive oxygen therapy can increase hypercarbia in blood which is detrimental.

Table 6.27: Differential diagnosis of acute exacerbation of COPD.

- Pneumonia
- Pneumothorax
- Left ventricular failure
- Pulmonary embolism
- Acute severe asthma
- Airways obstruction

- Antibiotics are given to treat respiratory infections.
- *Bronchodilators:* The dose and frequency of short-acting bronchodilators are escalated. These are administered initially by nebulization.
  Methyl xanthines like theophylline, aminophylline should not be used due to narrow therapeutic window.
- Short course of oral corticosteroid (Prednisolone 0.5 to 1 mg/kg for 5–7 days) hastens recovery and reduces chances of subsequent relapses.
- Diuretics are given in case of raised JVP and edema (signs of cor pulmonale).
- Mechanical ventilatory support (Noninvasive and invasive) may be required in patients with severe respiratory distress, severe hypoxia and hypercapnia.
- *Other treatment*:
  – Monitor fluid balance to prevent heart failure.
  – Consider heparin or LMW heparin for thromboembolism prophylaxis.
  – Identify and treat associated conditions like arrhythmias, cardiac failure, PE, etc.

Complications

The complications of COPD include:
- Pneumothorax due to rupture of bullae
- Respiratory failure (type II)
- Cor pulmonale.

Comorbidities in COPD

Many other diseases coexist with COPD either due to same risk factor like smoking or as a part of systemic inflammation.

Treatment of comorbidities is equally important as treatment of COPD. In general, the presence of comorbidities should not alter COPD treatment and comorbidities should be treated as per usual standards regardless of the presence of COPD. Common comorbidities are given in **Table 6.28**.

COR PULMONALE

Cor pulmonale is defined as dilation and hypertrophy of the right ventricle in response to diseases of the pulmonary vasculature and/or lung parenchyma. It does not include congenital heart disease and those diseases in which the right heart fails secondary to dysfunction of the left side of the heart. Common causes are chronic bronchitis, COPD,

Table 6.28: Comorbidities (GOLD 2021).

- Cardiovascular disease
  - Heart failure
  - Ischemic heart disease
  - Arrhythmias
  - Peripheral vascular disease
  - Hypertension
- Osteoporosis
- Anxiety and depression
- Lung cancer
- Metabolic syndrome and diabetes
- Gastroesophageal reflux
- Bronchiectasis
- Obstructive sleep apnea
- Cognitive impairment

PE and ILD. Dyspnea is the most common symptom. Signs include tachypnea, elevated JVP, hepatomegaly, and lower-extremity edema. Echocardiography, cardiac catheterization and imaging are required to diagnose it and to rule out other diseases. Treatment goal of cor pulmonale is to target the underlying pulmonary disease. It involves oxygenation, bronchodilators, diuretics and pulmonary vasodilators.

PULMONARY EOSINOPHILIA

Pulmonary eosinophilia or pulmonary infiltrates with eosinophilia (PIE) are distinct syndromes characterized by the presence of pulmonary infiltrate and eosinophilia (peripheral eosinophil count >500/µL). The most common cause of PIE in tropical countries is parasitic infestation and allergic bronchopulmonary aspergillosis (ABPA) in developed countries. Other causes of PIE are listed in **Table 6.29**.

Mechanism: Eosiophils release numerous soluble mediators, including granule-derived proteins, arachidonic acid metabolites, pro-inflammatory cytokines, superoxide anions, metalloproteases, and hydroxyl radicals that leads to tissue inflammation and injury.

Loeffler Syndrome (Simple Pulmonary Eosinophilia)

Immune hypersensitivity to ascaris lumbricoides causes Loeffler syndrome. Other parasitic infections including hookworms, strongyloides, trichinella spiralis, and toxocara canis and exposures to numerous drugs and other agents have also been recognized to induce a Loeffler-like syndrome.

The pulmonary manifestations begin approximately 9–14 days following ingestion and occur during the migration of larvae through the lung.

Clinical features: Patients usually present with low-grade fever, non-productive cough, dyspnea (mild to severe), chest discomfort on coughing or deep breathing, and, occasionally, hemoptysis.

Peripheral blood examination shows high eosinophil count. Ova in stool can be demonstrated after 6–8 weeks only.

Treatment: Usually self-limited, typically resolves in 1-2 weeks. Bronchodilators and rarely corticosteroids may be used. In cases due to ascaris, treatment with oral mebendazole (100 mg twice a day for 3 days or a single dose of 500 mg) should be given.

Tropical Eosinophilia

- Tropical eosinophilia is caused by filarial infection
- The manifestations are due to allergic and inflammatory reactions elicited due to clearance of microfilaria by the lungs
- The main presenting features are spasmodic cough that usually occurs at night, paroxysmal dyspnea, wheeze which may resemble status asthmaticus. Other organs like cardiac, pericardial, and CNS may be involved.
- Peripheral blood examination shows eosinophilia (> 3,000/µL) and X-ray chest generally reveals diffuse miliary opacities. Total serum IgE level (more than 1,000 U/mL) and anti-filarial antibody titer (IgE and IgG) are specifically elevated
- The treatment includes diethylcarbamazine (DEC) in dosage of 4–6 mg/kg body weight daily for 14–21 days. Alternative antifilarial drugs (e.g., ivermectin) or a trial of corticosteroids may be useful therapies for the chronic variant of the disease.

Acute Eosinophilic Pneumonia

Common in male with age of 20 and 40. It has been associated with patients of chronic smoker and with a history of chronic myelogenous leukemia, hematopoietic stem cell transplantation, HIV infection or hypersensitivity to inhaled agent.

Acute eosinophilic pneumonia (AEP) presents as ARDS with an acute illness with dyspnea, fever, nonproductive cough, tachypnea, pleuritic chest pain, and hypoxemia (arterial PaO_2 under 60 mm Hg).

Blood eosinophilia is usually absent at the onset of disease but there is striking eosinophilia (25%–55%) in BAL fluid. Serum IgE levels may be moderately elevated.

Chest radiology usually shows diffuse, symmetric alveolar and interstitial infiltrates resembling ARDS.

Table 6.29: Common causes of pulmonary eosinophilic disease.

Pulmonary eosinophilic syndromes of known cause
1. Parasitic-induced eosinophilic pneumonias (including Loeffler syndrome)
2. Drug- or toxin-induced eosinophilic pneumonias
3. Tropical pulmonary eosinophilia
4. Allergic bronchopulmonary mycosis

Pulmonary eosinophilic syndromes of unknown cause
1. Idiopathic acute eosinophilic pneumonia
2. Chronic eosinophilic pneumonia
3. EGPA (allergic granulomatosis and polyangiitis)
4. Idiopathic hypereosinophilic syndrome

Treatment: There is rapid dramatic responses to corticosteroid therapy, with methylprednisolone in doses of 60–125 mg administered every 6 hours and after resolution of respiratory failure, oral prednisone (in doses of 40–60 mg per day) may be continued for 2–4 weeks.

Chronic Eosinophilic Pneumonia

Common in female of age group 30–45 years, up to two-third patients have history of asthma.

Chronic eosinophilic pneumonia (CEP) typically has a subacute presentation including dyspnea, low-grade fevers, malaise, drenching night sweats, and moderate weight loss.

The majority (66%–95%) have peripheral blood eosinophilia (usually > 1,000/mm^3).

Chest radiology: Infiltrates are typically dense and patchy areas of airspace consolidation with ill-defined margins usually affecting the outer two-thirds of the lung fields called "photographic negative of pulmonary edema".

Treatment: Prednisone 0.5 mg/kg/d (40–60 mg a day) continued until 2 weeks after resolution of symptoms and radiographic abnormalities, generally for 4–6 weeks.

Allergic Bronchopulmonary Aspergillosis

It is a complex hypersensitivity reaction in response to colonization of the airways with *Aspergillus fumigatus* that occurs almost exclusively in patients with asthma or cystic fibrosis (CF).

Clinical features: Usually presents as difficult to control asthma and recurrent exacerbations. In severe cases fever, malaise, expectoration of brownish mucus plugs, and, at times, hemoptysis may occur.

Investigation: There is marked eosinophilia in blood and bronchoalveolar lavage (BAL). Total serum IgE and IgE specific for *Aspergillus* also increased. Diagnosis of ABPA is made according to International Society for Human and Animal Mycology (ISHAM) criteria (*see* **Table 6.30**).

Treatment: Depends on clinical staging (*see* **Table 6.31**).

Corticosteroids: Indicated in stage I or III include prednisone 0.5–1 mg/kg a day for 2 weeks, followed by 0.5 mg/kg every other day for 6–8 weeks. Steroids are tapered (by 5–10 mg every 2 weeks) over the ensuing 3 months.

Table 6.30: Diagnostic criteria of ABPA (ISHAM ABPA criteria).

1. Predisposing condition: Asthma OR cystic fibrosis
2. Obligatory criteria (both should be present):
   – Immediate cutaneous hypersensitivity reaction to *Aspergillus* antigens or *Aspergillus fumigatus*
   – Increased IgE levels > Total IgE >1,000 IU/mL
3. Other criteria (at least 2 out of 3):
   – Peripheral blood eosinophil count >500 cells/μL
   – Bronchiectasis on computed tomography of the chest
   – Presence of IgG antibodies against Af or precipitating antibodies

Table 6.31: Staging of ABPA for treatment purpose.

Stage 0: Asymptomatic
Stage 1: Acute
Stage 2: Response
Stage 3: Exacerbation
Stage 4: Remission
Stage 5a: Treatment dependent ABPA
     5b: Steroid dependent asthma
Stage 6: Advanced ABPA

Anti-fungal (DOC Itraconazole for 16 weeks): Indicated in those patient, who are unable to taper oral glucocorticoids, i.e., steroid dependent or having frequent exacerbation of ABPA.

Hypereosinophilic Syndrome

The diagnosis depends on the fulfillment of following criteria:
- Eosinophilia (>1,500/μL) for at least 6 months
- Lack of evidence of any detectable cause
- Sign and symptoms of multisystem organ dysfunction, such as involvement of heart, nervous system, lungs and liver.

The therapy includes the use of glucocorticoids and/or hydroxyurea.

PULMONARY EMBOLISM

Definition

Pulmonary embolism (PE) is defined as obstruction of the pulmonary artery or one of its branches by material (e.g., thrombus, tumor, air, amniotic fluid or fat) that originated elsewhere in the body. PE is an important cause of mortality in hospitalized patients. The most common source of emboli is proximal leg and pelvic deep vein thrombosis (DVT). **Table 6.32** shows important predisposing conditions for DVT. Other causes of PE are shown in **Table 6.33**.

Virchow's triad: This triad includes endothelial damage, hypercoagulability and venous stasis.

Table 6.32: Predisposing factors for DVT.

Genetic
- Factor V leiden
- Prothrombin gene mutation
- Protein C or protein S deficiency

Acquired
- Fracture of lower limb bone
- Hospitalization for heart failure/atrial fibrillation or myocardial infarction within 3 months
- Hip and knee replacement
- Previous History of VTE
- Smoking
- Oral contraceptive
- Pregnancy
- Surgery and trauma
- Long air travel
- Malignancies
- Antiphospholipids antibody syndrome

> **Table 6.33:** Causes of pulmonary embolism.
> 1. Deep vein thrombosis (in lower limb)
> 2. Nonthrombotic causes
>   a. Amniotic fluid embolism (tear of placental margin, fetal membrane leak)
>   b. Air embolism
>   c. Fat embolism (long bone fractures, blunt trauma)
>   d. Tumor embolism (choriocarcinoma)
>   e. Septic emboli (Infective endocarditis affecting tricuspid and pulmonary valves)

> **Table 6.34:** Differential diagnosis of pulmonary embolism.
> **Cardiac diseases**
> - Acute myocardial infarction
> - Acute left ventricular failure
> - Pericardial tamponade
> - Aortic dissection
>
> **Pulmonary diseases**
> - Pneumothorax
> - Pneumonia
> - Exacerbation of asthma or COPD
> - Primary pulmonary hypertension
>
> **Others**
> - Anxiety

Any of above feature can predispose to thrombus formation in large vein especially lower limb vein.

Clinical Syndromes

The PE can result in different syndromes depending upon the site, size and speed of onset of embolism. Dyspnea is the most frequent symptom and tachypnea is the most frequent sign.

Acute Massive Pulmonary Embolism

- This is due to the obstruction of main or proximal pulmonary artery leading to decreased cardiac output and right ventricular dilatation
- Presentations are sudden onset of severe dyspnea, apprehension, central chest pain, faintness and syncope
- Signs include tachycardia, tachypnea, cyanosis, hypotension, increased JVP, right-sided S3 and wide split P2.

Acute Small/Medium Pulmonary Embolism

- There is obstruction of segmental small pulmonary artery which often leads to peripheral pulmonary infarction
- Usual symptoms are dyspnea, pleuritic chest pain, fever, cough and hemoptysis
- Signs may include tachycardia, tachypnea, pleural rub, and features of pleural effusion
- Clinical features may be more severe if there is underlying cardiopulmonary disease.

Chronic Pulmonary Embolism

- Chronic occlusion of pulmonary microvasculature is generally asymptomatic initially. Later, it may produce pulmonary hypertension and right heart failure
- This can present as chronic exertional dyspnea
- Signs of pulmonary hypertension (loud P2) and right ventricular failure (raised JVP, RV heave, pedal edema) can be found.

Differential Diagnosis

The PE should be differentiated from conditions which present with acute dyspnea or chest pain as shown in **Table 6.34**.

Investigations

- *Chest X-ray:* Generally, the X-ray chest is normal in PE but it is helpful in ruling out other conditions like pneumothorax, pneumonia and heart failure. The findings in PE include peripheral wedge, shaped opacity also called Hamptom's hump (due to pulmonary infarction), local infiltrates, pleural effusion, pulmonary oligemia (Westermark's sign) and an enlarged right descending pulmonary artery (Palla's sign). *A normal X-ray chest along with acute dyspnea and hypoxemia suggests the diagnosis of PE.*
- *Electrocardiography:* The ECG findings are common. These are tachycardia (most common), right axis deviation, incomplete RBBB, nonspecific ST-T changes or more specifically $S_1Q_3T_3$ pattern or T wave inversion in V_1 to V_4.
- *Arterial blood gas analysis:* The values may reveal low PaO_2, normal to low $PaCO_2$ (type I respiratory failure), respiratory alkalosis initially and metabolic acidosis in severe cases.
- *D-dimer test:* D-dimer is a degradation product released into circulation when fibrin is thrombolysed by endogenous plasmin. The plasma level of D-dimer is raised in >90% cases of PE. However, it can also be high in other conditions like pneumonia, MI and sepsis. Hence, a raised value is not diagnostic of PE. *The low value of D-dimer excludes the diagnosis of PE* so it has very high negative predictive value.
- *Imaging:*
  - **Computed tomography pulmonary angiogram (CTPA):** Spiral CT of the chest with IV contrast has good sensitivity and specificity for the diagnosis of PE and is now the investigation of choice in patients with acute dyspnea
  - **Magnetic resonance (MR) imaging** with contrast is also increasingly being used for the diagnosis of PE
  - **Ventilation perfusion (V/Q) lung scanning,** a popular investigation in past, is now less commonly used. However, it may be useful when performed within 24 hours of presentation and in patients with no previous cardiopulmonary disease such as COPD, pneumonia, lung fibrosis, etc.

f. *Doppler ultrasonography:* This is done to detect deep vein thrombosis in the leg veins.
   1. *Compression ultrasound*: An incompressible vein is used as evidence of a clot-filled vein
   2. *The color Doppler mode of ultrasound*: The flow in arteries and veins can be identified by the direction of flow in relation to the ultrasound probe.

   The combination of compression and Doppler ultrasound is known as duplex ultrasound.
   For proximal DVT in the legs, duplex ultrasound has a sensitivity ≥ 95%, a specificity ≥ 97%.
g. *Echocardiography:* This is useful to exclude other conditions such as MI, pericardial tamponade and dissection of aorta. Echocardiography can diagnose right ventricular dysfunction and may detect major central PE.
h. *Pulmonary angiography:* This is the "gold standard" method for the definitive diagnosis of PE. However, in the current era, the CT pulmonary angiography has replaced pulmonary angiography as the former is less invasive.

Diagnosis

According to clinical features and severity of disease, PE can be classified in to 3 classes as given below:
1. *High-risk or massive PE*: Hemodynamically unstable patient may have any of following:
   a. Cardiac arrest: Need CPR
   b. Obstructive shock (systolic BP < 90 mm Hg even with adequate fluid administration) and end organ hypoperfusion (altered mental status, cold skin, oliguria, etc.)
   c. *Persistent hypotension*: (Systolic BP < 90 mm Hg or fall in systolic BP > 40 mm Hg for more than 15 minutes)
2. *Intermediate-risk or submassive PE*: Hemodynamically stable PE but there is associated right ventricular strain.
3. *Low-risk PE*: If there is no evidence of right ventricular strain

Wells score: This scoring is used to classify hemodynamic stable patient in to low, intermediate and high risk probability.

Characteristics	Score
Previous pulmonary embolism or deep vein thrombosis	1.5
Heart rate >100 beats/minute	1.5
Recent surgery or immobilization	1.5
Clinical signs of deep vein thrombosis	3
Alternative diagnosis less likely than pulmonary embolism	3
Hemoptysis	1
Cancer	1
Interpretation: • Low probability: 0–1 point • Intermediate probability: 2–6 points • High probability: 7 or more points	

Treatment

- *Supportive measures:* Important supportive measures include:
  - Relief from pain by nonsteroidal anti-inflammatory drugs or opiates
  - Oxygen therapy to maintain oxygen saturation over 90%
  - Dobutamine in patients having severe right heart failure and cardiogenic shock.
- *Anticoagulation:* Anticoagulation prevents additional thrombus formation. The already formed clot is eventually lysed by endogenous fibrinolytic mechanisms.
  Detail of anticoagulants and their mechanism of actions are given in **Table 6.35**. Novel oral anticoagulants (NOACs) include dabigatran, rivaroxaban, apixaban and edoxaban.
  a. *Heparins:* Low molecular weight heparin (LMWH), such as enoxaparin is given subcutaneously twice a day. Alternatively, unfractionated heparin can be used intravenously (bolus of 5,000–10,000 IU followed by a continuous infusion at the rate of 1,000 IU/hour). The dose of heparin is adjusted according to activated partial thromboplastin time (aPTT). The LMWH is preferred over unfractionated heparin because of ease of administration and no need for monitoring.
  b. *Oral anticoagulants:* Oral anticoagulant (warfarin) is also started simultaneously. The heparin is stopped after 5 days while the warfarin is continued. The dose of warfarin is adjusted according to prothrombin time and international normalized ratio (PT/INR).
  c. *Newer oral anticoagulants:* Dabigatran, rivaroxaban, apixaban, edoxaban.
  d. *Duration and complications:* The duration of anticoagulation therapy is generally up to 3 months if cause of DVT is reversible. However, patients with history of previous embolism or having underlying prothrombotic conditions should be given oral anticoagulant lifelong. The most common complication of anticoagulation therapy is hemorrhage.
3. *Thrombolytic therapy:* Thrombolysis is indicated in acute massive PE with right ventricular dysfunction or hypotension. Thrombolytic agent used is recombinant tissue plasminogen activator (r-tPA) or streptokinase.
4. *Embolectomy:* Open surgical or catheter embolectomy is indicated in patients with massive PE where thrombolysis is contraindicated because of high risk of intracranial hemorrhage.
5. *Inferior vena caval filters:* A filter is placed in inferior vena cava to prevent the passage of emboli from pelvic

Table 6.35: Anticoagulants.

1. Vitamin K antagonist (**Antifactor II, VII, IX, X**): Warfarin
2. Heparin and related drugs
   a. Heparin (**Antifactor II, X**)
   b. LMWH (**Antifactor X**): (Enoxaparin, Dalteparin, Tinzaparin)
   c. Synthetic heparin derivatives (**Antifactor X**) (Fondaparinux – longer acting)
3. Direct thrombin inhibitors (**Antifactor-II inhibitors**)
   a. Parenteral: Hirudin, lepirudin, argatroban, bivalirudin
   b. Oral: Dabigatran
4. Direct **factor Xa** inhibitors: Rivaroxaban, apixaban, edoxaban

and lower limb veins to the lungs. This is done in patients with recurrent emboli despite adequate anticoagulation or where anticoagulation is contraindicated because of bleeding.

Prevention of PE

The preventive measures include early mobilization after surgery, adequate hydration and prophylactic use of LMWH or warfarin in patients undergoing major surgery.

TUBERCULOSIS

Epidemiology: Tuberculosis is among the oldest infections in humans. Around one-third of the world population is infected with *M. tuberculosis*. According to WHO estimate 10 million cases of TB occurred worldwide in 2019, 95% of then in developing countries and 1.4 million people (including 2.08 lakh patients of HIV) died from TB in 2019. It is still a significant cause of morbidity and mortality in the developing countries. It usually affects the lungs, although other organs (extrapulmonary tuberculosis) are involved in up to one-third of cases. There is an increase in the incidence of tuberculosis because of HIV infection. Nowadays there is huge problem with development of drug resistant tuberculosis which causes tremendous increase in morbidity and mortality. According to WHO 2020 report, there were 10% increase of MDR tuberculosis in 2019 (2.06 lakh) as compared to 2018 (1.86 lakh) world widely.

Causative organism: It is caused by bacteria belonging to *Mycobacterium tuberculosis* complex.
- The most common agent of human disease is *M. tuberculosis*
- *M. bovis*, an important cause of infection in those who consume unpasteurized milk, is now uncommon.

On Gram staining, *Mycobacteria* are often neutral. Once stained, they cannot be decolorized by acid alcohol, hence labeled as AFB.

Transmission: Most commonly the infection is transmitted from infected patients to other persons through droplet nuclei released by coughing, sneezing or speaking. The patients having cavitary pulmonary disease most infectious (sputum contains 10^5–10^7 AFB/mL). Other rare routes of transmission are ingestion, through skin and transplacental.

Risk factors: The risk of acquiring infection is increased by factors like poverty and overcrowding. Patients with diabetes, silicosis, alcoholism or immunocompromised states are at a greater risk of acquiring tuberculosis. Health workers are also at increased risk as they may be exposed to TB patients.

Primary Tuberculosis

Primary tuberculosis occurs due to initial infection in lungs and occasionally in tonsils or intestine. The primary lesion in lungs, tonsils and intestine is almost always accompanied by the lymph node involvement such as mediastinal, cervical and mesenteric groups, respectively.

Pathology: The macrophages ingest bacilli and eventually are killed through cellular immune responses leading to tissue necrosis and caseation. Activated monocytes turn into epithelioid cells and form granuloma at the periphery of caseation. In the majority of cases, lesions heal by calcification. In some, the healing is incomplete and the bacilli may disseminate to different organs through the blood stream. Lesions in these organs may develop years later.

Tuberculosis can be pulmonary, or extrapulmonary or both. Pulmonary tuberculosis is more common than extrapulmonary. However, in patients with HIV disease, extrapulmonary form of tuberculosis is more commonly seen.

Pulmonary Tuberculosis

Pulmonary tuberculosis can be classified into:
a. Primary pulmonary tuberculosis.
b. Post-primary pulmonary tuberculosis (adult type, reactivation or secondary tuberculosis).

Primary Pulmonary Tuberculosis

The bacilli enter the lung parenchyma and cause a peripheral parenchymal lesion. The bacilli eventually travel to the mediastinal lymph nodes. This is known as *primary complex*.
- Middle and lower lobes of the lung are usually involved
- In most (80–90%), the primary complex heals within 4–6 weeks. The healed calcified peripheral parenchymal lesion is known as Ghon's lesion **(Fig. 6.18)**
- It usually affects children and remains asymptomatic in most. However, in some, particularly in immunocompromised individuals, the disease may progress in the following forms:
  – The parenchymal lesion may enlarge and cavitate (progressive primary tuberculosis).

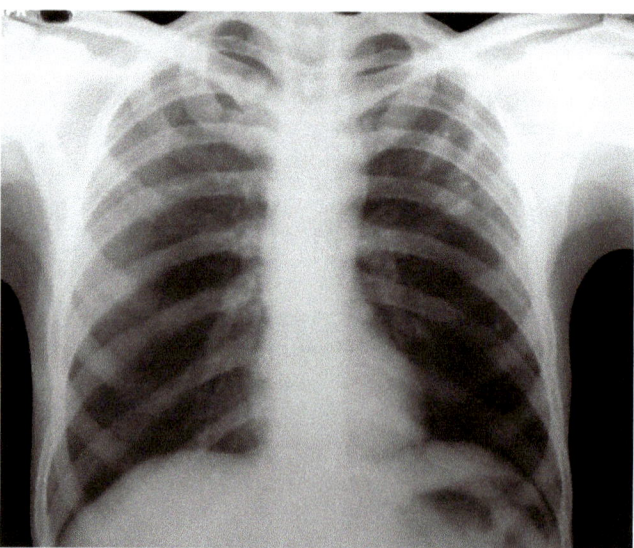

Fig. 6.18: X-ray chest showing Ghon's lesion.

- The disease may involve pleura and result into pleural effusion.
- Enlarged lymph node may compress bronchi and result in collapse (epituberculosis).
- Hematogenous dissemination is common and generally asymptomatic. However, occasionally it may lead to meningitis or miliary tuberculosis.
- Manifestations due to hypersensitivity reaction may occur in form of erythema nodosum or phlyctenular conjunctivitis.

Post-primary Pulmonary Tuberculosis

This is also known as adult-type, reactivation or secondary tuberculosis. It usually results from reactivation of latent infection and is localized to the upper lobes as growth of the mycobacteria is favored by high oxygen concentration. Parenchymal involvement may be in the form of small infiltrates, pneumonia, collapse, extensive cavitatory lesions or miliary lesions. The lesion may remit spontaneously or in some, it may progress to chronic fibrosis.

Clinical features: The patients initially present with symptoms like cough, malaise, loss of appetite, loss of weight, low grade fever with evening rise, night sweats and hemoptysis. The chest examination may be normal or may reveal inspiratory crackles, particularly after cough, and bronchial breathing over large cavities.

Other uncommon presentations may be in the form of pleural effusion, spontaneous pneumothorax and pyrexia of unknown origin (PUO).

Extrapulmonary Tuberculosis

Virtually any organ may be involved due to hematogenous spread of the infection. The occurrence of extrapulmonary form of tuberculosis has become more common with emergence of HIV disease. The most common extra-pulmonary site involved is lymph nodes. **Table 6.36** shows different forms of extrapulmonary tuberculosis.

Table 6.36: Forms of extrapulmonary tuberculosis.	
Tuberculous lymphadenitis	Painless enlargement of lymph nodes generally cervical, may be matted, may form sinus (scrofula) and collar stud abscess
Pleural tuberculosis	Pleural effusion, empyema, pneumothorax
Gastrointestinal	Most commonly ileocecal involvement, may present as abdominal pain, diarrhea, intestinal obstruction, ascites
Genitourinary	Hematuria, frequency, sterile pyuria, epididymitis, prostatitis, tubo-ovarian abscess, infertility
Pericardial	Pericardial effusion, constrictive pericarditis
Central nervous system	Meningitis, tuberculoma
Bone and joints	Spinal tuberculosis, arthritis

Miliary Tuberculosis

The miliary tuberculosis is a severe form of tuberculosis that results from hematogenous spread of tuberculous bacilli. This may be a form of primary tuberculosis or may occur due to reactivation of old foci. The lesions are characterized by granuloma (1–2 mm) that resembles millet seeds.

Clinical features: Besides constitutional symptoms like fever, weight loss and anorexia, patients may have hepatosplenomegaly and lymphadenopathy. The fundus examination may show choroidal tubercles.

Investigations: Chest X-ray shows miliary shadows **(Fig. 6.19)**. The hematological features include anemia, leukopenia or leukemoid reaction. The tuberculin skin test (PPD test) is negative in half of the patients. Liver or bone marrow biopsy may be required in some cases for the diagnosis.

HIV and Tuberculosis

Tuberculosis is the most common opportunistic infection in HIV infected individuals in India. The disease may appear at any stage of HIV disease.

Clinical presentation: The presentation is typical (upper lobe infiltrates and cavity) in early stages when the immunity is only partially compromised. However, in late stages, the presentation can be like primary tuberculosis. The extrapulmonary involvement is more common in HIV infected persons than in HIV negatives. *M. avium* complex (MAC) infection may occur when CD4 count becomes less than 50/cmm.

Diagnosis: The diagnosis of tuberculosis in HIV infected patients becomes difficult because of atypical clinical and radiological features. Moreover, the purified protein derivative (PPD) skin test and sputum smear for AFB are negative in most cases.

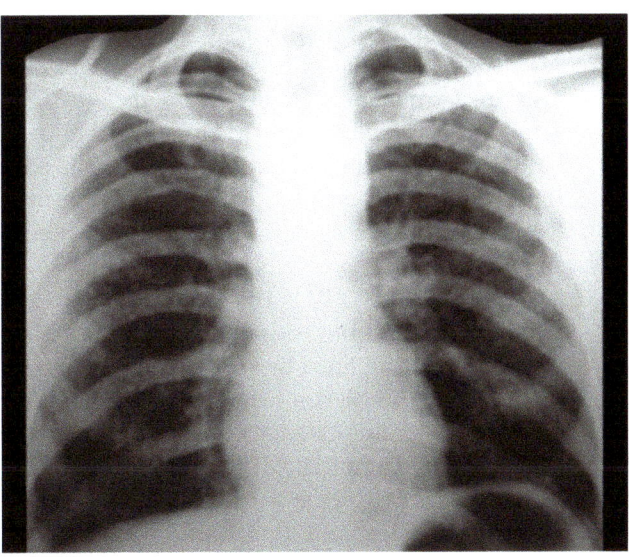

Fig. 6.19: X-ray chest showing miliary tuberculosis

Investigations

- *Demonstration of AFB*: The diagnosis of tuberculosis is based on the demonstration of AFB in the smear of the sputum or in other specimens such as tissue biopsy materials or body fluids. Sputum smear is typically positive when 5,000–10,000 organisms are usually present. *Ziehl-Neelsen or Auramine fluorescence* staining is usually done for this purpose. If the patient is not passing sputum, nebulization with hypertonic saline can be used to induce sputum expectoration. Samples can also be obtained by gastric lavage (in children), bronchoalveolar lavage (BAL) or transbronchial biopsy.
- *Culture methods*: It is gold standard test in diagnosis of tuberculosis. The culture provides confirmation of the diagnosis by the isolation and identification of *M. tuberculosis* from the specimen. Drug sensitivity can also be tested. Only 10–100 viable organisms are required to be culture positive. The growth on solid media (Löwenstein-Jensen media) is slow and may take 4–8 weeks. However, the time required for culture confirmation is shorter (2–3 weeks) when liquid media (BACTEC or MGIT-960) is used.
- *Molecular methods*: Nucleic acid amplification method provides diagnosis in hours but sensitivity is lower than culture and the cost is high. It is useful in cases with AFB negative pulmonary and extrapulmonary tuberculosis.
    a. *Gene expert:* It is cartridge based nucleic acid amplification test, it's commercial name is Gene Xpert (*Xpert® MTB/RIF*) and is World Health Organization (WHO) endorsed 2-hour test approved for use directly on raw sputum. It is specific for MTB complex and differentiates MTB from other mycobacteria. It can also be used on samples other than sputum [(CSF, gastric aspirate, lymph node aspirate and tissue (biospy sample)]. It has replaced microscopy as the 1st line diagnostic test specially in extrapulmonary tuberculosis, HIV patients, previous intake of anti TB drugs, contacts of chronic/MDR TB adults and pediatric population. This may be used to detect *Mycobacterium tuberculosis* as well as rifampicin resistance in a matter of hours (2 hours).
    b. TrueNat: It is similar to Gene Expert and is done on battery-powered portable machine developed in India. It also gives result in 2 hours and is approved for use in peripheral centers where there is no electric supply.
    c. *Line probe assay (LPA):* This is also nucleic acid amplification test but is done manually as DNA is extracted and amplified by PCR technique followed by detection of resistance by specific primers. It is of two type-1st line LPA which detect resistance to isoniazid and rifampicin (MDR TB) and 2nd line LPA which detect resistance to 2nd line drugs namely aminoglycosides and fluoroquinolones, hence combination of both LPA helps to detect XDR TB.

These tests have been approved for direct testing on smear positive specimens and on isolates from solid and liquid culture. Result of this test is available in approximately 48–72 hours. It can also differentiate MTB from other mycobacteria.

- *Interferon gamma release assays* (IGRAs) measure the release of interferon gamma (IFN-γ) from sensitized T cells in response to antigens. These tests are used to detect latent TB infection only (not active disease) like mantoux test. Unlike Mantoux test these have greater specificity as these antigens are not shared by BCG or atypical mycobacteria. These tests are better in situations where the prevalence of TB is low as in developed countries. The treatment of latent cases can prevent the development of active disease. Two most common test used for measurement of IFN-γ are T-SPOTTB and the Quantiferon–TB Gold assay. The exact advantage of these tests in high burden situation is not clear , hence are not recommended for diagnosis of TB in India.
- *Radiological tests:* The typical findings include infiltration of upper lobe with fibrosis and/or cavity **(Fig. 6.20)**. However, any type of radiographic pattern such as consolidation, collapse, pleural effusion or miliary can be seen in tuberculosis **(Figs. 6.21 to 6.23)**.
- *Tuberculin skin test:* PPD skin test (using Mantoux method or Heaf method) is positive (a) in persons infected with *M. tuberculosis,* (b) in persons sensitized by nontuberculous mycobacteria and (c) in those who have received BCG vaccination. A positive skin test does not tell about the active disease. A positive test in those who have not received BCG may suggest the diagnosis of tuberculosis. The test may be negative in miliary tuberculosis and in immunocompromised patients with tuberculosis.
- *Histopathological tests*: The fine needle aspiration cytology (FNAC) or biopsy specimens from the involved tissue may typically reveal caseous granuloma. AFB can

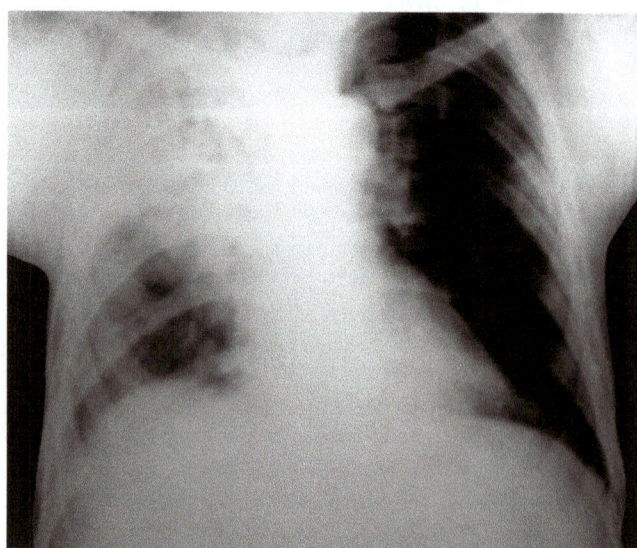

Fig. 6.20: X-ray chest showing right-sided infiltration and fibrosis of lung.

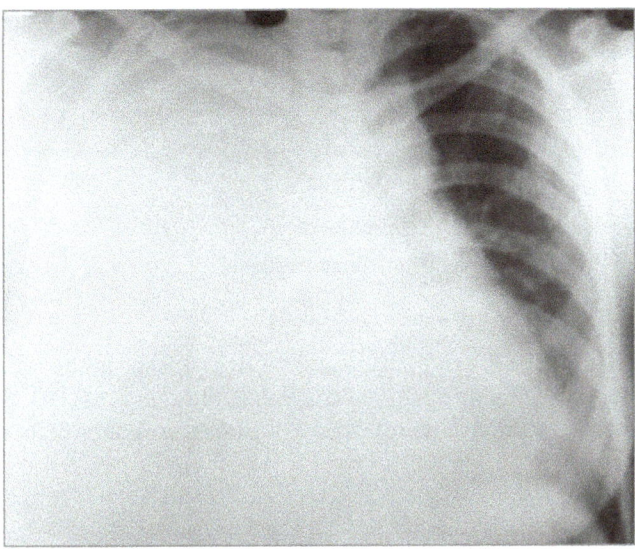

Fig. 6.21: X-ray chest showing right-sided massive pleural effusion with mediastinal shift.

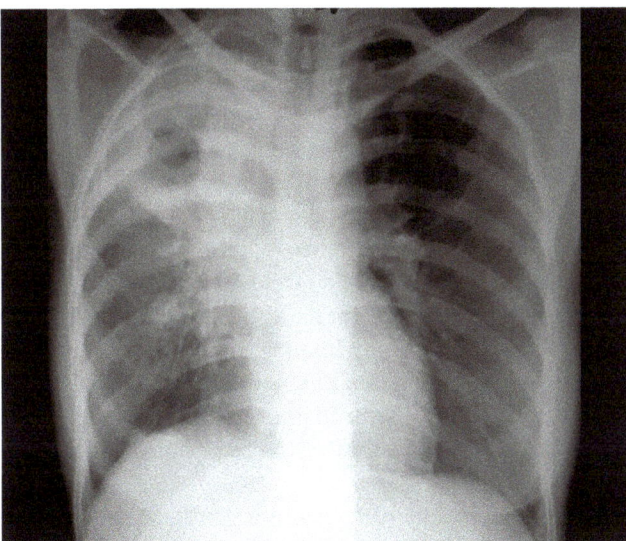

Fig. 6.22: X-ray chest: Right upper lobe fibro cavity lesion.

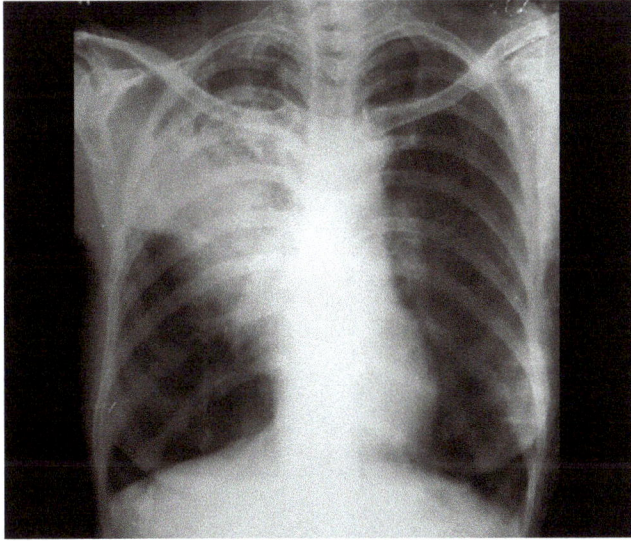

Fig. 6.23: X-ray chest: Right upper and middle lobe consolidation.

be demonstrated in tissue specimens. The tissue can be cultured to demonstrate mycobacteria.
- *Other tests*:
  – The hematological findings include anemia, raised ESR and C reactive protein
  – The fluid (pleural, pericardial, peritoneal) is exudative in nature and adenosine deaminase (ADA) level is elevated
  – Liver biopsy and bone marrow biopsy specimens may also be examined for the evidence of granuloma and AFB.

Treatment

The main aims of treatment of tuberculosis are:
- To cure the patients of tuberculosis.
- To decrease transmission of tuberculosis to others.
- To prevent relapse.
- To prevent morbidity and mortality from active tuberculosis.
- To prevent late effects of tuberculosis.
- To prevent emergence of DRTB.

Antitubercular Drugs

The antitubercular drugs are bactericidal or bacteriostatic in nature. The bactericidal drugs are used to rapidly reduce the number of viable organisms and render patients non-infectious. These also have sterilizing activity (kill all bacilli), hence, they prevent relapse. Bacteriostatic drugs are used along with the bactericidal drugs to prevent emergence of resistance.

First-line drugs: The first line drugs are rifampicin (R), isoniazid (H), pyrazinamide (Z) and ethambutol (E). Isoniazid and rifampicin are active against all population of TB bacilli while pyrazinamide and streptomycin are active against certain population of TB bacilli. In addition, pyrazinamide is active against bacilli in acid environment inside macrophages and has good CSF penetration. Streptomycin is particularly active against extracellular bacilli. The dosage and side effects of antitubercular drugs are given in **Table 6.37**.

Second line drugs: The second line drugs are less efficacious and more toxic. These are used when first line drugs fail.

Newer drugs:
- Bedaquiline, a diarylquinoline that inhibits mycobacterial ATP synthase has been associated when added to preferred background regimen with faster culture conversion in patients with multidrug resistant (MDR) TB. US-FDA approved in 2012 while Ministry of Health and Family Welfare (MOHFW) introduced in 2016 for treatment of MDR and XDR TB under National Tuberculosis Elimination Programme (NTEP).
- *Delaminid*: It is nitroimidazoles that inhibits mycolic acid synthesis and increases nitric oxide (NO) which damage DNA and inhibits ATP production. It is approved

Table 6.37: Antitubercular drugs and their dosage.

Drugs	Mode of action	Daily dose mg/kg	Common side effects
Isoniazid (H)	Bactericidal	5	Hypersensitivity, neuropathy, hepatitis
Rifampicin (R)	Bactericidal	10	Hepatitis, thrombocytopenia, flu-like symptoms, hypersensitivity, drug interactions
Pyrazinamide (Z)	Bactericidal	25	Gout, hepatitis, hypersensitivity
Ethambutol (E)	Bacteriostatic	15	Optic neuritis, hypersensitivity, color blindness for green
Streptomycin (S)	Bactericidal	15	Vestibular toxicity, deafness, hypersensitivity, renal toxicity

for treatment of MDR and XDR and included in NTEP by MOHFW, India in 2017.
- *Pretomanid:* Pretomanid was approved by US-FDA in August 2019 for treatment of TB. It is not available in India.

Treatment Regimen

The treatment consists of the intensive phase and the continuation phase. The response to therapy is monitored through clinical improvement, X-ray chest and culture or smear examination.

Intensive phase: The aim is to rapidly kill the bacilli, resolve symptoms and bring out sputum conversion (AFB negative) so that the patient becomes noninfectious. Generally, a fixed dose combination of 4 drugs is given daily for 2-3 months.

Continuation phase: The purpose is to eliminate the remaining bacilli from the lesion (sterilizing effect) so that relapse may not occur. This is generally given for 4-6 months.

The most commonly used regimen consists of a 2 months initial phase of RHZE followed by a 4 months continuation phase of HRE (2RHZE/4HRE).

Other Drugs/Therapy

- The supplementation of pyridoxine (10-25 mg/day) prevents isoniazid related neuropathy. It is given in those who are at high-risk of pyridoxine deficiency such as alcoholics, elderly, malnourished, diabetics, pregnant ladies and HIV patients
- Corticosteroids are useful if given with antitubercular drugs in seriously ill patients (miliary TB), and meningeal, pericardial or ureteric diseases to prevent adhesions
- Surgery may be needed in patients with massive and recurrent hemoptysis, constrictive pericarditis, lymph node suppuration, empyema and spinal cord compression.
- Pulmonary TB refers to disease involving lung parenchyma. Extrapulmonary TB refers to disease involving sites other than lung parenchyma. If both pulmonary and extrapulmonary sites are affected, it will be registered as pulmonary TB.

Directly Observed Treatment, Short Course

Patients swallow the drugs before a health personnel or some other responsible person. This ensures that the TB patient takes the right drugs, in the right dosage at the right intervals. Directly observed treatment, short course (DOTS) helps to improve cure rate and to reduce the chance of drug resistance.

Recent Changes in National Tuberculosis Elimination Programme

- Name of National TB Programme has been changed from RNTCP to National Tuberculosis Elimination Programme (NTEP)
- Category 2 and 3 have been abolished. Now category 1 includes all drug susceptible patients (DS-TB) and category 4 includes drug resistant patients (DR-TB).
- Now there is no intermittent regimen like twice or thrice a week. All doses should be given on daily basis.
- Drugs are given in fixed dose combination, means all 4 drugs are mixed in single tablet and number of tablets given according to weight bands **(Table 6.38)**.
- There is no extension in intensive phase.
- Treatment duration of all TB patients is 6 months except neurological TB, disseminated TB and musculoskeletal TB where 3-6 months extension can be given in continuation phase.
- After completion of treatment, patient needs to be clinically evaluated six monthly and/or by smear examination up to 24 months for relapse.

Complications of Pulmonary Tuberculosis

The complications of TB are given in **Table 6.39**.

Table 6.38: Fixed dose combinations of anti-tubercular drugs.

Weight category (2019)	Number of tables (FDCs)	
	Intensive phase: 4FDC (HRZE) 75/150/400/275	Continuation phase: 3FDC (HRE) 75/150/275
25–34	2	2
35–49	3	3
50–64	4	4
65–75	5	5
>75 kg*	6	6

*patients >75 kg may receive 5 tablets/day if they do not tolerate this dose.

Table 6.39: Complications of pulmonary tuberculosis.

Pulmonary complications
- Massive hemoptysis
- Aspergilloma
- Bronchiectasis
- Cor pulmonale
- Pleural calcification
- Bronchopleural fistula
- Obstructive airway disease

Extrapulmonary complications
- Amyloidosis
- Laryngitis
- Enteritis
- Empyema necessitans

Vaccination

Most countries recommend the use of *Bacillus Calmette Guérin (BCG)* vaccination. This contains attenuated strain of *M. bovis*.

- Intradermal route is recommended for the administration of the vaccine at the lower deltoid area
- In India, it is recommended to be administered to infants after birth or at the first contact of the infant with the health worker. The BCG vaccination is contraindicated in children with symptomatic HIV disease
- Ulceration at injection site and regional lymphadenopathy may occur in 1–10% of vaccinated persons
- The vaccination does not prevent infection or reactivation. However, it leads to inhibition of lympho-hematogenous spread of bacilli. Thus, highest efficacy of the BCG vaccine is in children with those forms of disease which involve hematogenous spread such as meningitis, miliary and disseminated TB. The vaccine provides about 70% protection for more than 10 years.

Chemoprophylaxis (Tuberculosis Preventive Treatment, TPT)

- Chemoprophylaxis has been applied in (a) tuberculin negative individuals to prevent occurrence of infection in high risk situations, (b) treating tuberculin positive cases to prevent disease
- In India, where a large majority of the population is tuberculin positive, it may be an expensive preposition. Programmatic management of tuberculosis preventive treatment (TPT) in India-2021 guidelines recommends TPT in people living with HIV and house hold contacts (<5 years of age) of pulmonary TB patients after ruling out active TB disease (testing for TBI is not required).
In household contacts of >5 years of age TPT is given to those having tuberculosis infection (TBI) after ruling out active disease, if tests for TBI are not available TPT must not be deferred. Patients on immunosupressive/anti-TNF therapy, patients having silicosis, patients on dialysis and patients planned for organ/hematologic transplant are given TPT if they have tuberculosis infection after ruling out active disease. Recommended tests for TBI are tuberculin skin test (TST) or interferon gamma release assay (IGRA).
- Isoniazid is given daily for 6 months in or combination of isoniazid plus rifapentine is given weekly for 3 months (12 doses).

Drug Resistant Tuberculosis

Resistance to TB drugs develops because of spontaneous point mutation in the *Mycobacterium genome*. It may be primary (patients infected with resistant bacilli and have not received TB drugs earlier) or secondary/acquired (resistance develops during treatment). Factors which favor the development of resistance are inadequate regimen, incomplete dosage or duration.

Types of Drug Resistant TB (DRTB)

- ***Mono-resistant TB (MR TB):*** A tuberculosis patient, whose biological specimen is resistant to one first-line anti-TB drug only.
- ***Isoniazid-resistant TB (HR TB):*** If specimen is resistance to isoniazid only.
- ***Poly-drug resistant TB (PDR TB):*** If specimen is resistant to more than one first-line anti-TB drug, other than both H and R.
- ***Rifampicin resistant TB (RR-TB):*** If specimen is resistant to rifampicin only.
- ***Multidrug resistant TB (MDR TB):*** Specimen is resistant to both rifampicin (R) and isoniazid (H) with or without resistance to other anti-TB drugs.
- ***Extensively drug resistant TB (XDR TB):*** A MDR TB patient whose biological specimen is additionally resistant to at least a fluoroquinolones (oflaxacin, levofloxacin, moxifloxacin) and a second line injectable drug (kanamycin, amikacin, capreomycin).

Diagnosis of DRTB

As per recommendation from programmatic management of DRTB 2019 (PMDT), all notified tuberculosis patients, pediatrics patients, extra pulmonary tuberculosis, HIV patients and contacts of known drug resistant TB should undergo molecular test [cartridge based nucleic acid amplification test (CB-NAAT) or TrueNat] to detect rifampicin resistance or rifampicin sensitive. Further testing should be done with LPA (first or second line) or liquid culture with drug sensitivity test to detect resistance to other anti-TB drugs.

Management of DRTB

Pretreatment Investigation

As second line anti-TB are less effective and have more side effect so few investigations are required to prevent toxicity and adverse drugs reactions of 2nd line anti-TB drugs **(Table 6.40)**.

Table 6.40: Pre-treatment evaluation.

- Complete blood count with hemoglobin and platelet count
- Renal function test
- Blood sugar
- Liver function test
- Thyroid function test
- Chest X-ray
- Urinary pregnancy test
- HIV test
- Serum electrolytes
- ECG
- Audiogram
- Ophthalmologist opinion to see uveitis
- Psychiatry evaluation

Treatment

According to PMDT 2019, there are three types of regimens used for treatment of DRTB.

- **Isoniazid (H): Mono resistant DRTB:** 6 months therapy needed with all oral second line drugs.
- **Shorter regimen:** This regimen should be offered to all MDR/RR-TB pulmonary and extrapulmonary TB except neurological TB and disseminated TB. It should not be used in pregnancy and previous history of any drug used from this regimen for more than 1 month.
  - If the intensive phase is prolonged, the injectable agent is only given three times a week in the extended intensive phase.
  - Linezolid dose is reduced to 300 mg/day after 6–8 months.
- **All oral longer regimen:** There is no contraindication for this regimen, it should be used in all DRTB patients where shorter regimen cannot be given.

Doses of second line anti-TB drugs: According to NTEP, all DRTB patients are given anti TB drugs according to their weight bands **(Table 6.41)**.

Regimens for DR-TB

Programmatic Management of Drug Resistant Tuberculosis in India-2021 guidelines recommends following regimens **(Tables 6.42 and 6.43)**.

1. Shorter (9–11 months) oral-bedaquiline containing MDR/RR-TB regimen (>5 years, >15 kg) consists of

Table 6.41: Drugs with dosage for adult with DRTB (Table taken from PMDT India 2019).

S. No.	Drugs	16–29 kg	30–45 kg	46–70 kg	>70 kg
1	Rifampicin (R)[1]	300 mg	450 mg	600 mg	600 mg
2	High dose H (H[h])	300 mg	600 mg	900 mg	900 mg
3	Ethambutol (E)	400 mg	800 mg	1,200 mg	1,600 mg
4	Pyrazinamide (Z)	750 mg	1,250 mg	1,750 mg	2,000 mg
5	Levofloxacin (Lfx)	250 mg	750 mg	1,000 mg	1,000 mg
6	Moxifloxacin (Mfx)	200 mg	400 mg	400 mg	400 mg
7	High dose Mfx (Mfx[h])	400 mg	600 mg	800 mg	800 mg
8	Bedaquiline (Bdq)	Week 0–2: Bdq 400 mg daily / Week 3–24: Bdq 200 mg 3 times per week			
9	Linezolid (Lzd)	300 mg	600 mg	600 mg	600 mg
10	Clofazimine (Cfx)	50 mg	100 mg	100 mg	200 mg
11	Cycloserine (Cs)[4]	250 mg	500 mg	750 mg	1,000 mg
12	Delamanid (Dlm)	50 mg twice daily (100 mg) for 24 weeks in 6–11 years of age / 100 mg twice daily (200 mg) for 24 weeks for ≥12 years of age			
13	Imipenem/cilastatin (Ipm/Cls)[4]	1,000 mg imipenem/1,000 mg cilastatin twice daily			
14	Meropenem (Mpm)[4]	1,000 mg three times daily (alternative dosing is 2,000 mg twice daily)			
15	Amikacin (Am)[2]	500 mg	750 mg	750 mg	1,000 mg
16	Capreomycin (Am)[2]				
17	Kanamycin (Km)[2]	500 mg	750 mg	750 mg	1,000 mg
18	Ethionamide (Eto)[4]	375 mg	500 mg	750 mg	1,000 mg
19	Na-PAS (60% weight/vol)[3,4]	10 gm	14 gm	16 gm	22 gm
20	Amoxyclave (Amx/Clv) (In child: WHO 80 mg/kg in 2 divided doses)	875/125 mg BD	875/125 mg BD	875/125 mg (2 morning + 1 evening)	875/125 (2 morning + 1 evening)
21	Pyridoxine (Pdx)	50 mg	100 mg	100 mg	100 mg

[1]For H mono/poly resistant TB
[2]For adult more than 60 years of age, dose of SLI should be reduced to 10 mg/kg (max up to 750 mg)
[3]In patient of PAS with 80% weight/volume the dose will be changed to 7.5 g (16–29 kg); 10 g (30–45 kg); 12 g (46–70 kg) and 16 g (>70 kg)
[4]Drugs can be given in divided doses in a day in the event of intolerance.

Table 6.42: Groups of second line anti-TB drugs.

GROUP A: Include all three medicines	1. Levofloxacin (Lfx) OR moxifloxacin (Mfx) 2. Bedaquiline (Bdq) 3. Linezolid (Lzd)
GROUP B: Add one or both medicines	4. Clofazimine (Cfz) 5. Cycloserine (Cs) OR Terizidone (Trd)
Group C: Add to complete the regimen and when medicines from Group A to B cannot be used	6. Ethambutol (E) 7. Delamanid (Dlm) 8. Pyrazinamide (Z) 9. Imipenem-cilastatin (Imp-Cln) OR Meropenem (Mpn) 10. Amikacin (Am) (OR Streptomycin) 11. Ethionamide (Eto) OR prothionamide (Pto) 12. P-aminosalicylicacid (PAS)

Table 6.43: Drug regimen for DRTB.

H mono/poly DR TB (R resistance not detected and H resistance)	
All oral H mono-poly DR-TB regimen	6 Lfx R E Z (Total duration: 6 months)
RR-/MDR-TB	
Shorter RR-/MDR-TB regimen	4–6 Mfxhd Km/Am Eto Cfz Z Hh E 5 Mfxhd Cfz Z E (IP: 4–6 months + CP: 5 months) *If the intensive phase is prolonged, the injectable agent is only given three times a week in the extended intensive phase. *Reduce Lzd to 300 mg/day after 6–8 months
All oral longer RR-/MDR-TB regimen	18–20 Bdq (6) Lfx Lzd Cfz Cs (Total duration: 18–20 months)

initial phase of 4–6 months and continuation phase of 5 months.

(4–6) Bdq$_{(6m)}$, Lfx, Cfz, Z, E, H, Eto/(5) Lfx, Cfz, Z, E

2. Shorter injection containing MDR/RR-TB regimen

   (4–6) Mfx^h, Km/Am, Eto, Cfz, Z, H^h, E//(5) Mfx^h, Cfz, Z, E

3. Longer oral M/XDR-TB regimen (18–20 months). It has no separate initial and continuation phase. All 5 drugs of group A and B are given initially. Four drugs are continued beyond 6–8 months. Pyridoxine should be given to all patients.

   (18–20) Lfx, Bdq$_{(6m\ or\ more)}$, Lzd, Cfx, Cs

4. Isoniazid (H) mono/poly DR-TB regimen (H resistance detected and R resistance not detected)

   (6–9) Lfx, R, E, H

New WHO recommendation

WHO has recently recommended regimen consisting of bedaquiline, pretomanid and linezolid (BPaL regimen) for 6–9 months for a defined group of MDR-TB patients.

RESPIRATORY FAILURE

Respiratory failure is defined as a condition in which lung function is inadequate to meet the metabolic requirement of the individual. The dysfunction can be in one or more components of the respiratory system such as airways, respiratory muscles, alveolar units and pulmonary vessels.

Respiratory failure manifests as hypoxemia ($PaO_2 < 60$ mm Hg) and/or hypercapnia ($PaCO_2 > 50$ mm Hg).

Clinical features of respiratory failure consist of those of underlying disease combined with manifestations of hypoxemia and hypercapnia **(Table 6.44)**.

Table 6.44: Clinical features of hypoxemia and hypercapnia.

Hypoxemia	
Symptoms	Dyspnea
Signs	Cyanosis, confusion, tachypnea, tachycardia, arrhythmias, flapping tremors (asterixis)
Hypercapnia	
Symptoms	Dyspnea, headache
Signs	Impaired sensorium, hypertension, tachycardia, tachypnea, papilledema, asterixis

Type I Respiratory Failure (Hypoxemic Respiratory Failure)

Type I respiratory failure may be acute, chronic or acute on chronic.

- *Acute:* This is characterized by low PaO_2 and normal or low $PaCO_2$. The important causes are pulmonary edema, pneumonia, ARDS, pneumothorax, PE and acute asthma. The management includes:
  - High concentration oxygen therapy
  - Prompt treatment of underlying disorders
  - Mechanical ventilation if no improvement.
- *Chronic:* There is low PaO_2 and normal $PaCO_2$. The important causes are emphysema and lung fibrosis. The treatment is directed toward underlying conditions.

Type II Respiratory Failure (Hypercapnic Respiratory Failure)

Type II respiratory failure may be acute, chronic or acute on chronic.

- *Acute:* There is hypoxia and hypercapnia. The latter can result into respiratory acidosis. Causes include:
  - Diminished respiratory drive (drugs, brainstem lesions)
  - Impaired respiratory muscles function (myasthenia gravis, myopathies, Guillain-Barré syndrome)
  - Asphyxia (inhaled foreign body, laryngeal edema)
  - Acute severe asthma.

  The treatment is aimed at reversal of precipitating events. The patient may need tracheostomy or mechanical ventilation. Respiratory stimulant (doxapram infusion) may be helpful in case the facilities for mechanical ventilation are not available.

- *Chronic:* This is characterized by the presence of hypoxemia, hypercapnea with near normal pH due to

compensatory rise in bicarbonate (HCO$_3$). The most important cause is COPD. The treatment is directed toward the cause. A controlled long-term oxygen therapy may be helpful.
- *Acute on chronic:* Any precipitating event such as acute infection, airways obstruction and cardiac failure can lead to acute deterioration in patients with chronic respiratory disease. The treatment consists of control of precipitating events and controlled low concentration oxygen therapy.

Type III Respiratory Failure

Type III respiratory failure can occur as a result of lung collapse, generally during perioperative period. That is why this is also called as *perioperative respiratory failure*. It can be avoided by frequent change in position and chest physiotherapy.

Type IV Respiratory Failure

Type IV respiratory failure occurs due to hypoperfusion of respiratory muscles in patients with shock. Respiratory failure occurs due to increased demand by respiratory muscles. The distribution of cardiac output to respiratory muscle is increased. However, respiratory failure may occur if the demand is not met with by the increased supply. Intubation and mechanical ventilation are helpful in the management of such condition.

PLEURAL DISEASES

Pleura consists of two layers. The parietal pleura lines the inner surface of the chest wall while visceral pleura covers the lung surface. There is a space between both layers of pleura which normally contains very thin layer of fluid (5–15 mL).

Pleurisy

Pleurisy is a term described when pleura is involved in any disease process. The inflammation in the pleura is also known as pleuritis.
- Common causes of pleurisy are viral infections, pneumonia, tuberculosis and malignancy
- The most important symptom of pleurisy is sharp and stabbing chest pain that worsens by coughing, sneezing or deep breathing (pleuritic pain)
- The clinical examination reveals pleural rub and other features of primary underlying disease. The disappearance of rub and chest pain suggests recovery or the development of pleural effusion
- The management of pleurisy includes treatment of the primary cause and the symptomatic control of pain. Analgesics and anti-inflammatory drugs are used for pain relief. Codeine is helpful in suppressing the cough and chest pain.

Table 6.45: Common causes of pleural effusion.

Transudative
- Congestive heart failure
- Cirrhosis with ascites
- Nephrotic syndrome

Exudative
- Tuberculosis
- Pneumonia
- Malignancy
- Pulmonary embolism
- Connective tissue diseases
- Pancreatitis

Pleural Effusion

Pleural effusion is defined as excessive accumulation of fluid in the pleural space. The collection of water like fluid is called hydrothorax and grossly purulent fluid is known as empyema. Presence of blood and lymphatic fluid in pleural space is called hemothorax and chylothorax, respectively. Important causes of pleural effusion are pneumonia, tuberculosis, cardiac failure, cirrhosis and malignancy. Other causes are mentioned in **Table 6.45**.

Clinical Features

Pleuritic chest pain often precedes the onset of effusion in case of pneumonia. Effusion due to other common causes like tuberculosis, lung malignancy and transudative effusion generally is not associated with pain. The most important symptom of pleural effusion is dyspnea and the severity depends on the rate and size of the accumulation of fluid. Symptoms of underlying disease occur frequently (*see* **Table 6.46**). Examination reveals diminished movements on the side of the effusion, mediastinal shift to the opposite side and stony dull note on percussion. Auscultation of the chest shows reduced or absent breath sounds.

Investigations

Chest X-ray reveals the presence of fluid and the evidence of underlying disease in the lungs (**Fig. 6.21**). Ultrasound is helpful to confirm the presence of fluid and to guide the aspiration. CT chest is usually required to diagnose the underlying pathology.

The aspiration of fluid confirms the diagnosis of pleural effusion. The biochemical, microbiological and cytological examination of the pleural fluid is helpful in knowing the underlying cause. The measurement of lactate dehydrogenase (LDH) and protein in the pleural fluid helps in differentiating transudative from exudative effusion effusion (**Table 6.47** Light's criteria). The biopsy of the pleura may be needed to diagnose the underlying cause.

Table 6.46: Clinical features and investigations in pleural effusion.

Cause of pleural effusion	Transudative/ Exudative	Clinical features	Investigation
Parapneumonic effusion/empyema	Exudative/pus	• High grade fever, chest pain, dyspnea of short duration 3–5 days • Tender percussion in empyema	• Pleural fluid: Low pH (<7.2), low sugar • May show micro-organism on culture
Tubercular effusion	Exudative	• Low grade fever, loss of appetite and loss of weight • Subacute: 10–15 days • Dyspnea in later stage	• Pleural fluid: High protein • High ADA (>40 IU/mL) • Coagulum may be seen • Rarely AFB positive
Malignant	Exudative	Mostly silent pleural effusion unless massive which causes dyspnoea. Clinical features suggestive of underlying malignancy may be seen	• Pleural fluid: Usually hemorrhagic color • Malignant cells present in around 50% cases • Pleural biopsy required for diagnosis
Chylothorax	Exudative	Mostly silent unless massive which causes dyspnea. Clinical features suggestive of underlying etiology like malignancy, lymphoma or trauma may be seen	• Pleural fluid: Milky in colour • High triglycerides > 120 mg/dL with low cholesterol < 200 mg/dL • (Reverse finding in pseudochylothorax)
Congestive cardiac failure	Transudative	• Usually B/L pleural effusion, dyspnea is out of proportion of pleural effusion • Signs of CHF like pedal edema, elevated JVP, congestive hepatomegaly seen	• Pleural fluid usually clear like water • Cardiomegaly on chest X-ray, serum NT pro-BNP will be increased • 2D-ECHO is confirmatory
Hemothorax	Exudative	• Dyspnea, chest pain if trauma • Clinical features suggestive of underlying etiology will be seen	• Bloody in color • Pleural fluid hematocrit > 50% of peripheral blood hematocrit

(JVP: jugular venous pressure; AFB: acid fast bacilli; ADA: adenosine deaminase; CHF: congestive heart failure; NT: N terminal)

Table 6.47: Light's criteria.

Presence of any one of following criteria shows exudative pleural effusion.
1. Pleural fluid to serum fluid protein > 0.5
2. Pleural fluid to serum LDH ratio > 0.6
3. Pleural fluid LDH > two third of upper limit of normal serum LDH

(LDH: lactate dehydrogenase)

Management

- *Therapeutic pleural aspiration*:
  - The aspiration of fluid may be required to relieve the dyspnea in cases with large effusion.
  - There is no need to do therapeutic aspiration in mild to moderate transudative pleural effusion and tubercular effusion.
- *Intercostal tube drainage (ICTD/thoracostomy)* required in following condition:
  - Empyema
  - Complicated parapneumonic pleural effusion (fluid pH < 7.2, presence of bacteria, etc.)
  - Recurrent malignant pleural effusion.
- *Treatment of underlying etiology*: Like anti-TB drugs for tuberculosis, antibiotics for parapneumonic effusion, treatment of CHF, nephrotic syndrome, etc.
- *Pleurodesis*: Sclerosing agents are injected to obliterate pleural space. These agents are talc powder, 10% povidone iodine, tetracycline, doxycycline, and bleomycin. Sclerosing agents produce inflammation in the pleura leading to adhesion and obliteration.

Pleurodesis is commonly done in recurrent malignant pleural effusion.
- *Other surgical interventions* like decortication, video assisted thoracoscopic surgery (VATS), etc. are done in complicated empyema where lung is trapped due to pleural thickening.

PNEUMOTHORAX

Presence of air in the pleural space is known as pneumothorax.

Classification

- *Spontaneous pneumothorax*:
  Primary: It can be without evidence of any overt lung disease. It is common in tall young males age between 20 and 40, smokers and those with apical subpleural blebs **(Fig. 6.24)**.
  Secondary: Pneumothorax developed due to underlying lung disease like COPD (most common), asthma, ILD, TB, necrotizing pneumonia, esophageal rupture, etc.
- *Traumatic pneumothorax*: It may be iatrogenic while inserting central line, mechanical ventilation or other procedures like pleural aspiration, pleural biopsy, etc. or due to trauma to the chest wall.

Types of Pneumothorax

- *Close type*: The communication between pleural space and lung seals off as the lung deflates and it does not reopen.

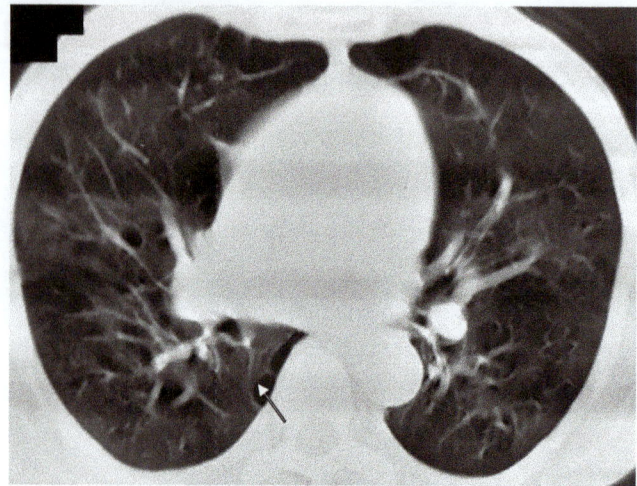

Fig. 6.24: CT scan thorax showing subpleural blebs which can rupture and cause pneumothorax.

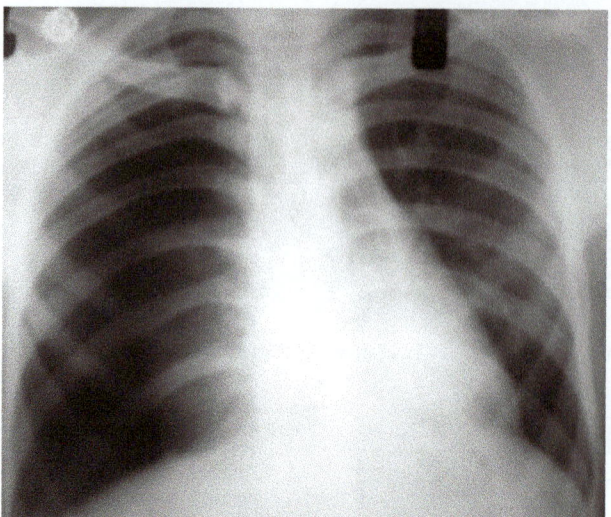

Fig. 6.25: Right-sided pneumothorax.

- *Open type:* The communication between pleural space and lung fails to seal off and air continues to transfer freely.
- *Tension pneumothorax:* The communication between pleural space and lung works as a one way valve that allows air to enter the pleural space during inspiration and coughing but prevents its escape.

Clinical Features

Most important symptoms of pneumothorax are sudden onset breathlessness and unilateral chest pain. Clinical signs are given in **Table 6.48**.

Investigations

Chest X-ray usually shows collapsed lung which has sharply defined edge with complete translucency without lung markings surrounding it. The shift of mediastinum to opposite side is seen **(Fig. 6.25)**.

Width of the rim of air surrounding the lung is use for classification of pneumothorax into small (<2 cm or amount of pneumothorax < 50%) and large (>2 cm or amount of pneumothorax >50%).

CT thorax: It is required to find out the underlying cause. CT scan can also help in differentiating pneumothorax from bullous disease **(Fig. 6.26)**.

Management

- *Primary spontaneous pneumothorax:* It can be initially managed by simple aspiration. Thoracoscopy with

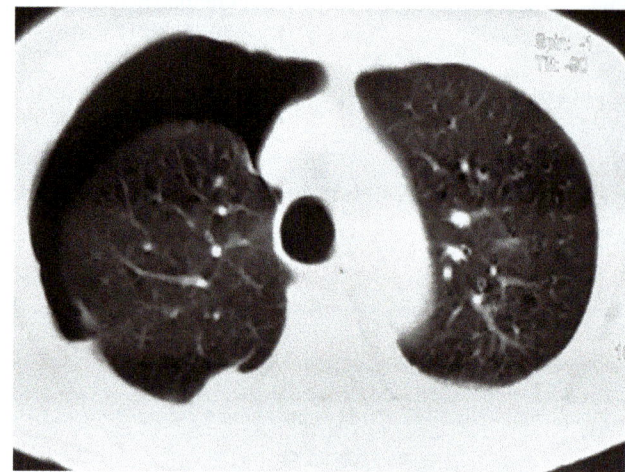

Fig. 6.26: CT scan thorax showing right sided pneumothorax.

stapling of blebs is indicated if lung expansion does not occur or patient develops recurrent pneumothorax.
- *Secondary spontaneous pneumothorax:* It is treated with tube thoracostomy with underwater seal drainage (ICTD). Alternatively, thoracoscopy with stapling of blebs can be performed.
- *Traumatic pneumothorax:* It should be treated with tubethoracostomy. Two tubes are needed in case of hemo-pneumothorax, one to be placed in upper part to drain air and another in lower part to drain blood.
- *Tension pneumothorax:* This is a medical emergency. A large bore needle should be inserted into pleural space through second anterior intercostals space. Later thoracostomy should be done and the needle removed.
- *Supportive treatment:* This includes oxygen inhalation and management of shock.
- *Pleurodesis:* Used in recurrent primary pneumothorax and in secondary pneumothorax even at 1st time occurrence.
- Treatment of underlying disease such as tuberculosis, COPD, ILD, etc.

Table 6.48: Signs of pneumothorax.

- Tachycardia, cyanosis, hypotension
- Decreased movement of chest wall on the side of lesion
- Mediastinal shift to opposite side
- Hyperresonant percussion note
- Decreased or absent breath sound
- Decreased or absent vocal fremitus and vocal resonance

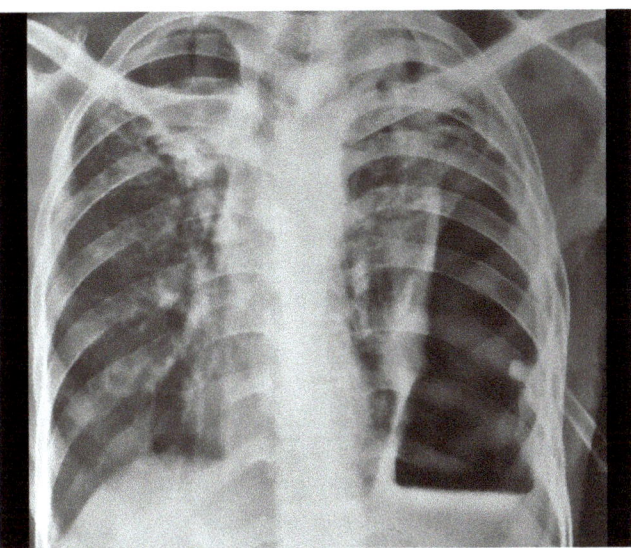

Fig. 6.27: X-ray chest showing left side pyopneumothorax with ICTD in situ. There is cavitatory lesion in right upper zone.

Complication of Pneumothorax

- *Pyopneumothorax:* More frequent in open type of pneumothorax **(Fig. 6.27)**.
- *Bronchopleural fistula (BPF):* There is communication between pleural cavity with alveoli specially in tuberculosis, severe trauma, etc. There will be bubbling in ICTD bag while deep respiration or coughing. Persistent BPF needs surgical treatment.
- *Subcutaneous or surgical emphysema:* Occurs when air leaks from side of ICTD. On examination there will be crepitation on palpation of chest wall. Usually it is self-resolving with oxygen supplementation and rarely requires subcutaneous surgical puncture to remove air.
- *Re-expansion pulmonary edema:* It occurs due to rapid expansion of lungs following ICTD or rapid pleural aspiration, usually self-limiting but rarely may be fatal.

INTERSTITIAL LUNG DISEASE

Interstitial lung disease is a group of diseases involving parenchyma of the lung, the alveoli, alveolar epithelium, capillary endothelium and spaces between these structures.

Classification

Interstitial lung disease is classified into two main types depending on the underlying histopathological changes.
- Predominant inflammation and fibrosis associated
- Predominant granulomatous reaction associated.

Pathogenesis

There are inflammatory changes in the air spaces and alveolar walls initially which gradually involve interstitium and vessels. Eventually, chronic inflammation leads to fibrosis. In granulomatous type, lymphocytes, macrophages and epithelial cells organize into discrete granuloma in the lung parenchyma.

Table 6.49: Clinical features of interstitial lung disease.

Symptoms
- Progressive dyspnea
- Dry cough (or minimal sputum)
- Fatigue, weight loss
- Chest pain, hemoptysis (uncommon)

Signs
- Tachypnea
- Cyanosis, clubbing (rare)
- Bilateral basal end inspiratory crackles
- Wheezes (occasional)
- Signs of cor pulmonale

Clinical Features

Progressive dyspnea is the most common presenting symptom whereas tachypnea and basal end inspiratory crackles is the important sign. Other symptoms and signs are given in the **Table 6.49**.

Common Causes of ILD

Important causes of ILD are:
- Idiopathic interstitial pneumonia
- *Occupational*: Fumes, gases, asbestos, organic and inorganic dust
- Sarcoidosis
- *Connective tissue diseases*: Systemic lupus erythematosus (SLE), rheumatoid arthritis
- Drugs and others.

Investigations

- *Chest X-ray:* The findings are nonspecific. Most common findings are bibasilar reticular pattern, nodular, and mixed pattern **(Fig. 6.28)**.

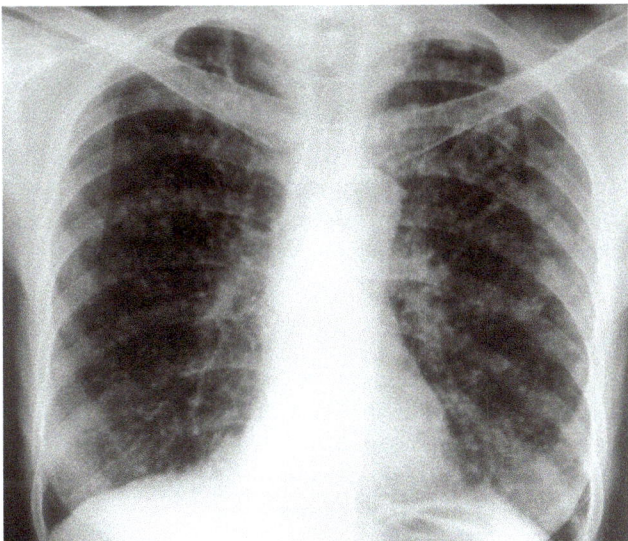

Fig. 6.28: Interstitial lung disease (X-ray showing reticulonodular shadows).

- *CT thorax:* High resolution CT scan confirms the diagnosis and can detect the disease in early stages.
- *Pulmonary function tests:* It reveals restrictive pattern. FEV_1 and FVC are reduced; FEV_1/FVC is usually normal or increased. Total lung capacity, functional residual capacity and residual volume are decreased.
- Arterial blood gas analysis may reveal hypoxia and respiratory alkalosis.
- *Bronchoalveolar lavage:* This may be helpful in the diagnosis of sarcoidosis.
- *Others:* ANA, rheumatoid factor, serum ACE level.

Treatment

The main goal of treatment is aggressive suppression of inflammation, oxygen supplementation, treatment of cor pulmonale and lung transplantation in advanced cases. Suppression of inflammation can be achieved by:
- Corticosteroids
- *Immunosuppressive drugs*: Cyclophosphamide, azathioprine.

LUNG CANCERS (BRONCHOGENIC CARCINOMA)

Lung cancer is the leading cause of death due to cancers worldwide. Smoking is causally associated with lung cancer; however, it can occur in nonsmokers also.

Etiology of Lung Cancers

The most common cause of lung cancer is cigarette smoking. Various carcinogens and tumor promoters are inhaled during smoking.
- In active smokers, the relative risk of developing lung cancer is 13 fold while it is 1.5 fold in passive smokers.
- The chance of developing cancer is even more in case a smoker has COPD.
- The chance of developing lung cancer depends on the amount and duration of cigarette smoking (cigarette pack years).
- The risk of lung cancers reduces following smoking cessation.

Apart from smoking, several other risk factors have been identified. These are occupational exposure to asbestos, arsenic, bischloromethyl ester, chromium, mustard gas, nickel and hydrocarbons (polycyclic aromatic).

Classification

The classification of lung cancers is mainly based on the cell types. Four major cell types constitute most of the primary lung cancers and these are:
1. Squamous (epidermoid) carcinoma
2. Small cell (oat cell) carcinoma
3. Adenocarcinoma
4. Large cell carcinoma

The most common type of lung cancer worldwide is adenocarcinoma. Adenocarcinoma is also common in nonsmokers, females and young patients. Squamous and small cell carcinomas are associated with heavy tobacco use. Other types include undifferentiated carcinoma, carcinoids and bronchial gland tumors.

For treatment and prognostic purposes the lung tumors are divided into, small cell lung cancer (SCLC) and non-small cell lung cancer (NSCLC).

Clinical Features

The symptoms and signs of lung cancers occur due to various factors/mechanisms, which are given below.
- *The presence of local tumor* growth (central or endobronchial) may lead to cough, hemoptysis, wheeze, stridor, dyspnea and postobstructive pneumonitis. Squamous cell and small cell carcinoma tend to occur centrally while adenocarcinomas often occur in more peripheral lung locations. Peripheral growth of the primary tumor may cause pain from pleural or chest wall involvement, dyspnea and features of lung abscess due to tumor cavitation. Patient may have clubbing (usually non-small cell carcinoma) and hypertrophic primary osteoarthtopathy.
- *Invasion or obstruction of nearby structures* can cause dyspnea (tracheal obstruction), dysphagia (esophageal compression), hoarseness of voice (recurrent laryngeal nerve palsy) and Horner's syndrome (enophthalmos, ptosis, miosis and ipsilateral loss of sweating over face). Local invasion of structures such as 8th cervical and 1st and 2nd thoracic nerves and destruction of first and second ribs by tumor in the apex of lung with shoulder pain is known as Pancoast's syndrome. Regional spread of tumor can cause superior vena caval obstruction (superior vana cava syndrome). Lymphatic obstruction may result in pleural effusion.
- Extrathoracic metastasis can occur at numerous sites like brain, bones, bone marrow, liver and lymph nodes giving rise to various symptoms and signs.
- Paraneoplastic syndromes occur due to biologically active hormones secreted by the tumor (especially small cell carcinoma). However, in many cases, the mechanism is unknown. Some of the important paraneoplastic syndromes found in lung cancers are hypercalcemia, hyponatremia, hypokalemia, hypertrophic pulmonary osteoarthropathy, peripheral neuropathies, cerebellar degeneration, venous thrombosis and Eaton lambert's syndrome.

Investigations

- X-ray chest reveals mass lesion which is generally central in squamous cell and small cell carcinoma and peripheral in adenocarcinoma and large cell carcinoma. Cavitary lesion can be seen in some cases of squamous cell and

large cell carcinoma. Other findings are mediastinal lymphadenopathy, lung collapse **(Figs. 6.29 and 6.30)** bone erosions and pleural effusion **(Fig. 6.31)**.
- CT scan helps in detecting the small size tumor and local and distant metastasis. These findings are helpful in staging the disease **(Fig. 6.32)**.
- Fiberoptic bronchoscopy is useful in cases of endobronchial growth where tumor tissue can be obtained for histological diagnosis **(Figs. 6.33 and 6.34)**.
- Diagnostic pleural tap, if effusion present.
- Fine needle aspiration cytology/biopsy of enlarged supraclavicular or cervical lymph nodes.
- Sputum examination for the presence of malignant cells.
- *Positron emission tomography scan (PET)*: Whole body PET scan is needed to see distant metastasis.
- *MRI brain:* It is needed to see micro-metastasis in case of small cell lung carcinoma prior to treatment.

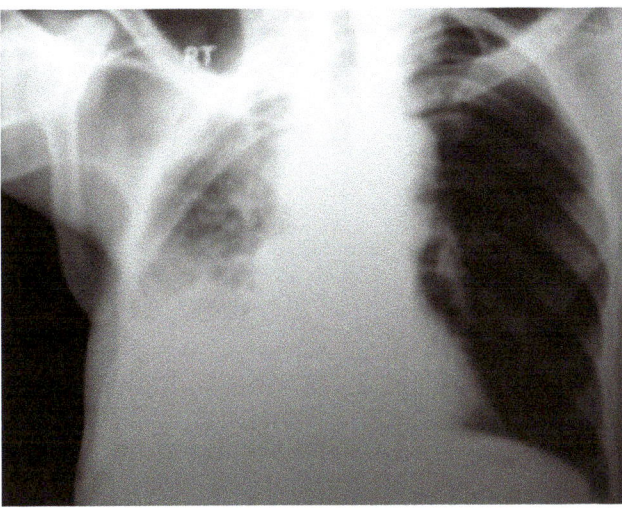

Fig. 6.31: Carcinoma right lung (X-ray showing collapse of lung with destruction of ribs).

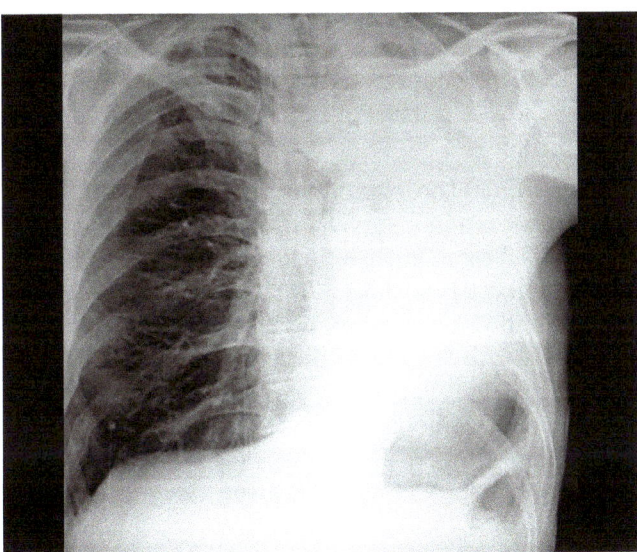

Fig. 6.29: X-ray chest shows complete collapse of left lung.

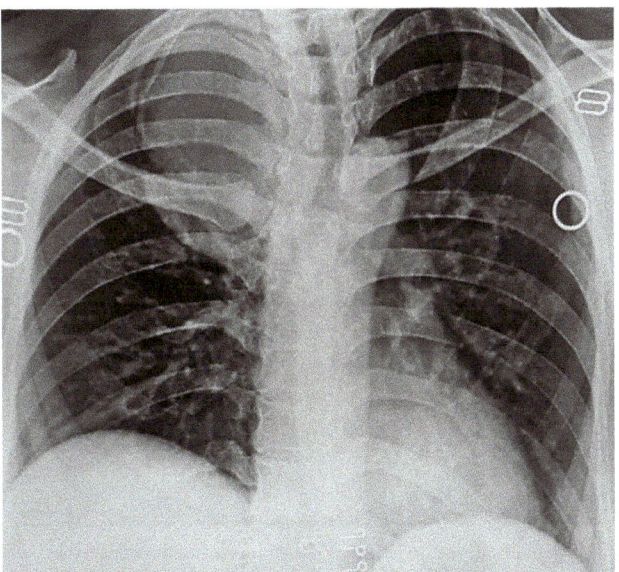

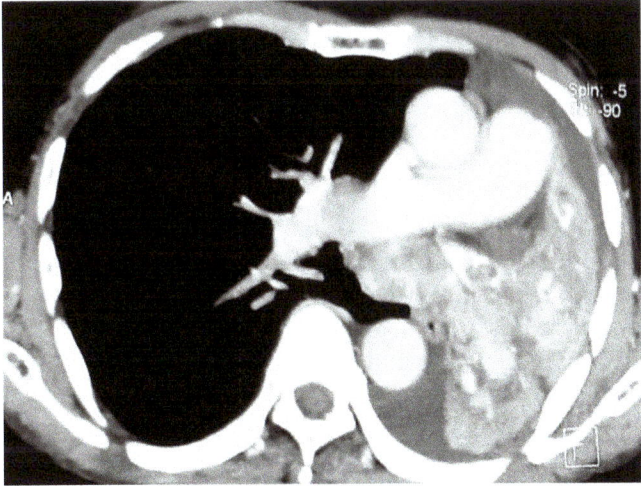

Fig. 6.30: Contrast enhanced CT thorax shows mass obstructing left main bronchus causing complete collapse of left lung.

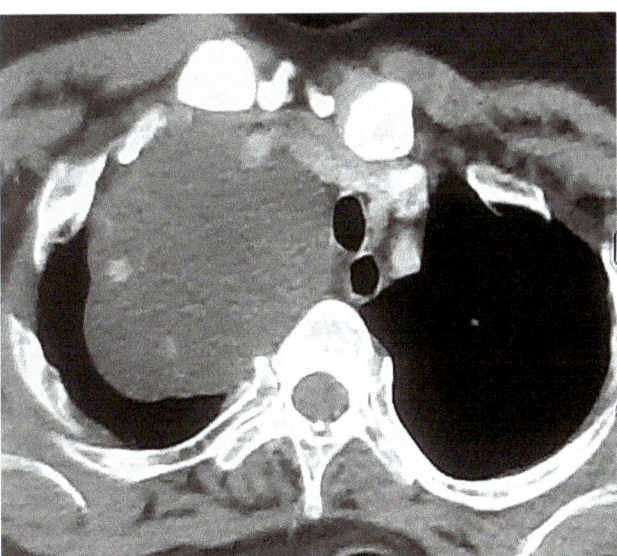

Fig. 6.32: Chest X-ray and HRCT thorax of a 26-year-old female shows large space occupying lesion in right side of thorax shifting trachea to left side. It was diagnosed as germ cell tumor by biopsy.

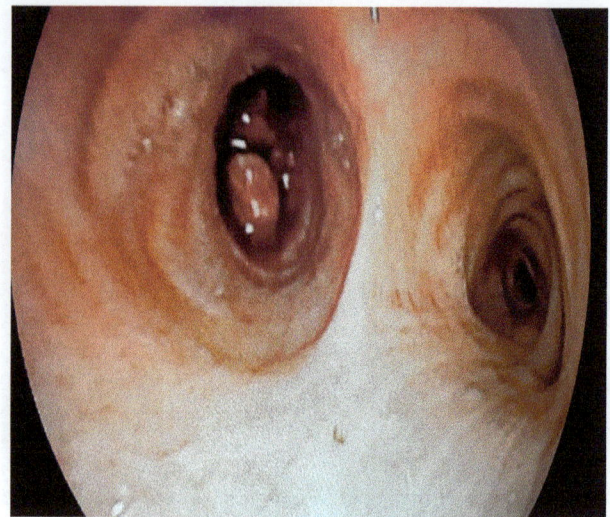

Fig. 6.33: Bronchoscopic view from carina shows mass obstructing left main bronchus.

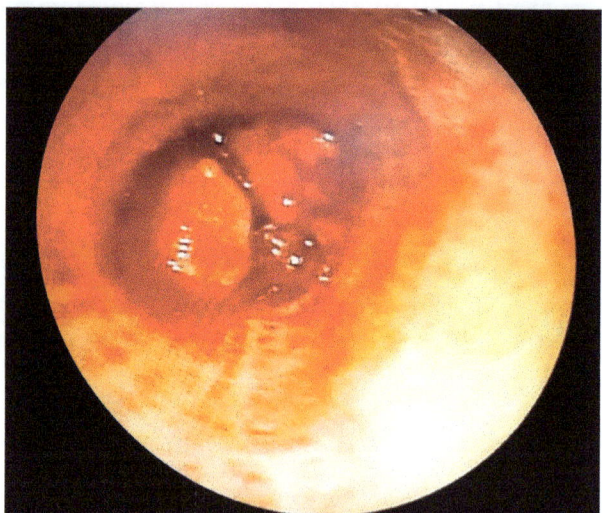

Fig. 6.34: Bronchoscopic view shows intrabronchial mass occluding left main bronchus.

Definitive diagnosis can only be made by biopsy followed by histopathological examination (HPE) and immunohistology. This is helpful to differentiate small cell carcinoma from non-small cell carcinoma.

Biopsy can be done by following methods:
- Image guided lung biopsy like CT guided biopsy or USG guided biopsy where lung mass is in peripheral location.
- Bronchoscopic biopsy like transbronchial lung biopsy, intrabronchial biopsy from intrabronchial lung mass.
- Mediastinal lung mass or lymphnode can be biopsied by mediastinoscopy or endobronchial lung ultrasound guided FNAC, etc.
- Thoracoscopic pleural biopsy can be done in case of pleural metastasis or undiagnosed pleural effusion.

Molecular test: Few mutations like epidermal growth factor receptors (EGFR), anaplastic lymphoma kinase (ALK), c-ROS oncogene 1 (ROS-1) can be detected. This allows targeted treatment with better response than what is obtained with standard chemotherapy alone, especially in cases of adenocarcinoma.

Management

Staging: TNM staging depends on extent of involvement of lung parenchyma (T1–T4), mediastinal lymphnode involvement (N1–N3) and metastasis (M1a–c) and according to involvement of TNM. NSCLC can be staged as 1,2,3,4, and SCLC as limited type (confined to thorax) and extensive type (outside thorax).

Following modalities of treatment are applied in patients with bronchogenic carcinoma:
- Surgery
- Chemotherapy
- Radiotherapy
- Palliative therapy

Surgery: Surgery offers best hope in patients with early stage disease (stage I and II), where the 5 year survival rates are more than 75% and 55%, respectively. However, surgery is not possible in majority of cases due to extensive spread of disease or presence of severe cardiac or renal disease or other comorbid illnesses.

Chemotherapy: The combination chemotherapy drugs can increase median survival in patients with small cell carcinoma, whereas, in general, chemotherapy is less effective in non-small cell bronchogenic carcinoma. The drugs used in combination chemotherapy in NSCLC are cisplatin/carboplatin with any one of these drugs like gemcitabine, docetaxel, paclitaxel, pemetrexete or vinorelbine. While in SCLC cisplatin/carboplatin are given with either etoposide or irinotecan.

Most of chemotherapies are given every 21 days (4–5 cycles).

Targeted drugs for non-small cell lung carcinoma (adenocarcinoma): Following drugs are very useful if lung tissue shows particular receptors in HPE specially in stage 4 carcinoma.
- *EGRF mutation:* Gefitinib, erlotinib, afatinib, osimertinib, etc.
- *ALK mutation:* Crizotinib, Ceritinib, alectinib, brigatinib, etc.
- *ROS-1 translocation:* Crizotinib.
- *K-RAS mutation:* Selumetinib.

Radiotherapy: The important role of radiotherapy in bronchogenic carcinoma is in the palliation of distressing complications such as superior vena caval obstruction, recurrent hemoptysis and pain due to chest wall infiltration or skeletal metastatic deposits. Radiotherapy when used along with chemotherapy in small cell carcinoma can improve the survival. It can also be helpful in patients with localized disease where surgery is not indicated due to various reasons.

Palliative therapy: This includes removal of obstruction of airways by endobronchial stenting or laser treatment through bronchoscopy. Effective pain management is also important in patients with advanced cancer.

SWINE INFLUENZA A (H1N1)—"SWINE FLU"

Introduction

Swine influenza A (H1N1) is a highly contagious acute respiratory illness of pigs caused due to one of the several strains of swine influenza A virus. Among humans, the virus is either transmitted by direct contact, i.e., through aerosols or through indirect contact, and also by the asymptomatic carrier pigs. The symptoms of swine influenza A in humans is similar to that of influenza namely chills, fever, sore throat, muscle pains, severe headache, coughing, weakness, and lethargy.

Pathogenesis

Its structure like envelope glycoproteins (the hemagglutinin and the neuraminidase) changes frequently. Minor change is called antigenic drift which causes outbreaks while major change is called antigenic shift which causes epidemic and pandemics.

The incubation period for swine influenza infection appears to range from 2 to 7 days and most patients with swine influenza infection might shed virus from 1 day before the onset of symptoms through 5–7 days after the onset of symptoms or until symptoms resolve. In young children and in patients who are immunocompromised or severely ill, the infectious period might be longer. The clinical spectrum of swine flu influenza ranges from self-limiting illness to severe acute respiratory failure and death.

Clinical Features

According to CDC, the symptom of swine influenza are:
- Fever
- Cough
- Sore throat
- Body aches
- Headaches
- Chills
- Fatigue.

In some cases, diarrhea and vomiting are the presenting complaint.

It has been noted that around 2% of infected individuals in some countries have developed severe disease, and that this has occurred most commonly in those aged 30–50 years. Many of these severe cases have other chronic health conditions; however, between a third and half of the serious cases have occurred in otherwise healthy, young-to-middle-aged people.

Laboratory Diagnosis

For the detection of swine influenza virus, a proper respiratory sample, i.e., a simple nose or throat swab is required.

Real-Time PCR

Real-time PCR is used to detect seasonal influenza A, B, H1, H3, and avian H5 serotypes.

Treatment

Two classes of antiviral medication are available for the treatment of seasonal human influenza: **Neuraminidase inhibitors** (oseltamivir and zanamivir) and **adamantanes** (rimantadine and amantadine). Presently government of India recommends TAMIFLU (Oseltamivir) as a drug of choice which is available at all government health bodies. Doses and schedule given in **Table 6.50**.

Vaccination

Vaccine is prescribed to be given annually. The composition of the vaccine is updated every year depending on the prevalent strains. Trivalent vaccine (2020–2021) contains:
- A/Guangdong-Maonan/SWL1536/2019 (H1N1)pdm09-like virus
- A/Hong Kong/2671/2019 (H3N2)-like virus
- B/Washington/02/2019 (B/Victoria lineage)-like virus.

Quadrivalent (four-component) vaccines, which protect against a second lineage of B viruses, contains above 3 viruses plus B/Phuket/3073/2013-like (Yamagata lineage) virus.

IMPLICATIONS ON DENTAL PRACTICE

- Elective dental care is deferred in acute respiratory infections including common cold, sinusitis, pneumonia and acute bronchitis.

Table 6.50: Antiviral drugs for swine flu.

Age group	Treatment	Chemoprophylaxis
Oseltamivir for adults	75 mg capsule twice/day for 5 days	75 mg capsule once/day
Oseltamivir for children (age 12 months/older) Weight 15 kg or less	60 mg per/day divided into two doses	30 mg once/day
Oseltamivir for children (age 12 months/older) Weight 15–23 kg	90 mg/day divided into two doses	45 mg once/day
Oseltamivir for children (age 12 months/older) Weight 24–40 kg	120 mg/day divided into two doses	60 mg once/day
Oseltamivir for children (age 12 months/older) Weight > 40 kg	150 mg/day divided into two doses	75 mg once/day

- General anesthesia should be avoided in presence of respiratory infections.
- Prolonged use of corticosteroid inhalers may lead to increased incidence of oral candidiasis. Patients are advised to rinse mouth with water after using inhalers.
- Use of decongestant and antihistaminics may cause oral dryness.
- Toothache may occur due to maxillary sinusitis. It should be differentiated from odontogenic infections. Pain in more than one tooth in the same maxillary quadrant suggests sinus infection.
- Mouth breathing due to chronic sinusitis may lead to oral dryness and oral diseases such as gingivitis.
- Poor oral health predisposes to the development of pneumonia due to aspiration of salivary secretion containing both aerobic and anaerobic bacteria. Colonization of dental plaque and oral mucosa with pathogens is more common among hospitalized patients. Hence, regular use of chlorhexidine gluconate mouth washes is recommended in hospitalized patients.
- Inhalation of tooth or fragments or rarely endodontic instruments can cause lung abscess.
- Numerous dental products and materials such as toothpaste, tooth enamel dust, methyl methacrylate may exacerbate the asthma.
- Elective dental procedure should only be done when asthma is well-controlled. Patients are asked to bring the asthma medication with them.
- The history of allergy to aspirin or NSAIDs should always be asked in asthmatic patients as these agents may precipitate asthmatic attacks.
- Use of beta blockers may preferably be avoided in asthmatic patient.
- If the patient develops acute asthmatic attack during dental procedure, the procedure is stopped and all intraoral devices are removed. The patient is placed in comfortable position and the patency of airways is ensured. Oxygen is given and beta 2 agonists are administered through nebulization. Medical assistance may be called for.
- Drug interactions should be taken in mind. For example, macrolide antibiotics (erythromycin, clarithromycin) may increase the level of theophylline. Use of epinephrine containing local analgesics may precipitate arrhythmias if patient is taking theophylline or beta agonists.
- Aminoglycoside group of drugs (streptomycin, amikacin) can enhance the activity of neuromuscular blocking drugs and increase the weakness in myasthenic patients.
- Long-term use of beta 2 agonists may cause reduced salivary flow and increased incidence of caries and candidiasis. Fluoride supplement is advised for all asthmatic patients particularly those taking beta 2 agonists. Ipratropium can also cause dry mouth.
- There is association between oral infections and exacerbation of COPD. Therefore, maintenance of good oral hygiene is must in these patients.
- Patients with COPD are better treated in upright position as they may become more breathless if laid flat. Patients may not be able to tolerate rubber dam.
- Special caution is needed during dental procedures in patients with PE who are on oral anticoagulants. In such patient, prothrombin time and INR are estimated before the procedure. A level of INR <2.5 is safe for dental care including simple extraction.
- Tuberculosis is unlikely to be transmitted to the dental staff unless the patient is having active pulmonary tuberculosis or the dental staff is immunocompromised. Hence, dental treatment is best deferred until the active tuberculosis has been treated.
- Patient with tuberculosis and HIV infection can have oral lesions in the form of chronic oral ulcerations and candidiasis.
- Mycobacteria are resistant to many disinfectants. Hence, heat sterilization should be used.
- The drug interaction with antitubercular agents must be considered while prescribing the dental treatment.
- Rifampicin can cause red saliva.

SELF ASSESSMENT

Multiple Choice Questions

1. Following part of lung is mostly involved in lung abscess:
   A. Middle lobe of the lung
   B. Posterior segment of lower lobe
   C. Superior segment of lower lobe and posterior of upper lobe
   D. Posterior segment of upper lobe and superior of lower lobe
2. Following are causes of cavity in lung, *except*:
   A. Lung abscess
   B. Tuberculosis
   C. COPD
   D. Wegener's granulomatosis
3. Which is not a clinical manifestation of lung abscess?
   A. Clubbing
   B. Chest pain
   C. Copious amount of sputum
   D. Episodic dyspnea with wheeze
4. Kussmaul's breathing is seen in:
   A. Metabolic alkalosis   B. Respiratory alkalosis
   C. Metabolic acidosis   D. Respiratory acidosis
5. Polycythemia is seen in:
   A. Emphysema   B. Pleural effusion
   C. Bronchial asthma   D. Lung abscess
6. Stony dull note on percussion is present in:
   A. Pleural effusion   B. Pneumothorax
   C. Pulmonary fibrosis   D. Bronchial asthma
7. Following is the sign of consolidation:
   A. Bronchial breath sound
   B. Increased vocal fremitus
   C. Whispering pectoriloquy
   D. All of above

CHAPTER 6: RESPIRATORY DISEASES

8. Most common source of PE is:
   A. Splenic vein
   B. Arteriovenous fistula
   C. Leg and pelvic veins
   D. Subclavian vein
9. Peripheral neuropathy can be caused by:
   A. Isoniazid
   B. Rifampicin
   C. Ethambutol
   D. Streptomycin
10. Hepatitis can be caused by:
    A. Rifampicin
    B. Isoniazid
    C. Pyrazinamide
    D. All of the above
11. Significant improvement in FEV_1 after bronchodilator inhalation is seen in:
    A. COPD
    B. Bronchiectasis
    C. Bronchial asthma
    D. None of the above
12. Following indicates severe asthma, *except*:
    A. Pulsus paradoxus
    B. Cyanosis
    C. $PaO_2 > 80$ mm Hg
    D. Silent chest
13. Clubbing can be found in all, *except*:
    A. Lung abscess
    B. Lung cancer
    C. Pneumonia
    D. Bronchiectasis
14. Hemoptysis can be present in:
    A. Pulmonary tuberculosis
    B. Chronic bronchitis
    C. Mitral stenosis
    D. All the above
15. Tropical pulmonary eosinophilia is associated with:
    A. Aspergillus infection
    B. Nitrofurantoin
    C. Filaria
    D. Malaria
16. Fibro-cavitatory lesion is feature of:
    A. Primary tuberculosis
    B. Post-primary tuberculosis
    C. Miliary tuberculosis
    D. All of above
17. Following can be used in the treatment of pulmonary edema, *except*:
    A. Morphine
    B. Furosemide
    C. Beta blockers
    D. Nitrates
18. The most common symptom in PE is:
    A. Chest pain
    B. Fever with chills
    C. Dyspnea
    D. Hemoptysis
19. Following is preferred for the definitive diagnosis of acute PE:
    A. D-dimer test
    B. Arterial blood gas analysis
    C. Ventilation perfusion scan
    D. Spiral CT
20. Following can be found in pulmonary infarction:
    A. Dyspnea
    B. Pleuritic chest pain
    C. Hemoptysis
    D. All the above
21. Following are the causes of type I respiratory failure, *except*:
    A. Pneumonia
    B. Pulmonary embolism
    C. Respiratory muscle paralysis
    D. Pulmonary edema
22. Domiciliary oxygen therapy is indicated in:
    A. Pneumonia
    B. COPD
    C. Pulmonary eosinophilia
    D. None of the above
23. Following drugs are used in patients with eosinophilia, *except*:
    A. Prednisolone
    B. Hydroxyurea
    C. Diethyl carbamazine
    D. Nitrofurantoin
24. Hyper-resonant note and absent breath sounds are features of:
    A. Pleural effusion
    B. Pneumothorax
    C. Pneumonia
    D. Pulmonary fibrosis
25. "Blue bloater" is associated with:
    A. Emphysema
    B. Chronic bronchitis
    C. Pulmonary fibrosis
    D. Bronchial asthma
26. Bedaquiline is used in treatment of:
    A. MDR-Tuberculosis
    B. Drug resistant malaria
    C. Enteric fever
    D. Meningitis
27. Which of the following is not a part of COPD management?
    A. PDE 5 inhibitor (roflumilast)
    B. Infuenza vaccine
    C. Pneumococcal vaccine
    D. Rituximab (anti CD20)
28. According to recent GOLD guidelines, COPD patients are divided into:
    A. 4 groups (A, B, C, D)
    B. 3 groups (A, B, C)
    C. 4 groups (1, 2, 3, 4)
    d. 2 groups (early, late)
29. All of the following are taken into consideration to group COPD patients, *except*:
    A. Degree of airflow limitation
    B. Risk of exacerbation
    C. Severity of symptoms
    D. Vaccination status
30. According to National TB Treatment Guidelines, patients are currently divided into:
    A. 2 categories
    B. 3 categories
    C. 4 categories
    D. 5 categories
31. Which of the following is used in treatment of acute pulmonary edema?
    A. Furosemide
    B. Thiazide
    C. Indapamide
    D. Spironolactone
32. Which of the following is the preferred therapy during acute asthmatic attack?
    A. IV aminophylline
    B. Nebulization with beta 2 agonists
    C. Oral deriphyllin
    D. Inhaled anticholinergics
33. Investigation of choice in asthma is:
    A. Spirometry
    B. CT scan Thorax
    C. Chest X-ray
    D. Clinical examination is sufficient
34. Drug of choice in stable COPD is:
    A. Tiotropium
    B. Inhaler Budesonide
    C. Oral Salbutamol
    D. Oral theophylline
35. Drug of choice in asthma is:
    A. Inhaled Formoterol
    B. Inhaled salbutamol
    C. Inhaled corticosteroid
    D. Oral theophylline
36. Light's criteria used to differentiate exudative pleural effusion from transudative pleural effusion. It all includes all parameters, *except*:
    A. Pleural fluid protein to serum protein ratio > 0.6
    B. Pleural fluid LDH to serum LDH ratio > 0.6

C. Pleural fluid protein to serum protein ratio > 0.5
D. Pleural fluid LDH is more than two third of upper limit of normal serum LDH

37. What is common cause of chylothorax?
    A. Trauma
    B. Hodgkin's lymphoma
    C. Abdominal surgery
    D. All of the above

38. Which is new upcoming drug for drug resistant tuberculosis?
    A. Kanamycin
    B. Levofloxacin
    C. Ethionamide
    D. Pretomanid

39. First line anti-TB drugs are given for 6 months. In which condition duration of ATT is prolonged by 3–6 months?
    A. Tuberculosis abdomen
    B. Pericardial effusion
    C. TB lymphadenopathy
    D. Musculoskeletal TB

40. Indication of thrombolysis in PE is:
    A. Young patient with pneumonia
    B. Patient has chest pain
    C. Recurrent thromboembolism
    D. Systolic BP < 90 mm Hg

41. Gene Xpert test for drug resistant tuberculosis is use to detect resistance of:
    A. Rifampicin
    B. Isoniazid
    C. Both isoniazid and rifampicin
    D. All fine line drugs

42. Bronchovocation test or bronchial challenge test to diagnose suspected asthma in:
    A. Pediatric age group
    B. Occupational asthma
    C. In suspected asthma where spirometry is normal
    D. Elderly people.

43. Asthma control is assessed by:
    A. Night time system
    B. Limitation of physical activity
    C. Frequency of SOS salbutamol use
    D. All of the above

44. What are the comorbidies of COPD?
    A. Osteoporosis
    B. Metabolic syndrome
    C. Ischemic heart disease
    D. All of the above

45. What is the modality of treatment of COPD which halt disease progression?
    A. Smoking cessation
    B. Anticholinergic drugs
    C. Inhaled steroid
    D. Pulmonary rehabilitation

46. Following drugs are used as targeted drugs in non-small cell lung carcinoma is:
    A. Erlotinib
    B. Crizotinib
    C. Osimertinib
    D. All of the above

47. Nosocomial pneumonia occurs after how much time following admission to hospital?
    A. After 48 hours
    B. After 72 hours
    C. After 24 hours
    D. After 2–4 hours

48. Following drug is included in group of newer oral anticoagulant drugs:
    A. Dabigatran
    B. Rivaroxaban
    C. Apixaban
    D. All of the above

Fill in the Blanks

1. Enlargement of_____secondary to lung disease is called cor pulmonale.
2. Foul smelling sputum suggests infection due to _____ organisms.
3. Pink frothy sputum can be present in _____.
4. Most common cause of CAP is _____.
5. Most common cause of HAP is _____.
6. Barrel-shaped chest is seen in _____.
7. FEV_1/FVC ratio is_____in COPD.
8. Interrupted brief explosive sounds on lung auscultation is known as_____.
9. Continuous musical adventitious lung sound is called _____.
10. Inspiratory sound heard in case of tracheal obstruction is called_____.
11. Healed calcified parenchymal lesion in primary tuber-culosis is called as_____lesion.
12. Cyclical waxing and waning of respiration intervened with a short period of apnea is known as _____ breathing.
13. The most common cause of chronic type II respiratory failure is_____.
14. The drug of choice in tropical pulmonary eosinophilia is_____.
15. Pink puffers are associated with the disease _____.
16. Pleural rub is a sign of_____.
17. Nasal or bleating sounds on lung auscultation are called_____.
18. Normal partial pressure of oxygen in arterial blood (PaO_2) is_____.
19. Normal partial pressure of carbon dioxide in arterial blood ($PaCO_2$) is_____.
20. Normal arterial blood pH is_____.
21. Chylothorax pleural fluid has more_____while pseudochylothorax has more_____.
22. Multi drug resistant TB bacilli is resistant to_____ and_____drugs.
23. Primary tuberculosis usually heals by_____while post primary TB is healed by_____.
24. In diagnosis of bronchial asthma, spirometry finding called Reversible obstruction in spirometry procedure means change in FEV_1 of _____% and FVC _____mL.
25. Bronchial thermoplasty is bronchoscopic procedure used in_____.
26. Bronchodialator of choice in Group C COPD is_____.
27. _____carcinoma of lung is common in Asian female.
28. Paraneoplastic syndromes are common in_____carcinoma of lung.
29. Pleural effusion in tuberculosis is_____type while in CHF it is_____type.

CHAPTER 7

Renal Diseases

STRUCTURE AND FUNCTIONS OF NORMAL KIDNEYS

Anatomically, each kidney has an outer cortex and an inner medulla **(Fig. 7.1)**. The basic functional unit of the kidney is the nephron. The nephron consists of the glomerulus, Bowman's capsule and the renal tubule. Each kidney has around 1 million nephrons. The renal tubule is again composed of several segments—proximal tubule, loop of Henle, distal tubule and the collecting duct **(Fig. 7.1)**. The cortex consists mostly of glomeruli and proximal tubules, and the medulla consists of parallel arrays of loops of Henle and collecting ducts. The kidney is the primary regulator of the normal body fluid composition, which includes the balance of water, acid-base balance and electrolyte concentrations, including sodium, potassium, calcium and phosphorus. The kidney is responsible for excretion of endogenous nitrogenous wastes and exogenous drugs and toxins. The kidney also helps in long-term maintenance blood pressure, and is a producer of important hormones: Renin (for blood pressure control), erythropoietin (for production of red blood cells) and activated vitamin D (for bone health). Major functions of the kidney are summarized in **Table 7.1**.

SYNDROMES IN NEPHROLOGY

Patients with renal disease present with certain features to the clinician which are popularly called as syndromes, as

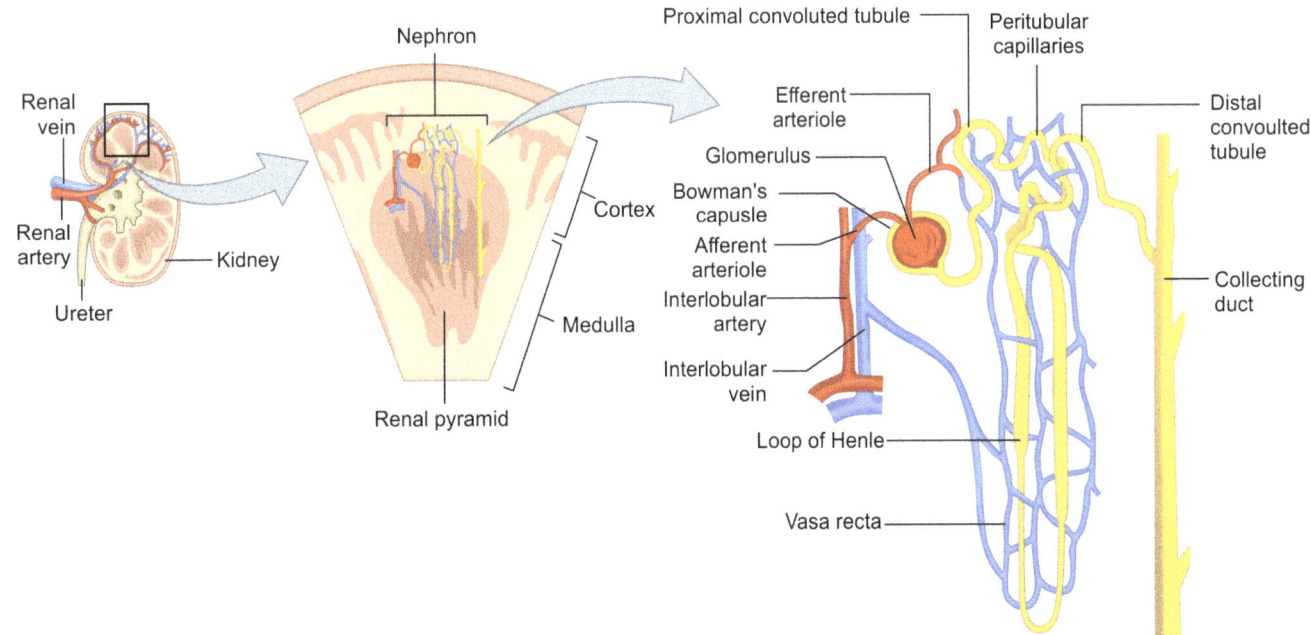

Fig. 7.1: Structure of nephron.

Table 7.1: Major functions of normal kidney.

- Maintenance of normal body water and electrolyte balance
- Maintenance of acid-base balance
- Excretion of endogenous and exogenous waste products
- Long-term regulation of blood pressure
- Production of hormones—renin, erythropoietin and 1,25 dihydroxy vitamin D

Table 7.2: Renal syndromes.

Syndrome	Clinical and laboratory findings
Nephrotic syndrome	Edema, proteinuria > 3 g/day, hypoalbuminemia, hyperlipidemia
Acute nephritis	Edema, hypertension, hematuria, oliguria, azotemia
Rapidly progressive renal failure	Edema, azotemia, progressive loss of renal function over days to weeks, with normal kidney sizes on imaging
Acute kidney injury	Oliguria, anuria, azotemia, documented decline in renal function within 2–7 days
Chronic kidney disease	Azotemia of >3 months, edema, hypertension, anemia, bone pains, small kidneys on imaging
Asymptomatic urinary abnormalities	Proteinuria, microscopic hematuria in the absence of any symptoms
Nephrolithiasis	Renal colic, hematuria, history of previous stone passage in urine, stone seen on earlier X-ray or ultrasound
Urinary tract obstruction	Oliguria, anuria when both kidneys are obstructed, flank tenderness, full urinary bladder on abdominal palpation, azotemia

Table 7.3: Commonly used terminologies.

Term	Description
Oliguria	Decreased urine output; adults < 400 mL/day; children < 0.5 mL/kg/hr
Anuria and absolute anuria	Profound decrease in urine output; adults < 100 mL/day; absolute anuria: 0 mL/day
Polyuria	Increased urine output; adults > 3 liters/day; children > 4 mL/kg/hr
Hematuria	Presence of 5 or more red blood cells in urine; gross (visible to naked eye) and microscopic
Proteinuria	Urinary protein excretion > 150 mg/day
Microalbuminuria	Urinary protein, mainly albumin excretion in the range of 30–300 mg/day; a feature of early diabetic kidney disease
Nocturia	Increased frequency of urination at night
Pollakiuria	Increased daytime frequency of urination
Azotemia	Increased values of nitrogenous wastes in the body, viz., serum urea and creatinine values
Uremia	Symptoms associated with azotemia—nausea, anorexia, metallic taste, generalized weakness, itchiness, restlessness, hiccups
Renal colic	Sudden onset of severe pain beginning in the flank region, radiating to the ribs or the groin region, can occur in one or both sides

these help in localizing the nature, duration and diagnostic approach to the underlying renal disease **(Table 7.2)**. **Table 7.3** is a glossary of terms used in **Table 7.2**, and includes terminology used to describe alterations in volume, composition and diurnal variability in urine.

INVESTIGATIONS IN RENAL DISEASE

Upon suspecting the presence of renal disease in a patient, it is common to order investigations to assess kidney structure and function, by blood and urine tests, and kidney imaging by ultrasound and other modalities, before proceeding for a renal biopsy in selected cases. **Table 7.4** summarizes investigations routinely performed in nephrology practice.

- *Estimation of glomerular function rate (GFR):* As the main function of the kidneys is filtration, the most widely accepted test of kidney function is the GFR which assesses the average filtration capacity of the nephrons of both kidneys. The normal GFR is approximately 130 mL/min/1.73 m² for men and 120 mL/min/1.73 m² for women, with variations based on age, body size, diet, pregnancy and other factors. The various methods for assessing GFR in clinical practice are summarized in **Table 7.4**.
- *Urine examination:* It is one of the key tests used to evaluate kidney disease. It includes examination of physical characteristics such as color, turbidity, odor and specific gravity, chemical characteristics such as presence of blood, glucose and protein, and microscopic analysis of the urine sediment to look for cells and crystals. Abnormalities in the physicochemical and microscopic analysis of urine during "routine screening" done at schools, army and job recruitments, can sometimes uncover underlying kidney disease. Some important abnormalities in urinalysis are summarized in **Table 7.4**.
- *Imaging:* Imaging evaluation of the kidneys often provides important information with regard to nature and duration of renal disease. Commonly utilized imaging modalities and their special uses in nephrology are summarized in **Table 7.4**.
- *Serum biochemistry:* The estimation of blood urea, serum creatinine, blood sugar and electrolytes, mainly sodium and potassium are important.
- *Renal biopsy:* Light microscopy, electron microscopy, and immunofluorescence of the biopsy specimen are helpful in the diagnosis, prognosis and treatment of various disorders **(Table 7.4)**.
- *Others:* Other investigations may be required in specific situations to know the etiology of renal diseases such as antinuclear antibody (ANA) in SLE, serum protein electrophoresis in myeloma and serum IgA level in IgA nephropathy.

NEPHROTIC SYNDROME

The nephrotic syndrome is defined by the presence of proteinuria of more than 3–3.5 g/day, hypoalbuminemia,

Table 7.4: Key investigative modalities.

Assessment of GFR

Measured GFR—by clearance of inulin, radio-isotope based methods—iothalamate, iohexol, ethylenediaminetetraacetic acid	Gold standard is inulin clearance (difficult in clinical practice) Measured GFR by radio-isotope methods is used in special situations (kidney donation, amputees, etc.)
Estimated GFR—based on serum creatinine (Cockcroft-Gault, MDRD, CKD-EPI equations); serum cystatin C (CKD-EPI equation)	Most commonly used in clinical practice are MDRD and CKD-EPI equations of estimated GFR Cockcroft-Gault equation is used for drug dosing

Urinalysis and urine microscopy

Changes in color	White urine in chyluria; red/brown urine in porphyria, beet intake and hematuria; yellow urine in jaundice; purple urine in infection with *E.coli*, *Pseudomonas*
Changes in odor	Sweet/fruity odor in ketosis; mousy odor in phenylketonuria; ammoniac odor in urease-producing bacterial infection
Changes in specific gravity	Fixed specific gravity of 1.010 with chronic kidney disease; high specific gravity with iodinated contrast media exposure
Presence of protein in urine by dipstick	Semiquantitative technique and has high specificity for urine albumin; raised in nephrotic states, acute and chronic glomerulonephritis, diabetic nephropathy
Presence of blood in urine by dipstick	Indicates hematuria; also raised in hemolysis, muscle injury or excess vitamin C intake
Presence of glucose in urine by dipstick	Seen in uncontrolled diabetics with high blood glucose levels; renal glucosuria is a condition with urine glucose excretion with normal blood glucose levels
Nitrite detection in urine	Detects presence of bacteria with nitrate reductase activity such as *E. coli* and *Klebsiella* (common causes of UTI)
Leukocyte esterase in urine	Detects presence of leukocytes in urine, indicating UTI; falsely negative when taking antibiotics such as imipenem, cephalexin, tobramycin and amoxicillin-clavulanate
Presence of erythrocytes in microscopy	Irregularly shaped (dysmorphic) RBCs in urine indicate hematuria due to glomerulonephritis; regularly shaped (isomorphic) RBCs indicate bleeding from urinary system such as due to renal, ureteric stones, malignancies
Presence of leukocytes in microscopy	Indicate UTI; can also be seen in acute interstitial nephritis, glomerulonephritis, acute rejection in transplant patients
Hyaline casts in urine	Can occur normally in concentrated or acidic urine, can occur in acute kidney injury
Granular casts in urine	Occur in acute tubular necrosis, commonly along with epithelial casts
WBC casts in urine	Found in acute interstitial nephritis and acute pyelonephritis (infections of the kidney)
Crystals in urine	Crystal examination is essential for evaluation of renal stone disease; rhomboid uric acid crystals are found in acidic urine; calcium oxalate crystals are bipyramidal; triple phosphate crystals are coffin-lid like

Imaging in renal disease

Ultrasound	Most common method of assessing kidney size, position; also, a screening investigation for urinary tract obstruction, renal stones, cysts, malignancies; color Doppler imaging is used for assessing renal arteries and veins
Intravenous urography	Useful in evaluation of urinary tract obstruction, stone disease, in patients with normal renal function; involves administration of intravenous contrast
Computed tomography	Is used commonly for evaluation of suspect renal masses, ectopic (malpositioned) kidneys, renal stones, and upper UTIs; can be performed with or without intravenous contrast
Magnetic resonance imaging	Useful in evaluation of urinary tract obstruction or malignancies, especially in those with contraindications to contrast or where radiation exposure is to be avoided
Nuclear scintigraphy	Provides accurate assessment of renal function and for evaluating renal blood flow; less useful in patients with moderate or severe renal dysfunction

Renal biopsy

Indications for renal biopsy	• Nephrotic syndrome in adults and in selected cases in children • Nonrecovering acute kidney injury • Cases of systemic lupus erythematosus (SLE), small-vessel vasculitis, Goodpasture disease, diabetes mellitus with atypical features • Persistent proteinuria in nondiabetic more than 1 g/day • Isolated persistent microhematuria (RBCs in urine microscopy) • Unexplained cause for chronic kidney disease (when kidney sizes are normal)

Contd...

Contd...

	• Familial kidney disease (to evaluate for cause) • Renal dysfunction in postrenal transplant patients
Techniques for renal biopsy	• Most commonly used is the percutaneous biopsy technique done by nephrologists and/or radiologists—performed usually under ultrasound guidance • Other techniques include laparoscopic, open and transjugular renal biopsies (used very rarely)

(GFR: glomerular function rate; UTI: urinary tract infection; RBCS: red blood cells; WBC: white blood cell; MDRD: Modification of Diet in Renal Disease; CKD-EPI: Chronic Kidney Disease Epidemiology Collaboration)

Table 7.5: Primary and secondary nephrotic syndromes.

Idiopathic or primary nephrotic syndrome (% in incidence in adults):
- Minimal change disease (10–15%)
- Focal segmental glomerulosclerosis (20–25%)
- Membranous nephropathy (25–30%)
- Membranoproliferative glomerulonephritis (5–10%)

Secondary nephrotic syndrome:
- *Metabolic:* Diabetes mellitus (common), obesity
- *Autoimmune:* Systemic lupus erythematosus (common), rheumatoid arthritis
- *Infection:* HIV, Hepatitis B, malaria
- *Drugs:* Gold, mercury, penicillamine, NSAIDs
- *Malignancy:* Lymphoma, leukemia, solid tumors
- *Hereditary:* Alport syndrome, Fabry disease
- *Miscellaneous:* Pregnancy (in relation with pre-eclampsia, common), reflux nephropathy

(HIV: human immunodeficiency virus; NSAIDs: nonsteroidal anti-inflammatory drugs)

edema and hyperlipidemia. If the nephrotic syndrome is part of another systemic illness such as diabetes mellitus, systemic lupus erythematosus (SLE), amyloidosis and malignancies, it is called secondary, whereas, if no underlying systemic illness is found, it is known as primary or idiopathic nephrotic syndrome. Various primary and secondary etiologies for nephrotic syndrome are presented in **Table 7.5**.

Pathophysiology

- The primary defect in the nephrotic state lies in the excessive urinary protein losses. The protein loss in minimal change disease is quite selective and mostly albumin loss, however, in certain other primary and secondary nephrotic states [especially in those with inflammation of glomeruli, viz., glomerulonephritides such as membranoproliferative glomerulonephritis (MPGN), SLE], the protein loss may not be selective. The urinary protein loss is attributable to the breakage of the glomerular filtration barrier.
- Hypoalbuminemia is secondary to reduced hepatic albumin synthesis, ongoing urinary protein losses and albumin redistribution.
- Edema in nephrotic syndrome is explained by two differing hypotheses, the primary over-fill versus the primary under-fill theory. The over-fill theory states that the urinary protein losses trigger the kidneys to retain excessive salt and water from the distal nephron segments, thereby causing over-fill of the intravascular compartment—higher hydrostatic pressures leading to the edematous state. The under-fill theory states that the excessive urinary protein losses lead to hypoalbuminemia, which lowers the plasma oncotic pressures, which then leads to interstitial edema. Current thinking suggests that both these mechanisms may be contributing to edema formation.
- Hyperlipidemia in nephrotic state is secondary to increased hepatic lipid synthesis and reduced lipid breakdown and manifests primarily as increase in low-density lipoprotein (LDL) cholesterol and sometimes, increase in serum triglycerides levels as well.
- Other notable consequences of the nephrotic syndrome include hypercoagulable state; increased occurrence of deep and renal vein thrombosis and pulmonary thromboembolism.
- *Hypothyroidism:* Due to loss of thyroid-binding protein.
- Iron unresponsive microcytic hypochromic anemia due to (loss of iron-binding protein transferring.
- Increased secondary infections due to altered serum immunoglobulin levels.

Clinical Features

Patients with nephrotic syndrome typically present with periorbital edema, more pronounced in the morning hours after waking **(Figs. 7.2 and 7.3)**. Gradually, edema involves the whole of the body, also known as anasarca. More pronounced fluid retention involves formation of ascites and

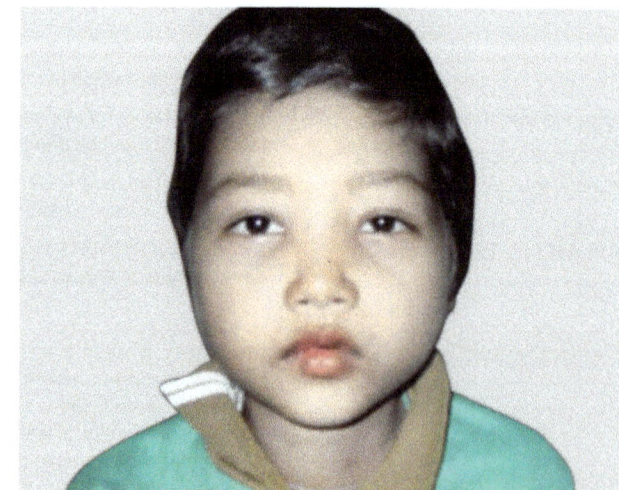

Fig. 7.2: A child with periorbital puffiness secondary to nephrotic syndrome.

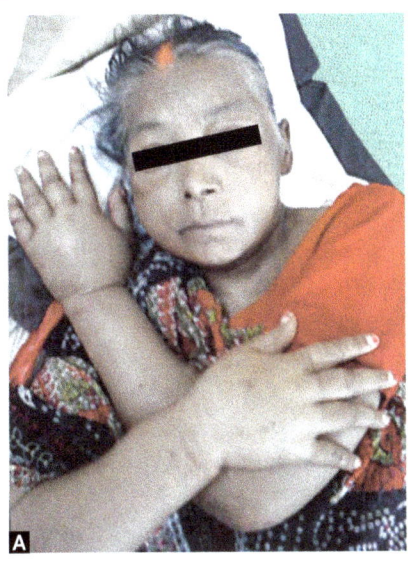 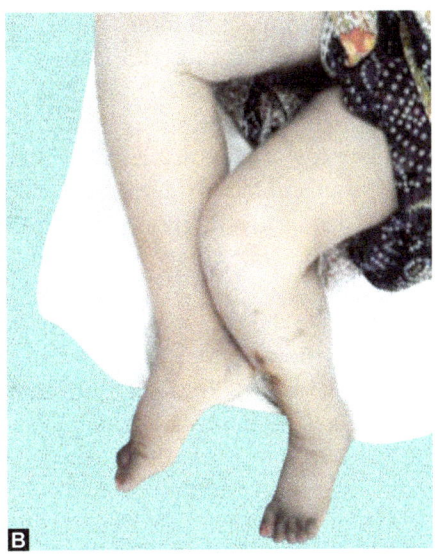

Figs. 7.3A and B: Anasarca secondary to nephrotic syndrome in adult.

pleural effusions (fluid accumulation in the peritoneal and pleural cavities, respectively). Pronounced weight gain, often as much as 10% of the body weight may occur with the onset of nephrotic syndrome. Rarely, the first clue to an underlying state may be the occurrence of an apparently unprovoked thromboembolic event. Hypertension is common, especially with secondary causes, and those with some associated renal dysfunction. White nails are typically found in severe cases, with profound hypoalbuminemia. Presence of erythema and tenderness in the lower limbs should alert the examiner to the possibility of local cellulitis or deep vein thrombosis in the nephrotic patient.

Investigations

- Laboratory investigations typically reveal low serum albumin levels (<3.5 g/dL, but often much lower), 24-hour urinary protein excretion exceeding 3 g/day and serum cholesterol exceeding 200 mg/dL.
- Serum urea and creatinine measurements are commonly in the normal range, unless the patient has associated glomerulonephritis or acute kidney injury (AKI).
- Common screening tests that are routinely performed during the evaluation of nephrotic states, include fasting blood sugar and HbA1c to look for underlying diabetes mellitus, viral markers (for HIV, hepatitis B and C).
- Antinuclear antibodies to screen for SLE. Complement levels (C3, C4) are usually low in patients with MPGN, SLE and infection associated glomerulonephritides.
- Ultrasound examination usually reveals normal sized kidneys, with normal corticomedullary differentiation, unless complicated by AKI. Large kidney sizes with nephrotic syndrome are typically seen in HIV associated nephropathy and renal amyloidosis.
- Kidney biopsy is performed in most cases of nephrotic syndrome in adults, except in clinically unambiguous diabetic nephropathy and pre-eclampsia.

Treatment of Nephrotic Syndrome

- *Nonpharmacologic measures:* Patients with nephrotic syndrome are advised to follow sodium restriction (<2 g/day), protein intake of 0.8 g/kg/day (with additional protein to cover ongoing protein losses) and strict smoking cessation.
- *Blood pressure control and renin-angiotensin system (RAS) inhibition:* The goal blood pressure in patients with nephrotic states is approximately 130/80 mm Hg or less, and is preferably lowered using RAS inhibitors (captopril, perindopril, losartan, telmisartan). Beyond BP control, RAS inhibitors have far-reaching benefits in proteinuria-lowering and consequently slowing progression of renal disease in several causes of nephrotic syndrome.
- *Lipid lowering drugs, aspirin and anticoagulation:* Lipid lowering therapies such as statins are prescribed in resistant nephrotic states to ameliorate hyperlipidemia, and addition of aspirin to statins confers protection in adult nephrotics judged to be at higher risk of cardiovascular events. Need for chronic anticoagulation (warfarin, acecoumarin) is warranted primarily in membranous nephropathy (MN) (with serum albumin < 2.5 g/dL), other resistant nephrotic states (with serum albumin < 2 g/dL) and in patients who have already suffered an episode of thromboembolism (as secondary thromboprophylaxis).
- *Diuretic therapy:* Loop diuretics such as furosemide and torsemide are commonly prescribed for amelioration of edema, often in combinations with distal-acting diuretics such as amiloride, spironolactone and metolazone.

Disease-specific Therapies

- Steroids, primarily prednisolone have demonstrated efficacy in several primary and secondary nephrotic states, either solely or in combination with other immunosuppressive medications. Steroids cause remission in

85–90% of childhood cases of nephrotic syndrome. Steroids are central to management of adult minimal change disease, focal segmental glomerulosclerosis (FSGS), MN, MPGN, IgAN, SLE-associated nephrotic states as well. High dose and long duration steroid use is associated with development of typical Cushingoid facies (moon face, fat deposition in the neck), striae in the abdomen, muscle weakness, peptic ulcers, osteoporosis and a heightened risk of infections.

- Cyclophosphamide is an alkylating agent, that is administered in either oral or intravenous form, in the treatment of frequent relapsing, steroid dependent nephrotic children, as well as in the management of MN and lupus nephritis. Cyclophosphamide use is associated with anemia, leukopenia, thrombocytopenia, oral mucositis, heightened infection risk, alopecia, hemorrhagic cystitis and lowered sperm and oocyte counts.
- Cyclosporine and tacrolimus (otherwise known as calcineurin inhibitors or CNIs) are immunosuppressive drugs with selective efficacy on T-lymphocytes as well as podocyte-modulating action. These drugs have demonstrated efficacy in the management of steroid-resistant and steroid-dependent nephrotic syndrome in children, as well as in the management in isolation/conjunction with steroids in FSGS and MN. Side effects of CNIs include hypertension, renal dysfunction, gingival hyperplasia (with cyclosporine), tremors (with tacrolimus), heightened infection risk and electrolyte abnormalities.
- Mycophenolate mofetil is an antiproliferative drug, that acts by selective inhibition of nucleic acid synthesis by de novo pathway, specifically used by lymphocytes. This drug finds use in the management of lupus nephritis, and C3 GN, a subtype of MPGN. Side effects of this drug include cytopenias and a heightened risk of infections. It is also a pregnancy class E drug (should not be used in pregnant women), and utmost care in females of reproductive age group to avoid pregnancies.
- Rituximab, a monoclonal antibody against CD 20, has profound anti B-cell proliferative effect. Rituximab has been successfully used in cases of steroid and CNI-resistant nephrotic syndrome in children and in the management of MN. Rituximab is administered via intravenous route, weekly or fortnightly, with effects lasting up to 6 months. Apart from infusion reactions, heightened infection risk including tuberculosis, risk of anaphylaxis, other rare side effects include polymorphic leukoencephalopathy, a debilitating neurologic disorder.

ACUTE AND RAPIDLY PROGRESSIVE GLOMERULONEPHRITIDES

Acute nephritic syndrome is characterized by a triad of edema, hematuria and hypertension. Other features of this syndrome include features of azotemia (nausea, vomitings,

Table 7.6: Differences between nephrotic and nephritic syndrome.

Nephrotic syndrome	Nephritic syndrome
Insidious onset	Relatively sudden onset
Greater degree of edema	Lesser degree of edema
Hypertension less common	Hypertension more common
Urine Protein +++/ ++++ Urine RBCs +/−	Urine Protein ++ Urine RBCs always +++
Renal dysfunction uncommon	Renal dysfunction common
Hypoalbuminemia always present	Serum albumin levels may be normal or slightly low

Table 7.7: Etiology of acute nephritic syndrome and rapidly progressive glomerulonephritis.

Acute nephritis	Rapidly progressive glomerulonephritis
• Poststreptococcal glomerulonephritis • Other infection-related glomerulonephritis • IgA nephropathy • Lupus nephritis	• *Type I:* Linear staining on immunofluorescence: Anti-GBM nephritis, Goodpasture disease (alongwith lung hemorrhage) • *Type II:* Granular staining on immunofluorescence (immune complex): Lupus nephritis, IgA nephropathy, poststreptococcal glomerulonephritis • *Type III:* Mild or absent staining on immunofluorescence (pauci-immune): Granulomatosis with polyangiitis (Wegener's granulomatosis), microscopic polyangiitis, renal limited ANCA vasculitis

(ANCA: anti-neutrophil-cytoplasmic-antibody; GBM: glomerular basement membrane)

generalized weakness) occurring over a short period of time, usually within a week. When features of azotemia occur in a progressive manner over days to weeks, the condition is denoted as rapidly progressive glomerulonephritis (RPGN). Occurrence of RPGN correlates with the presence of numerous crescents on kidney biopsy, a term denoted as crescentic glomerulonephritis. **Table 7.6** denotes the differences in the clinical and laboratory features of the nephrotic and the acute nephritic syndromes.

The various glomerular diseases which present as acute nephritic syndrome and RPGN are presented in **Table 7.7**.

Pathophysiology

In acute nephritic syndrome, glomerular lesions usually result from either in situ formation or deposition of circulating immune complexes. The prototype of acute nephritis is poststreptococcal glomerulonephritis (PSGN). Certain streptococcal strains are nephritogenic—their proteins tend to generate antibody formation, alternate complement pathway activation and subsequent deposition of these complement bound antigen-antibody complexes to the subepithelial portion of the glomerular basement membrane. This deposition incites glomerular inflammation—proliferation of leukocytes, mesangial and endothelial cells within glomerular capillaries (endocapillary proliferation), and in some cases, there is proliferation of parietal epithelial cells and inflammatory cells in the Bowman's space outside of the capillary (extracapillary proliferation), which leads to the formation of crescents—a pathognomonic feature in biopsies of patients with RPGN. In other cases, anti-glomerular basement membrane antibodies (anti-GBM disease), interaction with anti-neutrophil cytoplasmic antibodies [renal and systemic anti-neutrophil-cytoplasmic-antibody (ANCA) vasculitis] or a type III hypersensitivity reaction might underlie the development of glomerular inflammation and subsequent crescent formation. Early crescents are usually cellular and partial or circumferential, and over days to weeks, fibroblast influx occurs into the extracapillary space leading to fibro cellular and fibrous crescents, and finally when the glomerular inflammation progresses unabated, the glomeruli undergo global sclerosis and irreversible damage.

Clinical Features

Poststreptococcal glomerulonephritis typically presents in children 2-4 weeks after an episode of pharyngitis (postpharyngitic hematuria) or skin infection, with abrupt onset of edema, hypertension and smoky or cola colored urine. IgA nephropathy, on the other hand, presents as episodic hematuria often within 24 hours of pharyngitis (synpharyngitic hematuria). Patients with Goodpasture disease present with cough, breathlessness and hemoptysis (signifying lung hemorrhage) along with gross or microscopic hematuria and features of azotemia. Renal and systemic ANCA vasculitis occurs predominantly in older adults, with nonspecific features such as fever, malaise, weight loss, upper respiratory (sinusitis, rhinitis) and lower respiratory (cough, hemoptysis and infiltrates on chest radiograph) involvement along with progressive renal dysfunction over days to weeks. Due to insidious onset and nonspecific features, a proportion of these patients are picked up in advanced uremia. SLE afflicts young women more commonly, and lupus nephritis is typically evident in the first few years of disease itself. In previously undiagnosed cases presenting as acute nephritis or RPGN, the presence of oral ulcers, hair loss, butterfly rash on cheeks (malar rash), joint pains raise the possibility of underlying lupus nephritis.

Investigations

Aside from the typical findings of acute nephritic syndrome in urine examination (outlined in **Table 7.6**), PSGN is characterized by hypocomplementemia (low C3, C4 levels) and elevated antistreptolysin O (ASO) titers in postpharyngitic cases. Routinely, renal biopsy is not performed for cases of PSGN unless the patient has atypical clinical or laboratory features such as nephrotic proteinuria, persistent renal failure and hypocomplementemia or older age at presentation. The pathologic correlate of PSGN is the presence of diffuse proliferative glomerulonephritis (DPGN).

In adults with a presentation of either acute or RPGN, it is usual to order for serologies such as ANA, ANCA and anti GBM antibodies, in addition to tests for HIV, hepatitis B and C viruses, complement levels and coagulation profile. In the absence of contraindications, a renal biopsy is performed in cases of RPGN as urgently as feasible. This facilitates early and effective treatment strategies, and minimizes irreversible renal damage.

Treatment of Glomerulonephritides

- Most cases of PSGN resolve spontaneously, however, antihypertensives for BP control during the acute phase, diuretics for management of fluid overload and pulmonary edema, and treatment of any ongoing streptococcal infection (with oral or intravenous penicillin) are mandated. In the rare cases of PSGN which are complicated by crescents (not spontaneously recovering), a course of steroids may be justified.
- The episodic hematuria in IgA nephropathy is usually self-resolving, and courses of steroid with or without cyclophosphamide are reserved for patients presenting with RPGN.
- In the case of Goodpasture disease (or anti-GBM disease), early and very aggressive treatment may be instituted with pulse intravenous methylprednisolone and cyclophosphamide, with or without plasma exchange for removal of the disease-causing antibodies and control of lung hemorrhage and renal failure.
- Renal and systemic ANCA vasculitis is also managed on somewhat similar lines as anti GBM disease, with the addition of rituximab in certain cases.
- In the case of hepatitis B, C associated glomerulonephritis, management primarily focusses on administering antivirals (such as lamivudine, entecavir for hepatitis B infection, and sofosbuvir, daclatasvir, ribavirin for hepatitis C infection).
- Lupus nephritis is managed with steroids in addition to mycophenolate mofetil, cyclophosphamide, tacrolimus or rituximab, as per specific clinical indications (which are beyond the purview of this text).

ACUTE KIDNEY INJURY

Definition

Acute kidney injury is a combination of pathophysiological processes marked by fall in GFR over a span of hours to days. It results in accumulation of metabolic waste products like urea and creatinine, impaired regulation of fluid, electrolytes and acid-base abnormalities.

Although the term "injury" implies parenchymal damage, the decline in renal functions may not be associated with parenchymal damage in early phase of obstructive causes or reduced intravascular volume.

Table 7.8: Causes of acute kidney injury.	
Prerenal acute kidney injury	
Hypovolemia	Blood loss; gastrointestinal losses—diarrhea, vomiting; fluid loss in third space like in nephrotic syndrome, cirrhosis, pancreatitis; renal loss due to overt diuresis
Hypotension	Shock, congestive heart failure, valvular defects
Impaired renal autoregulation	Drugs such as NSAIDs, ACE inhibitors
Intrinsic acute kidney injury	
Glomerular	Rapidly progressive glomerulonephritis
Tubular	• Ischemic injury due to hypotension, hypovolemia • Nephrotoxic agents such as antibiotics, radiocontrast dyes, chemotherapeutic drugs, drug abuse • Endogenous toxins such as hemoglobin, myoglobin leading to pigment nephropathy, hyperuricemia, paraproteinuria
Interstitium	• Allergic due to drugs • Infections • Autoimmune • Infiltration by malignant cells
Postrenal acute kidney injury	
Upper urinary tract	• Tumor invasion in the intra-abdominal or retroperitoneal space • Retroperitoneal fibrosis • Traumatic injury • Renal stones, clots • Strictures
Lower urinary tract	• Prostate hypertrophy • Calculi • Tumor • Posterior urethral valve, stricture • Functional disorder due to neurogenic bladder

(NSAIDs: nonsteroidal anti-inflammatory agents; ACE: angiotensin-converting enzyme)

Acute kidney injury as defined by the Kidney Disease Improving Global Outcomes (KDIGO) initiative, is an increase in serum creatinine by ≥0.3 mg/dL within 48 hours or to ≥1.5 times baseline, known or presumed to have occurred within the prior 7 days.

It can be oliguric or nonoliguric. Usually, oliguric kidney failure is associated with higher mortality.

The various causes of AKI have been enumerated in **Table 7.8**.

The classification scheme for the severity stages of AKI based on serum creatinine, urine output in a specified time duration has been illustrated in **Table 7.9**.

Pathophysiology

The pathophysiology of AKI is complex and still incompletely known. However, for simplicity and understanding, the following flow chart describes the evolution and progression of acute tubular necrosis (the pathologic correlate of AKI) as a result of ischemia (decreased renal blood flow), which is one of the commonest causes of AKI (**Fig. 7.4**). Broadly, AKI progresses through four stages: *Initiation, extension, maintenance and recovery*, which take place over 10–14 days.

Management

Evaluation in a patient of AKI involves a thorough history and physical examination, followed by urine and blood investigations, imaging and if needed a kidney biopsy.

History and Examination

- Possible dehydration via diarrhea, vomiting will point towards a prerenal cause. Low blood pressure, tachycardia, dry mucous membrane will further support a prerenal cause of AKI.
- A history of colicky flank pain radiating towards groin, passage of urinary stone, poor urinary flow will suggest an obstructive cause.
- Cola colored or sometimes reddish urine will point towards a glomerular cause.
- Concomitant purpuric rashes can raise the possibility of allergic interstitial nephritis.
- A detailed medication history can throw light on the likelihood of a drug related AKI.

Table 7.9: Severity staging of AKI.						
AKI staging criteria						
RIFLE	By rise in s. creatinine values	AKIN	By rise in s. creatinine values	KDIGO	By rise in s. creatinine values	Urine output common to all
Risk	≥50%	Stage 1	≥0.3 mg/dL or 50%	Stage 1	≥0.3 mg/dL or 50%	<0.5 mL/kg/hr for >6 hours
Injury	≥100%	Stage 2	≥100%	Stage 2	≥100%	<0.5 mL/kg/hr for >12 hours
Failure	≥200%	Stage 3	≥200%	Stage 3	≥200% or increase in serum creatinine to >4 mg/dL or initiation of renal replacement therapy	<0.5 mL/kg/hr for >24 hours or anuria for >12 hours
Loss	Complete loss of renal functions >4 weeks					
End-stage	Complete loss of renal functions >3 months					

(AKIN: Acute Kidney Injury Network; KDIGO: Kidney Disease Improving Global Outcomes)

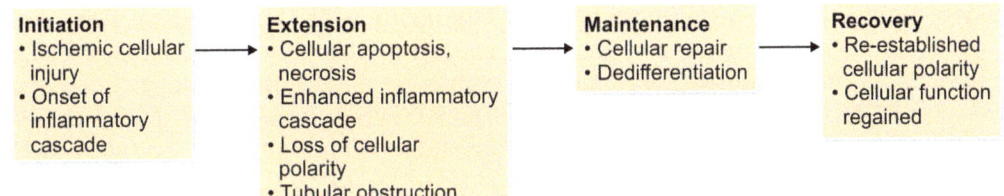

Fig. 7.4: Schema of pathophysiology of ischemic acute kidney injury.

- Ophthalmic evaluation can show signs of atheroembolism.

Investigations

- *Urine examination* is an invaluable tool to identify the cause and localization of the site of tissue injury. Protein excretion of ≤1 g/day is usually seen in ischemic acute tubular necrosis. Proteinuria of >1 g/day and dysmorphic RBCs in the urine will point towards a glomerular cause. Urinary sediments showing muddy brown casts relates to acute tubular necrosis while white blood cell casts are seen in interstitial nephritis, pyelonephritis and sometimes in glomerulonephritis. Crystals of uric acid and oxalate can also be seen in urine which are linked to acute urate nephropathy and ethylene glycol toxicity respectively.
- *Use of biomarkers in detection of AKI:* Structural damage to the kidney generally precedes the manifested decline in GFR by the traditional biomarker such as s. creatinine. Hence, early detection of the injury by biomarkers can provide a basis for an early intervention. New tubular injury markers include Kidney injury molecule-1, neutrophil gelatinase-associated lipocalin (NGAL), liver-type fatty acid-binding protein (L-FABP), tissue inhibitor of metalloproteinase-2 (TIMP-2), insulin-like growth factor-binding protein 7 (IGFBP-7) and IL-18. Of these a combination of TIMP-2 and IGFBP-7 has shown promise in early detection of AKI in sepsis patients. However, optimal use of these biomarkers in AKI is still a matter of debate.
- *Radiological examination:* Ultrasonographic evaluation is the commonly used screening test to check for the kidney size, echogenicity of cortex, medulla and veracity of the pelvicalyceal system. Computed tomography may be required in certain cases of obstructive renal injury.
- *Kidney biopsy:* It is reserved for suspected cases of intrinsic AKI other than ischemic or toxic injury ones where a specific targeted therapy can alter the course of the disease. **Table 7.9** provides an overview of management of complications of AKI.

Obstructive causes need appropriate measures to relieve obstruction. Drug doses should be modified according to the GFR. Choice of dialysis modality in the form of intermittent hemodialysis (IHD), sustained low-efficiency dialysis (SLED), continuous renal replacement therapy (CRRT) or peritoneal dialysis needs to be individualized to the patient's need and supportive infrastructure.

Absolute indications of renal replacement therapy (RRT) are:
- Volume overload not responsive to diuretic therapy
- Hyperkalemia not responding to medical treatment
- Metabolic acidosis
- Uremic symptoms such as encephalopathy, seizures, pericarditis and bleeding
- Removal of dialyzable toxins (e.g., lithium)

Table 7.9: Treatment of acute kidney injury and its complications.

Complications	Management
Hypervolemia	Salt restriction to <5 g a day, water restriction, loop diuretics, ultrafiltration through dialysis
Hyponatremia	Restriction of free water intake and hypotonic solutions
Hyperkalemia	Stop causal drugs such as potassium sparing diuretics, restrict potassium rich diet; calcium gluconate (if ECG changes present), inhalation beta agonists, insulin with dextrose, potassium binding resin, loop diuretics if nonoliguric and renal replacement therapy
Hyperphosphatemia	Dietary restriction and binding agents such as calcium acetate, sevelamer carbonate and lanthanum carbonate
Hypocalcemia	Oral or intravenous replacement if symptomatic
Hypermagnesemia	Antacids containing magnesium to be discontinued
Metabolic acidosis	Sodium bicarbonate if pH < 7.15, renal replacement therapy (RRT)
Hyperuricemia	Severe cases associated with cell lysis treated with intravenous fluids (if nonoliguric), rasburicase and allopurinol
Nutrition	<ul><li>Nonhypercatabolic and not requiring RRT should have dietary protein intake of 0.8–1.0 g/kg body wt./per day</li><li>Hypercatabolic and RRT requiring should have dietary protein intake of 1.0–1.5 g/kg body wt./per day</li><li>Caloric intake should be 20–30 kcal/kg body weight</li><li>Enteral feeding is preferred whenever possible</li></ul>
Anemia and bleeding	Blood transfusion may be required when hemoglobin is <7 g/dL. Bleeding usually responds to desmopressin and RRT

Outcome: Kidneys have the ability to recover even after cases of severe injury requiring dialysis. Occurrence of in-hospital AKI lengthens the hospital stay and increases the mortality as well. Around 5–10% cases of AKI may not recover completely and require long term management to slow the progression of renal dysfunction.

CHRONIC KIDNEY DISEASE

Chronic kidney disease (CKD) is defined as abnormalities of kidney structure or function or GFR <60 mL/min/1.73 m² for 3 months or more. The abnormalities include albuminuria (≥30 mg/g), presence of urinary sediments, abnormalities due to tubular dysfunction, histological abnormalities, structural defects in imaging or a kidney transplant. CKD affects around 5–10% of world population.

Glomerular filtration rate can be estimated from serum creatinine by using certain equations, such as the Modification of Diet in Renal Disease (MDRD) Study equation, Cockcroft-Gault formula or the CKD-EPI (Chronic Kidney Disease Epidemiology Collaboration) equation. The CKD severity is classified as per the level of GFR and albuminuria (**Table 7.10**).

Causes: The various causes of CKD have been enumerated in **Table 7.11**.

Other risk factors for CKD include small for gestation birth weight, obesity, advanced age, African race (*APOL1* gene), family history of kidney disease, an earlier history of AKI and anomalies of kidney and urinary tract.

Pathophysiology

Figure 7.5 presents a simplified flow diagram describing the progressive nature of CKD.

Table 7.10: Stages of chronic kidney disease.

GFR stages	GFR (mL/min/ 1.73 m²)	Terms
G1	≥90	Normal or high
G2	60–89	Mildly decreased
G3a	45–59	Mildly to moderately decreased
G3b	30–44	Moderately to severely decreased
G4	15–29	Severely decreased
G5	<15	Kidney failure
Albuminuria stages	**AER (mg/day)**	**Terms**
A1	<30	Normal to mildly increased
A2	30–300	Moderately increased
A3	>300	Severely increased

(AER: albumin excretion rate; GFR: glomerular filtration rate)

Table 7.11: Etiology of chronic kidney disease.

Diabetes mellitus	
Hypertension	
Chronic glomerulonephritis	Primary: FSGS, IgA nephropathy, MPGN, membranous nephropathy
	Secondary (with systemic disease): SLE, amyloidosis, pauci-immune glomerulonephritis
Hereditary	Polycystic kidney diseases, medullary cystic disease
Chronic tubulointerstitial nephritis	Sarcoidosis; drug related, e.g., NSAIDs, Infections: CMV, leptospirosis; Idiopathic
Obstructive uropathy	Vesicoureteric reflux, renal/ureteric calculi, benign prostatic hyperplasia
Vascular	Fibromuscular dysplasia, atherosclerosis causing renal artery stenosis

(FSGS: focal segmental glomerulosclerosis; MPGN: membranoproliferative glomerulonephritis; SLE: systemic lupus erythematous; NSAIDs: nonsteroidal anti-Inflammatory drugs; CMV: cytomegalovirus)

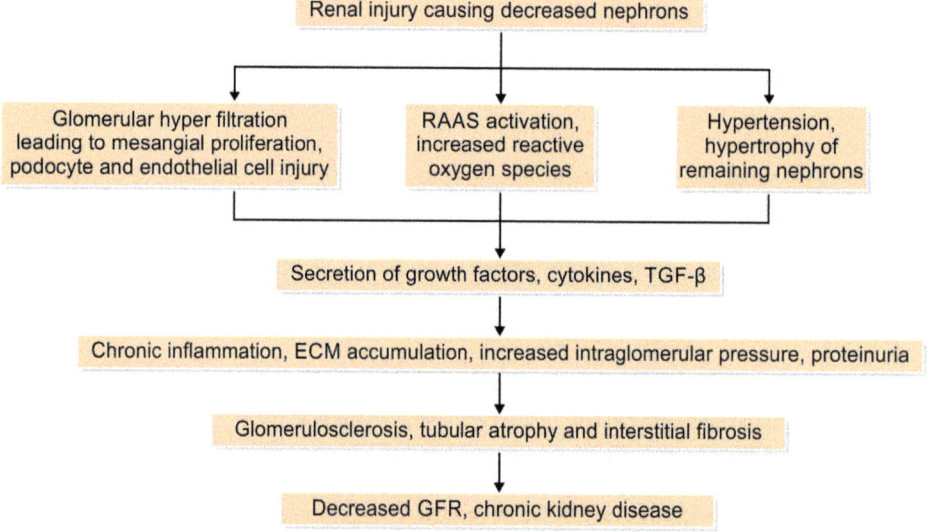

Fig. 7.5: Pathophysiology of chronic kidney disease.
(RAAS: renin-angiotensin-aldosterone system; TGF: transforming growth factor; ECM: extracellular matrix; GFR: glomerular filtration rate)

Investigations

Symptoms of renal failure are often late to occur and by the time patient becomes symptomatic, a substantial amount of renal function is already lost. Usually the symptomatology consists of anorexia, nausea, pedal edema, pruritus and breathlessness. Investigations include renal function tests, hemoglobin, viral markers (hepatitis B, C and HIV) and urine examination. Serum calcium, phosphorus, vitamin D level and intact parathyroid hormone (PTH) levels also need to evaluated. Imaging gives an idea about the kidney size or any structural abnormality. Other additional investigations are guided by the systemic findings or suspicion of any acute precipitating factor.

Clinical Features and Management

Metabolic Disorders

Commonly seen abnormalities are sodium retention and excess extracellular fluid retention due to impaired excretion. Hyperkalemia either due to its excess intake, concomitant intake of drugs such as RAS inhibitors or hyporeninemic hypoaldosteronism in diseases such as diabetes.

Metabolic acidosis is primarily due to impaired ammonia production in the tubules in the early stages of the kidney disease. In the later stages many organic anions accumulate which lead to high anion gap metabolic acidosis.

Dietary salt restriction and use of diuretics greatly helps in the management of hypervolemia. Dilutional hyponatremia responds well to fluid restriction. Restriction in the dietary intake of potassium rich food along with potassium excreting diuretics and potassium binding resins are the corner stones in the management of hyperkalemia. Alkali therapy is needed to prevent a fall in bicarbonate concentration below 22 mEq/L. Poor response to the above management is an indication for dialysis.

Mineral Bone Disorder

It is a systemic disorder of mineral and bone metabolism due to CKD manifested by (1) abnormalities of calcium, phosphorus, PTH or vitamin D metabolism, (2) abnormalities of bone turnover, mineralization, volume, growth or strength and (3) vascular or soft tissue calcification.

There is phosphate retention due to declining GFR; decreased serum calcium ion and 1,25-dihydroxyvitamin D (calcitriol) concentration and increased fibroblast growth factor 23 (FGF23) concentration (phosphatonin).

Secondary hyperparathyroidism due to phosphate retention leads to high bone turnover (Osteitis fibrosa cystica). Excess suppression of PTH by high intake of calcium or vitamin D can lead to low turnover bone disease. Patients may experience bone pain and increased incidence of fractures.

Vascular and soft tissue calcifications can lead to calcific uremic arteriopathy.

Management includes dietary phosphate restriction, use of phosphate binding agents. Elevated PTH levels can be taken care by calcitriol. Cinacalcet acts on calcium sensing receptors thereby lowering elevated PTH levels. Dialysis can help in removing excess phosphate.

Cardiovascular Complications

Chronic kidney disease, with its high burden of vascular disease risk factors is associated with a number of adverse cardiovascular events. The risk factors for ischemic vascular disease include hypertension, diabetes, dyslipidemia, vascular calcification and a chronic inflammatory state.

Cardiomyopathy, diastolic dysfunction, left ventricular hypertrophy all contribute to the high incidence of congestive heart failure in CKD patients.

Pericarditis characterized by chest pain with a distinct rub on auscultation is mostly seen in patients with advance degree of uremia. It usually responds well to heparin free dialysis. Sometimes a massive pericardial effusion with tamponade effect requiring pericardial drainage can also be seen.

Hypertension usually requires salt restriction and antihypertensive agents. ACE inhibitors or angiotensin-receptor blockers (ARBs) are the preferred drugs. A blood pressure of ≤130/80 mm Hg is targeted. Excess fluid removal by dialysis is an important aspect of managing hypertension in end stage renal disease patients. Use of Aspirin and statins is guided by the cardiac and lipid status of the CKD patients. Lifestyle changes are also advocated to such patients.

Neurologic Complications

Cognitive dysfunction, dementia, sleep disturbances, encephalopathy, seizures, peripheral and autonomic neuropathies are the features of neurological involvement in CKD patients.

An individualized approach is advised in the management of these complications. It involves the use of aspirin, antiepileptics, replacement of water soluble vitamins in dialysis patients and optimizing dialysis therapy.

Hematological Complications

Anemia of normocytic and normochromic nature is common and present from the early stages of CKD. Causes include iron, vitamin B_{12} and folate deficiency; chronic inflammation; decreased red blood cell survival duration; decreased production of erythropoietin and hyperparathyroidism. Use of erythropoiesis stimulating agents has greatly decreased the need of blood transfusion. Correction of the deficient factor is required for the optimum response. A hemoglobin of approximately 11 g/dL is targeted.

Chronic kidney disease patients exhibit abnormalities in their hemostatic response that increases the risk of bleeding. The defects include impaired platelet adhesion and aggregation, malfunction of platelet glycoproteins such as GPIIb/IIIa resulting in prolonged bleeding time. Use of desmopressin or estrogen can help manage this. In advanced stages of renal failure dialysis can also be helpful.

Miscellaneous

Chronic kidney disease affects the functionality of multiple organ systems. Dysgeusia, gastritis, peptic ulcer disease and constipation are often seen in these patients. Glucose metabolism is impaired and insulin levels are moderately raised. Infertility, spontaneous abortions, menstrual irregularities affect women with CKD. Pruritus, darkening of skin tone owing to deposition of urochromes mark the dermatological manifestations. Along with medical therapy, dialysis is known to improve these abnormalities.

Smoking cessation, weight loss in obese patients and dietary modifications go a long way in slowing the rate of loss of renal functions. Dietary approach for the CKD patients has been described in **Table 7.12**.

RENAL REPLACEMENT THERAPY

It is required in symptomatic CKD patients usually when GFR goes below 10 mL/min/1.73 m² along with the indications listed above. Three forms of RRT are available:
1. Hemodialysis **(Fig. 7.6)**
2. Peritoneal dialysis
3. Renal transplantation.

Table 7.12: Dietary recommendations for chronic kidney disease.

Asymptomatic early stages of CKD	Protein: 0.8 g/kg/day; calories: 30–35 kcal/kg/day. In case of proteinuria can add 1 g protein for each gram of protein lost
Symptomatic, advance stage CKD (not requiring dialysis)	Protein: 0.6 g/kg/day; calories: 30–35 kcal/kg/day
Dialysis patients	Protein: 1.2–1.4 g/kg/day; calories: 30–35 kcal/kg/day

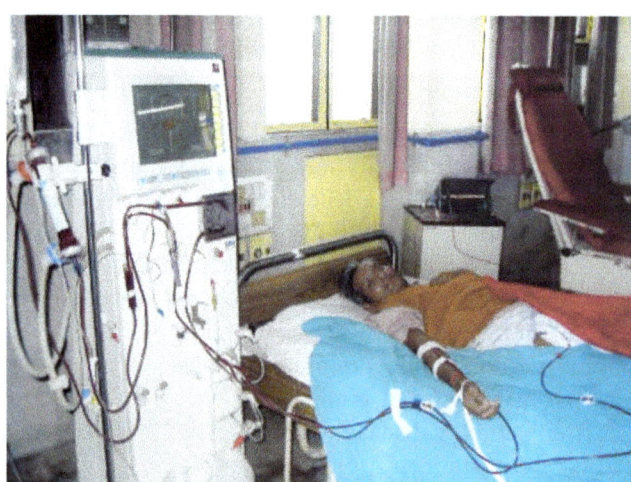

Fig. 7.6: A patient with end stage renal disease undergoing hemodialysis.

Depending upon his lifestyle, social and financial support, patient chooses a particular modality. By far renal transplantation is the best form of replacement therapy which offers the opportunity to reverse most of the uremia related organ dysfunction.

IMPLICATIONS ON DENTAL PRACTICE

- Xerostomia, uremic fetor and metallic taste sensation are common oral manifestations of advanced renal disease, especially those starting on dialysis.
- Renal osteodystrophy, a manifestation of mineral bone disorder in CKD, often causes tooth mobility, malocclusion, jaw fractures, and abnormal bone healing after tooth extraction.
- Lower rates of caries have been observed in patients with CKD as urea has antibacterial and antiplaque activity.
- Elective dental procedures must be planned preferably on nondialysis days, as the risk of bleeding may be higher immediately after hemodialysis sessions secondary to heparin use.
- Elective dental procedures are avoided during AKI, unless the dental problem is causative to systemic sepsis.
- Pain management in patients with underlying kidney disease, should avoid NSAIDs such as diclofenac, aceclofenac, ibuprofen and naproxen, and other drugs of this group. Paracetamol and tramadol are preferred analgesics in this patient population.
- Aminoglycoside antibiotics such as amikacin, streptomycin and kanamycin should be avoided in patients with CKD and AKI.
- Patients who are renal transplant recipients are immunocompromised due to the use of immunosuppressive medications, and therefore, prone to severe and disseminated infections.
- Some renal transplant recipients receive cyclosporine which causes gingival hyperplasia.

SELF ASSESSMENT

1. **Most common type of acute renal failure is:**
   A. Renovascular B. Prerenal
   C. Postrenal D. Drug induced
2. **The nephrotic syndrome in adult is mostly due to:**
   A. Minimal change disease
   B. Membranous glomerulonephritis
   C. Goodpasture's disease
   D. Wegner's granulomatosis
3. **Dysmorphic red blood cells in urine are found in:**
   A. Bladder cancer B. Renal stone
   C. Glomerulonephritis D. Prostatism
4. **Prerenal ARF can occur in:**
   A. Massive blood loss
   B. Severe diarrhea
   C. Heart failure
   D. All of the above

5. Which of the following is usually not a feature of minimal change disease?
   A. Massive proteinuria B. Hypoproteinemia
   C. Oliguria D. Hyperlipidemia
6. The most important abnormality in ARF is:
   A. Ketosis B. Metabolic acidosis
   C. Metabolic alkalosis D. All of the above
7. The most important electrolyte disturbance in renal failure is:
   A. Hyponatremia B. Hypernatremia
   C. Hypokalemia D. Hyperkalemia
8. Amount of protein normally excreted in urine per day is:
   A. 1 g B. 500 mg
   C. 150 mg D. No protein is present
9. Microalbuminuria is defined as excretion of following amount of albumin daily:
   A. Less than 30 mg B. 30–300 mg
   C. 300–650 mg D. More than 650 mg
10. Following is the most common systemic cause of nephrotic syndrome:
    A. SLE B. Diabetes mellitus
    C. Leukemia D. Gold therapy
11. The most common cause of death in ARF is:
    A. Infections B. Pulmonary edema
    C. Hypertension D. Hypocalcemia
12. Following feature is specific for chronic renal failure:
    A. Hyperkalemia B. Acidosis
    C. Oliguria D. Small contracted kidneys
13. Following are the features of CRF:
    A. Hypercalcemia and hyperphosphatemia
    B. Hypocalcemia and hypophosphatemia
    C. Hypocalcemia and hyperphosphatemia
    D. Hypercalcemia and hypophosphatemia
14. The key component of nephrotic syndrome is:
    A. Anasarca B. Hypoalbuminemia
    C. Massive proteinuria D. Hyperlipidemia
15. The following is not seen in nephritic syndrome:
    A. Hematuria B. Oliguria
    C. Proteinuria D. None of the above
16. Insulin is used in the treatment of:
    A. Hyperkalemia B. Hypercalcemia
    C. Hypernatremia D. Hypermagnesemia
17. Following are present in case of nephrotic syndrome:
    A. Massive proteinuria B. Hyperlipidemia
    C. Renal vein thrombosis D. All of the above
18. Most common cause of nephrotic syndrome in children is:
    A. Minimal change disease
    B. Membranous glomerulopathy
    C. Diabetes mellitus
    D. Amyloidosis
19. Which of the following is the functional unit of the kidney?
    A. Glomerulus B. Nephron
    C. Renal pelvis D. Renal tubule
20. What degree of proteinuria constitutes nephrotic syndrome?
    A. > 150 mg/day B. > 1 g/day
    C. > 3 g/day D. > 300 mg/day
21. What constitutes the triad of nephritic syndrome?
    A. Proteinuria, hematuria, hypertension
    B. Hematuria, hypertension, nocturia
    C. Azotemia, proteinuria, hypertension
    D. Edema, hypertension, hematuria
22. Which group of drugs is commonly used to reduce urinary protein in patients with nephrotic syndrome?
    A. RAS inhibitors – ramipril, losartan
    B. Diuretics – furosemide, spironolactone
    C. Immunosuppressive – cyclophosphamide
    D. Calcium and vitamin D
23. Which of the following medication does not usually cause AKI?
    A. Amikacin B. Diclofenac
    C. Radiocontrast dyes D. Paracetamol
24. What is the usual time taken for AKI to resolve?
    A. 48 hours B. 7 days
    C. 10–14 days D. 28 days
25. What is the commonest cause of CKD worldwide?
    A. Renal stone disease
    B. Diabetes mellitus
    C. Primary hypertension
    D. FSGS
26. Which of the following represent common electrolyte abnormalities in CKD?
    A. Hypercalcemia and hyponatremia
    B. Hypocalcemia and hyperkalemia
    C. Hypokalemia and hyponatremia
    D. Hyperphosphatemia and hypercalcemia
27. Which of the following is a correct dietary advice given to patients with CKD who are not on dialysis?
    A. High energy and fat intake
    B. Low energy and low fiber intake
    C. Low protein and high fiber intake
    D. High fat and fiber intake
28. Which of the following drugs causes gingival hyperplasia?
    A. Cyclophosphamide B. Cyclosporine
    C. Tacrolimus D. Rituximab

Fill in the Blanks

1. The amount of proteinuria in nephrotic syndrome is more than _____ per day.
2. The oliguria is defined as urine output less than _____ per day.
3. The retention of nitrogenous waste products due to renal insufficiency is called _____.
4. Normal level of blood urea is _____.
5. Normal serum creatinine level is_____.
6. Normal level of serum total protein and albumin is _____.
7. In end-stage renal disease, the GFR is _____/minute.

CHAPTER 8

Nervous System

EXAMINATION OF CRANIAL NERVES

A basic knowledge of cranial nerves is desirable for dental practitioners since patients may present with a number of symptoms pertaining to the oromaxillary area. There are 12 cranial nerves. These are named as follows:

   I   Olfactory
   II Optic
   III Oculomotor
   IV Trochlear
   V   Trigeminal
   VI Abducent
   VII Facial
   VIII Vestibulocochlear
   IX Glossopharyngeal
   X   Vagus
   XI Accessory
   XII Hypoglossal

Olfactory Nerve

Olfactory nerve, which carries the sensation of smell, arises in the olfactory mucous membrane from receptor nerve cells, situated in upper part of the nasal cavity. The nerve fibers pass through the cribriform plate of the ethmoid bone and enter the olfactory bulb in the cranial cavity. Olfactory tract connects the olfactory bulb to the olfactory area of the cerebral cortex.

The presentation of olfactory nerve damage may be lack of smell sense (anosmia) or altered sense of smell (parosmia). Hallucination of smell may occur as aura of temporal lobe seizure. Important causes of anosmia are given in **Table 8.1**.

Common substances such as clove oil, peppermint oil, soap or fruits are used to test the sense of smell. Each nostril is tested separately. However, local causes like sinusitis, etc,. should be ruled out before contributing the dysfunction due to the neurological cause.

Table 8.1: Important causes of anosmia

- Sinusitis and other local nasal disorders
- Head injury
- Subfrontal meningioma
- Bacterial meningitis
- Covid 19 infection

Optic Nerve

The optic nerve is the nerve of sight. It is composed of the axons of the cells in the ganglionic layer of the retina. The optic nerve emerges from the back of eyeball and passes through optic canal to enter in the cranial cavity where it unites with the opposite optic nerve to form the optic chiasma. From the optic chiasma fibers run in optic tract **(Fig. 8.1)**. The fibers from the medial half of retina cross the midline in optic chiasma and enter the optic tract of opposite side, while the

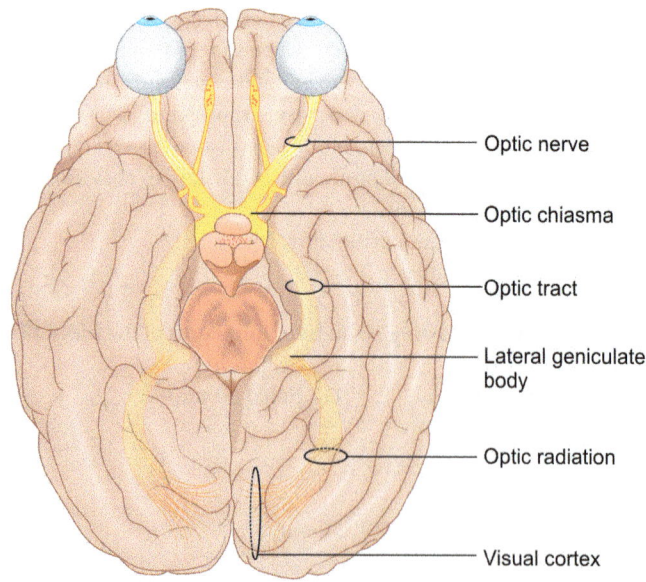

Fig. 8.1: Optic nerve course.

fibers from the lateral half of each retina pass in the optic tract of the same side. Most of the fibers in the optic tract end by synapsing with nerve cells in lateral geniculate body. The axons of nerve cells in lateral geniculate body pass as the optic radiation to the visual cortex of the cerebral hemisphere.

Few fibers from the optic tract pass to prerectal nucleus and superior colliculus and are concerned with light reflexes. Following are different components of optic nerve testing:
- Visual acuity
- Visual fields
- Color vision
- Pupillary examination.

Visual Acuity

Visual acuity is measured by Snellen's chart **(Fig. 8.2)**. Patient is placed at a distance of 6 meters and asked to read letters on the chart. This tests the distant vision. Normal eye can read down the letters up to seventh line from top (visual acuity 6/6). In case of very poor visual acuity (1/60) when patient is not able to read the top letters from a distance of 1 meter, other tests are performed. These are counting fingers (CF), hand movements (HM), perception of light (PL) or no perception of light (no PL).

Near vision is tested with the help of test types of varying sizes from the ordinary reading distance. The near vision is recorded as the smallest type patient can read comfortably. Smallest print is N5.

Visual Field

Different methods to test visual field are: (a) confrontation test using a finger, (b) red pin confrontation test, and (c) perimetry. When the size of test object is 5 mm, the field of vision is 100 degrees laterally, 60 degrees medially, 60 degrees superiorly and 75 degrees inferiorly.

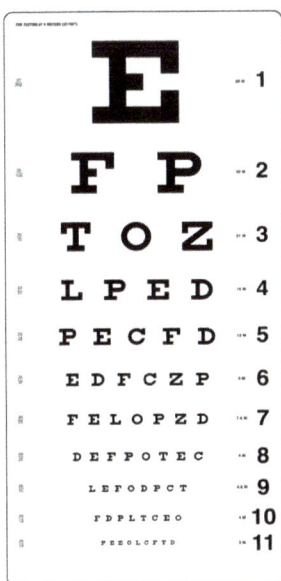

Fig. 8.2: Snellen's chart.

Scotoma is known as a zone of loss of vision in the visual field. The scotoma can be central or paracentral. Important cause of unilateral central scotoma is optic neuritis. Unilateral paracentral scotomas are due to vascular disease (retinal embolism or retinal artery branch occlusion). Bilateral paracentral scotomas are due to vitamin B_{12} deficiency or alcoholism. Glaucoma can cause comma-shaped defect in visual field (paracentral 'arcuate' scotoma) due to damage of nerve fibers in retina or optic nerve.

Loss of vision in one half of visual field is known as hemianopia. When vision is lost in same half of visual fields in both eyes it is known as homonymous. Right homonymous hemianopia means right half of the field in both eyes is affected. Quadrantanopia is a term used to describe blindness in one quadrant of visual field. Loss of vision in outer half of field (temporal halves) in both eyes is known as bitemporal hemianopia. Binasal hemianopia is loss of visual field in inner or nasal halves of visual fields. Hemianopia may occur due to lesions in optic nerve or chiasma (incongruous) or postgeniculate lesions (congruous). Bitemporal hemianopia is due to damage of fibers in optic chiasma derived from the nasal part of each eye due to pituitary tumors, inflammatory and traumatic lesions extending out of sella turcica. Binasal hemianopia is due to bilateral lesion of outer aspect of optic chiasma.

Color Vision

Color vision is tested using Ishihara's pseudoisochromatic plates consisting of multicolor dots outlining certain digits **(Fig. 8.3)**. Most common color vision anomaly is red green deficiency, which is inherited as sex-linked recessive condition. Acquired causes of defective color vision are macular and optic nerve disease.

Pupillary Examination

The pupillary light reflex consists of optic nerve fibers as afferent component and parasympathetic fibers in oculomotor nerve as efferent. The light shown in one eye results in constriction of pupil in the same eye (direct pupillary reaction) as well as in other eye (consensual pupillary reaction). The absence of direct pupillary light reaction but the presence of consensual reaction indicates the lesion of the optic nerve in that eye. This is performed using swinging light test (swinging torch test). The size of pupils is noted. The pupil can be smaller or larger in size due to various causes **(Table 8.2)**.

Accommodation Reflex

Pupillary accommodation reflex includes meiosis (pupils become smaller) and convergence of the eyes on accommodating for the near objects. This is impaired in the lesions of third nerve and in autonomic neuropathies.

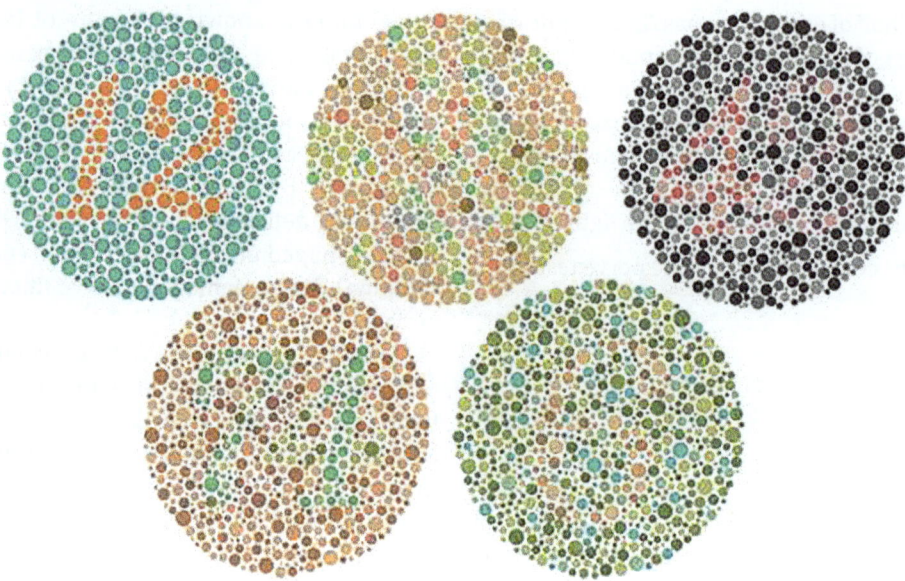

Fig. 8.3: Ishihara plate.

Table 8.2: Causes of smaller or larger pupils.		
	Unilateral	**Bilateral**
Dilated	• III nerve compression by cerebral mass, posterior communicating artery aneurysm, uncal herniation • II nerve lesion (Marcus Gunn pupil), dilatation in abnormal eye detected by Swinging torch reflex • Anticholinergic drugs: Atropine, tropicamide eye drops	• Midbrain damage by supratentorial mass • Anticholinergic drugs: Atropine, tropicamide eye drops • Direct ocular trauma
Small pupil (Constricted)	• Horner's syndrome (Disease of sympathetic efferents) • Mechanical: Iritis or trauma • Pharmacological: Pilocarpine eye drops	• Metabolic encephalopathies • Deep hemispheric lesions (hydrocephalus, thalamic hemorrhage) • Argyll Robertson pupil (Syphilis) • Pharmacological: Pilocarpine eye drops
Pinpoint (<1 mm)		• Narcotic or barbiturate overdose • Pontine hemorrhage • Organophosphorus and carbamate poisoning

Argyll Robertson pupil: The pupil is small and irregular. Accommodation reflex is present while there is no light reflex. This is seen in neurosyphilis.

Adie pupil (Tonic pupil): There is absence or delayed pupillary constriction to light or to accommodation. It is of little clinical significance.

Horner's syndrome: This is due to paralysis of cervical sympathetic nerve. Sympathetic nerve fibers originating in the lower cervical and upper thoracic region of the spinal cord pass through the ophthalmic division of the fifth cranial nerve to the eye. Sympathetic activity mediates pupillary dilatation and elevation of the upper lid through the contraction of smooth muscles of levator palpebrae superioris. Features of Horner's syndrome are:
- Pupillary constriction
- Slight drooping of the upper lid (ptosis)
- Absence of pupillary dilatation in the dark
- Loss of ciliospinal reflex
- Impaired sweating of the face on the side of lesion.

Oculomotor Nerve

The oculomotor nerve after emerging from the anterior surface of midbrain passes forward between the posterior cerebral and superior cerebellar arteries and continues in the middle cranial fossa in the lateral wall of cavernous sinus. It then passes through superior orbital fissure to enter the orbital cavity. The oculomotor nerve supplies the following muscles of the eye:
- Levator palpebrae superioris
- Superior rectus
- Inferior rectus
- Inferior oblique.

It also supplies the ciliary muscles and constrictor pupillae muscles of the iris.

The functions of the oculomotor nerve are:
- Lifting the upper eyelid
- Turning the eye upward, downward and medially
- Constriction of pupil
- Accommodation of the eye.

The test is done by asking patient to look in different directions. Horizontal and outward movement of eyeball is called abduction, whereas horizontal inward movement is termed adduction. Vertical upward movement is termed elevation and downward is termed depression. Superior and inferior recti act as elevator and depressor alone when the eye is in abduction. Inferior and superior oblique act as elevator and depressor, respectively, when eye is in adduction.

Lower motor neuron lesion (infranuclear lesion) of III, IV and VI cranial nerves leads to weakness of individual or group of muscles. While upper motor neuron lesions (supranuclear lesion) lead to paralysis of conjugate movement of the eye.

The infranuclear lesion of the oculomotor nerve may lead to following abnormalities:
- No movement of eyeball in medial and upward direction, movement is possible in lateral direction and slightly downwards
- Lateral and downward displacement of the eye
- Dilatation of the pupil
- Loss of accommodation reflex of the pupil.

Trochlear Nerve

The trochlear nerve leaves the midbrain and passes forward in middle cranial fossa in the lateral wall of the cavernous sinus. It then passes through superior orbital fissure to enter the orbital cavity. It supplies the superior oblique muscle of the eyeball and helps in turning the eyeball downward and laterally.

Infranuclear lesions of the trochlear nerve may result in impaired downward movement when eyeball is in medial position.

Trigeminal Nerve

Trigeminal nerve is the largest cranial nerve. It has a sensory root and a small motor root. It leaves the anterior side of pons and passes through the posterior cranial fossa to reach the apex of petrous temporal bone in the middle cranial fossa. Here, the sensory root forms the trigeminal ganglion. The three divisions, namely ophthalmic (V1), maxillary (V2) and mandibular (V3) arise from the ganglion.

- The ophthalmic division is sensory and supplies skin of forehead and scalp as far as the vertex, the conjunctiva of the eye, cornea, the upper eyelid, lacrimal gland, the mucous membranes of the paranasal sinuses, the nasal cavity and the skin of nose as far as the tip.
- The maxillary division is also sensory and it passes through foramen rotundum to supply the skin overlying the maxilla, upper lip, the lower eyelid and its conjunctival surface, the teeth of upper jaw, the maxillary sinus, the palate, and the mucous membrane of the nose.
- The mandibular division is both motor and sensory. These roots pass through the foramen ovale. The sensory fibers supply the skin of the lower part of cheek, the skin over the mandible, the lower lip and the side of the head. It also supplies the teeth of lower jaw, temporomandibular joint, mucous membrane of the cheek, the floor of the mouth and the anterior part of the tongue **(Fig. 8.4)**.

The motor fibers supply:
- Muscles of mastication
- Mylohyoid muscle
- Anterior belly of the digastric muscle
- Tensor veli palatini of the soft palate
- Tensor tympani of the middle ear.

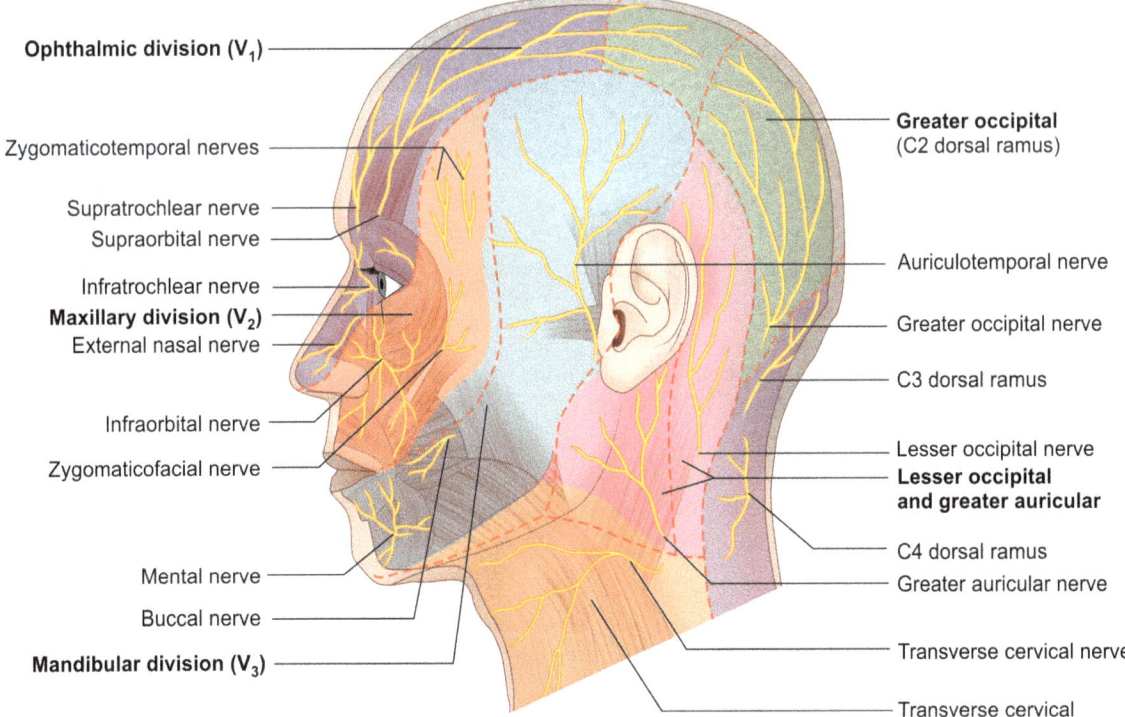

Fig. 8.4: Areas supplied by different divisions of the trigeminal nerve.

The sensory component of the trigeminal nerve is examined by testing the touch, pain and cold sensations in the areas supplied. The lesion of the whole trigeminal nerve leads to loss of sensations in the skin and mucous membrane of the face and nasopharynx. Lacrimal and salivary secretions may be diminished. *Trophic ulcers may develop in the mouth, nose and cornea. Lack of salivary secretion may also alter taste perception.*

The motor component of trigeminal nerve is tested by asking the patient to clench the teeth. Normally, temporal and masseter muscles become prominent which can be easily palpable. Muscles do not become prominent on the paralyzed side. While opening the mouth, jaw deviates to the paralyzed side. This is because of uninhibited action of lateral pterygoid muscles which push the jaw to the paralyzed side.

Corneal reflex: The corneal reflex may be absent either due to lesion of Vth nerve (afferent component of the reflex) or due to facial nerve (efferent component of the reflex).

This is tested by touching the lateral edge of cornea with a fine cotton wisp. Normally, this leads to the blinking of the eyes. Alternatively, it can be tested by lightly blowing puff of air into each cornea.

Abducens Nerve

The Abducens nerve emerges between the pons and the medulla oblongata and passes forward in the middle cranial fossa along with internal carotid artery through the cavernous sinus. It then passes through superior orbital fissure to enter the orbital cavity.

It supplies the lateral rectus muscle and its function is to turn the eyeball laterally.

Infranuclear lesions of the VIth nerve may result in inability to move eye outward **(Fig. 8.5)** with diplopia (double vision) and convergent squint because of unopposed action of medial rectus.

Facial Nerve

Facial nerve emerges as two roots between the pons and the medulla oblongata and passes laterally in the posterior cranial fossa with the VIII nerve and enters the internal acoustic meatus in the petrous part of temporal bone. The nerve then enters the facial canal and laterally through the inner ear. It emerges from the canal through the stylomastoid foramen. The nerve then passes through the parotid gland and divides into branches which innervate the muscles of the face and scalp except the *levator palpebrae superioris*. It also supplies the platysma, stylohyoid, posterior belly of the diagastric and the stapedius muscle of the middle ear.

The facial nerve controls facial expression, salivation and lacrimation. It also carries the taste sensation from the anterior two-third of the tongue, floor of the mouth and the palate. The taste fibers pass from the lingual nerve (a branch of fifth cranial nerve) into the chorda tympani, to join the facial nerve above stylomastoid foramina. The sensory component of facial nerve carries sensations from the part of the skin of external ear. Examination of the facial nerve is described under 'facial nerve palsy'. Innervation of tongue is given in **Table 8.3**.

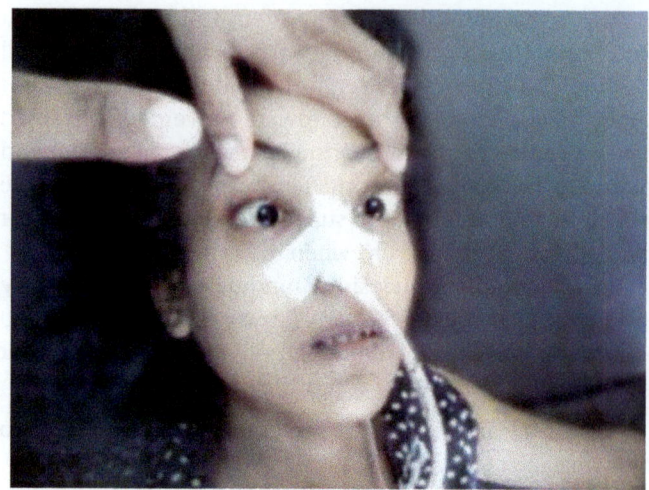

Fig. 8.5: Right VI nerve palsy. There is no lateral movement of right eyeball while looking towards right side.

Taste sensation examination: Patient is asked about the loss or change in the taste. The examination is done by applying solutions one-by-one on the surface of protruded tongue. The solutions generally used for different taste modalities are sugar (sweet), common salt (salt), citric acid (sour) and quinine (bitter). The patient is asked to indicate the nature of taste while tongue is still protruded. This is to differentiate the impairment of taste sensation in anterior or posterior parts of the tongue.

Ageusia is defined as loss of taste sensation **(Table 8.4)**.

Table 8.3: Innervation of the tongue.

Sensory	Taste
Anterior two-third—V nerve	Anterior two-third—VII nerve
Posterior one-third—IX nerve	Posterior one-third—IX nerve

Table 8.4: Causes of loss of taste (ageusia)/alteration in taste.

- Aging > 60 years
- Nasal and sinus problems
  - Alergies, sinusitis, nasal polyps
  - Common cold, flu, covid 19, salivary glands infection
- Dental problems
  - Gingivitis, periodontal diseases
- Cigarette smoking
- Head or facial injury mass
- Alzheimer's disease
- Parkinson's disease
- Zn, Vit B_{12} deficiency
- Damage to nerve of taste sensation (Herpes zoster, Cerebello-pontine tumor (meningioma, neuroma)
- Polyneuropathies: Diphtheria, porphyria, lupus amyloidosis
- Drugs: Ampicillin, metronidazole, quinolones, tetracycline, antipsychotics, antiparkinsonism

Vestibulocochlear Nerve

Vestibulocochlear nerve consists of vestibular and cochlear fibers. These fibers leave the brain between the pons and the medulla oblongata. After crossing the posterior cranial fossa it enters the internal acoustic meatus with the facial nerve. The vestibular fibers originate from the vestibule and semicircular canals and are concerned with the sense of position and movements of head. The cochlear fibers originate from the cochlea to the internal ear and are concerned with hearing.

Important symptoms of vestibular dysfunction are vertigo, giddiness and unsteadiness. In vertigo, external objects seem to move around the patient. Auditory manifestations include tinnitus, hyperacusis and auditory hallucination and delusion. Tinnitus means persistent ringing in the ears. In hyperacusis, there is excessive sensitivity to sound and it occurs due to paralysis of stapedius muscle.

Tests of Hearing

- Hearing is tested by producing whispered and conventional voice at varying distances.
- Hearing may also be tested using vibrating tuning fork (512 Hz). Rinne test and Weber test are used to diagnose sensory neural and conductive hearing loss.
- Audiometry is used to measure the extent of hearing loss and to locate the site of lesion.

Tests of Vestibular Functions

- Eye movements are observed in all gazes to find out nystagmus.
- Positional testing.
- Caloric test.

Glossopharyngeal Nerve

Glossopharyngeal nerve has both motor and sensory components. It emerges from the anterior surface of the medulla oblongata and passes laterally in the posterior cranial fossa. It then passes through the jugular foramen and descends through the upper part of neck to the tongue. The motor fibers supply the stylopharyngeus muscle, parasympathetic fibers supply the parotid gland and sensory fibers carry general sensations and taste sensation from the posterior part of the tongue and pharynx. It also innervates carotid body and carotid sinus.

The function of this nerve is to assist swallowing and promoting salivation.

The loss of taste sensation in the posterior part of the tongue occurs, if the glossopharyngeal nerve is damaged.

Vagus Nerve

The vagus nerve has both motor and sensory components. It emerges from the anterior surface of the medulla oblongata and passes laterally in the posterior cranial fossa. It then passes through the jugular foramen and descends through the neck along with carotid arteries and internal jugular vein within the carotid sheath. After passing through the mediastinum, it pierces the diaphragm and terminates in the abdomen.

Vagus nerve innervates the heart and great vessels, the larynx, trachea, bronchi, lungs and alimentary canal (from pharynx to splenic flexure of colon). It also supplies liver and pancreas and other glands associated with alimentary canal.

Accessory Nerve

The accessory nerve is a motor nerve and has cranial root and a spinal root. The cranial root emerges from the anterior surface of the medulla oblongata and runs laterally in the posterior cranial fossa. The spinal root arises from nerve cells in the anterior column of the upper five segments of the cervical part of the spinal cord. The nerve ascends through the spinal cord and enters the skull through the foramen magnum and joins the cranial root.

The two roots leave the cranium through the jugular foramen and separate. The cranial root is distributed to muscles of the soft palate, pharynx through branches of vagus nerve (pharyngeal plexus). It also supplies the muscles of larynx except the cricothyroid muscle. The spinal root supplies the trapezius and sternocleidomastoid muscles.

Examination of IX, X, and XI Cranial Nerves

Due to common innervations of various structures by IX, X and XI cranial nerves, symptoms are generally common and overlapping.

Palatal paralysis: Unilateral paralysis of palate may not lead to symptoms or symptoms are very minimal. However, bilateral paralysis of palate may produce following:

- There is regurgitation of fluid during swallowing through the nose. This is due to paralysis of soft palate
- Patient is not able to pronounce the words which require closure of nasopharynx. For example, 'egg' and 'rub' are pronounced as 'eng' and 'rum', respectively
- Dysphagia (difficulty in swallowing) for solid foods may occur in lower motor neuron lesion and markedly for liquids in upper motor neuron lesion.

Examination of palatal movement is performed by asking the patient to say 'ah'. In case of bilateral paralysis there is no movement of the palate. Palate will remain flat and immobile on the side of paralysis and median raphe is pulled toward the other side in case of unilateral lesion.

Palatal reflex: It may be impaired in the lesion of IX or X cranial nerves. Normally there is reflex contraction of the palate when the back of the pharynx is tickled.

Laryngeal paralysis: The innervation of larynx is given in **Table 8.5**.

Table 8.5: Innervation of larynx.	
Superior laryngeal branch	• Sensory: Larynx above the level of vocal cords • Motor: Cricothyroid muscle
Recurrent laryngeal branch	• Sensory: Larynx below the level of vocal cords • Motor: All laryngeal muscles except cricothyroid

- Bilateral damage of superior laryngeal branch of vagus nerve leads to hoarse voice
- Unilateral paralysis of recurrent laryngeal nerve (branch of vagus nerve) leads to hoarse speech and bovine cough (patient cannot cough clearly and effectively). Bilateral paralysis may cause stridor or respiratory obstruction.

Laryngoscopic examination reveals characteristic features of vocal cord paralysis.

Examination of spinal part of accessory nerve: Trapezius and sternomastoid muscles are tested for the evidence of lesion in the spinal part of the XI nerve. Patient is asked to shrug the shoulder against resistance for testing trapezius muscle. There is weakness in the rotation of chin toward the opposite side in sternomastoid paralysis.

Hypoglossal Nerve

The hypoglossal nerve is a motor nerve. It emerges from the anterior surface of the medulla oblongata and passes laterally in the posterior cranial fossa. It then passes through the hypoglossal canal and runs downward and forward in the neck. The hypoglossal nerve innervates the muscles of the tongue except the palatoglossus muscle and controls the movements and shape of the tongue.

The hypoglossal nerve is examined by asking the patient to protrude the tongue, move the tongue from side-to-side and to lick each cheek with the tongue. In unilateral lesion, the tongue deviates to the paralyzed side on protrusion. Presence of wasting or fasciculations on the tongue indicates lower motor neuron lesion of the hypoglossal nerve.

■ EXAMINATION OF A COMATOSE PATIENT

Consciousness: It is a state when patient is aware of self and the environment. The person is able to respond to internal as well as external changes/needs.

Sleep: This is a normal variation in consciousness. Patient can be aroused to a normal state of consciousness either spontaneously or by external stimuli from the state of sleep.

Confusional state: It is an altered state of consciousness characterized by clouded alertness and disorientation. *Delerium* is a confusional state with marked agitation.

Drowsiness: It is like light sleep, which cannot be easily aroused and the alertness can only be maintained for brief period. Once awakened, patient is usually disoriented and tends to fall asleep despite verbal stimulation.

Stupor: It is a condition where arousal can occur only by vigorous stimuli and arousal is brief and incomplete.

Coma: It is a state of persistent loss of consciousness, where patient is unarousable and unable to respond to external events or inner needs like hunger. The coma indicates disorders of arousal mechanisms in the brain.

Pathophysiology of Coma

Alertness is maintained by proper functioning of reticular activating system (RAS) that contains brainstem, ascending projections and the cortex. Hence, coma occurs due to:
- Effect on RAS and its projections.
- Involvement of both cerebral hemispheres.
- Suppression of reticulocerebral functions by drugs, toxins or metabolic factors, such as hypoglycemia, uremia, anoxia or hepatic failure.

Unilateral lesions like stroke and tumor generally do not alter consciousness unless they produce mass effect to compress opposite hemisphere or brainstem. Subtentorial lesions produce coma by compressing the brainstem.

Causes: They can be classified into metabolic or diffuse causes and structural causes. Structural causes can be supratentorial or infratentorial. Important causes of coma are given in **Table 8.6**.

Diagnosis

Early diagnosis of underlying cause is of vital importance. The diagnosis is based on history, general physical and neurological examination and the laboratory investigations.

Table 8.6: Important causes of coma.
Metabolic causes: • Hypoglycemia • Hypoxemia or hypercapnea • Hypothermia • Hypercalcemia • Hypernatremia or hyponatremia • Liver failure • Renal failure • Diabetic ketoacidosis CNS infection/inflammation Drugs and toxins Sepsis Postictal state or subclinical seizure Hypertensive encephalopathy Hypothyroidism Head injury Structural lesions: • Stroke • Brain abscess • Brain hematoma • Hydrocephalus • Brain tumor • Venous thrombosis

History

The following points must be taken to ascertain the cause of coma:
- History of trauma.
- Ingestion of drugs or toxins.
- Presence of chronic disease of liver, kidneys, heart or lungs.
- Diabetes.
- Circumstances and preceding symptoms like fever, seizures, headache, vomiting, etc.

General Physical Examination

- Presence of fever suggests a systemic infection, meningitis, encephalitis or brainstem fever.
- Hypothermia can be observed in alcoholism, barbiturate poisoning, hypothyroidism, hypoglycemia and circulatory failure.
- Severe hypertension indicates hypertensive encephalopathy or cerebral hemorrhage.
- Hypotension indicates sepsis, heart failure, internal hemorrhage, alcoholism and barbiturate poisoning.

Neurological Examination

The level of consciousness can be assessed by Glasgow Coma Scale. The score ranges from 3 (unresponsive) to 15 (normal) **(Table 8.7)**.

The type of neurological presentation may indicate the underlying causes:
- Hemiplegia (weakness of half of body) indicates stroke.
- Myoclonus; metabolic encephalopathy.
- Asterixis (flapping tremor); metabolic encephalopathy; drug intoxication.
- Decorticate rigidity (flexion of elbow and wrist with supination of arm); lesion rostral to midbrain.
- Decerebrate rigidity (extension of elbow and wrist with pronation of arm); lesion in midbrain or caudal diencephalon.
- Unilaterally dilated pupil signifies third cranial nerve damage whereas bilaterally dilated or unresponsive pupils suggests severe midbrain lesion, atropine or methyl alcohol intoxication, and severe anoxic encephalopathy. Bilaterally small or pin-point pupils are seen in narcotic overdose, metabolic encephalopathy and thalamic or pontine lesions.
- Conjugate horizontal deviation of eye balls on one side indicates damage to pons on other side or frontal lobe lesion on the same side (eyes look toward a hemispheric lesion and away from a brainstem lesion). Eyes turned down and inward indicates midbrain lesion.
- Moving the head from side-to-side and observing eye movement: Movement of eyes opposite to the direction of head movement is called Doll's eye phenomenon (Oculocephalic test). This is suppressed in awake patient while is present in comatosed patient with intact brainstem oculomotor function.
- Caloric stimulation test: The external auditory canal is irrigated with cold water, which leads to tonic deviation of eye balls to the side of cold water irrigation and nystagmus in the opposite side. Loss of this reflex suggests brainstem damage.
- Cheyne-Stokes breathing is seen in bilateral hemispheric damage whereas Kussmaul's breathing suggests metabolic acidosis.
- Presence of herniation must be recognized and managed promptly otherwise it may lead to irreparable brain damage and death. Herniation occurs due to shift in brain tissue due to edema or mass lesions.

Investigations

The following laboratory investigations are helpful in making the diagnosis of a patient with coma:
- Complete blood count.
- Blood sugar, blood urea, serum sodium and potassium, serum calcium.
- Liver function tests, serum ammonia level, serum ethanol.
- Thyroid function tests.
- Imaging of brain (CT, MRI).
- Cerebrospinal fluid (CSF) examination.
- Electroencephalography (EEG).

Management

Patient should be admitted in intensive care unit. Following are important steps in the management of coma:

General

- Maintenance of airway, breathing and circulation.
- Maintain normal body temperature.

Table 8.7: Glasgow Coma Scale.

Eye opening:	
Spontaneous	4
To voice	3
To pain	2
None	1
Best verbal response:	
Oriented	5
Confused	4
Inappropriate words	3
Unintelligible sounds	2
None	1
Best motor response:	
Obeys command	6
Localizes pain	5
Normal withdrawal	4
Flexor response	3
Extensor response	2
None	1

- Administration of oxygen.
- Mechanical ventilation.

Medications

- Administration of IV thiamine 100 mg.
- Administration of dextrose 50 mL (50%).
- Rapid correction of causative factors like hypotension, hypoglycemia, hypoxia, hypercalcemia, hypercapnea and hyperthermia.
- IV naloxone for opiate intoxication and flumazenil for benzodiazepine intoxication.
- Intravenous antibiotics in case of meningitis, septicemia.
- Management of increased intracranial pressure: (a) IV mannitol, (b) hyperventilation, (c) dexamethasone.

Operative Management

- Surgical evacuation of hematoma or hemorrhage.
- Shunt for hydrocephalus.
- Surgery for structural lesion.

Brain Death

A state of cessation of cerebral function while somatic function is maintained by artificial means and the heart continues to pump. Three essential elements are required for clinical diagnosis of brain death.
- Widespread **cortical** destruction reflected by deep coma and unresponsiveness to all stimuli including visual, auditory or painful stimuli. There is no spontaneous movement or any motor response to noxious stimuli.
- **Brainstem** damage shown by absence of pupillary response, loss of oculovestibular, corneal or gag reflexes.
- Destruction of **medulla** manifested by complete apnea.

Ancillary diagnostic tests, although not required in most cases may be helpful in diagnosing brain death. These tests are:
- EEG: Absence of brain-derived electrical activity.
- Radionuclide brain scan: Absence of cerebral blood flow.
- Somatosensory-evoked potentials: Absence of cortical and subcortical responses with intact peripheral nerve responses.
- Conventional angiography: Absent cerebral blood flow.

EPILEPSY

Epilepsy is defined as any disorder characterized by recurrent seizures due to chronic underlying process. A single seizure is not epilepsy.

Seizure: This is a transient clinical event due to abnormal paroxysmal excessive discharges from a group of central nervous system neurons. The seizure may present in form of motor, sensory, autonomic or psychic manifestations.

Convulsion: The motor form of seizure is called convulsion.

Classification

Seizures may be of two major types (**Table 8.8**):
1. *Partial seizure:* In this condition seizure activity is restricted to localized part of one cerebral hemisphere.
2. *Generalized seizure:* It involves both cerebral hemispheres diffusely and simultaneously.

Partial Seizures

Simple partial seizures are those where consciousness is preserved whereas it is impaired in complex partial seizures. Partial seizures may spread diffusely throughout the cortex and result in secondary generalized seizures. The manifestations depend on the area of the brain involved and may be in the form of motor, sensory, autonomic or psychic symptoms.

Simple Partial Seizures

Various presentations of simple partial seizures are:
- *Focal motor*: The jerky movements of limbs or other parts of the body depending upon the area of the motor cortex involved.
- *Somatosensory*: Localized paresthesias if sensory cortex is involved.
- *Special sensory*: Involvement of visual, auditory, olfactory and gustatory regions of the brain can lead to light flashes, buzzing, unusual odor (burning rubber) or epigastric sensations.
- *Autonomic*: Flushing, sweating and piloerection are due to autonomic involvement.

Table 8.8: Classification of seizures [2010 International League Against Epilepsy classification (ILAE Classification)].

Focal seizures
- With intact awareness (simple partial)
  - Focal motor
  - Focal sensory
- With impaired awareness (complex partial)
- Evolving to a bilateral, convulsive seizure (secondarily generalized seizure)
  - Tonic
  - Clonic
  - Tonic–clonic

Generalized seizures
- Tonic–clonic (in any combination)
- Absence
  - Typical
  - Atypical
  - Absence with special features
- Clonic
- Tonic
- Atonic
- Myoclonic
- Myoclonic absence
- Eyelid myoclonia

Unknown
- Epileptic spasms

- *Psychic*: Illusions, hallucinations, affective disturbances and *déjà vu* can be the manifestations of simple partial seizures.

  Partial motor seizures may present with additional characteristic features like:
  - Abnormal movements beginning in a restricted region like fingers may spread to involve larger part of the limb. This is known as **Jacksonian march**.
  - Weakness in the involved parts following motor seizures may occur for minutes or last for hours. This is called **Todd's paralysis**.
  - Rarely focal motor seizures may continue for hours or days (*epilepsia partialis continua*).

Complex Partial Seizures

Complex partial seizures are characterized by focal seizure activity accompanied with impaired consciousness.
- They arise generally from the temporal or frontal lobes
- The complex partial seizure begins with the aura (in form of simple partial seizure) and is the same (stereotypic) every time in a particular patient.
- The patient stares blankly (blackouts) and has involuntary automatic behavioral movements (*automatism*) such as chewing, lip smacking, emotion display or running.
- The patients do not respond to visual or verbal commands during the seizure and become drowsy following seizures.
- There is amnesia about the recollection of ictal (seizure) phase.

Primary Generalized Seizures

Tonic-Clonic Seizures

Tonic-clonic seizures (grand mal, primary generalized seizures) may occur abruptly without warning or there may be some premonitory symptoms. There is sudden loss of consciousness and the patient may fall on the ground and sustain injuries.

Tonic phase: The initial phase is characterized by increased muscle tone throughout the body. Cyanosis, impaired respiration, pooling of secretions in the oral cavity occurs because of tonic contractions of muscles of respiration. Increased tone in laryngeal muscles may cause 'ictal cry'. Tongue bite may occur due to contraction of jaw muscles. Increased sympathetic manifestations such as tachycardia, hypertension and dilatation of the pupils may also occur.

Clonic phase: Tonic phase lasts for a minute and is followed by 'clonic phase' characterized by jerky movements for a few minutes. Subsequently, the patient goes in a state of muscular flaccidity and unresponsiveness (postictal phase). There may be bladder or bowel incontinence.

Patient gradually regains consciousness over minutes to hours and may have postictal headache, confusion, muscle ache and fatigue for hours. Postictal period is defined as the time between the end of seizure and the return to baseline mental status.

The presence of aura suggests partial seizure with secondary generalization. An aura is a simple partial seizure manifesting as sensory, autonomic or psychic symptoms.

Absence Seizures (Petit Mal)

- This occurs in childhood and ceases after 20 years of age
- This is characterized by brief lapses of sensorium with loss of postural control
- These are too subtle to be noticed or referred to as day dreaming
- The attacks are much briefer (seconds) and more frequent than complex partial seizures
- There is no postictal confusion
- There may be mild motor movements like blinking of eyes, chewing and hand clonus
- This is associated with characteristic EEG pattern.

Causes of Seizures

The etiology depends on the age of the patient. A list of causes of seizures is given in **Table 8.9**.
- Hypoxia, metabolic derangements, congenital defects and birth trauma are important causes of seizures in neonates
- Febrile seizures are more common in early childhood
- Head trauma is common cause of seizures in young adults
- In older people, cerebrovascular disease, tumors and degenerative disorders are important causes of seizures
- Metabolic and electrolyte imbalance, drugs and systemic illnesses can cause seizures at any age.

Investigations

- *EEG*: This may help in the diagnosis and classification of seizure disorders. Characteristic EEG changes in petit mal seizures (3 Hertz spike and wave activity) differentiate it from complex partial seizures.
- *Brain imaging*: CT or MRI is indicated in patients with focal seizures, focal neurological signs or if age of onset is more than 20 years **(Fig. 8.6)**.
- *Metabolic*: Serum electrolytes, urea, calcium, blood glucose and liver function tests are done to rule out any metabolic cause.
- *Other tests*: Blood count, ESR, X-ray chest, CSF examination, ANA and other specific tests may be needed to diagnose infective or inflammatory causes.

Differential Diagnosis

The seizures should be differentiated from transient ischemic attacks (TIA), syncope and pseudoseizures. Pseudoseizures do not occur during sleep and are not associated with unconsciousness, cyanosis, incontinence and tongue bite. There are no postictal headache, confusion

Table 8.9: Causes of seizures.

Idiopathic

Genetic
- Neurofibroma
- Inborn errors of metabolism

Trauma
- Birth trauma
- Head injury

Metabolic
- Alcohol withdrawal
- Hypoglycemia
- Hypocalcemia
- Hyponatremia
- Hypoxia
- Renal failure
- Liver failure

Intracranial space occupying lesions
- Tuberculoma
- Neurocysticercosis
- Brain abscess
- Brain tumor
- Vascular malformations

Cerebrovascular diseases
- Hemorrhage
- Emboli

Infections
- Encephalitis
- Meningitis
- HIV
- Toxoplasmosis

Inflammatory
- SLE
- Sarcoidois
- Degenerative
- Alzheimer's disease

Drugs
- Lignocaine
- Quinolones
- Penicillins
- Theophylline
- Chloroquine, Mefloquine
- Psychotropic agents

Febrile seizures

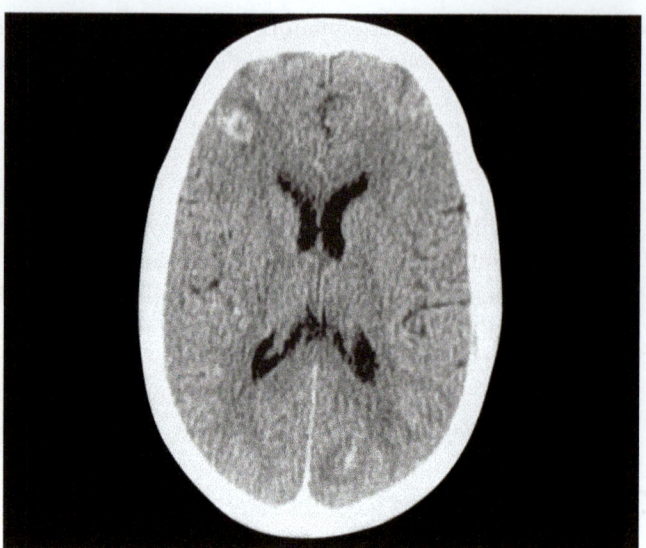

Fig. 8.6: CT head showing solitary ring lesion (tuberculoma).

and focal neurological deficit. EEG changes and high serum prolactin level are features of "true" seizures and not found in pseudoseizures. Pseudoseizures may occur in hysterical reactions and malingering and may be precipitated by emotional stress.

Management

General Precautions

- The patient should refrain from working with dangerous equipment and should avoid swimming, fishing or cycling
- He should also avoid any activity such as driving where loss of consciousness is dangerous. The patient should avoid working near fire or at a height
- These precautions should be taken until a good control of seizures is obtained.

Immediate Care of Seizures

- The patient is shifted to a safer place, away from danger (water, fire and machine)
- The patient is turned to the semiprone position to prevent aspiration
- The patient should not be left alone until full recovery from seizures as there may be drowsiness and confusion in the postictal stage or the seizures may reoccur
- Nothing should be given by mouth until the patient has fully recovered
- If convulsions continue for a prolonged duration (>5 minutes) or reoccur without the patient regaining consciousness, hospitalization is a must.

Treatment of the Underlying Condition

If the cause of seizures is a metabolic abnormality (electrolyte abnormality or glucose abnormality) it should be corrected effectively. Correctable causes for seizures (hyponatremia, hypoglycemia, alcohol withdrawal, drug toxicity, etc.) do not require long-term antiepileptic therapy. In case of drug-induced seizures, the offending drug should be withdrawn. Structural CNS lesions like brain tumor, abscess and vascular malformation must be treated appropriately. The antiepileptic treatment may not be required once the underlying condition has been well-treated.

Avoidance of Precipitating Factors

Seizures may be precipitated by specific trigger factors such as sleep deprivation, alcohol withdrawal, mental stress, physical exhaustion, flickering lights (TV or monitor), music, loud sounds and drug abuse. Such situations should be avoided.

Table 8.10: The antiepileptic drugs.

Drug	Daily dose (adult)	Important side effects
Phenytoin	300–400 mg	Ataxia, diplopia, drowsiness, gingival hyperplasia, folate deficiency, osteomalacia
Carbamazepine	200–2000 mg	Ataxia, diplopia, drowsiness, blood dyscrasia, hepatotoxicity, hyponatremia
Valproic acid	400–2000 mg	Rashes, liver damage, drowsiness, blood dyscrasia
Phenobarbital	60–180 mg	Ataxia, confusion, drowsiness, rash
Clonazepam	1–12 mg	Ataxia, drowsiness
Gabapentin	300–2400 mg	Ataxia, drowsiness
Lamotrigine	25–500 mg	Ataxia, drowsiness, diplopia, rash
Ethosuximide	500–1500 mg	Ataxia, rash, blood dyscrasia
Primidone	250–1000 mg	Ataxia, confusion, drowsiness, rash, megaloblastic anemia
Topiramate	200–600 mg	Ataxia, confusion, drowsiness, renal stones
Tiagabine	32–56 mg	Ataxia, confusion, drowsiness, paraesthesia, depression
Oxcarbazepine	900–2400 mg	As for carbamazepine
Levetiracetam	1000–3000 mg	Sedation, fatigue, psychosis
Zonisamide	200–400 mg	Sedation, headache, psychosis, renal stone
Felbamate	2400–3600 mg	Insomnia, dizziness, aplastic anemia, hepatic failure
Lacosamide	200–400 mg	Dizziness, ataxia, diplopia
Rufinamide	800–3200 mg	Sedation, fatigue, dizziness, ataxia
Clobazam	10–40 mg	Fatigue, sedation, ataxia
Brivaracetam	100–200 mg	Fatigue, dizziness, ataxia, mood changes

Antiepileptic Drug Therapy

A single unprovoked seizure is not an indication to start antiepileptic therapy as about two-third of these patients will not have seizure. A diagnosis of epilepsy is made after two or more unprovoked seizures. Drug treatment to prevent seizures is indicated in patients with recurrent seizures of unknown etiology or when known cause of seizures cannot be reversed. Choice of medicine depends on the type of seizures **(Tables 8.10 and 8.11)**.

- Treatment should be initiated with a single drug
- Dose of the drug should be gradually increased until seizures are controlled or side effects appear. If seizures are not controlled by a single drug, a second drug is added while the first drug is gradually withdrawn. In most patients, seizures can be controlled by a single drug. In some, a combination of two or more drugs is required to control the seizures.
- If seizures are refractory to medical treatment, the patient may benefit from surgical interventions.

Monitoring

Patient should be monitored for the side effects of the medication. Blood counts, liver function tests and renal function tests are done at regular intervals. Serum level of drug can be measured to guide appropriate dosage and to check the compliance.

Duration of Therapy

Treatment should be continued until there have been no seizures for at least 2-3 years. The dosage of the drugs should be tapered and withdrawn gradually over 2-3 months.

Status Epilepticus

This can be convulsive (tonic clonic) or nonconvulsive type.

Convulsive status epilepticus refers to continuous seizure activity or intermittent seizures with impaired consciousness in interictal period. Practically, seizure activity lasting for more than 5 minutes should be managed as status epilepticus.

Nonconvulsive status epilepticus is defined as impairment or loss of consciousness with electrographic (ECG) seizure activity and clinically absent or subtle motor activity. These patients do not present with convulsions, but

Table 8.11: The choice of antiepileptic drugs.

Type of epilepsy	Drug(s) of choice
Partial or secondary generalized seizures	Carbamazepine Lamotrigene Levetiracetam Phenytoin Valproic acid
Primary generalized seizures	Valproic acid Lamotrigine
Absence seizures	Valproic acid Ethosuximide
Myoclonic	Valproic acid Clonazepam Lamotrigene Topiramate

with a fluctuating abnormal mental status, confusion and impaired responsiveness. The treatment approach is same as convulsive status epilepticus.

Causes

Abrupt drug (antiepileptic drugs) withdrawal or non-compliance is the most common cause of the status epilepticus. Other causes are metabolic disorders, intracranial infections and structural lesions of the brain.

Management

The status epilepticus should be treated as emergency **(Table 8.12)**. The patient should be hospitalized.
- Airway is maintained and oxygen is administered.
- Intravenous line is started, a blood sample is withdrawn for laboratory analysis and intravenous dextrose (50% dextrose 25-50 mL) is promptly given. The initial laboratory tests include glucose, electrolytes, calcium, urea, creatinine, liver transaminases and complete blood count.
- Intravenous diazepam (10 mg) or lorazepam (4 mg) is given slowly in 2 minutes. This can be repeated once after 15 minutes if seizures are not controlled. Metazolam 0.2 mg/kg or clonazepam 0.015 mg/kg can also be used.
- If seizures continue beyond 30 minutes: (a) intravenous phenytoin (20 mg/kg) at a rate not more than 50 mg/minute is given. Alternatively, fosphenytoin can be given in a doses of 20 mg/kg PE (phenytoin equivalents) IV. One should monitor for cardiac arrhythmia and hypotension; (b) In patients taking valproate and who may be having subtherapeutic levels, valproate 20–30 mg/kg can be given intravenously. Lacosamide 400 mg IV or levetiracetam 20-30 mg/kg IV may also be given.

- If seizures coninue, the patient is in refractory status epilepticus. An additional dosage of 5-10 mg/kg of phenytoin or 10 mg/kg PE of fosphenytoin may be repeated. Alternatively, valproate 20-30 mg/kg IV given over 15 minutes.
- If there is no access to intensive care unit (ICU), phenobarbitone (IV 20 mg/kg) at a rate not more than 50 mg/minute is given if seizures are still uncontrolled. An additional dose of 5-10 mg/kg may be repeated if needed. Respiratory depression and hypotension are important adverse events.
- Uncontrolled seizures are finally managed by admission in ICU and general anesthesia and neuromuscular blockade along with ventilatory support. Anesthetic agents used are midazolam, propofol and pentobarbitone.
- Once the status is controlled, long-term antiepileptic medications are started.
- The underlying cause is identified if any and treated accordingly.

Complications

Important complications of status epilepticus are cardio-respiratory dysfunction, hyperthermia, rhabdomyolysis and irreversible neurological damage.

MENINGITIS

Meningitis means inflammatory changes in the meninges and the subarachnoid space. Involvement of brain parenchyma along with meninges is known as meningoencephalitis. It may result in altered consciousness, seizures, raised intracranial pressure and stroke.

Causes: Meningitis is generally due to infective causes. These could be viruses, bacteria or fungi. The noninfective causes of meningitis are SLE, sarcoidosis, or neoplastic invasion. Bacterial meningitis is the most common suppurative CNS infection.

Meningitis can be classified into three main categories **(Table 8.13)**:
- Acute purulent (pyogenic, septic, bacterial)

Table 8.12: Drugs used in status epilepticus.

Drugs	Dosage
Diazepam	10 mg slow IV in 2 minutes
Lorazepam	4 mg slow IV in 2 minutes
Phenytoin	20 mg/kg IV infusion, 50 mg/minute, repeat 10 mg/kg
Fosphenytoin	20 mg/kg PE IV infusion, 150 mg/minute, repeat 10 mg/kg PE
Valproate	20–30 mg/kg IV
Phenobarbital	20 mg/kg IV infusion, 50 mg/minute, repeat 10 mg/kg
Midazolam	0.2 mg/kg IV bolus, followed by infusion 0.1 mg/kg/hour
Propofol	1–2 mg/kg IV load, followed by infusion 2 mg/kg/hour
Pentobarbital	5 mg/kg IV load, followed by infusion 1 mg/kg/hour
Levetiracetam	20–30 mg/kg IV
Clonazepam	0.015 mg/kg IV
Lacosamide	400 mg IV

Table 8.13: Types of meningitis.

- **Acute meningitis**
  Bacterial meningitis
  Viral meningitis
- **Subacute meningitis**
  Tuberculosis
  Fungal
  Spirochetal (syphilis)
- **Chronic meningitis**
  Infections (tuberculosis, syphilis, fungal)
  Malignancies (metastatic cancers, leukemia, lymphoma, melanoma)
  Autoimmune disorders (sarcoidosis, SLE, Behcets syndrome)
  Chemicals (injections in subarachnoid space, resection of tumors

- Viral (aseptic)
- Chronic meningitis (tuberculous, fungal).

Acute Bacterial Meningitis

The organisms responsible for acute bacterial meningitis are variable and may differ with the age of the patients. The most common organisms in adults are *S. pneumoniae* (50 %), *N. meningitides*, group B streptocci, *H. infuenzae* and *Listeria monocytogenes*. A list of various organisms responsible for acute meningitis is given in **Table 8.14**.

Bacterial meningitis is either secondary to bacteremic illness or due to spread of infection from adjacent structures like ear, sinus, nose or fractured skull. Old age, alcoholism, diabetes, splenectomy are additional risk factors. Meningococcal meningitis results from airborne infection that initially leads to nasopharyngeal colonization.

Pathology

- Pia-arachnoid is congested and infiltrated with inflammatory cells
- The pus may form in the subarachnoid space which may lead to adhesions
- Adhesions may result in obstruction to CSF flow (hydrocephalus) and cranial nerve damage
- Cerebral infarction may occur due to obliterative endarteritis
- Cerebral edema can lead to raised intracranial pressure (ICP) and coma.

Clinical Manifestations

The classical triad is fever, headache and neck rigidity. The majority of patients develop impairment in sensorium. Nausea, vomiting and photophobia are also common. Patients with meningococcal meningitis may develop rash and adrenocortical failure with shock *(Waterhouse-Friderichsen syndrome)*. Other features are seizures and signs of raised ICP **(Table 8.15)**.

Table 8.14: Causes of bacterial meningitis.

Neonates
- Gram-negative bacilli
- Group B streptococci
- Listeria monocytogenes

Children
- H. influenzae
- S. pneumoniae
- N. meningitidls

Adults
- S. pneumoniae
- N. meningitidis
- H. influenzae
- Listeria monocytogenes

Elderly
- S. pneumoniae
- N. meningitidis
- Listeria monocytogenes
- Gram-negative bacilli

Posttraumatic/Postsurgical
- S. aureus

Table 8.15: Signs of meningitis.

Signs of meningeal irritation
- Neck rigidity
- Kernig's sign
- Brudzinski's sign

General
- Skin rashes (meningococcal)
- Shock (meningococcal)

Signs of raised ICP
- Altered consciousness
- Papilledema
- Sixth nerve palsy
- Dilated pupil
- Cushing's reflex (bradycardia, hypertension)

Others
- Focal neurological signs

Signs of Meningeal Irritation

- **Neck rigidity** is the pathognomonic sign of meningeal irritation **(Figs. 8.7A and B)**. This is demonstrated as an increased resistance to passive flexion of the neck. Other causes of neck rigidity are diseases of the cervical spine, posterior fossa tumor and subarachnoid hemorrhage.
- **Kernig's sign** is elicited when the patient is lying supine. The thigh is flexed on the abdomen with the knee flexed

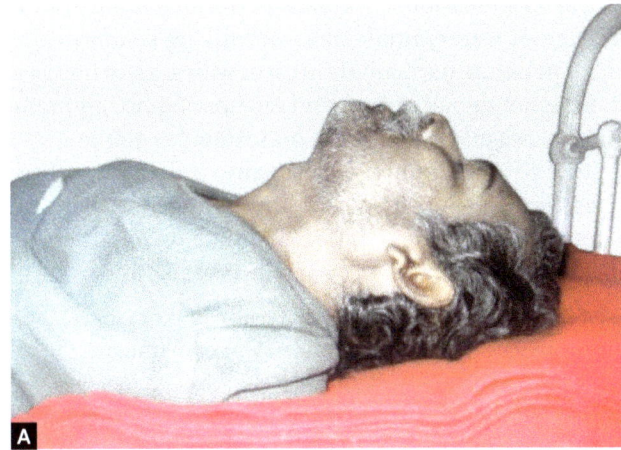

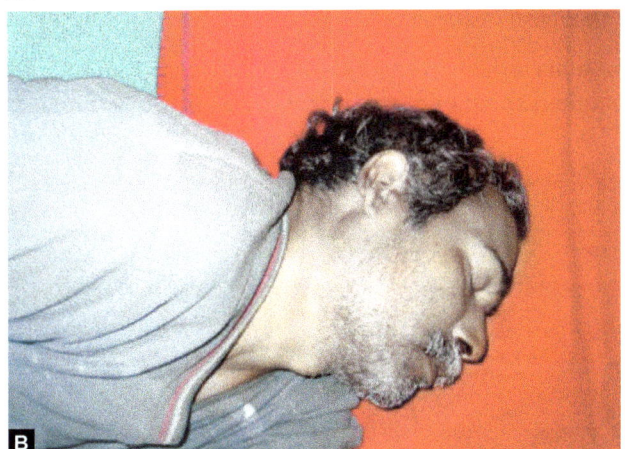

Figs. 8.7A and B: Neck rigidity: (A) Supine, (B) Lateral position.

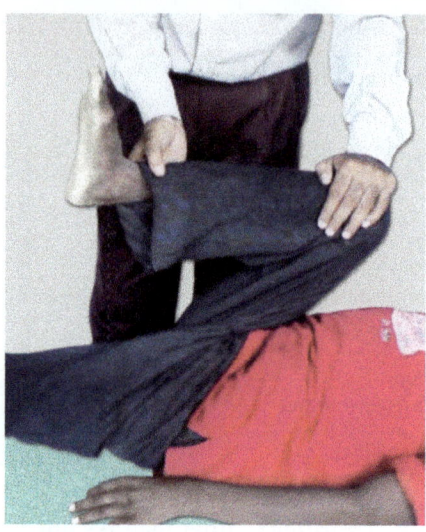

Fig. 8.8: Elicitation of Kernig's sign.

(Fig. 8.8). Passive extension of the knee causes pain and spasm of the hamstrings. This is due to irritation of meninges in the lower spine.
- **Brudzinski's sign** is elicited when the patient is in a supine position. Passive flexion of the neck results in a spontaneous flexion of hips and knees.

Investigations

CSF examination: Diagnosis is made by lumbar puncture and CSF examination. CT scan is performed to rule out the presence of intracranial space-occupying lesion prior to lumbar puncture particularly in cases with signs of increased ICP, focal neurological signs and seizures. Lumbar puncture in such cases may lead to fatal brainstem herniation.

The CSF is examined for pressure, cell count, protein, glucose, smear stain for bacteria and culture. PCR may rarely be needed. The findings of CSF examination of normal and patients with meningitis are given in **Table 8.16**.

Blood examination: There is generally leukocytosis. Blood culture may be helpful in the detection of organism.

Treatment

Antimicrobial Treatment

Acute bacterial meningitis is an emergency. Antimicrobial treatment should be started as soon as possible. Prognosis depends on early initiation of antimicrobial treatment. Drugs are given intravenously and for prolonged period. The dosage of antimicrobials used in treatment of bacterial meningitis is given in **Table 8.17**.

When lumbar puncture cannot be done or attempt to obtain CSF has failed, antimicrobials are given intravenously after obtaining a blood sample for culture. However, CSF should be obtained as soon as possible.

Empirical treatment is started before the CSF culture and Gram stain report is available. It is directed against the most common microorganisms present in a particular age group (**Table 8.18**). Antimicrobials used against specific organisms in meningitis are given in **Table 8.19**.
- Ceftriaxone or cefotaxime provides adequate coverage against *S. pneumoniae*, *H. infuenzae*, Group B streptococci and *N. meningitidis*
- Vancomycin is added to cover cephalosporin resistant *S. pneumoniae*
- Ampicillin is added to cover *L. monocytogenes* in patients less than 3 months of age or more than 55 years and also in immunocompromised patients
- Ceftazidime is active against *P. aeruginosa* and is preferred over ceftriaxone or cefotaxime in hospital-acquired meningitis, posttraumatic and postsurgical meningitis.

Duration of Therapy

The duration of antibiotic therapy depends on the type of organism. A one-week therapy is given in case of *H. influenzae*

Table 8.17: Drugs and their dosage used in bacterial meningitis.

Agent	Daily adult dose, frequency of administration
Ceftriaxone	4 g/day, 12 hourly
Cefotaxime	12 g/day, 4 hourly
Ceftazidime	6 g/day, 8 hourly
Cefepime	6 g/day, 8 hourly
Ampicillin	12 g/day, 4 hourly
Penicillin G	20–24 million units/day, 4 hourly
Vancomycin	2 g/day, 12 hourly
Cefepime	6 g/day, 8 hourly
Metronidazole	1.5-2 g/day, 8 hourly
Meropenem	3 g/day, 8 hourly

Table 8.16: CSF examination findings.

	Normal	Bacterial	Tubercular	Viral
Color	Clear, water-like	Turbid	Straw color, Cob web formation	Clear
Cell count	0–5 cells/mm^3	200–20,000	100–5,000	10–2,000
Cell type	All lymphocytes	Mainly polymorphs	Mostly lymphocytes (polymorphs predominate in acute stage)	Mostly lymphocytes
Protein	15–45 mg/dL	High	High	Mildly increased
Glucose	50–70% of blood glucose	Low	Low	Normal
Other findings	—	Gram stain	AFB stain, mycobacterial culture positive	Viral isolation, PCR/culture positive

Table 8.18: Empirical choice of antibiotics in bacterial meningitis.	
Neonates and infants < 3 months	Ampicillin + ceftriaxone, cefotaxime
Children and adults	Ceftriaxone, cefotaxime or cefepime + vancomycin
Adults > 55 years	Ampicillin + ceftriaxone, Cefotaxime or cefepime + vancomycin
Hospital-acquired meningitis Posttraumatic or postsurgical, Immuncompromised patients	Ampicillin + ceftazidime or meropenem + vancomycin

Table 8.19: Choice of antibiotics for specific microorganisms.	
Organisms	Antibiotics
1. **N. meningitidis** Penicillin sensitive Penicillin resistant	Penicillin G or ampicillin Ceftriaxone or cefotaxime or cefepime
2. **S. pneumoniae** Penicillin sensitive Penicillin resistant	Penicillin G Ceftriaxone or cefotaxime, vancomycin
3. **Gram-negative bacilli**	Ceftriaxone or cefotaxime
4. **H. influenzae**	Ceftriaxone or cefotaxime or cefepime
5. **Pseudomonas spp**	Ceftazidime, cefepime or meropenem
6. **S. arueus** Methicillin sensitive Methicillin resistant	Naficillin Vancomycin
7. **Listeria monocytogenes**	Ampicillin + gentamicin
8. **Anaerobic organisms**	Metronidazole

and *N. meningitidis* infection. *S. pneumoniae* needs antibiotic therapy for two weeks whereas *L. monocytogenes* and gram-negative bacilli infections require a 3-week therapy.

Adjunctive Therapy

The use of dexamethasone has decreased morbidity and mortality in pneumococcal meningitis in adults. This is also beneficial in pneumococcal and *H. influenzae* meningitis in infants and children. Ten milligrams of dexamethasone is given 15–20 minutes before or concurrent with the first dose of antibiotic. Therapy is continued at the same dosage every 6 hours for 4 days.

Supportive Therapy

Patients with raised intracranial pressure (ICP) are managed in intensive care unit. Intravenous mannitol, hyperventilation and elevation of patient's head to 30 degree are measures to reduce ICP.

Prevention of Meningococcal Infection

- Persons in close contact with patients of meningococcal meningitis should be given oral rifampicin for 2 days (adult: 600 mg 12 hourly, children: 10 mg/kg 12 hourly). Alternatively, adults can be given single dose of ciprofloxacin (750 mg), azithromycin (500 mg) or intramuscular ceftriaxone (250 mg)
- Vaccines are available against meningococci of group A and C and *H. influenza*.

Complications

Sensorineural hearing loss, decreased intellectual functions, seizures, memory impairment and gait disturbances are the main complications of bacterial meningitis.

Viral Meningitis

Involvement of meninges may occur in viral infections which primarily affect other organs. Most common viruses are enteroviruses (coxsackie, echo, polio virus). Others are mumps, measles, influenza, herpes zoster, herpes simplex, HIV, EBV and hepatitis.

- Headache is the main feature
- Neck rigidity is generally present. Kernig's and Brudzinski's signs are usually absent
- Seizures and focal neurological deficit generally do not occur
- Sensorium may be mildly altered
- Other features are fever, myalgia, malaise, anorexia, vomiting and abdominal pain
- CSF examination reveals a rise in cell count, mostly lymphocytes, slightly increased protein and normal sugar **(Table 8.16)**.

Treatment is supportive. However, acyclovir may be useful in severe cases of herpes simplex, varicella zoster or EBV meningitis. The course is generally benign and self limiting.

Subacute/Chronic Meningitis

The patients with subacute/chronic meningitis present insidiously. Common pathogens are *Mycobacterium tuberculosis*, atypical mycobacteria, fungi (*Cryptococcus, histoplasma*) and spirochetes (*Treponema pallidum*).

Tuberculous Meningitis

Meningeal involvement by the *Mycobacterium tuberculosis* may occur through hematogenous spread in cases of primary or postprimary pulmonary disease. The rupture of the brain tubercle into the subarachnoid space may also cause meningitis. The meninges, especially at the base are covered with exudates and tubercles.

Clinical Features

The onset of symptoms is insidious; in some it may be acute. Patients have headache, vomiting, low grade fever and alteration in sensorium. Signs of meningeal irritation are present. Other signs are cranial nerve (oculomotor) palsies,

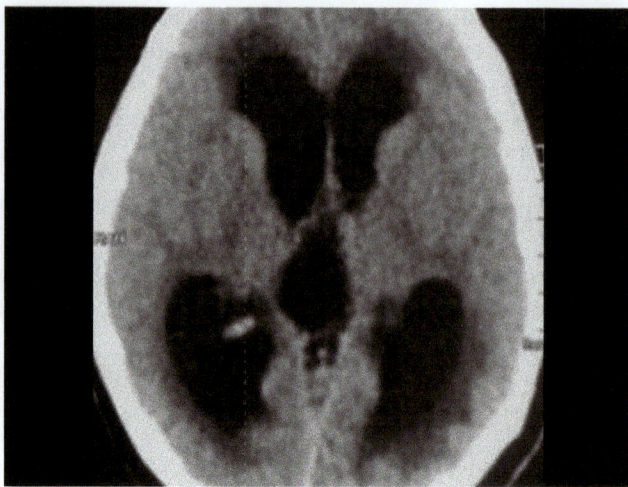

Fig. 8.9: CT scan head showing dilatation of ventricle suggestive of hydrocephalus.

papilledema and focal neurological deficit. Hydrocephalus is a common complication **(Fig. 8.9)**.

Investigation

- CSF examination
    - The CSF is straw-colored clear but when allowed to stand, a fine clot (spider web) is formed
    - There is high lymphocyte count, high protein and low glucose
    - In acute cases, polymorphs may predominate
    - The AFB stain may be positive. Culture for AFB is positive in 80% cases **(Table 8.16)**.
- CT or MRI brain may show meningeal enhancement or hydrocephalus.

Treatment

Antitubercular treatment should be started as soon as possible **(Table 8.20)**. A combination of rifampicin, isoniazid, pyrazinamide and ethambutol or streptomycin is given for 8 weeks. Rifampicin, isoniazid and ethambutol are continued for the next 7-10 months. Pyridoxine is added to prevent isoniazid toxicity, addition of steroids for initial few weeks increases survival and reduces complications. Mortality is high if treatment is delayed.

Table 8.20: Treatment of tubercular meningitis in adults.	
Drugs	**Dosage**
Rifampicin	10 mg/kg/day
Isoniazid	300 mg/day
Pyrazinamide	30 mg/kg /day in divided doses
Ethambutol	15-25 mg/kg/day
Sreptomycin	0.75-1.0 g IM daily
Pyridoxine	20-40 mg/day
Dexamethasone	12-16 mg per day for 3 weeks, then tapered over 3 weeks

Complications

Complications like hydrocephalus, focal deficits and cranial nerve palsies may occur. These are seen more commonly in cases where treatment is delayed.

Fungal Meningitis

Fungal meningitis usually occurs in the immunocompromised individuals. Its incidence has gone up due to emergence of HIV disease. Cryptococcal meningitis is an important opportunistic infection in HIV patients. Biochemical and cytological findings in CSF are similar to that of tuberculous meningitis. The diagnosis can be confirmed by microscopy (India ink preparation for Cryptococcus) and specific serological tests. The treatment of cryptococcal meningitis in HIV inection is amphotericin B plus flucytosine for at least 2 weeks, followed by oral fluconazole for a minimum of 8 weeks. HIV infected patients may require lifelong fluconazole 200 mg/day as maintenance therapy.

HEADACHE

Headache is one of the most common symptoms. In most cases, it is benign in nature. Occasionally, it may be the manifestation of serious illness such as brain tumor, intracranial hemorrhage, meningitis and temporal arteritis. Pain producing intracranial structures are the scalp, dural sinuses, middle meningeal artery, falx cerebri and proximal parts of large pial arteries.

Pathological Basis of Headache

- The distension, stretching and irritation of the pain sensitive intracranial structures such as dura mater and proximal parts of the blood vessels cause headache
- Brain parenchyma, cerebral ventricles, choroids plexus, pial veins are insensitive to pain
- Inflammation and trauma to cranial and cervical muscles and irritation of cranial and spinal nerves may also lead to headache.

Classification

The headache is classified as primary and secondary **(Table 8.21)**. Secondary headache has underlying cause and the clinical features vary accordingly. The mechanism of primary headache is poorly known and it is probably due to disturbances in serotonergic neurotransmission.

Approach to a Case of Headache

A detailed history is important in the case of headache. The onset, severity and the site of headache are important.
- Acute severe headache may suggest subarachnoid hemorrhage or meningitis

Table 8.21: Causes of headache.
Primary headache disorders • Migraine • Tension-type headache • Trigeminal autonomic cephalgias including Cluster headache
Secondary headache *Intracranial causes* • Subdural and intracerebral hematoma • Subarachnoid hemorrhage • Brain abscess, meningitis, encephalitis • Obstructive hydrocephalus • Vasculitis • Benign intracranial hypertension (Pseudotumor cerebri) • Cerebral ischemia or infarction *Extracranial causes* • Giant cell arteritis (temporal arteritis) • Sinusitis • Glaucoma • Optic neuritis • Dental diseases • Temporomandibular joint disease • Disease of cervical spine *Systemic causes* • Fever, hypoxia, hypercapnia, hypertension, anemia, allergy • Drugs (nitrates) • Depression

Table 8.22: Symptoms that suggest a serious underlying disorder.
• First severe headache • Worst headache ever • Abnormal neurologic examination • Fever or systemic signs • Vomiting preceding headache • Pain increased by cough, lifting and bending • Pain that disturbs sleep • Onset after 55 years of age • Associated local tenderness

- Subarachnoid hemorrhage presents as sudden onset severe headache that reaches maximal intensity within seconds or few minutes (thunderclap headache)
- Hemicranial headache is a feature of migraine
- Inquiry should be made about precipitating factors like alcohol, emotional stress, foods or medications
- Chewing movements may exacerbate the pain due to temporomandibular joint disease, trigeminal neuralgia and glossopharyngeal neuralgia
- Rebound headache occur in the setting of chronic use of pain killers or narcotics
- Temporal arteritis is characterized by dull unilateral headache in patients of more than 60 years of age. Temporal artery is thick and palpable. Other associated features are jaw claudication, low grade fever, an elevated ESR and C reactive protein
- Depression can cause chronic treatment resistant headache. A detailed history and other signs of depression suggest the diagonosis.

Cranial CT or MRI is indicated if the onset of headache is at middle age, progressive headache that disturbs sleep, or is associated with neurological symptoms or signs. Symptoms that suggest a serious underlying disorder are given in **Table 8.22**.

Migraine

Migraine is a common cause of headache and it is more common in females. It is defined as episodes of unilateral throbbing headache, nausea and vomiting and/or symptoms of neurological dysfunctions. Following are different types of migraine:

- *Classical migraine:* Headache is characteristically associated with premonitory sensory, motor or visual symptoms (aura).
- *Common migraine:* There is headache without aura. It is most frequent type of migraine.
- *Migraine equivalent:* Rarely migraine can present with focal neurological deficit without headache.
- *Complicated migraine:* Migraine with transient focal neurological features or that leaves a persistent neurological deficit is called complicated migraine.

The headache typically starts with nonspecific prodromal symptoms like malaise and irritation followed by an aura of a focal neurological event. There is severe throbbing hemicranial headache with nausea, vomiting, photophobia and phonophobia. The patient prefers to be in quiet and darkened room and to go to sleep. The aggravating factors for the headache are menses, red wine, hunger, lack or excess of sleep, alcohol, emotional or physical stress, perfumes and oral contraceptive pills. The deactivators or relieving factors are sleep, pregnancy and drugs such as triptans. Family history of migraine is often present.

The most common aura is visual, which is in the form of scotomas, hallucinations and fortification spectra. The latter is *pathognomonic* for migraine and is characterized by silvery zigzag lines marching across the visual fields for 20–25 minutes.

Variants of Migraine

Basilar migraine: The neurological symptoms are in the form of vertigo, diplopia and dysarthria. These symptoms are followed by headache and impaired sensorium. Transient blindness may also occur, particularly in young females.

Ophthalmoplegic migraine: This is characterized by pain around the eye, nausea, vomiting and diplopia. Diplopia is due to transient external ophthalmoplegia mainly involving third cranial nerve and rarely sixth nerve.

Familial hemiplegic migraine: In this variant attack of migraine is associated with lateralized weakness as aura. It is inherited as autosomal dominant pattern.

Facial migraine (Carotidynia, lower-half headache): The pain occurs repeatedly in jaw, neck and periorbital area. There may be an associated throbbing headache. The pain is

Table 8.23: Drugs used in treatment of acute migraine.

Drug	Dosage	Maximum dose
Analgesics		
Acetminophen	500–650 mg q6–8 h	
Ibuprofen	400 mg q4–6 h	
Naproxen	220–550 mg bd	
Aspirin	325–650 mg q4–6 h	
5–HT 1 agonists		
Sumatriptan	50–100 mg tablet at onset, may repeat after 2 h	200 mg/day
	5–20 mg as nasal spray, may repeat after 2 h	40 mg/day
	6 mg SC, may repeat after 1 h	12 mg/day
Zolmitriptan	2.5 tablet at onset, may repeat after 2 h	10 mg/day
	5 mg as nasal spray, may repeat after 2 h	10 mg/day
Naratriptan	2.5 mg tablet at onset, may repeat after 4 h	5 mg/day
Rizatriptan	5–10 mg tablet at onset, may repeat after 2 h	30 mg/day
Almotrptan	12.5 tablet at onset, may repeat after 2 h	25 mg/day
Frovatriptan	2.5 tablet at onset, may repeat after 2 h	5 mg/day
Eletriptan	20–40 at onset, may repeat after 2 h	80 mg/day
Ergotamine	2 mg sublingual tablet at onset and q half an hour	3/day, 5/week
Ergotamine 1 mg, caffeine 100mg	1–2 tablet at onset, then 1 tablet q half an hour	6/day,10/week
Dihydroergotamine	0.5 mg nasal spray followed by second spray after 15 min	1 mg/day
	1 mg IV, IM, SC at onset, then q 1 h	3mg/d,6mg/wk
Dopamine Antagonists		
Metoclopramide	5–10 mg orally, 10 mg IV	
Prochlorperazine	10–25 mg or 10 mg IV	
Domperidone	10 mg orally	

accompanied with tenderness and prominent pulsations of cervical carotid artery. There may be soft tissue swelling over the artery. The condition is more common in older patients and it is generally precipitated by *dental trauma*.

Pathophysiology of Migraine

The mechanism of migraine is multifactorial and complex. It has definite genetic predisposition and is influenced by strong environmental components. Headache and related symptoms are caused by dilatation of the extracranial vessels whereas focal neurological dysfunctions are due to intracranial vasoconstriction. Neurotransmitters such as serotonin and dopamine are implicated in the genesis of the migraine. Other possible mechanisms are activation of dorsal raphe neurons in upper brainstem.

Treatment

Avoidance of trigger factors: The trigger factors are identified and best avoided. Alcohol, red wine, chocolate are avoided. Adequate sleep should be ensured. Meals should not be missed.

Treatment of acute attack
- Rest in a quite darkened room is helpful.
- Analgesics (aspirin, paracetamol and other NSAIDs) are usually effective if taken early at the onset of headache. This is often combined with dopamine antagonists (metoclopramide, domperidone, prochlorperazine). Drugs used in the treatment of acute attack are given in **Table 8.23**.
- Severe attacks may be treated with triptans (sumatriptan, zolmitriptan) and ergotamine. These are 5-HT (serotonin) agonists and are potent constrictors of extracranial vessels. Triptans can be given orally, subcutaneously or intranasally. The usual dose of sumatriptan is 6 mg subcutaneously repeated at one hour (not more than two doses per day) or 25-100 mg orally which may be repeated at 2 hours (maximum 200 mg/day). These are contraindicated in patients with coronary artery disease, uncontrolled hypertension and in hemiplegic and basilar migraine. Triptans can be combined with naproxen. They are avoided in pregnancy.
- Ergotamine is best effective when taken early during prodromal phase. The initial dose is 1-2 mg orally which may be repeated at every 30 minutes to a maximum of 10 mg per day or 16 mg per week. It is contraindicated in coronary artery disease and pregnancy. This is given orally often in combination with 100 mg caffeine. Dihydroergotamine (DHE) can be given parenterally (1-2 mg IM, SC) at the onset of the headache. Intravenous DHE (1 mg) along with prochlorperazine (5-10 mg) is effective during severe attacks.
- Narcotic analgesics (meperidine) can be used in severe acute attacks. However, this should not be used for chronic headaches to prevent addiction and tolerance.

Table 8.24: Prophylactic therapy of migraine.	
Drug	Dosage (daily)
Propranolol	80–320 mg
Amitriptyline	10–50 mg (at night)
Dothiepin	25–75 mg at night
Sodium valproate	400–1000 mg
Gabapentin	900–3600 mg
Topiramate	25–200 mg
Flunarizine	5–15 mg
Methysergide	4–8 mg
Verapamil	80–240 mg
Botulinum toxin A	IM injection by trained clinician
Metaprolol	50–200 mg
Nortryptiline	25–75 mg
Venlafaxine	75–150 mg
Pizotifen	2–8 mg
Candesartan	4–24 mg
Neuromodulation	
Riboflavin	400 mg

Prophylactic therapy: This is necessary if migrainous headache occurs more than 3 times a month or if attacks are unresponsive to abortive therapy and significant disability is associated with attacks. The drugs are taken daily. It may take 2–6 weeks before the drugs are effective. A prolonged treatment is required. Once the response is obtained, the dose can be tapered and withdrawn. The common drugs used for prophylaxis are given in **Table 8.24**. Most patients respond to low dose amitriptyline, propranolol or valproate.

Tension Headache

This is a very common type of headache which is experienced by the majority of the population at some time or the other.
- The headache is constant, generalized and may continue for weeks or months
- It is commonly described as a dull, tight, pressure or band-like sensation
- Pain is less noticeable when the patient is busy and becomes worse at the end of the day
- Emotional stress, noise and fatigue may precipitate the headache
- Unlike migraine, there is no photophobia, nausea, vomiting or focal neurological symptoms.

This responds poorly to analgesics. Management of underlying anxiety or depression often helps. Relaxation techniques like massage, hot baths and biofeedback are also helpful.

Cluster Headache (Migrainous Neuralgia)

- It is common in middle-aged males and there is no family history
- The pain occurs periodically at a specific time of the day, generally in the early morning. The pain is severe and lasts for 30–90 minutes. There is unilateral periorbital pain associated with nasal congestion, lacrimation, rhinorrhea or redness of the eye
- Horner's syndrome may occur during the attack
- Patients may remain asymptomatic for weeks or months before another bout of headache (cluster) occurs
- Alcohol triggers the attack.

Treatment of acute attack with oral drugs is unsatisfactory. Inhalation of 100% oxygen (7 L/minute for 15 minutes) is the most effective modality of treatment for acute attack. Subcutaneous sumatriptan (6 mg) may be effective.

Preventive therapy is generally effective. The drugs used are propranolol, amitriptyline, valproate, verapamil, cyproheptadine. Lithium carbonate and prednisolone are also effective.

Headache Due to Raised Intracranial Pressure

Headache due to raised intracranial pressure is worse in the morning upon waking and improves as the patient becomes upright. It may be associated with vomiting. It may worsen on bending forward, coughing or straining. The headache is relieved by simple analgesics.

Intracranial mass lesions and hydrocephalus are main causes of raised intracranial pressure. It is rare for mass lesion to present with severe headache alone; seizure or focal neurological deficits are usual presenting features.

FACIAL PAIN

The pain in the facial area may be due to various causes. Most cases are due to dental problems, trigeminal neuralgia, postherpetic neuralgia and atypical facial pain. Provocation of pain due to hot, cold or sweet foods is typical of dental origin. The stimulation by cold stimulus repeatedly induces dental pain whereas pain cannot be repeatedly induced in case of neuralgias. A list of important causes is given in **Table 8.25**.

Trigeminal Neuralgia

Trigeminal neuralgia *(tic douloureux)* occurs in middle-aged or elderly patients, more commonly in females. Pain occurs

Table 8.25: Causes of facial pain.
- Trigeminal neuralgia
- Atypical facial pain
- Postherpetic neuralgia
- Glossopharyngeal neuralgia
- Other causes:
  - Glaucoma
  - Sinusitis
  - Mastoiditis
  - Dental problems
  - Temporomandibular joint disease
  - Jaw pain due to angina pectoris
  - Giant cell arteritis

in the facial region supplied by second and third divisions of the trigeminal nerve.

Pathogenesis

There is demyelination of the trigeminal nerve root at the point of their entry into the pons. The demyelination is commonly due to the compression mainly by aberrant blood vessels (superior cerebellar artery, tortuous vein). In a few patients, it may occur due to multiple sclerosis or brainstem tumor.

Clinical Features

Trigeminal neuralgia is characterized by episodes of sudden, severe, sharp lancinating pain in the area of lips, gums, cheek and chin. The pain lasts for a few seconds or sometimes persists for a minute or two. The pain is so severe that patients may flinch as if a motor tic (hence called tic douloureux). The pain is triggered by chewing, speaking, smiling and touching trigger zones in the trigeminal territory. There is a tendency for remissions and relapses.

Examination does not reveal any neurological sign. Presence of neurological signs and sensory loss suggest multiple sclerosis or posterior fossa tumor.

Investigations

CT and MRI may be needed to detect the underlying cause such as multiple sclerosis and tumors. High resolution MR angiography is helpful in visualizing aberrant vessels.

Treatment

Medical: The drug of choice is carbamazepine (up to 1200 mg/day) or oxcarbazepine. If not controlled, other drugs such as phenytoin (300–400 mg daily), topiramate (50 mg twice daily), lamotrigene (400 mg daily) or gabapentin (up to 2400 mg/day) are tried alone or in combination. Baclofen (10–20 mg thrice a day) may be used alone or in combination with carbamazepine or phenytoin.

Surgical: This is tried when medical treatment fails.
- The most common therapy is heat lesion of the trigeminal ganglion or nerve *(radiofrequency thermal rhizotomy)*
- Injection of *alcohol* in Meckel's cave has been practiced in the past. Excessive damage of the nerve may lead to loss of sensation in the face (anesthesia dolorosa)
- *Posterior craniotomy and microvascular decompression* is quite effective and generally done in younger patients
- *Gamma radiosurgery* to the trigeminal root is a recent noninvasive effective tool to treat trigeminal neuralgia.

Atypical Facial Pain

Atypical facial pain occurs usually in middle-aged depressed females. It is a constant pain often burning type which is centered on the maxilla, but may spread to the rest of the face on the affected side. Sometimes it may involve other side of the face, neck or back of the head. Tricyclic antidepressant, analgesics, carbamazepine or phenytoin may be tried. The response to therapy is poor.

Glossopharyngeal Neuralgia

Glossopharyngeal nerve (IX cranial nerve) supplies taste sensation to the posterior one-third of the tongue and sensation to the posterior pharynx (along with X nerve). Glossopharyngeal neuralgia is similar in quality to trigeminal neuralgia but is less common. Pain occurs on one side of the throat in the area of tonsillar fossa which may radiate to the ear. In some the pain may remain localized in the ear. The pain may be initiated by swallowing, coughing, chewing or yawning. Pain may be accompanied by syncope in some cases. Sensory and motor examination is normal. No cause is demonstrable in most cases; however, multiple sclerosis may be responsible for the pain in some.

Medical treatment is the same as for trigeminal neuralgia. Carbamazepine or *oxcarbazepine* is the drug of choice. Microvascular decompression and partial rhizotomy can be done in refractory cases.

Postherpetic Neuralgia

Postherpetic neuralgia is the complication of *herpes zoster* (shingles) infection. It occurs more commonly in elderly patients when first division of trigeminal nerve is involved **(Fig. 8.10)**. Pain is continuous and burning in character throughout the affected territory of trigeminal nerve. Even a light touch may precipitate the pain. Pain may last for years. Simple analgesics may be helpful. Phenytoin (300 mg/day), carbamazepine (up to 1,200 mg/day), gabapentin (up to 3,200 mg/day) may be tried if analgesics fail to control the pain. Tricyclic agents (amitryptiline) alone or along with phenothiazine are often effective in severe cases.

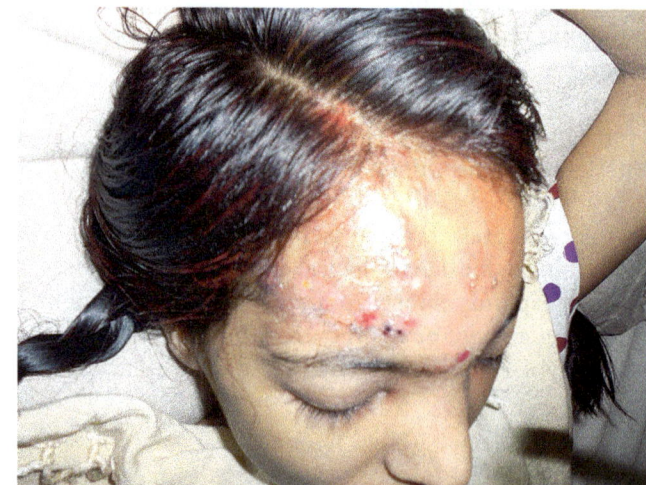

Fig. 8.10: Herpes zoster involving first division (ophthalmic) of trigeminal nerve.

FACIAL NERVE PALSY

The facial nerve (VII cranial nerve) arises from the pons, passes through the facial canal and exits from the skull though stylomastoid foramina. It then passes through the parotid gland and subsequently divides into branches **(Fig. 8.11)**. It provides motor innervation to all muscles of the facial expression and the stapedius. Through its branch, the chorda tympani, it carries taste sensation from the anterior two-third of the tongue. It also carries cutaneous impulses from the anterior wall of the external auditory canal (see also 'examination of the cranial nerve').

Features of Facial Nerve Palsy

The findings of motor lesion of unilateral facial nerve are as follows:
- There is loss of facial expression at the side of the palsy.
- Furrows of the forehead are absent
- The eye is more widely open and the eyelids do not close completely on the side of lesion **(Fig. 8.12)**
- There is drooping of the corner of the mouth. When the patient is asked to smile or show his teeth, the angle of the mouth at the side of the lesion does not move **(Fig. 8.13)**
- There is loss of nasolabial fold on the affected side **(Fig. 8.13)**
- On attempted closure of the eyelids, the eye ball on the paralyzed side rolls up (Bell's phenomenon). It is a normal phenomenon which is preserved and can be visualized in facial nerve paralysis
- Food collects between teeth and the lips
- Saliva dribbles from the angle of the mouth on the paralyzed side
- The patient is unable to whistle or blow
- If the nerve to stapedius is damaged, there is hyperacusis (sensitivity to loud sounds).

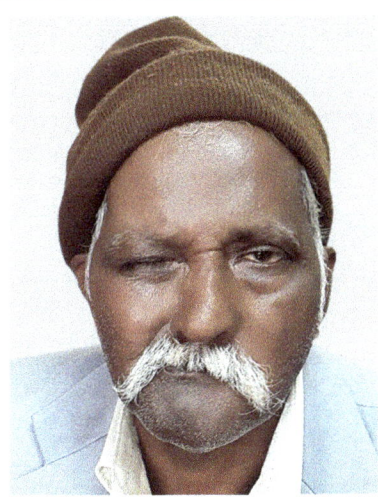

Fig. 8.12: Left sided infranuclear palsy of VII cranial nerve showing loss of nasolabial fold, drooping of angle of mouth and lack of closure of eye on left side.

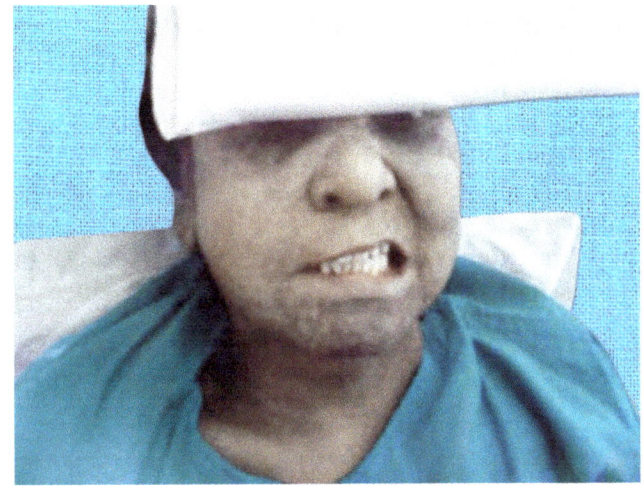

Fig. 8.13: Facial nerve palsy (There is loss of nasolabial fold and drooping of angle of mouth on right side).

There is loss of taste in the anterior two-third of the tongue on the same side. There is no sensory loss over the face.

Causes of Facial Nerve Palsy

The involvement of facial nerve at its origin in the pons or at any site throughout its course may lead to infranuclear facial palsy (lower motor neuron type). The causes of the lesion at different sites are given in **Table 8.26**. Important causes of supranuclear palsy are cerebral thrombosis, cerebral embolism, cerebral hemorrhage and brain tumor.

Melkersson-Rosenthal syndrome is triad of recurrent facial nerve palsy, recurrent facial edema and plication of tongue.

Ramsay Hunt syndrome is a complication of herpes zoster infection of geniculate ganglion associated with facial palsy and vesicular eruption in external auditory canal and pharynx.

Facial diplegia is bilateral facial infranuclear palsy seen in Guillain-Barré syndrome and sarcoidosis.

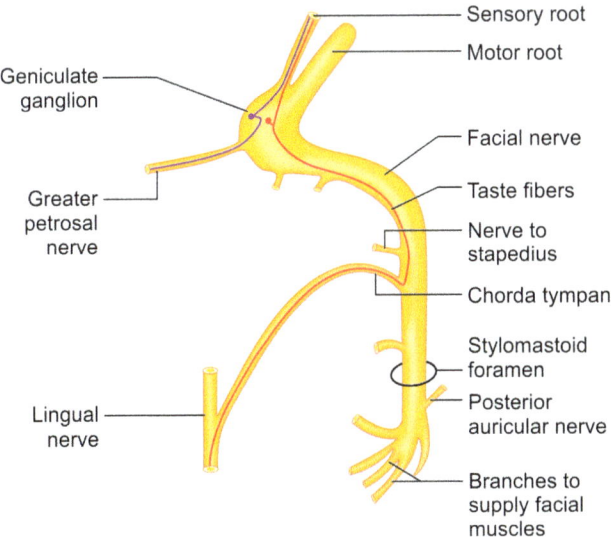

Fig. 8.11: Pathway of VII cranial nerve.

Table 8.26: Causes of infranuclear facial nerve palsy.	
Pons	Infarction, tumor, multiple sclerosis
Cerebellopontine angle	Acoustic neuroma
Temporal bone	Chronic suppuratve otitis media (CSOM), cholesteatoma, Bell's palsy, Ramsay Hunt syndrome, dermoid, carotid body tumor
Outside skull	Parotid lesions, trauma, lymph node swelling
Others	Guillain-Barré syndrome, sarcoidosis (Uveoparotid fever, Heerfordt syndrome), diabetes mellitus, leprosy, lyme disease, Melkersson-Rosenthal syndrome

Table 8.27: Features of supranuclear and infranuclear facial palsy.	
Supranuclear facial palsy	Infranuclear facial palsy
Upper motor neuron lesion	Lower motor neuron lesion
Upper part of face relatively spared	Whole face involved
May be associated with aphasia	Aphasia not present
Usually accompanied with hemiplegia on same side (un-crossed hemiplegia)	May be accompanied with hemiplegia on opposite side (crossed hemiplegia)
Taste sensation not involved	Taste sensation may be involved
Emotional facial movement preserved	Emotional facial movement not preserved

Localization of the Site of Lesion in Infranuclear Facial Palsy

- *Lesion outside the stylomastoid foramina:*
  - If the lesion of the facial nerve is outside the stylomastoid foramen, only motor manifestations are present.
  - Taste is not involved as chorda tympani joins the facial nerve in the facial canal before the facial nerve emerges from the stylomastoid foramen.
  - There is no hyperacusis.
- *Lesion in the temporal bone:*
  - The lesion of the facial nerve in facial canal near the middle ear may cause hyperacusis in addition to loss of taste.
  - Other cranial nerves (auditory and vestibular) are also involved if the lesion is near the internal auditory meatus.
- *Lesion in the pons:* In the pontine lesion, sixth cranial nerve may also be involved and there may be hemiplegia of the opposite side (crossed hemiplegia).

If the recovery of motor function is incomplete, aberrant regeneration can cause synkinesis, i.e., movement of one muscle can cause movement of another or all muscles; for example, closure of eye can cause deviation of the angle of the mouth. Lacrimal gland fibers may join with fibers of other muscles so that while eating, tears may also flow *(crocodile tears)*. Orbicularis oculi fibers may join with orbicularis oris resulting in the closure of eyelids when the mouth is opened *(jaw winking)*.

Supranuclear Facial Palsy

The damage of corticonuclear fibers from motor cortex to facial nucleus may cause supranuclear facial palsy (upper motor neuron type). The infranuclear facial paralysis must be differentiated from supranuclear type of facial palsy **(Table 8.27)**.

In supranuclear facial palsy, the upper part of the face (frontalis, orbicularis oculi) is involved to a lesser extent than the lower part of the face whereas whole of the face is equally involved in infranuclear facial palsy. This is because upper part of the face is innervated by both motor cortices whereas the lower part of the face is innervated by the opposite hemisphere only.

- Supranuclear facial palsy is often associated with paralysis of the arm and leg of the same side or aphasia
- The taste sensation in the anterior two-third of the tongue is not involved in supranuclear type
- Emotional facial movements are also preserved in supranuclear type
- In supranuclear type, the lesion is on the opposite side of the palsy whereas it is on the same side of the palsy in infranuclear type
- Important causes of supranuclear palsy are cerebral thrombosis, cerebral embolism, cerebral hemorrhage and brain tumor.

Bell's Palsy

This is the most common type of facial palsy. It is a type of idiopathic infranuclear (lower motor neuron type) facial palsy, the cause of which is not known. The site of involvement is facial canal. Bell's palsy has been associated with reactivation of herpes simplex type I infection, but its causal role is not established.

Clinical Features

Onset is abrupt or subacute and the maximum weakness occurs in 48 hours. Pain around the ear may occur prior to or along with the weakness. Motor manifestations are the same as described earlier. Bell's phenomenon is present. There is loss of taste in the anterior two-thirds of the tongue on the same side. Hyperacusis occurs on the side of lesion if nerve to stapedius is also involved. There may be diminished salivation and tear secretion.

Investigations

MRI may show swelling and enhancement of geniculate ganglion and facial nerve. EMG has prognostic value.

Treatment

Most patients have complete recovery without treatment because lesion is mild and limited to conduction block only.

Symptomatic: This includes massage of the facial muscles and protection of the eye during sleep to prevent corneal damage. A lubricating eye drop is used to avoid dryness.

Specific: Administration of glucocorticoids with or without acyclovir improves the outcome. The dose of prednisolone is 60–80 mg daily for 5 days and then tapered over the next 5 days. Acyclovir is given in a dosage of 400 mg 5 times daily for 10 days. Combination of prednisolone with acyclovir is more effective than prednisolone alone.

Cosmetic surgery is helpful in restoring symmetry of the face in patients with permanent paralysis.

Prognosis

Over 80% of the patients recover completely in a few weeks time. Patients with complete paralysis have a less favorable prognosis than those with incomplete paralysis.

CEREBROVASCULAR DISEASES

Cerebrovascular diseases mainly include ischemic stroke, hemorrhagic stroke and vascular anomalies such as intracranial aneurysms and arteriovenous malformation. The incidence of cerebrovascular diseases increases with age.

- *Stroke or cerebrovascular accident* are characterized by abrupt onset of symptoms and neurologic deficits attributable to focal vascular cause
- Ischemia may be transient and there may be recovery from the neurological deficit within few hours but always within 24 hours. This is known as *Transient ischemic attack (TIA)*. TIAs are usually embolic. TIA is a risk factor for future stroke
- A reversible ischemic neurological deficit (RIND) is similar to TIA persisting for >24 hours but resolves within a week
- In some patients, the deficit continues to worsen after about 6 hours of the onset (***stroke-in-evolution***).

Causes

Stroke may be ischemic (thrombotic and embolic) or hemorrhagic. Important causes of stroke are given in **Table 8.28**. Risk factors for stroke are given in **Table 8.29**.

Clinical Manifestations

There is an acute onset of neurological dysfunction. The presentation is variable and depends upon the vessel involved. Patients generally present with headache, sudden loss of consciousness and seizures.

- Involvement in the carotid artery area (anterior circulation) leads to hemiplegia (weakness of upper and lower limbs of one side) and cortical sensory loss on the opposite side of the involved hemisphere
- Aphasia (loss of speech) may occur in left hemispheric involvement
- Vertebrobasilar strokes (posterior circulation) produce unilateral or bilateral motor sensory deficits of cranial nerves and brainstem signs. Symptoms like vertigo, nausea, vomiting, dizziness, dysarthria, ataxia are more common in posterior circulation strokes
- Sudden onset of severe headache and neck rigidity suggests subarachnoid hemorrhage.

Table 8.28: Causes of stroke.

Ischemic stroke
Thrombosis
- Lacunar infarction
- Large vessel thrombosis

Embolic
- From artery
  - Carotid bifurcation
- Cardioembolic
  - Atrial fibrillation
  - Myocardial infarction
  - Infective endocarditis
  - Valvular lesions

Others
- Hypercoagulable states
- Vasculitis
- Meningitis

Hemorrhagic
- Hypertension
- Trauma
- Anticoagulant therapy
- Aneurysm
- AV malformation
- Blood dyscrasias
- Brain tumor

Table 8.29: Risk factors for stroke.

- Hypertension
- Heart diseases (AF, CHF, IE)
- Diabetes mellitus
- Smoking
- Hyperlipidemia
- Age (old age)
- Gender (male)
- Previous vascular event (MI, stroke, peripheral embolism)

(AF, atrial fibrillation; CHF, congestive heart failure; IE, infective endocarditis; MI, myocardial infarction)

Investigations

- CT or MRI head is performed to diagnose the type (ischemic or hemorrhagic) and site of lesion **(Figs. 8.14, 8.15A and B)**
- Other tests done are carotid Doppler (to diagnose carotid stenosis), echocardiography (to rule out cardiac lesions) and CSF analysis
- Complete blood count, platelet count, PT, APTT and electrolytes are also performed

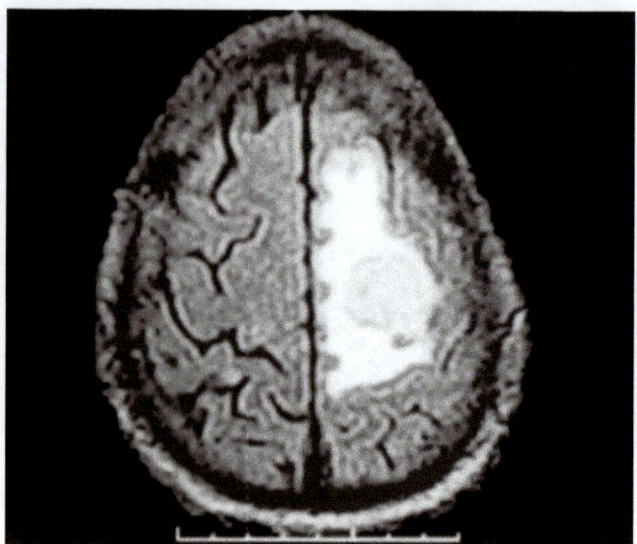

Fig. 8.14: MRI brain showing intracerebral hemorrhage.

- Tests such as blood sugar, lipid profile and ECG are done to find out the presence of risk factors
- Specific tests may be needed to diagnose an uncommon underlying cause.

Treatment

Following are the main components of management of ischemic stroke:
- *Medical support:* The patient should be urgently hospitalized. The medical management includes control of blood pressure, maintenance of fluid and electrolytes and control of intracranial pressure (with IV mannitol).
- *Thrombolysis:* This is indicated in early ischemic stroke within 3 hours of onset of symptoms. Recombinant tissue plasminogen activator (rTPA) is used for thrombolysis.
- *Endovascular mechanical embolectomy:* It is indicated in patients with large vessel intracranial occlusion within 6 hours of stroke onset, when there is contraindication to using thrombolysis or there is failure to achieve recanalization with thrombolytics.

- Aspirin in doses of 160–325 mg daily is indicated for acute and long-term management of ischemic stroke.
- Anticoagulation is required to prevent recurrent embolic strokes. Warfarin is used for chronic anticoagulation and the target INR should be 2–3 (in case of prosthetic valve 2.5–3.5). Direct-acting oral anticoagulants (DOACs) are as effective as warfarin for stroke prevention in patients with atrial fibrillation. Different DOACs are dabigatran, rivaroxaban, apixaban and edoxaban. Generally monitoring is not required in case of DOACs therapy.
- Carotid endarterectomy is indicated in patients with >70% carotid stenosis. It decreases the risk of stroke and death.
- Modification of risk factors includes the control of blood pressure, blood sugar, serum lipids and cessation of smoking.
- Physiotherapy and rehabilitation.

Management of Hemorrhagic Stroke

Patients should be admitted in intensive care unit for monitoring and supportive care. The details are given in **Tables 8.30 and 8.31**.

IMPLICATIONS ON DENTAL PRACTICE

- In patients of epilepsy, fixed prosthesis is placed rather than removable appliances because latter may dislodge during the seizure.

Table 8.30: Management of Intracerebral hemorrhage.
• Control of blood pressure by IV agents like labetalol
• Thrombocytopenia is to be managed by platelet transfusion
• Coagulopathies are managed with fresh frozen plasma (FFP), Vit K or specific agents as needed
• Decompression surgery may be needed in some cases to reduce mass effect and prevent herniation
• Ventricular drainage may be required in acute hydrocephalus in cases of intraventricular hemorrhage
• Surgical evacuation may ne required in patients with cerebellar hemorrhage with acute hydrocephalus or brainstem compression.

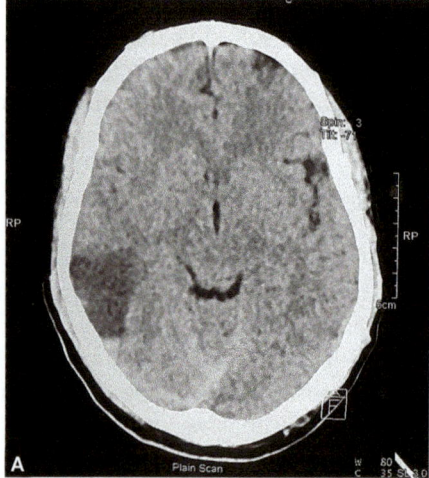 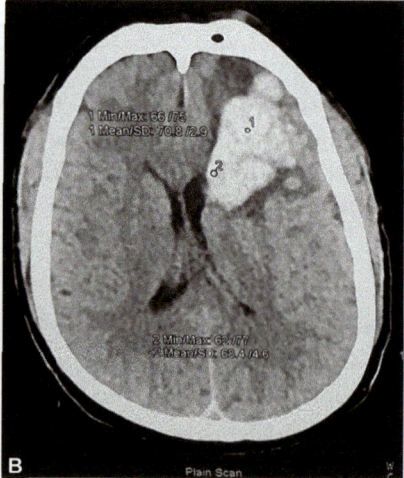

Figs. 8.15A and B: (A) CT scan head showing brain infarction; (B) CT scan head showing intracerebral hemorrhage.

Table 8.31: Management of subarachnoid hemorrhage.

- Bed rest is advised to conscious patients, exertion or straining should be avoided.
- Headache should be treated by analgesics.
- Control of blood pressure (systolic < 140 mmHg)
- Anticonvulsants are given to prevent seizures
- Nimodipine 60 mg 4 hourly is given for 3 weeks to prevent arterial spasm
- Intraventricular cerebrospinal fluid shunting is done in patients with acute hydrocephalus
- Monitoring of serum sodium (renal salt wasting can cause hyponatremia)
- Clipping of the aneurysm or coil embolization is done to prevent further hemorrhage

- Gingival growth occurs in patients taking phenytoin.
- There is no need to increase the dose of anticonvulsant therapy in well-controlled epilepsy prior to dental treatment. Routine use of sedation is not indicated.
- Seizure may occur during the dental procedures. Hence, one should be aware of the management of patients during seizures.
- Drugs may precipitate seizures or may interfere with the anticonvulsant drugs. Avoidance or the dose adjustment of the drugs may be required.
- Accumulation of food debris in the vestibule and the plaque on the teeth may occur on the affected side in cases of facial palsy. Saliva may trickle from the angle of mouth and lead to angular stomatitis.
- There is loss of taste in the anterior two-third of the tongue on the same side and there may be diminished salivation and tear secretion in Bell's palsy.
- CSF leak (CSF rhinorrhea) and recurrent bacterial meningitis may occur as a result of maxillofacial fracture involving the cribriform plate of the ethmoid.
- Patients with maxillofacial injuries should be given prophylactic antibiotics because of risk of bacterial meningitis.
- Patients with trigeminal neuralgia may develop oral complications as they may be reluctant to brush their teeth.
- Migrainous neuralgia must be differentiated from pain of dental origin by careful history and examination.
- Elective dental care should be deferred for 6 months in a patient with stroke since there is a risk of developing another stroke.
- Stroke should be considered in patients who develop sudden loss of consciousness or neurological deficits during dental surgery.

SELF ASSESSMENT

Multiple Choice Questions

1. **Which is true in Bell's palsy?**
   A. Is lower motor neuron lesion
   B. Is always bilateral
   C. May be caused by a cerebellopontine angle tumor
   D. All of the above

2. **Sodium valproate is an:**
   A. Antiepileptic drug   B. Antihypertensive drug
   C. Antithyroid drug   D. Antidiabetic drug

3. **Most effective drug for trigeminal neuralgia is:**
   A. Carbamazepine   B. Clonazepam
   C. Phenobarbitone   D. Ibuprofen

4. **The most common cause of facial nerve palsy, proximal to its branching in parotid is:**
   A. Bell's palsy   B. Ramsay-Hunt syndrome
   C. Acoustic neuroma   D. Brainstem diseases

5. **CSF glucose levels are normal in following type of meningitis:**
   A. Tubercular   B. Bacterial (pyogenic)
   C. Viral   D. Fungal

6. **Marked increase in polymorphs in CSF is a feature of which type of meningitis?**
   A. Pyogenic   B. Tubercular
   C. Viral   D. Fungal

7. **Which of the following is a cause of upper motor neuron facial palsy?**
   A. Bell's palsy
   B. Sarcoidosis
   C. Chronic suppurative otitis media (CSOM)
   D. Sroke (Cerebrovascular accident)

8. **In status epilepticus, the initial drug to be given is:**
   A. Phenytoin   B. Diazepam
   C. Phenobarbitone D. Carbamazepine

9. **Drug of choice for partial seizures is:**
   A. Phenytoin   B. Clonazepam
   C. Carbamazepine D. Gabapentin

10. **Which one is not true about trigeminal neuralgia:**
    A. Mainly occurs in middle-aged and elderly
    B. Pain lasts only for few seconds
    C. Ophthalmic division of trigeminal nerve is most commonly involved
    D. Neurological examination is normal (no motor or sensory deficit)

11. **Probable site of lesion in Bell's palsy is?**
    A. Within parotid gland   B. Brainstem
    C. Cerebellopontine angle D. Within facial canal

12. **Which one is not true about Bell's palsy:**
    A. Presence of hyperacusis
    B. Taste sensation is impaired
    C. Spontaneous recovery is common
    D. Treatment of choice is carbamazepine and acyclovir

13. **Side effects of phenytoin do not include:**
    A. Osteomalacia   B. Gum hypertrophy
    C. Folate deficiency D. Blindness

14. **Following is not seen in upper motor neuron facial lesion:**
    A. Loss of nasolabial fold
    B. Inability to blow or whistle
    C. Loss of wrinkles over forehead
    D. Dribbling of saliva on the side of palsy

15. **Ramsay-Hunt syndrome is characterized by all, except:**
    A. Presence of vesicles over external auditory canal
    B. Ipsilateral facial nerve palsy
    C. Cause is herpes simplex of geniculate ganglion
    D. Lower motor type of lesion

16. Which of the following opportunistic meningeal infection is commonly seen in AIDS?
    A. Cryptococcus   B. Candida
    C. Aspergillus   D. Histoplasma
17. Drugs useful in treatment of status epilepticus are all, *except*:
    A. Phenytoin   B. Phenobarbitone
    C. Clonazepam   D. Midazolam
18. Tongue bite, incontinence of urine or stools, cry and cyanosis are features of:
    A. Petit mal seizures   B. Grand mal seizures
    C. Myoclonic seizures   D. Partial seizures
19. Jacksonian march is seen in:
    A. Simple partial seizures   B. Petit mal seizures
    C. Grand mal seizures   D. Complex partial seizures
20. Neck rigidity, altered sensorium and skin rashes suggest:
    A. Meningococcal meningitis
    B. Pneumococcal meningitis
    C. *H. influenzae* meningitis
    D. Tubercular meningitis
21. Neck rigidity is present in:
    A. Posterior fossa tumor
    B. Meningitis
    C. Subarachnoid hemorrhage
    D. All of the above
22. Gum hypertrophy can occur with the use of:
    A. Calcium channel blockers
    B. Phenytoin
    C. Cyclosporine   D. All of the above
23. The consciousness is not impaired in:
    A. Grand mal seizures   B. Status epilepticus
    C. Simple partial seizures D. Complex partial seizures
24. All are features of common migraine, *except*:
    A. Unilateral headache   B. Visual symptoms
    C. Vomiting   D. Premonitory symptoms (Aura)
25. Which one is not true about "Cluster headache"?
    A. It is common in males
    B. Pain occurs periodically at a specific time of the day
    C. Severe pain lasting about 24–48 hours
    D. Pain is associated with nasal congestion and lacrimation
26. Which one is not effective in acute attack of migraine:
    A. Sumatriptan   B. Paracetamol
    C. Amitriptyline   D. Ergotamine
27. Most common cause of pyogenic meningitis in children is:
    A. *S. pneumonae*   B. *N. meningitidis*
    C. *H. influenzae*   D. *Listeria monocytogenes*
28. All of the following are used for prophylaxis of migraine, *except*:
    A. Topiramate   B. Valproate
    C. Gabapentin   D. Levetiracetam
29. Most common organism causing community acquired meningitis in adults is:
    A. *S. peumoniae*   B. *H. infuenzae*
    C. *N. meningitidis* D. *Listeria monocytogenes*
30. CSF examination of suspected meningitis patient shows protein = 412 mg %, glucose = 442 mg %, cell count of 314/ cubic mm with polymorphs 92%. Most likely diagnosis of:
    A. Acute bacterial meningitis
    B. Acute viral meningitis
    C. Tuberculous meningitis
    D. Cryptococcal meningitis
31. "Thunderclap headache" is a feature of:
    A. Migraine   B. Subarachnoid hemorrhage
    C. Cluster headache   D. Trigeminal neuralgia
32. Which of the following drug is not used in status epilepticus?
    A. Lorazepam   B. Phenytoin
    C. Midazolam   D. Gabapentin

Fill in the Blanks

1. Weakness of the involved part following motor seizure is called _____.
2. Tic douloureux is _____.
3. Anesthesia dolorosa is a complication of _____.
4. Most frequent type of migraine is _____.
5. The cell count in the normal CSF is _____.
6. Spider web is formed in the CSF of patients with _____ meningitis.
7. India ink preparation is used to diagnose _____ infection.
8. Hyperacusis is due to paralysis of _____ muscle.
9. Taste sensation from anterior two-third of the tongue is carried by _____ nerve.
10. Complex partial seizures generally arise from _____ lobes.
11. Rifampicin is used for the prophylaxis of _____.
12. Waterhouse-Friedreichsen syndrome is a complication of _____.
13. Most effective modality of treatment in cluster headache is _____.
14. Sumatriptan is contraindicated in patients with _____ and _____.
15. Recurrent meningitis can result from fracture of _____.

CHAPTER 9

Endocrine and Metabolic Disorders

THYROID DISORDERS

Anatomy of thyroid gland: The thyroid gland is situated in the neck anterior to the thyroid cartilage. It weighs around 15–20 g in the adult. The thyroid gland has two lobes, the right and the left, joined by an isthmus.

Physiology: It secretes mainly thyroxin (T_4) and a small amount of triiodothyronine (T_3).
- T_3 is the active form of the hormone. Most of the T_4 is converted into T_3 in peripheral tissues such as liver, muscles and kidneys.
- Thyroid hormones are carried in plasma, predominantly in the bound form with a plasma protein [thyroid binding globulin, (TBG)], while only a small amount circulates unbound (free hormone).
- Only the free form can enter cells and exerts its metabolic action.

Regulation of thyroid hormone secretion: The production of thyroid hormones is stimulated by the thyroid stimulating hormone (thyrotropin, TSH), released by the anterior pituitary in response to the hypothalamic thyrotropin releasing hormone (TRH). There is a negative feedback effect of thyroid hormone on the pituitary gland so that TSH secretion is suppressed if the level of thyroid hormone is raised or *vice versa* (**Fig. 9.1**).

Hypothyroidism

Hypothyroidism is more common in females. It can be due to either:
- Primary disorders of the thyroid gland (primary hypothyroidism), or
- Decreased TSH secretion by the pituitary gland (secondary hypothyroidism).

Causes of hypothyroidism are given in **Table 9.1**. The most common cause of hypothyroidism worldwide is iodine deficiency. However, in areas where iodine deficiency is not

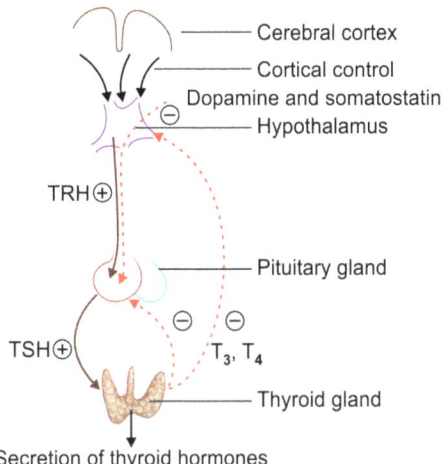

Fig. 9.1: Feedback control of thyroid hormone.

Table 9.1: Causes of hypothyroidism.

Primary hypothyroidism
- Spontaneous atrophic
- Post-thyroidectomy
- Following ^{131}I administration for hyperthyroidism
- Congenital
- Goitrous
- Hashimoto's thyroiditis
- Iodine deficiency
- Infiltrative disorders (sarcoidosis, amyloidosis, Riedel's thyroiditis)
- Drug induced (Lithium, amiodarone, methimazole, carbimazole, propylthiouracil)
- Genetic enzyme defects (Dyshormonogenesis)

Secondary hypothyroidism
- Hypopituitarism
- Post-surgery
- Post-radiation
- Pituitary tumor
- Sheehan's syndrome
- Infiltrative disorders
- Disorders of hypothalamus

present, the important causes are autoimmune thyroiditis (Hashimoto's thyroiditis) and iatrogenic.

Autoimmune hypothyroidism is initially associated with goiter, which later becomes atrophic (atrophic thyroiditis). It is also associated with other autoimmune disorders.

Clinical Features

Table 9.2 shows important symptoms and signs in hypothyroidism.

Common symptoms in hypothyroidism are a dry coarse skin, weakness, tiredness, cold intolerance, puffy face, edema in hands and feet, constipation, weight gain and a hoarse voice **(Fig. 9.2)**. Prolonged hypothyroidism results in the deposition of hydrophilic mucopolysaccharides in tissues. This causes non-pitting edema (myxedema).

Investigations

- Thyroid function tests **(Table 9.3)**:
  - High serum TSH is the earliest and most sensitive indicator of primary hypothyroidism.
  - The serum TSH level is low in secondary hypothyroidism.
  - Serum T_4 is low.

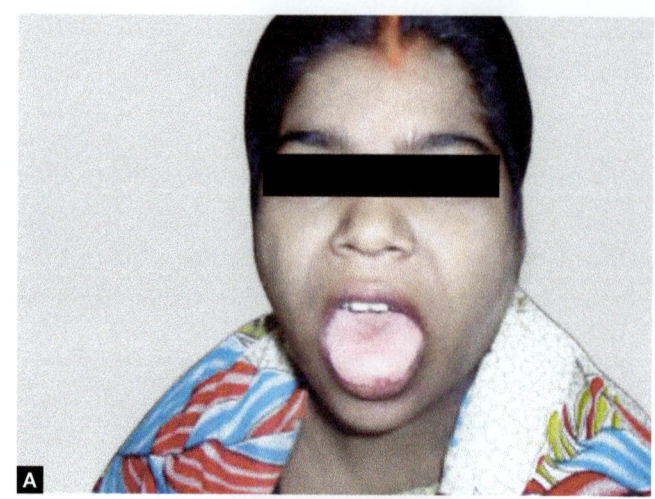

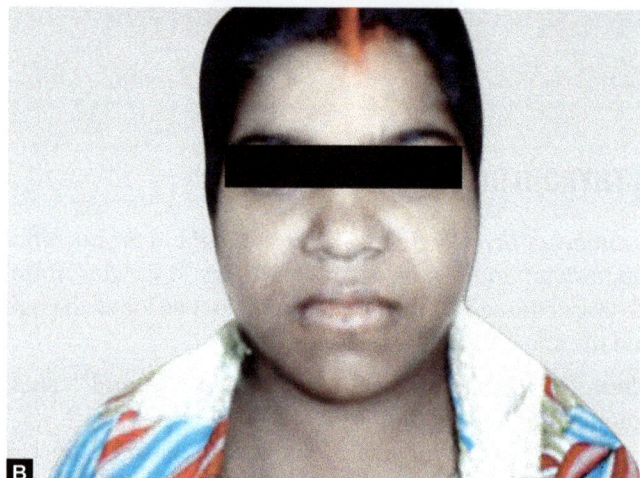

Figs. 9.2A and B: (A) Enlarged tongue in hypothyroidism; (B) Facial puffiness and pallor in hypothyroidism.

Table 9.2: Clinical features of hypothyroidism.

General
- Weakness, tiredness
- Cold intolerance
- Dry coarse skin
- Pallor
- Hair loss
- Puffy face, hand, and feet (Myxedema)
- Weight gain, poor appetite
- Hypothermia
- Goiter
- Hoarse voice

Gastrointestinal
- Constipation
- Large tongue

Reproductive
- Menorrhagia
- Amenorrhea
- Infertility
- Galactorrhea

Nervous system
- Poor memory
- Poor concentration
- Carpal tunnel syndrome
- Delayed relaxation of deep reflexes

Cardiovascular
- Bradycardia
- Hypertension
- Ischemic heart disease
- Pericardial effusion

Respiratory
- Pleural effusion
- Sleep apnoea

Table 9.3: Interpretation of thyroid function tests.

TSH	T_4	T_3	Most likely diagnosis
High	Low	Low	Primary hypothyroidism
Low/normal	Low	Low	Secondary hypothyroidism
Mildly high	Normal	Normal	Subclinical hypothyroidism
Low	High	High	Primary thyrotoxicosis
Low	Normal	High	Primary T_3 toxicosis
Low	Normal	Normal	Subclinical hyperthyroidism
High	High	High	Secondary thyrotoxicosis

- Serum T_3 levels is low but is not reliable for the diagnosis of hypothyroidism.
- High serum TSH and normal serum T_4 indicates subclinical or mild hypothyroidism.
- High titer of antibodies against thyroperoxidase (TPO) and thyroglobulin are found in patients with Hashimoto's thyroiditis and atrophic thyroiditis.
- Other findings are anemia (normocytic or macrocytic), high serum cholesterol and triglycerides, increased serum creatine kinase and LDH, hyponatremia, and low voltage ECG.

Treatment

- Hypothyroidism should be treated with oral levothyroxine. The treatment is generally started with low dose (50–100 µg daily) and gradually increased
- In elderly, a smaller starting dose (25 µg) is preferred to avoid cardiac side effects
- TSH is monitored periodically and the dose of thyroxine is adjusted accordingly
- The ideal goal is to maintain TSH at the lower half of the reference range
- Treatment is needed lifelong.

Myxedema Coma

This is a rare presentation of hypothyroidism. The clinical features are altered sensorium, hypothermia, hypoglycemia, hypoventilation, hypoxia, hypercapnia, hyponatremia, and hypotension. Convulsions may occur. Coma is induced by infection, cold exposure and systemic illness. This is more commonly seen in the elderly. It has a high mortality rate despite intensive treatment.

Treatment

- The treatment includes intravenous administration of levothyroxine (T_4), 400 µg as a loading dose followed by 50–100 µg daily.
- If parenteral T_4 is not available, T_3 can be given intravenously in the dosage of 10–25 µg, 8 hourly. T_4 can also be given through nasogastric tube.
- Supportive measures include external warming, use of broad-spectrum antibodies, and correction of hypoglycemia and hyponatremia.
- As there is impaired adrenal reserve in severe hypothyroidism, 50–100 mg hydrocortisone is also given every 6 hourly.

Congenital Hypothyroidism

Congenital hypothyroidism occurs in about 1 in every 4000 newborns. Thyroid gland dysgenesis is the most common cause of neonatal hypothyroidism (85%). Dyshormonogenesis and TSH-receptor antibody mediated hypothyroidism are other causes.

Clinical features: The infants appear normal at birth. Only 10% can be diagnosed clinically. Important clinical features are given in **Table 9.4**. Cretinism is severe hypothyroidism

Table 9.4: Clinical features of congenital hypothyroidism.

- Feeding problems
- Prolonged jaundice
- Hypotonia
- Enlarged tongue
- Delayed physical growth and development
- Mental retardation
- Short stature
- Umbilical hernia
- Other features as seen in adult patients with hypothyroidism

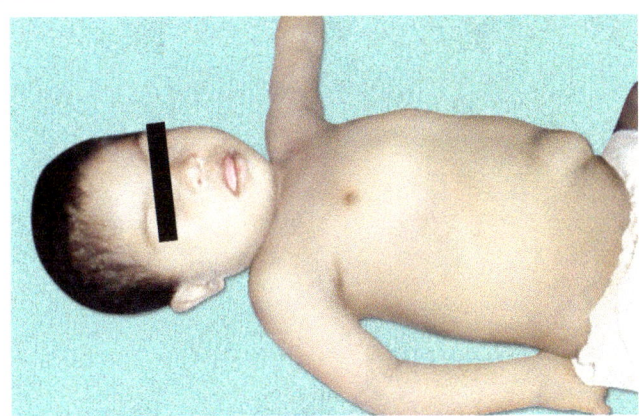

Fig. 9.3: Cretinism.

beginning in infancy. This is marked by mental retardation **(Fig. 9.3)**. Permanent neurological damage occurs if treatment is delayed. Congenital malformations are also common in congenital hypothyroidism.

Diagnosis: This is made by the estimation of serum TSH levels and T_4 levels. Serum T_4 is low while TSH is high. In developed countries, routine screening of the TSH levels is performed in the newborn.

Treatment: It includes administration of levothyroxine. The dose is adjusted according to the TSH levels.

Hyperthyroidism

A state of excessive thyroid hormone due to hyperfunction of the thyroid gland is called hyperthyroidism. Thyrotoxicosis is defined as clinical manifestations due to excessive thyroid hormones. The main causes of hyperthyroidism are Graves' disease, toxic multinodular goiter and toxic adenomas **(Figs. 9.4A and B)**. Other causes are given in **Table 9.5**.

Graves' Disease

Graves' disease (Basedow's disease) is the most common cause of thyrotoxicosis (60–80%).

- It is more common in females and occurs generally between 20–40 years of age.
- Graves' disease is an autoimmune disorder with genetic predisposition. The antibodies (TSH-R antibodies) bind TSH receptors on thyroid follicular cells and stimulate thyroid hormone production and goiter formation.
- It can be accompanied by other autoimmune diseases like pernicious anemia, myasthenia gravis and diabetes mellitus.
- Graves' disease is characterized by diffuse enlargement of the thyroid gland, infiltrative ophthalmopathy (exophthalmos) and pretibial myxedema (dermopathy).

Clinical Features

- Important manifestations are weight loss with increased appetite, sweating, palpitation, tremors, and nervousness.

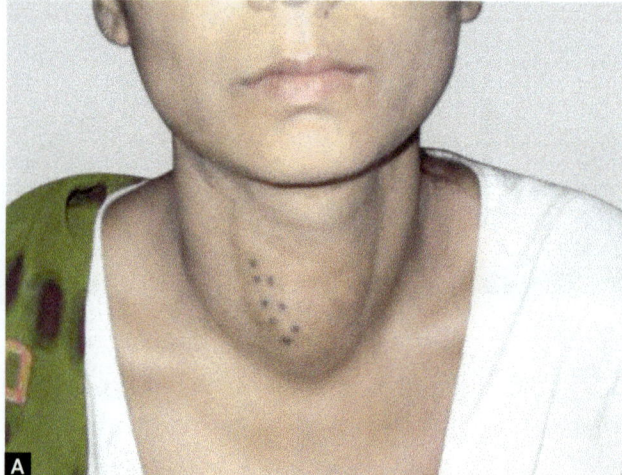

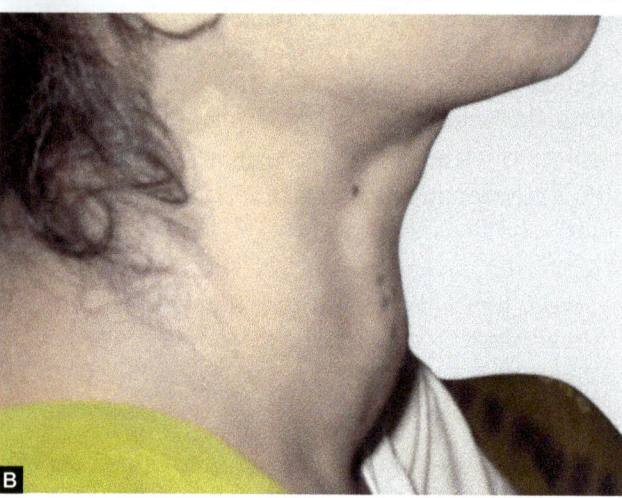

Figs. 9.4A and B: Enlarged thyroid gland.

Table 9.6: Clinical features of thyrotoxicosis.

Symptoms
- Weight loss with increased appetite
- Heat intolerance and sweating
- Nervousness and restlessness
- Palpitation
- Diarrhea
- Oligomenorrhea, amenorrhea
- Muscle cramps and weakness
- Anginal chest pain

Signs
- Tachycardia, atrial fibrillation
- Fine finger tremors
- Moist warm skin
- Goiter
- Hyper-reflexia
- Proximal myopathy
- Lid lag and lid retraction
- Clubbing
- Bruit over thyroid gland*
- Ophthalmopathy*
- Dermopathy*

*Features of Grave's disease

Table 9.5: Causes of thyrotoxicosis.

Primary hyperthyroidism
- Graves' disease
- Multinodular goiter
- Toxic adenoma (solitary nodule)
- Subacute thyroiditis (de Quervain's)
- Iodide induced (Jod-Basedow disease)
- Drugs–amiodarone
- Radiographic contrast media
- Excessive iodine ingestion
- Struma ovarii (ovarian teratoma producing thyroid hormone)
- Functioning thyroid carcinoma metastasis

Secondary hyperthyroidism
- TSH secreting pituitary tumor
- Pregnancy and trophoblastic tumors

Thyrotoxicosis without hyperthyroidism
- Thyrotoxicosis factitia (ingestion of excess thyroid hormone)

The signs are tachycardia, atrial fibrillation, lid retraction, wide palpebral fissure, and exophthalmos. Other clinical features of thyrotoxicosis are given in **Table 9.6**.

b. Ophthalmopathy is present in 20–50% patients of Graves' disease. It may precede the development of thyrotoxicosis or may develop after successful treatment of hyperthyroidism in Graves' disease. It usually consists of chemosis, scleral injection, periorbital edema and proptosis. Proptosis may cause corneal drying and damage. In severe cases exophthalmos, diplopia and optic nerve compression may occur.

c. Dermopathy occurs in about 5% of patients with Graves' disease. Purple or pink patches over anterior and lateral aspect of the leg (pretibial myxedema) are commonly seen.

d. Thyroid acropachy is unusual feature of Graves' disease and manifests as digital clubbing and swelling of fingers and toes.

Laboratory Findings in Hyperthyroidism

- Serum total and unbound (free) T_3 and T_4 are increased and TSH level is suppressed. Serum TSH is the best initial diagnostic test; normal TSH levels exclude clinical hyperthyroidism. In some cases, only T_3 levels are raised whereas T_4 is normal (T_3 toxicosis, **Table 9.3**).
- TSH-R antibodies levels are increased in about 75% of cases of Graves' disease.
- ESR may be increased in subacute thyroiditis.
- The uptake of radioactive iodine by thyroid is high in Graves' disease and toxic nodular goiter, whereas it is low in subacute thyroiditis.
- Ultrasonography of thyroid gland reveals diffuse enlargement of thyroid gland. It helps in differentiating Graves' disease from nodular goiter.

Treatment

The hyperthyroidism of Graves' disease is treated by antithyroid drugs, radioactive iodine (^{131}I) or subtotal thyroidectomy. The choice of treatment depends on the cause and severity of hyperthyroidism, the patient's age and clinical situation.

- *Antithyroid drugs:* The most commonly used drugs are **carbimazole, methimazole** and **propylthiouracil**.
  - These drugs reduce the synthesis of thyroid hormones by inhibiting the iodination of tyrosine. These drugs also reduce the thyroid antibody levels.
  - These are used in young adults and in patients with mild thyrotoxicosis and small goiter.
  - The drugs are given (carbimazole 5-40 mg/day, propylthiouracil 100-200 mg every 6-8 h) for prolonged periods of about 1-2 years. Relapse occurs in about 50% patients with hyperthyroidism after stopping treatment.
  - Rash, fever, arthralgia are common side effects. Agranulocytosis is an uncommon and serious side effect.

  Propranolol is used to control adrenergic symptoms (tachycardia, tremor, sweating and anxiety) that occur due to hyperthyroidism of any origin. It has no effect on thyroid hormone synthesis and secretion and the usual dose is 20-40 mg every 6 hours.

b. *Radioactive iodine* (^{131}I): It causes progressive destruction of thyroid cells. It can be used as initial treatment or for relapses after stopping antithyroid drugs or after surgery. This treatment is contraindicated in pregnancy and breast feeding. The majority of patients develop hypothyroidism following radioactive iodine therapy. Hence, a long-term follow-up with measurement of thyroid hormones and TSH is necessary.

c. *Thyroid surgery (Subtotal thyroidectomy):* This is indicated in cases of relapse after antithyroid drugs and in young males with large goiter or severe hyperthyroidism. This is also preferred in pregnant women or in those who plan pregnancy. Before surgery, the patient is made euthyroid by antithyroid drugs. Ipodate sodium or iopanoic acid 500 mg twice daily can be added to fast achieve euthyroid status. Potassium iodide is then added 1-2 weeks before surgery. Both drugs are discontinued after surgery. Complications of surgery are recurrent laryngeal nerve palsy and hypoparathyroidism. However, recurrence of hyperthyroidism or development of hypothyroidism may occur.

Thyroid Crisis

This is a severe form of thyrotoxicosis which can occur during stressful illnesses, thyroid surgery or radioactive iodine administration. It is most commonly precipitated by infection. It may manifest as high fever, delirium, tachycardia, vomiting, diarrhea, cardiac arrhythmia, and myocardial infarction. In elderly, heart failure may occur. The mortality rate is high.

Treatment

- Patients should be rehydrated and given broad-spectrum antibiotics if infection is suspected.
- Propranolol is given orally 80 mg 6 hourly or 1-5 mg intravenously 6 hourly.
- Patient is also given carbimazole 40-60 mg daily or methimazole 20 mg every 6 hourly. Alternatively propylthiouracil 150-250 mg every 6 hours may be given.
- Ipodate sodium (500 mg orally per day) is very effective in bringing the T_3 levels to normal if given within 1 hour after the first dose of anti-thyroid drug. This is a radiographic contrast medium which inhibits the release of thyroid hormones and peripheral conversion of T_4 to T_3.
- Hydrocortisone (300 mg) is given as IV bolus followed by 100 mg every 8 hours.

CALCIUM METABOLISM

The total amount of calcium is about 2% of the body weight. Most of it (99%) is in the bones.

- Normal total serum calcium level is 9-10.5 mg/dL (2.2-2.6 mmol/L). Half of this is present in free form (ionized calcium) and the remainder is bound with proteins mainly albumin. The total serum calcium level is low in conditions in which hypoalbuminemia exists, however, free calcium level is normal.
- Ionized calcium is responsible for the physiological functions of the calcium such as nerve function and muscle contraction.

Regulation of Calcium Metabolism

The calcium metabolism is regulated chiefly by the parathyroid hormone (parathormone) and vitamin D.

Parathyroid hormone (PTH): Serum calcium level is principal regulator of parathyroid hormone release. Low serum calcium level stimulates parathyroid hormone secretion. Parathyroid hormone maintains serum calcium level by the following mechanisms:
- It promotes resorption of calcium from bones
- It promotes absorption of calcium from renal tubules
- It stimulates the synthesis of 1,25-dihydroxy-cholecalciferol by the kidneys and thus indirectly promotes the absorption of calcium from the intestine.

Vitamin D: It enhances the absorption of calcium and phosphate from the gut.

Hypocalcemia

Hypocalcemia is defined as serum calcium level below 9 mg/dL with normal serum albumin level or an ionized calcium of less than 4.2 mg/dL. The important causes of hypocalcemia are chronic renal failure, vitamin D deficiency, and hypoparathyroidism **(Table 9.7)**.

- Calcium chelators (citrates) present in the transfused blood may lead to hypocalcemia following multiple blood transfusions.

Table 9.7: Causes of hypocalcemia.

- Chronic renal failure
- Vitamin D deficiency
  - Decreased intake
  - Decreased exposure to sunlight
  - Malabsorption
  - Decreased production of active forms
- Hypoparathyroidism
- Pseudohypoparathyroidism
- Multiple blood transfusions
- Hyperphosphatemia
- Hypomagnesemia
- Acute pancreatitis
- Low serum albumin (free calcium is normal)

- Hypomagnesemia causes decreased secretion of PTH and inhibits the action of vitamin D and PTH on bones leading to hypocalcemia.
- Pseudohypoparathyroidism is characterized by tissue resistance to the action of parathyroid hormone with normal or increased secretion of parathyroid hormone.

Manifestations

Hypocalcemia causes increased excitability of peripheral nerves leading to tetany. Triad of manifestations of hypocalcemia is carpopedal spasm, convulsions and laryngeal spasm. Other features are muscle spasm, perioral and limb paresthesia.

In carpopedal spasm **(Fig. 9.5)**, there is flexion of metacarpophalangeal joints, extension of interphalangeal joints of fingers and thumb and apposition of thumb (**main d'accoucheur**).

Prolonged hypocalcemia as in hypoparathyroidism may cause cataract, basal ganglia calcification, raised intracranial pressure, papilledema, and psychosis.

Tetany which is not obvious *(Latent tetany)* can be detected by eliciting **Trousseau's sign** and **Chvostek's sign**.

- Trousseau's sign is the appearance of carpal spasm within 3 minutes when sphygmomanometer cuff on the upper arm is inflated more than systolic blood pressure **(Fig. 9.5)**.
- Chvostek's sign: Contraction of facial muscles in response to tapping over the branches of facial nerve as they emerge from the parotid gland is called Chvostek's sign.

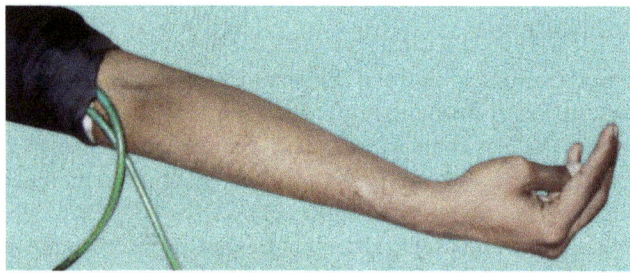

Fig. 9.5: Elicitation of Trousseau's sign.

Investigations

- Serum calcium is low.
- Total serum calcium is normal but ionized calcium is low in alkalosis. In hypoalbuminemia, total serum calcium is low but ionized calcium is normal **(Table 9.8)**.
- Serum phosphorus is elevated in most of the causes of hypocalcemia except in vitamin D deficiency where it is low.
- Serum parathyroid hormone level is elevated except in hypoparathyroidism and magnesium deficiency **(Table 9.8)**.
- Serum magnesium is measured to rule out hypomagnesemia.
- The ECG may show prolongation of QT interval. Arrhythmias may occur.

Treatment

Treatment of severe symptomatic hypocalcemia: Calcium gluconate 2 g, equivalent to 180 mg elemental calcium (20 mL of 10% calcium gluconate) should be given intravenously in 10–15 minutes. This should be followed by infusion of 60 mL of 10% calcium gluconate in 500 mL dextrose water slowly in 4–6 hours. Subsequently the infusion rate should be adjusted to maintain serum calcium level between 8 and 9 mg/dL. Magnesium should also be corrected if low.

The underlying cause should be treated and long-term therapy started.

Long-term treatment:
- Oral calcium supplement is given in the dosage of 1–2 g elemental calcium daily. The preferred salt is calcium carbonate which is the least expensive and is well tolerated. The calcium when given with food is well absorbed. The goal is to maintain serum calcium level between 8 and 8.5 mg/dL. At this level, the symptoms of hypocalcemia do not occur and the chance of hypercalciuria is minimal.
- The vitamin D is supplemented in the dosage of 400–1000 units per day. The dose of active form of vitamin D (1,25-dihydroxycholecalciferol, calcitriol) is 0.25–0.5 µg daily.

Table 9.8: Laboratory findings in hypocalcemia.

	Total serum calcium	Ionized serum calcium	Serum phosphate	Serum PTH
Hypoalbuminemia	Low	Normal	Normal	Normal
Alkalosis	Normal	Low	Normal	Normal
Osteomalacia (Vit D deficiency)	Low	Low	Low	High
Chronic renal failure	Low	Low	High	High
Hypoparathyroidism	Low	Low	High	Low
Pseudohypoparathyroidism	Low	Low	High	High

Hypercalcemia

Hypercalcemia is defined as serum calcium level above 10.5 mg/dL with normal serum albumin or an ionized calcium of more than 5.2 mg/dL. Important causes of hypercalcemia are given in **Table 9.9**.
- Primary hyperparathyroidism and malignancy account for 90% of all the cases of hypercalcemia.
- Hypercalcemia in malignancy may occur due to: (a) metastasis in bone, (b) increased bone resorption due to increased osteoclast activating factor (OAF), and (c) production of PTH related peptide (PTHrP).
- Sarcoidosis may cause hypercalcemia by increased production of vitamin D_3 by granulomatous tissue.
- Increased bone turnover in hyperthyroidism may lead to hypercalcemia.
- Prolonged immobilization may cause hypercalcemia due to continuing bone resorption in the absence of normal postural stimuli for bone formation.
- Milk alkali syndrome is due to ingestion of large amount of calcium and absorbable antacids such as milk or calcium carbonate.

Clinical Features

The symptoms generally occur if serum calcium level is more than 12 mg/dL. Symptoms are more marked if hypercalcemia develops rapidly.
- Gastrointestinal manifestations are anorexia, nausea, vomiting, peptic ulcer and constipation.
- Renal symptoms include polyuria, polydipsia, renal colic and nephrolithiasis.
- Neurological presentations are confusion, depression, drowsiness, stupor and coma.
- Ectopic calcification may occur in soft tissue if serum calcium level is more than 13 mg/dL.

Investigations

Serum calcium and serum PTH levels are measured.

Table 9.9: Important causes of hypercalcemia.

Primary hyperparathyroidism
- Parathyroid adenoma
- Parathyroid hyperplasia
- Parathyroid carcinoma

Malignancy
- Tumors producing PTH-related proteins (malignancy of lung, ovary, kidney)
- Hematological malignancies (Myeloma, lymphoma, leukemia)

Other causes
- Sarcoidosis
- Vitamin D excess
- Hyperthyroidism
- Lithium and thiazide use
- Milk alkali syndrome
- Immobilization

- High PTH level is present in primary hyperparathyroidism while it is low in malignancies where parathyroid hormone-related protein (PTHrP) is raised.
- Other tests are done to detect the presence of malignancies if suspected.
- Measurement of thyroid hormones and vitamin D levels may be required.
- ECG findings include short QT interval and ventricular arrhythmias.

Treatment

- Restoration of extracellular fluid volume is done with 0.9% saline. Three to four liters of fluid may be needed in the first 24 hours.
- Saline diuresis is induced by giving an infusion of saline which promotes the excretion of calcium. Frusemide may be added in case of renal impairment or heart failure.
- Bisphosphonate (60–90 mg pamidronate or zoledronate 4 mg) is given intravenously. It inhibits bone resorption. This is the drug of choice in malignancies. Monoclonal antibody Denosumab can be given to patients of malignancy-associated hypercalcemia which is refractory to bisphosphonates. This is antibody against RANKL and inhibits osteoclastic activity.
- Calcitonin (IM or SC) may be given particularly when there is renal failure. It inhibits bone resorption and promotes calcium excretion.
- Oral glucocorticoids are effective in hypercalcemia due to hematological malignancies, sarcoidosis and vitamin D toxicosis.
- Hemodialysis may be needed in cases of renal failure and heart failure.
- The underlying cause should be treated. Parathyroidectomy is done in primary hyperthyroidism.
- Cinacalcet, a calcimimetic agent is recommended in symptomatic primary hyperparathyroidism who are not candidates for surgery.

PARATHYROID DISORDERS

There are four parathyroid glands situated posterior to the thyroid gland. These produce parathyroid hormone (PTH) which is a peptide comprising of 84 amino acids. The secretion of PTH is regulated by the ionized calcium levels in serum. The important physiological roles of PTH are:
- It promotes resorption of calcium from bones
- It promotes absorption of calcium from renal tubules
- It stimulates the synthesis of 1,25-dihydroxy-cholecalciferol by the kidneys, thus indirectly promoting the absorption of calcium from the intestine.
- It inhibits the absorption of phosphate by the renal tubules.

Hypoparathyroidism

Important causes of hypoparathyroidism are post-thyroidectomy, after parathyroid gland surgery, hemochromatosis and hypomagnesemia.

- Hypoparathyroidism can also be hereditary such as in **Di George syndrome**. This is characterized by hypocalcemia, cardiovascular and facial anomalies.
- Hypoparathyroidism can be a manifestation of polyglandular autoimmunity type I in which other features are candidiasis, Addison's disease and vitiligo.
- Pseudohypoparathyroidism is a condition in which the production of PTH is normal, but there is tissue resistance to PTH. This is associated with structural abnormalities such as short stature and short fourth metacarpal.
- Pseudopseudohypoparathyroidism is characterized by the presence of structural abnormalities as seen in pseudohypoparathyroidism but normal calcium and PTH levels.

Clinical Features

The manifestations of hypoparathyroidism are due to hypocalcemia (see hypocalcemia).

Investigations

- Serum calcium is low, serum phosphate is high, and serum alkaline phosphatase is normal.
- The PTH level is low. It is normal or high in pseudohypoparathyroidism.
- Magnesium level is measured to rule out hypomagnesemia.

Treatment

- Treatment of hypoparathyroidism includes supplementation of calcium and vitamin D.
- Recombinant human parathyroid hormone (rhPTH) is recommended in patients not adequately responding to calcium and vitamin D therapy. It is given as subcutaneous injection. However it is highly expensive and has been reported to increase risk of osteosarcoma in animal studies.
- Recently transplantation of parathyroid tissue removed from prior surgery has been shown to be beneficial in some.

Hyperparathyroidism

Primary hyperparathyroidism is caused by hypersecretion of PTH. In majority of cases, this is due to autonomous hypersecretion of PTH. Primary hyperparathyroidism (adenoma or hyperplasia) may be familial and part of multiple endocrine neoplasia (MEN types 1, 2a).

Secondary hyperparathyroidism is characterized by the hypersecretion of PTH due to stimulation by hypocalcemia (**Table 9.10**). There is hyperplasia of all parathyroid glands.

Table 9.10: Types of hyperparathyroidism.

Primary hyperparathyroidism
- Parathyroid adenoma (80%)
- Parathyroid hyperplasia of two or more glands
- Parathyroid carcinoma

Secondary hyperparathyroidism
- Chronic renal failure
- Malabsorption
- Osteomalacia and rickets

Tertiary hyperparathyroidism

In **tertiary hyperparathyroidism** hyperplastic parathyroid glands (as in case of secondary hyper-parathyroidism) may result in adenoma formation and autonomous PTH secretion.

Clinical Manifestations

Majority of patients may be asymptomatic. However, symptoms are generally due to hypercalcemia (see hypercalcemia). Bone resorption occurs due to excessive PTH activity. This may lead to demineralization, pathological fractures and generalized cystic bone lesions (**osteitis fibrosa cystica**). This can also present as "**brown tumors**" (cysts of the jaw).

Investigations

- In primary hyperparathyroidism serum PTH level is elevated, serum calcium is high and phosphate is low. Serum alkaline phosphatase is raised if bone disease is present.
- In secondary hyperparathyroidism, PTH level is elevated. Serum calcium is low and phosphate is high.
- Bone X-ray may show demineralization, subperiosteal erosions, resorption of terminal phalanges and loss of lamina dura of the teeth. Skull X-ray may reveal pepper-pot appearance.
- Radioimaging and ultrasound neck are needed to localize and diagnose parathyroid tumors.

Treatment

Parathyroidectomy is recommended for patients with symptomatic hyperparathyroidism. Medical management of hypercalcemia is described elsewhere (see hypercalcemia).

PITUITARY GLAND

Anatomy: The pituitary gland is situated in the sella turcica. The gland is connected to the hypothalamus with pituitary stalk or infundibulum. The pituitary gland has two lobes, anterior and posterior. Portal vessels carry blood from the hypothalamus to the anterior lobe while the posterior lobe receives nerve fibers from the hypothalamus.

Physiology: The anterior lobe of pituitary gland secretes growth hormone (GH), prolactin (PRL), adrenocortico-

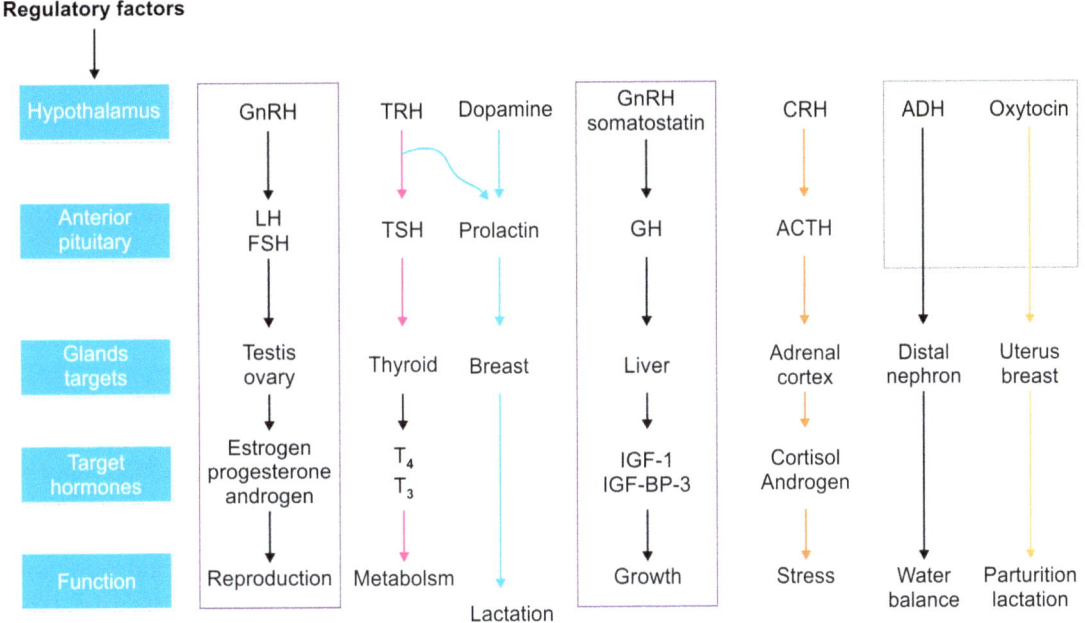

Fig. 9.6: Pituitary hormones.
(ADH: antidiuretic hormone; GnRH: gonadotropin-releasing hormone; GHRH: growth hormone-releasing hormone; TRH: thyrotropin-releasing hormone; TSH: thyroid-stimulating hormone; LH: luteinizing hormone; FSH: follicle stimulating hormone; GH: growth hormone; ACTH: adrenocorticotropic hormone; IGF: insulin growth factor; T_3: trioidothyronine; T_4: thyroxine)

tropic hormone (ACTH), thyroid stimulating hormone (TSH), follicle stimulating hormone (FSH) and luteinizing hormone (LH). The secretion of these hormones is controlled by the hypothalamus. The hypothalamus stimulates or inhibits the secretion of anterior pituitary hormones through the release of substances in the portal vessels **(Fig. 9.6)**.

Anti-diuretic hormone (ADH) and oxytocin are synthesized in the hypothalamus and transported through the nerve axons to the posterior pituitary.

Hypopituitarism

Hypopituitarism may be caused by hypothalamic dysfunction or pituitary disease. There may be single or multiple hormonal deficiencies.

Important causes of hypopituitarism are pituitary adenoma, granulomas, apoplexy (Sheehan's syndrome), metastatic carcinoma and brain tumors, such as craniopharyngioma and meningioma. Pituitary tumor can be a part of MEN (multiple endocrine neoplasia, type I).

Other causes are trauma, surgery, radiation, encephalitis, hemochromatosis and stroke.

Clinical Features

The clinical manifestations are variable and depend upon the deficient hormones and the underlying cause. Panhypopituitarism means absence of all anterior pituitary hormones. With progressive lesions of the pituitary, the deficiency of GH occurs first and TSH deficiency occurs in the last. Important clinical features are given in **Table 9.11**.

Table 9.11: Clinical features of hypopituitarism.

Hormone	Clinical features
GH deficiency	Short stature, lethargy, asthenia, small heart, central obesity
Gonadotropins (FSH, LH) deficiency	Hair loss, decreased libido, amenorrhea, infertility, osteopenia
ACTH deficiency	Weakness, fatigue, weight loss, hypotension, pallor
TSH deficiency	Fatigue, weakness, weight gain, hyperlipidemia, cold intolerance
ADH deficiency	Thirst, polyuria

Other manifestations are due to the underlying cause. For example, tumor may produce headache, visual field defects, diplopia and hyperprolactinemia.

Investigations

- Visualization of the pituitary region is best done with the help of MRI.
- Levels of pituitary hormones are low in the serum.
- Levels of hormones produced by target glands on which pituitary hormones act are also low.
- Stimulation tests are performed to detect the deficiencies of these hormones.

Treatment

- *Removal of underlying cause:* Trans-sphenoidal surgery of pituitary tumor can correct hypopituitarism. Radiation therapy with gamma knife or X-ray may also be helpful.
- *Substitution therapy:* Substitution therapy with hormones may be needed life long.

- Cortisol replacement is done by giving hydrocortisone or prednisolone in case of ACTH deficiency. Mineralocorticoid replacement is not required.
- Levothyroxine (25–300 μg/day) is given to maintain serum T4 to the upper limit of the reference range. TSH level is not helpful for monitoring the therapy.
- Human growth hormone is given subcutaneously to correct its deficiency.
- Sex hormone replacement is indicated if there is gonadotropin deficiency.

Acromegaly

Acromegaly is caused by an excess of growth hormone secreted by pituitary adenoma. In most cases the adenoma is more than 1 cm in diameter (macroadenoma).

Clinical Features

If the growth hormone excess occurs early in life, i.e., before the fusion of epiphyses, tall stature and gigantism will result. In adult life, after closure of epiphyses, acromegaly results (**Figs. 9.7A and B**).

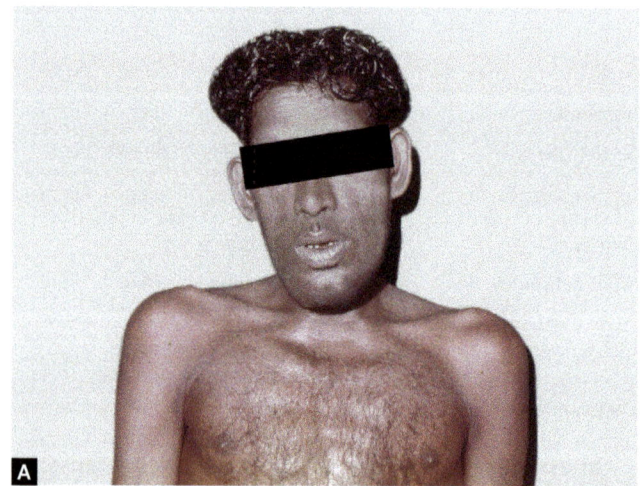
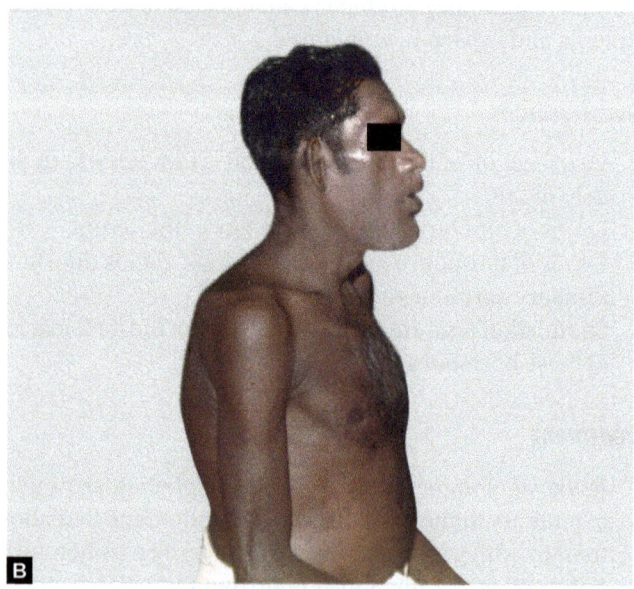

Figs. 9.7A and B: Acromegaly.

- Most common symptoms are headache and sweating.
- Head size increases and mandible becomes more prominent. It leads to prognathism and malocclusion.
- Tooth spacing is widened.
- Tongue is hypertrophied (macroglossia).
- Hands are enlarged and feet are widened.
- There may be hypertension, cardiomegaly, and diabetes mellitus.
- Expansion of macroadenoma may lead to local complications including hypopituitarism.

Investigations

- Serum GH is measured during oral glucose tolerance test. In normal subjects, plasma GH is suppressed to below 2 mU/L. Failure of suppression of GH level or paradoxical rise suggests acromegaly.
- Assessment of other pituitary functions is also done.
- Serum insulin like growth factor I (IGF-I) is elevated.
- Plasma glucose is high.
- MRI demonstrates pituitary tumor. X-ray of skull may reveal enlarged sella.

Treatment

- *Surgical:* Trans-sphenoidal surgery is the first line of treatment. External radiotherapy (gamma knife, heavy particle radiation) is given to patients not responding to surgery.
- *Medical:* Somatostatin analogs injections (octreotide, lanreotide, pasireotide) are used to treat patients with persistent acromegaly after surgery. These can be used as primary therapy also. Growth hormone receptor antagonist (pegvisomant) can be used subcutaneously to block the effects of GH.

Addison's Disease

Adrenal cortex secretes three major classes of steroids:
a. Glucocorticoids (cortisol)
b. Mineralocorticoids (aldosterone)
c. Adrenal androgens.

Adrenal medulla secretes catecholamines. Hypothalamic-pituitary-adrenal axis controls the secretion of glucocorticoids and adrenal androgens through adrenocorticotropic hormone (ACTH). Mineralocorticoid secretion is under control of rennin-angiotensin-aldosterone system.

Adrenal disorders mainly include: (a) hypofunction (adrenal insufficiency), and (b) hyperfunction (Cushing syndrome).

Adrenal insufficiency may result from either due to disease of adrenal glands (primary adrenal failure, Addison's disease) or due to ACTH deficiency caused by disorders of pituitary gland or hypothalamus (secondary adrenal failure). Secondary adrenal failure may also occur due to chronic glucocorticoid therapy that suppresses ACTH secretion. In primary adrenal failure, there is inadequate secretion of

Table 9.12: Causes of Addison's disease.

- Autoimmune
- Tuberculosis
- Histoplasmosis
- HIV/AIDS
- Bilateral adrenalectomy
- Intra-adrenal hemorrhage (Waterhouse-Friedrichsen syndrome)
- Amyloidosis
- Drugs (etomidate, ketoconazole, metyrapone)
- Hemochromatosis
- Metastatic carcinoma
- Lymphoma
- Congenital adrenal hyperplasia

both cortisol and aldosterone with increased level of ACTH, whereas in secondary adrenal failure, there is deficiency of cortisol alone with decreased ACTH level.

Etiology

The most common cause of Addison's disease is autoimmune adrenalitis. This may be associated with other autoimmune disorders like hypothyroidism. Other important causes are tuberculosis, HIV/AIDS, and histoplasmosis **(Table 9.12)**.

Clinical Features

The clinical features are generally non-specific. Important symptoms include anorexia, nausea, vomiting, weight loss, weakness and fatigue. Patient may have postural hypotension and hyponatremia. Although presentation is usually chronic, patient may present acutely as shock triggered by surgery, illness, or injury. Other features are hyperpigmentation due to increased secretion of ACTH, volume depletion and hyperkalemia **(Figs. 9.8 and 9.9)**.

Diagnosis

Tests for primary adrenal insufficiency:
- Random plasma cortisol level is usually low. Its level may be normal.
- ACTH stimulation test: Cortisol level fails to increase in response to exogenous ACTH or cosyntropin (synthetic ACTH).
- ACTH level: This is high in Addison's disease.
- Plasma rennin activity is high with low or low-normal aldosterone level.
- There may be hyponatremia and hyperkalemia.

Tests to ascertain the cause of adrenal failure:
- Measurement of antibodies against steroid secreting cells

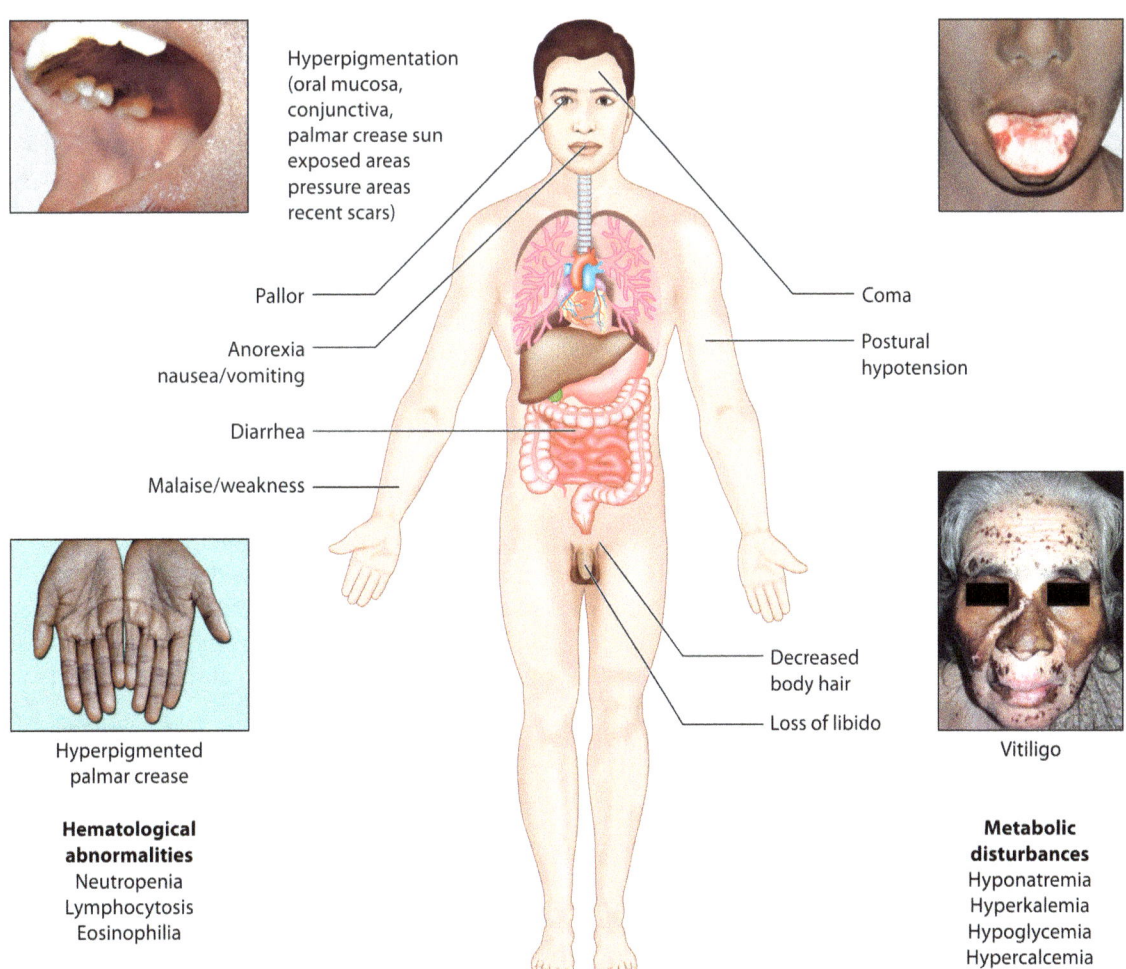

Fig. 9.8: Features of Addison's disease.

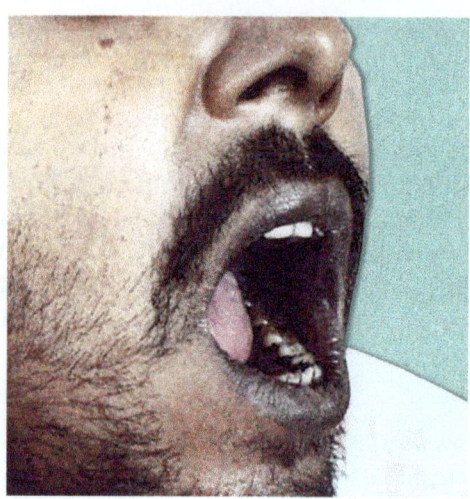

Fig. 9.9: Pigmentation of oral mucosa (Addison's disease).

- Tests for tuberculosis
- CT/MRI to identify metastatic malignancy
- Elisa for HIV.

Treatment

- ***Immediate treatment:*** In case of adrenal crisis, patient should be admitted and managed urgently. Inj. Hydrocortisone 100 mg I.V. is administered 8 hourly. Intravenous fluid (dextrose saline) is infused until hypotension is corrected. Patient is later maintained on oral prednisolone. Precipitating cause should be treated.
- ***Maintenance therapy:*** All patients will require cortisol replacement with prednisolone. The dose of prednisolone should be kept to a minimum to avoid the side effects. Most will need aldosterone replacement therapy with fludrocortisone. Usually a dose of 7.5–15 mg/day of prednisolone is required. However, a higher dose may be needed in case of intercurrent stress, severe illness, or surgery. The maintenance dose of fludrocortisone is generally 0.05 to 0.2 mg daily. Salt intake is increased.
- ***An identification tag is provided.*** Patient should bear identification tag containing his medical diagnosis.

Cushing's Disease

Cushing's disease is due to hypersecretion of ACTH by the pituitary gland and it is the most common cause of Cushing's syndrome. **Cushing's syndrome** is defined as a state of cortisol excess due to any cause.

ACTH causes increased production of corticosteroids by the adrenal cortex. Cushing's disease is usually because of benign small pituitary adenoma (microadenoma).

Clinical Features

The manifestations include central obesity, thin extremities, plethoric "moon face", and "buffalo hump". Other features are purple striae over abdomen and thigh, easy bruisability, acne, hypertension, osteoporosis, muscle wasting, hyperglycemia, impaired wound healing and psychosis. The tendency to infections is increased **(Fig. 9.10)**.

Investigations

- Overnight dexamethasone suppression test, 24 hours urinary free cortisol measurement and plasma ACTH level are important tests performed to diagnose Cushing's disease.
- Cushing's disease must be differentiated from other causes of hypercortisolism such as exogenous glucocorticoid, adrenal tumor secreting cortisol independent of ACTH, and ectopic production of ACTH by non-pituitary tumors (small lung cell carcinoma).
- MRI is needed to detect underlying cause such as tumors of pituitary and adrenal glands.

Treatment

- Patients are treated by trans-sphenoidal resection of pituitary adenoma.
- Medical treatment with drugs that inhibit corticosteroid synthesis is given before surgery. The drugs are metyrapone, aminoglutethimide and ketoconazole. Pasireotide can be beneficial as it suppresses ACTH secretion by the tumor.
- Patients who fail to respond to pituitary surgery undergo pituitary irradiation or bilateral adrenalectomy.

Diabetes Insipidus

This disorder is characterized by increased thirst and the passage of an increased amount of dilute urine. It is caused by the deficiency of antidiuretic hormone (vasopressin, ADH) or by resistance to the effects of ADH.

Diabetes insipidus can be classified into two types:
1. Central diabetes insipidus (deficient ADH).
2. Nephrogenic diabetes insipidus where ADH secretion is normal but renal tubules are unresponsive to ADH.

Causes of diabetes insipidus are given in **Table 9.13**.

Clinical Manifestations

The patient has excessive thirst. The volume of ingested fluid may reach upto 20 liters a day (polydipsia). The patients passes large amount of dilute urine (polyuria). If the fluid intake is not maintained as in an unconscious patient, the problems of hypernatremia and dehydration may occur.

Investigations

- Plasma osmolality is increased and the urine is dilute (low specific gravity and low osmolality).
- Water deprivation test is used for the diagnosis of diabetes insipidus.
- In central type of diabetes insipidus, serum ADH is low and the urine osmolality improves on desmopressin (DDAVP) administration.

CHAPTER 9: ENDOCRINE AND METABOLIC DISORDERS

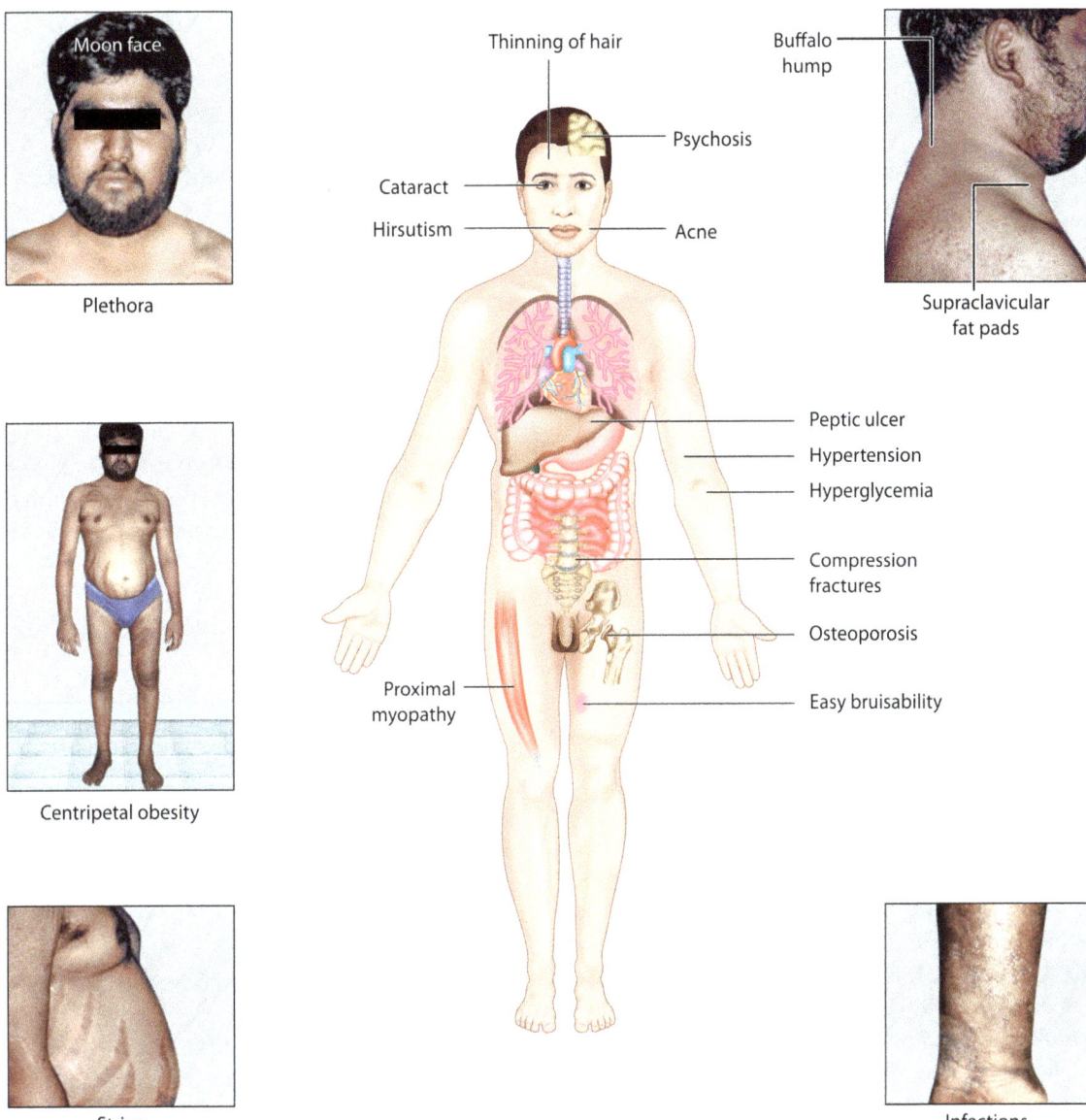

Fig. 9.10: Features of Cushing's disease.

Table 9.13: Important causes of diabetes insipidus.
Central
• Hypothalamic or pituitary stalk lesion
– Tumor, head injury, surgery, meningitis, encephalitis
• Genetic
• Idiopathic
Nephrogenic
• Genetic
– X-linked recessive
• Acquired
– Metabolic—hypokalemia, hypercalcemia
– Drugs—demeclocycline, lithium, methicillin
– Heavy metals
– Others—pyelonephritis, amyloidosis, sickle cell anemia, polycystic kidney disease

- On the contrary, serum ADH level is normal and there is no response to DDAVP in nephrogenic diabetes insipidus.
- MRI is useful in locating the hypothalamic or pituitary tumor.

Treatment

- DDAVP, an analog of ADH is the drug of choice in central type of diabetes insipidus. This is given orally, intranasally or parenterally.
- Thiazide, amiloride and indomethacin are helpful in nephrogenic diabetes insipidus.

DIABETES MELLITUS

Diabetes mellitus (DM) is a metabolic disorder characterized by hyperglycemia due to absolute or relative deficiency of insulin.

Classification

Two broad categories of DM are type 1 and type 2. Other types include gestational diabetes mellitus, and diabetes due to drugs, pancreatic diseases and genetic

Table 9.14: Classification of diabetes mellitus.

- **Type 1 diabetes mellitus**
  A. Immune mediated
  B. Idiopathic
- **Type 2 diabetes mellitus**
- **Other specific types:**
  a. Genetic defects of beta cell function: Maturity onset diabetes of the young (MODY)
  b. Genetic defects in insulin action
  c. Diseases of pancreas: Pancreatitis, neoplasia, hemochromatosis, pancreatectomy
  d. Endocrinopathies: Acromegaly, Cushing's syndrome, hyperthyroidism-pheochromocytoma, glucagonoma
  e. Drugs and chemicals: Thiazides, corticosteroids, phenytoin, thyroid hormone
  f. Infections: Congenital rubella, coxsackie, cytomegalovirus
  g. Uncommon forms of immune-mediated diabetes
  h. Genetic syndromes: Down's syndrome, Klinefelter's syndrome, Turner's syndrome
- **Gestational diabetes mellitus**

syndromes **(Table 9.14)**. The prevalence of DM has risen over past decades. Type 2 DM is more common.

Type 1 Diabetes Mellitus

This form of diabetes is immune mediated in 90% of cases (type 1 A). It occurs most commonly in children and young adults. It also includes latent autoimmune diabetes of adulthood (LADA). In 10% cases, it is idiopathic (type 1B).

In this disorder, there is virtually no circulating insulin. Pancreatic beta cells fail to respond to insulinogenic stimuli. Exogenous insulin is therefore required to control hyperglycemia and prevent ketosis.

Type I A diabetes is a T-cell mediated autoimmune disease and may be associated with other autoimmune diseases like thyroid disease, Addison's disease, vitiligo and pernicious anemia. Autoimmune process is triggered by infectious or environmental stimuli in genetically susceptible individuals. Possible triggers are viral infections (coxsackie, rubella), bovine milk protein and nitrosourea compounds.

These patients have normal beta cell mass at birth which gradually declines over months or years due to immunologic destruction. Pancreatic islets are infiltrated with lymphocytes (insulinitis).

In many patients immunologic markers appear before diabetes manifests clinically. Immunological markers are islet cell antibodies (ICA), insulin antibodies (IAA), antibodies against glutamic acid decarboxylase (GAD), zinc transporter 8 (ZnT8) and tyrosine phosphatase (IA-2). These antibodies can be used for screening siblings of the patients.

HLA-DR3 and/or HLA-DR4 haplotypes are associated with the type 1 DM. Risk of developing DM is increased 10 fold in the relatives of type 1 DM patients. HLA-DQ genes are specific markers for type 1 susceptibility.

Type 2 Diabetes Mellitus

Type 2 diabetes mellitus is a disease of middle aged and elderly. It is polygenic and multifactorial in origin involving genetic and environmental factors. There are three basic pathophysiological abnormalities in type 2 DM:
- Impaired insulin secretion
- Insulin resistance (inability of insulin to act on target tissues mainly liver and muscles)
- Increased hepatic glucose production.

Most of the patients are obese and insulin resistant. Insulin resistance increases with age, sedentary lifestyle, and abdominal-visceral obesity.

In addition, there is impairment of beta cell function. Diabetes occurs only when insulin secretion is not adequate to meet the requirement. There is hyperglycemia but endogenous insulin prevents the development of ketoacidosis. Hyperglycemia worsens insulin resistance and beta cell response to glucose (glucose toxicity) and both improve when glucose is normalized with the treatment.

Many biologic products are secreted by adipocytes that modulate insulin secretion, insulin action, and body weight. Leptin and adiponectin improve insulin sensitivity while tumor necrosis factor alpha and resistin interfere with insulin action.

In the early stages, glucose remains normal, despite insulin resistance, because beta cells compensate by increasing insulin secretion. Gradually there is decline in the insulin secretion and overt hyperglycemia occurs. There is also an increased output of glucose from liver which contributes to fasting hyperglycemia.

Genetic factors are important in the development of type 2 diabetes. The concordance rate in twins is 100%. Several genes are involved. Individuals with family history of diabetes are at increased risk of developing diabetes, if both parents have diabetes, the risk is 40%.

Clinical Features

The classical symptoms are polyuria, thirst (polydipsia), nocturia, and rapid weight loss despite good appetite. These are seen in type 1 DM.

Polyuria is due to osmotic diuresis secondary to hyperglycemia. Thirst is due to hyperosmolality of the plasma. Weight loss is due to depletion of glycogen and triglycerides, increased lipolysis and increased protein catabolism and loss of muscle mass.

Other symptoms are tiredness, fatigue, and irritability. Blurring of vision, frequent infections, and slow healing of wounds may also be present. The infections include bacterial and fungal infections of skin and genitalia.

The patients with type 2 DM may be asymptomatic when they are diagnosed during routine laboratory tests. The patients are obese or have high waist circumference They may present with the features of chronic neurological,

CHAPTER 9: ENDOCRINE AND METABOLIC DISORDERS

Table 9.15: Clinical features of type 1 and type 2 diabetes mellitus.

	Type 1	Type 2
Onset (age)	<30 years	>30 years
Body habitus	Lean	Obese
Ketoacidosis	Common	Rare
Family history	Uncommon	Yes
Autoantibodies	Present	No
Other autoimmune diseases	Yes	No
Complications at diagnosis	No	May be present
Insulin therapy	Must	May be needed
Polyuria, polydipsia, polyphagia, weight loss	Common	Less common

cardiovascular, ophthalmic and renal complications **(Table 9.15)**. Chronic skin infections, generalized pruritus and fungal vaginitis are common. Some patients may have hyperkeratotic dark skin in axilla, groin and nape of neck (Acanthosis nigricans). This is indicative of insulin resistance.

Females who have unexplained fetal loss or deliver large babies should be screened for DM.

The patients may present with acute complications such as diabetic ketoacidosis (DKA), hyperglycemic hyperosmolar state (HHS) or features of chronic complications.

Diagnostic Criteria

Diagnosis of DM is made if any of the following criteria is present **(Table 9.16)**:

- If fasting plasma glucose is ≥**126 mg/dL.** Fasting means no caloric intake for at least 8 hours (this should be confirmed by a repeat test)
- If random plasma glucose is ≥**200 mg/dL** in presence of symptoms of DM. Random means without regards to the time since last meal.
- If oral glucose tolerance test shows plasma glucose of ≥**200 mg/dL at 2 hours** after glucose load equivalent of 75 gm anhydrous glucose dissolved in water.
- If glycosylated hemoglobin (HbA1c) is >**6.5%**.

Impaired fasting glucose (IFG) is defined as fasting plasma glucose levels between 100 mg/dL and 125 mg/dL. Fasting plasma glucose of < 100 mg/dL is considered normal.

Impaired glucose tolerance (IGT) is defined as plasma glucose levels between 140 mg/dL and 199 mg/dL, 2 hours after 75 g glucose load. Patients with IFG or IGT are at substantial risk for developing type 2 DM and cardiovascular disease.

Prediabetes is classified as impaired fasting glucose or impaired glucose tolerance or glycosylated hemoglobin is between 5.7 to 6.4%. Prediabetics are at increased risk of developing cardiovascular complications.

Investigations

Urine Test

The urine is tested for the presence of glucose, ketones, and protein. Presence of albumin (>30 mg/d) in urine or spot urine albumin:creatinine ratio of >30 mcg albumin per mg of creatinine suggests nephropathy.

Blood Tests

The plasma glucose tests are performed for the diagnosis of DM (see above). The fasting plasma glucose is done after overnight fast (at least 8 hours fast). The random test is defined as without regard to time since the last meal.

Oral glucose tolerance test (OGTT) is performed by giving 75 g glucose dissolved in water and measuring plasma glucose after 2 hours. The persons should be on unrestricted carbohydrate diet for 3 days before the test.

The criteria for the diagnosis of DM in pregnancy (gestational diabetes) are different and more stringent.

Glycated Hemoglobin (HbA1c) Measurement

HbA1c is formed by the non-enzymatic condensation of glucose molecules with free amino groups of hemoglobin. It provides an accurate measure of glucose control over a period of 8–12 weeks. The major form of glycated Hb is HbA1c which normally comprises of 2–4% of total Hb. The measurement of HbA1c should be made at 3-4 months interval and the therapy is adjusted accordingly **(Table 9.17)**.

Serum Fructosamine Measurement

Serum fructosamine is formed by non-enzymatic glycation of serum proteins, mainly albumin. Its level reflects the glycemic control for the preceding 2 weeks. This is particularly useful for the assessment of the glycemic control in diabetic women who have recently become pregnant.

Table 9.16: Criteria for diagnosis of diabetes.

Test	Normal	Prediabetes	Diabetes
Fasting plasma glucose (mg/dL)	<100	100–125	≥126
Plasma glucose 2 hours after glucose load	<140	140–199	≥200
HbA1c (%)	<5.7	5.7–6.4	>6.5

Table 9.17: Conditions affecting glycated Hb.

- Hemoglobinopathies
- Recovery from acute blood loss
- Anemia
- Blood transfusion
- Pregnancy
- IV iron and Erythropoietin therapy in renal failure
- Vitamin C and E
- Post-splenectomy

Self Monitoring of Blood Glucoses

Glucometers are available for the measurement of capillary blood glucose. The test can be performed by the patients themselves at home.

Continuous Blood Glucose Monitoring System

The blood glucose can be monitored continuously throughout 72 hours with the help of a subcutaneously placed sensor. This is useful in the detection of asymptomatic hypoglycemia.

C –peptide Measurement

C-peptide is indicative of endogenous insulin secretion. Serum C-peptide is low in long standing type 1 DM whereas it is high in severe insulin resistance (type 2 DM). It is also helpful in the diagnosis of spontaneous hypoglycaemia.

Other Tests

Serum lipids are routinely measured. Patients with type 2 DM may have dyslipidemia characterized by high triglycerides, low HDL cholesterol, and presence of small dense LDL particles. These patients are more susceptible to atherosclerosis.

Type 1 diabetics have raised triglycerides and LDL cholesterol but normal HDL cholesterol.

Blood urea, serum creatinine, electrolytes, liver function tests are also performed.

Complications of Diabetes

The complications of DM may be classified as acute or chronic. The complications are listed in **Table 9.18**.

Mechanisms of diabetic complications are complex. However, increased metabolism of glucose to sorbitol via the polyol pathway, glycation of structural proteins and deposition of advanced glycation end products in various tissues, and free radical mediated damage are some of the key pathogenetic mechanisms. Hyperglycemia leads to increased formation of diacylglycerol and activation of protein kinase C. Various functional abnormalities in diabetes have been linked to the protein kinase C activity.

Diabetic Ketoacidosis

This is a serious complication seen more frequently in type 1 DM and less frequently in type 2 DM. Diabetic ketoacidosis (sDKA) is caused by insulin deficiency often in association with stress and activation of counter-regulatory hormones. The stress conditions include infections, trauma, myocardial infarction and surgery.

The biochemical abnormalities are hyperglycemia, ketosis and metabolic acidosis. Hyperglycemia leads to osmotic diuresis, dehydration and electrolyte loss. Insulin deficiency and elevated glucagon, growth hormone and catecholamines lead to increased lipolysis from adipose tissue and increased synthesis of ketone bodies in the liver.

Table 9.18: Complications of diabetes mellitus.

Acute complications
- Diabetic ketoacidosis (DKA)
- Hyperglycemic hyperosmolar state (HHS)

Chronic complications
- Microvascular
  - Retinopathy
  - Neuropathy
  - Nephropathy
- Macrovascular
  - Coronary artery disease
  - Cerebrovascular disease
  - Peripheral vascular disease
- Non-vascular
  - Gastrointestinal (gastroparesis, diarrhea)
  - Genitourinary
  - Dermatologic
- Infectious
  - Cataract and glaucoma
- Miscellaneous (multiple etiology)
  - Diabetic foot **(Fig. 9.11)**
  - Erectile dysfunction

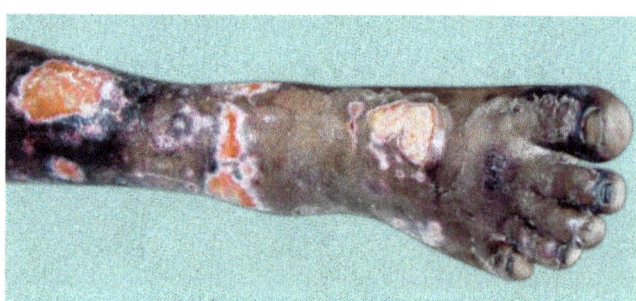

Fig. 9.11: Diabetic foot.

Clinical Features

The usual clinical manifestations are nausea, vomiting and abdominal pain. Patients may have respiratory distress, shock, confusion and coma. Examination reveals the presence of dehydration, rapid and deep breathing (Kussmaul's breathing), and fruity breath odor. There may be tachycardia and hypotension.

Investigations

Plasma glucose is very high. Arterial blood gas measurement shows metabolic acidosis. Urine examination reveals positive ketone test. Hyponatremia, hyperkalemia, azotemia and hyperosmolality are the other findings. Urine culture, blood culture, blood counts and X-ray of chest should be done to detect the evidence of infections. ECG is performed to rule out cardiac events.

Management

This is the medical emergency. The patient is hospitalized. The essential components of treatment are:

- Intravenous saline is initially given to correct dehydration. Once blood glucose level falls to 250 mg/dL, the fluid is changed to 5% dextrose solution.
- Intravenous infusion of regular insulin is administered until the ketoacidosis is corrected.
- Potassium and phosphate are replaced as needed.
- Sodium bicarbonate is generally not required. However, it is given if blood pH is less than 7.0.
- Antibiotics are given to treat infections.
- The electrolytes, blood glucose, blood urea, serum creatinine, arterial blood gases are periodically monitored.

Hyperglycemic Hyperosmolar State (HHS) (Non-ketotic Hyperosmolar Diabetic Coma)

This is characterized by severe hyperglycemia, hyperosmolality and dehydration without ketoacidosis. Ketoacidosis is generally absent because residual insulin secretion is adequate to inhibit lipolysis and ketogenesis.

It is a complication of type 2 DM. The precipitating factors include stress, infections, drug non-compliance, stroke and alcohol. The onset is insidious. The usual symptoms are polyuria, weight loss, drowsiness and altered sensorium. Severe dehydration, hypotension and tachycardia are the usual clinical findings. Thromboembolic complications are common.

Laboratory findings include marked hyperglycemia (>600 mg/dL), plasma osmolality greater than 350 mOsm/L, absence of ketonemia, pH >7.3 and prerenal azotemia. Lactic acidosis may occur in some patients.

Treatment includes fluid replacement, insulin therapy, and management of electrolytes especially potassium and phosphates. The requirement for insulin is less in HHS than in DKA.

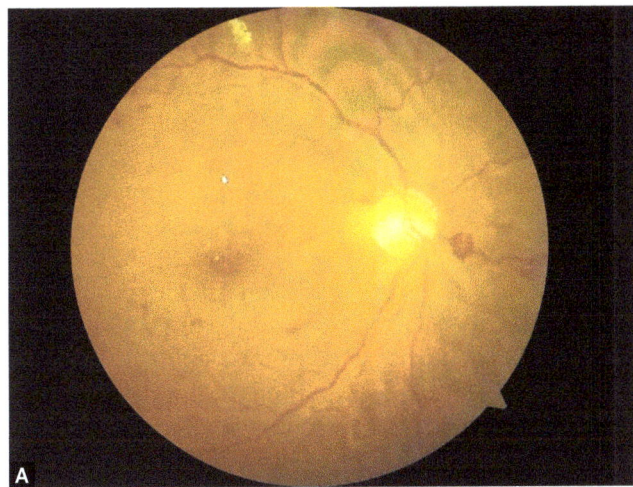
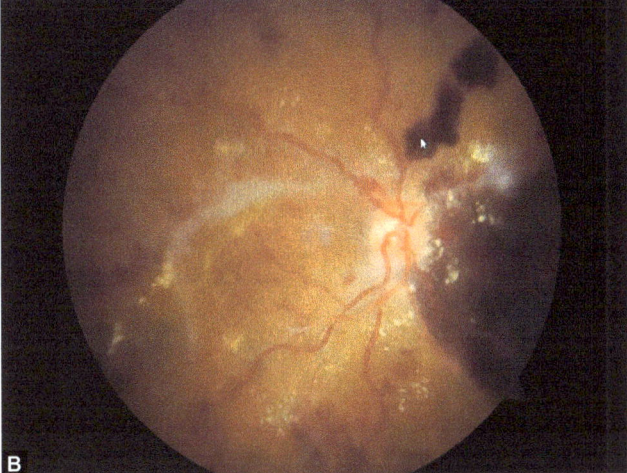

Figs. 9.12A and B: (A) Non-proliferative diabetic retinopathy; (B) Proliferative diabetic retinopathy.

Chronic Complications

Ocular Complications

These are important causes of blindness in the diabetics in developed countries. Diabetic retinopathy is an important ocular complication of DM. This generally develops after 10 years of the disease and almost all patients have retinopathy after 20 years of the disease. Duration of the disease and degree of the glycemic control are important predictors of this complication.

The diabetic retinopathy has two stages; non-proliferative (background or simple retinopathy) and proliferative retinopathy. Simple retinopathy is characterized by microaneurysms, retinal hemorrhages, exudates and cotton wool spots. New vessel formation in addition to changes seen in simple retinopathy occurs in proliferative retinopathy **(Figs. 9.12A and B)**.

Other ocular complications are macular edema, premature cataract and glaucoma.

Prevention is the most desired way to control the complications. Comprehensive eye examination is recommended at the time of diagnosis in type 2 DM and within 5 years after the onset of type 1 DM. Strict control of blood sugar and blood pressure prevents the development or slow the progression of retinopathy. Regular eye examination is recommended. The treatment of proliferative retinopathy and macular edema is laser photocoagulation or intravascular injection of anti-vascular endothelial growth factor. Intake of aspirin for cardioprotection is not contraindicated in patient with retinopathy.

Diabetic Nephropathy

This is the leading cause of end stage renal disease (ESRD). About 30–40% patients with type 1 DM and 15–20% patients with type 2 DM develop nephropathy after 20 years. The early manifestation of nephropathy is the onset of microalbuminuria. Microalbuminuria is defined as the urinary excretion of 30–300 mg albumin per day. Presence of albumin (>30 mg/d) in urine or spot urine albumin:creatinine ratio of >30 mcg albumin per mg of creatinine suggests nephropathy. It progresses to overt proteinuria (>300 mg/day) in few years.

- Intensive control of blood sugar and blood pressure is an effective way to reduce the progression of microalbuminuria to overt nephropathy.

- Urinary albumin measurement and estimated glomerular filtration rate (eGFR) should be done in all patients in type 2 DM annually whereas these are recommended to be done after 5 years of diagnosis in patients with type 1 DM.
- Dietary protein restriction may be beneficial in some patients.
- Angiotensin converting enzyme (ACE) inhibitors or angiotensin II receptor blockers (ARB) reduces the progression of overt nephropathy. Serum potassium and creatinine should be periodically monitored.
- Sodium-glucose cotransporter 2 inhibitor (SGLT 2) is beneficial in type 2 DM patients with nephropathy. This retards the progression of nephropathy and also reduces cardiac complications.
- Glucagon-like peptide-1 (GLP 1) receptor agonists are also useful in reducing renal and cardiovascular complications.

Diabetic Neuropathy

This may be sensory, motor, autonomic or combined. It may manifest as polyneuropathy or mononeuropathy. Neuropathy occurs in 50% cases with long standing DM. The presence of neuropathy is a risk factor for foot trauma, ulceration and arthropathy. Cranial nerves may also be involved. The most commonly affected nerves are 3rd and 6th cranial nerves. Autonomic neuropathy may manifest as postural hypotension, resting tachycardia, nocturnal diarrhea, impotency and urinary bladder dysfunctions. Hyperhidrosis or anhidrosis may occur.

The neuropathy may be asymptomatic. Annual examination of lower extremities for the touch and vibration sensations is recommended.

Painful neuropathy is treated with tricyclic antidepressants (nortryptyline, amitriptyline) or anticonvulsants (carbamazepine, gabapentin, and phenytoin). Pregabalin (75–300 mg) or duloxetine is also used in diabetic neuropathy. Topical use of capsaicin or 5% lidocaine patch may be beneficial.

Blood glucose should be controlled strictly. Alcohol should be avoided and vitamins (B_{12}, B_6, and folate) are replaced if deficient.

Macrovascular Complications

Various risk factors for the macrovascular disease include insulin resistance, hyperglycemia, microalbuminuria, hypertension, hyperlipidemia, smoking, and obesity.

Following are ways to minimize macrovascular complications;
- Optimal glycemic control
- Control of blood pressure to less than 130/80 mmHg (120/80 mmHg in patients with proteinuria). First line antihypertensive agents are ACE inhibitors or ARBs. Serum potassium level should be monitored.
- Dyslipidemia is managed with statins (target LDL level <100 mg/dL, Triglyceride <150 mg/dL). If patient has cardiovascular disease along with DM, the ideal goal is LDL < 70 mg/dL. In case, statin fails to achieve the goal, other agents such as ezetimibe or PCSK9 inhibitor can be added. High intensity statin (atorvastatin 40–80 mg daily or rosuvastatin 20–40 mg daily) is therapy recommended in all diabetic patients aged between 45 years and 70 years with cardiovascular disease risk. In others, moderate intensity statin therapy is recommended.
- Aspirin may be given as primary prevention if patient has increased cardiovascular risk and is more than 50 years of age.
- Cessation of smoking
- Weight reduction

Management of Diabetes

Ideal goals of the glycemic control in patients with DM are as follows, however, these goals are individualized.
- Average preprandial glucose values 80–130 mg/dL
- Bedtime glucose value of 100–140 mg/dL
- Peak postprandial glucose less than 180 mg/dL
- The level of HbA1c less than 7%.

The management of patients with DM includes:
- Diet control
- Exercise
- Education
- Medications for glycemic controls
- Treatment of associated conditions like hypertension, dyslipidemia, obesity and cardiovascular disease
- Detection and management of diabetes-related complications.
- Prophylactic vaccines for influenza, pneumococcus, human papillomavirus, and hepatitis B

Diet Modification

The diet is modified in such a way that it helps in maintenance of ideal body weight and provides essential nutrients. The caloric intake is optimized. Protein and fat should provide 15–20% and less than 30% of the total caloric intake respectively. Saturated fat should provide less than 10% of the total caloric intake. Cholesterol intake is restricted to less than 300 mg per day. Intake of dietary fibers is increased. Carbohydrate intake is individualized based on glycemic control, plasma lipids and body weight. Use of sweeteners is acceptable. Low glycemic index foods are preferred as they result in lower rise in blood glucose after meals. Low glycemic index foods (value less than 55) are fruits, vegetables, legumes, grainy breads, lentils and pasta.

Exercise

It provides multiple benefits;
- It improves insulin sensitivity

- Lowers plasma glucose
- Reduces blood pressure
- Improves dyslipidemia
- Lowers cardiovascular risk
- Enhances weight loss
- Maintain muscle mass.

Moderate to vigorous intensity aerobic exercises are recommended. Aerobic exercise for 150 minutes or more spread over at least 3 days per week is advised. There should not be a gap of more than 2 days consecutively. In addition, 2–3 sessions of resistance exercises per week is also recommended. In general exercise is planned under medical supervision.

Education

The education of patients on different aspects of the disease is very important. They should be educated about the diet, exercise, self-monitoring of blood glucose and urinary glucose and ketones. Patients should be warned about the symptoms and dangers of hypoglycemia. They are trained in foot and skin care and about insulin injections. Patients should be told about hazards of smoking and persuaded to stop it.

Pharmacological Management

If glycemic control is not achieved by non-pharmacological means such as diet control, and increased physical activities in 3–4 weeks, pharmacological therapy is indicated. Pharmocological therapy consists of oral and parenteral drugs.

Glucose Lowering Agents

Most oral glucose lowering agents require some pancreatic function for their glucose lowering effects, hence they are generally used in type 2 DM. Insulin is ultimately required in advanced stage of type 2 DM. Oral glucose lowering agents are classified into various groups **(Table 9.19)**.

The treatment should be started with lower dosage and increased slowly to the optimal dose in several days or weeks.

Some of these agents are available in extended release forms. Hence, these need to be administered less frequently.

Insulin secretagogues: These agents stimulate insulin secretion by pancreatic beta cells. Important side effects are weight gain and hypoglycemia. Sulfonylurea should be given 30 to 60 minutes before meals. Non-sulfonylureas are given with each meal to reduce meal related increase in blood glucose. These should not be given if a patient is observing fast.

Biguanides: Biguanides reduce hepatic glucose production and improve glucose utilization in peripheral tissues. These are taken with food. They also improve lipid profile and promote weight loss. Side effects are diarrhea, anorexia, nausea and lactic acidosis. They do not result in hypoglycemia. Metformin is contraindicated in renal insufficiency, heart failure, liver disease, severe hypoxia and other conditions associated with the acidosis.

Alpha glucosidase inhibitors: They reduce postprandial hyperglycemia by delaying glucose absorption. These are given with the first bite during meal. Side effects are diarrhea and flatulence. These agents can also be used in type 1 DM.

Table 9.19: Glucose lowering agents (Anti-diabetic drugs).

Drugs	Daily dose
ORAL	
Insulin secretagogues	
Sulfonylureas	
• Glipizide	2.5–40 mg in 1 or 2 divided doses
• Gliclazide	40–320 mg in 2 divided doses
• Glimepiride	1–8 mg, single dose
• Glibenclamide (glyburide)	2.5–10 mg in 1 or 2 divided doses
Non-sulfonylureas:	
• Repaglinide	0.5–4 mg three times before meals
• Mitiglinide	5–10 mg three times before meals
• Natiglinide	60–120 mg three times before meals
Biguanides:	
Metformin	500–2000 mg in 2–3 divided doses
Alpha glucosidase inhibitors	
Acarbose	75–300 mg in 3 divided doses
Miglitol	75–300 mg in 3 divided doses
Voglibose	0.6–0.9 mg in 3 divided doses
Thiazolidinediones	
Pioglitazone	15–45 mg, single dose
Incretins	
DDP-IV inhibitors	
Sitagliptin	100 mg OD
Vildagliptin	50 mg BD
Saxagliptin	5 mg OD
Linagliptin	5 mg OD
Alogliptin	25 mg OD
Teneligliptin	20–40 mg OD
Bile acid sequestrant	
Colesevelam	3 tablets of 625 mg twice a day
Dopamine receptor agonist	
Bromocriptine mesylate	0.8–4.8 mg once daily
SGLT$_2$ inhibitors	
Dapagliflozin	5–10 mg once daily
Canagliflozin	100–300 mg one daily
Empagliflozin	10–25 mg once daily
Remogliflozin	100 mg twice daily
Ertugliflozin	15 mg once daily
GLP-1 receptor agonist	
Semaglutide	14 mg once weekly
PARENTERAL	
Insulin (*see* Table 9.20)	
Incretins	
GLP-1 receptor agonist	
Exenatide	5–10 mcg BD
Exenatide, extended release	2 mg once weekly
Liraglutide	0.6–1.8 mg once daily
Dulaglutide	0.75–4.5 mg once weekly
Lixisenatide	20 mcg daily
Semaglutide	1 mg once weekly
Amylin analog	
Pramlintide	15–120 mcg three times before meals

Thiazolidinediones: Thiazolidinediones enhance insulin sensitivity in muscle, adipose tissue and liver, hence reduce insulin resistance. These can cause hepatotoxicity and fluid retention hence, are not given in cases of liver disease and congestive heart failure. They may increase the risk of fracture in women. Rosiglitazone is not available now. Pioglitazone should be used in low doses (15 mg/ day).

Incretins

The glucose-dependent insulinotropic polypeptide (GIP) and glucagon-like peptide (GLP-1) are two major incretin hormones released in response to ingestion of meal. In the fasting stage, their levels are low but after eating a meal their secretion increases rapidly.

- GIP is a peptide (42 amino acid) secreted by endocrine K cells in proximal gastrointestinal tract
- GLP-1 is a peptide (30–31 amino acid) secreted from L cells in the distal gastrointestinal tract.

They mediate their actions by binding and activation of receptors (GLP-1R and GIP-R) located in several tissues, including alpha and beta cells in the pancreas.

GIP and GLP-1 stimulate glucose dependent insulin release from beta cells. They contribute 60–70% of the total postprandial insulin response in healthy individuals (Incretin effect). This incretin effect is markedly decreased in diabetic patients due to low levels of postparandial incretin hormones. GLP-1 also suppresses hepatic glucose output by inhibiting glucagon response from alpha cells in a glucose dependent manner.

After secretion these are rapidly metabolized by the enzyme dipeptidyl peptidase (DPP-4). The plasma half-life of these incretins is short (2–5 minutes). Following degradation, the metabolites are eliminated from the kidneys.

Agents that either have similar action as GLP-1 or increase GLP-1 activity are available for use in diabetes. Two major strategies have been developed to increase the effects of incretins:

1. *Incretin mimetics (GLP-1 analogs, GLP-1 receptor agonists):* These agents that mimic the action of GLP-1 on glucose control. These are resistant to endogenous DPP-4, thus have prolonged GLP-1 like action and improve glycemic control by reducing glucose concentration by following mechanisms:
   - Beta cell effect; enhancement of glucose dependent insulin secretion and restoration of first phase insulin response
   - Suppression of elevated glucagon secretion
   - Slowing of gastric emptying
   - Reduction of food intake.

   GLP-1 receptor agonists also result into weight loss. Some of these agents have cardiovascular benefits and slow down the progression of renal damage. These are indicated as an adjunct therapy to improve glycemic control in patients with type 2 DM who are taking metformin, sulfonylurea or combination of both but have not achieved glycemic control. Major side effects include nausea, vomiting, and diarrhea. There is an increased risk of pancreatitis with the use of GLP-1 receptor agonists. These should not be used in patients with personal or family history of medullary thyroid carcinoma or MEN syndrome type 2.

   Exenatide: Exenatide is a 39 amino acid peptide and exhibits same glucoregulatory effects as the human incretin hormone GLP-1. It is given in dosage of 5–10 mg subcutaneously twice daily. Now it is also available in extended release form. Extended release form is given in a doses of 2 mg once weekly.

   Liraglutide: Liraglutide is soluble fatty acid GLP-1 analog. It has a long half life of approximately 12 hours. It is given as subcutaneous injection once a day. The dose of Liraglutide is 0.6–1.8 mg daily.

   Dulaglutide: It is given as subcutaneous injection once weekly and has been recently approved for use in diabetes mellitus.

   Semaglutide: It is synthetic analog of GLP-1 which is given as 0.25 to 1 mg subcutaneous weekly. Oral form is also available.

   Lexisenatide: The dose ranges from 10–20 mcg once daily subcutaneously.

2. *Incretin enhancers (DPP-4 inhibitors):* These are oral anti-diabetic drugs and act by inhibiting DPP-4 (dipeptidyl peptidase) enzyme. By inhibiting the DPP-4, the endogenous levels of incretins (GLP-1) are increased. These are indicated as an adjunct therapy to improve glycemic control in patients with type 2 DM who are taking metformin, sulfonylurea or combination of both but have not achieved glycemic control. Recently they have been approved for use as first line agents either alone (monotherapy) or in combination with metformin. These can be used in combination with metformin, sulfonylurea and insulin They are weight neutral having no effect on body weight. Major side effects include nasopharyngitis, dizziness, headache, diarrhea, and constipation. Pancreatitis has been reported in rare cases.

   Various DPP-4 inhibitors are:
   - Sitagliptin is used orally in dosage of 100 mg daily.
   - Vildagliptin is used orally in dosage of 50 mg twice daily.
   - Saxagliptin is used orally in dosage of 2.5–5.0 mg once daily.
   - Linagliptin is used orally in dosage of 5 mg once daily.
   - Alogliptin is used orally in dosage of 25 mg daily.
   - Tenegliptin is used orally in dosage of 20–40 mg daily.

   No dose adjustment of Linagliptin is required in patients with renal failure. The dosage of other gliptins is adjusted in renal failure and they are used in reduced doses.

SGLT 2 Inhibitors

Glucose is filtered by renal glomeruli and reabsorbed in the proximal tubules by the action of sodium- glucose – cotransporters (SGLT). SGLT2 is involved in reabsorption of glucose in the proximal tubules. Dapagliflozin, cangliflozin, empagliflozin, remogliflozin and ertugliflozin are SGLT2 inhibitors and all are given orally. These agents prevent reabsorption of glucose in tubules and consequently lead to glycosuria. They reduce risk for all-cause and cardiovascular mortality as well as slow down the progression of renal disease. They also cause modest weight loss of 2–4 Kg. The main side effects are increased incidence of urinary tract infection and genital fungal infections. The usual dose of dapagliflozin is 10 mg daily (5 mg in hepatic disease), canagliflozin is 100-300 mg once daily, empagliflozin 10–25 mg once daily, and remegliflozin 100 mg twice daily. These drugs can be used as monotherapy or in combination with other drugs or insulin.

Pramlintide

It is an amylin analog given as injection. It suppresses glucagon secretion, delays gastric emptying and decreases appetite. Pramlintide is used in patients with type 1 and insulin treated type 2 diabetes mellitus to improve glucose control by blunting postprandial blood glucose. The dose is 15-120 mcg before each meal. Side effects include nausea, vomiting and diarrhea.

Other Drugs

Bromocriptine (dopamine receptor agonists) in doses of 0.8–4.8 mg once daily has been used in patients with diabetes who do not achieve glucose control with other oral drugs.

Colesevelam hydrochloride is a bile acid sequestrant and has glucose lowering properties. It can be used as monotherapy or in conjunction with metformin or sulfonylureas in doses of 3 tablets of 625 mg twice daily. Its major side effect is constipation. It should not be used in patients with high triglycerides.

Insulin

Human insulin is produced through recombinant DNA technology. Bovine and porcine insulins are now rarely used. Insulins are divided into various groups based on the onset and duration of action **(Table 9.20)**. Insulin is indicated in type 1 DM and in type 2 DM where glucose control is not achieved with oral agents. Insulin is usually given subcutaneously in abdomen, thighs, buttocks and upper arms. However, regular insulin can also be given intravenously. Insulin pumps can be used for continuous subcutaneous delivery. Insulin pen injector devices are also available which cause lesser pain.

Inhaled insulin (Technosphere insulin) is recombinant human regular insulin as a dry powder formulation that can be inhaled before meals. Inhaled insulin taken before meals may improve glucose control without increasing risk of hypoglycemia or weight gain. They are not indicated in asthma, chronic obstructive pulmonary disease, and in patients who smoke or who recently have stopped smoking. Spirometry is recommended to rule out chronic lung disease before initiating inhaled insulin therapy.

Insulin lispro, aspart, glulisine, glargine, degludec, and detemir are genetically modified insulin analogs. Insulin is

Table 9.20: Types of insulin.

Insulin preparations	Onset (in h)	Peak (in h)	Duration (in h)
Ultrashort acting			
Insulin lispro, insulin aspart, insulin glulisine	<0.25	0.5–1.5	3–4
Short acting			
Regular insulin	0.5–1	2–3	6–8
Intermediate acting			
NPH (neutral protamine hagedorn)	2–4	6–12	10–16
Lente insulin	3–4	6–12	12–18
Long acting			
Ultralente insulin	4–6	10–16	18–20
PZI (protamine zinc insulin)	3–8	14–24	24–36
Insulin glargine	2–4	—	20–24
Insulin detemir	1–4	—	12–24
Insulin degludec	2–4	—	24

Combination
Premixed insulins
70/30, 70% NPH and 30% regular
50/50, 50% NPH and 50% regular
75/25, 75% protamine lispro and 25% lispro
70/30, 70% Insulin degludec and 30% insulin aspart
Premixed insulin/GLP 1 RA products
Glargine/lixisenatide
Degludec/liraglutide

available in the concentration of 40 U/mL (U-40) or 100 U/mL (U-100). Concentrated insulin preparations are now also available. U-500 regular insulin is five times more concentrated than U-100 regular insulin.

Regular U-500 has delayed onset and longer duration of action and can be given as two or three daily injections. Rapid-acting U 200 insulin lispro (200 units/mL) has also been approved.

U-300 glargine and U-200 degludec are three and two times as concentrated as their U-100 formulation and have longer duration of action. Higher doses of basal insulin can be administered with less volume.

Complications of insulin therapy include hypoglycemia, insulin allergy, weight gain, insulin resistance due to antibodies and lipodystrophy at injection sites.

Insulin Regimens

Various insulin regimens are followed in order to achieve the uniform glycemic control.

- Basal-bolus regimen: Long acting insulin is given once a day (basal insulin) usually at bed time and short/ultra short acting insulin is used before each meals (bolus insulin). Basal insulin requirement is fulfilled by long acting or intermediate acting insulin. These are often combined with the regular, lispro or aspart insulin to mimic physiological release of insulin with meals. The preparation containing lispro or aspart insulin is injected just before or after the meals while those with the regular insulin is given 30–45 minutes prior to meal. Generally total dose of insulin required is 0.5–1.0 unit/kg/day

which is divided into multiple doses. 40–50% of the daily requirement is given as basal insulin.
- Twice daily premixed insulin regimens: It includes twice daily injection of intermediate insulin mixed with short acting insulin. Two-third of the total dose is given before the morning meal and remaining one-third before the evening meal.
- Continuous subcutaneous insulin infusion (CSII) is another regimen delivered by programmable pump.

Management Steps in Diabetic Patients

The steps in the management of diabetic patients depend upon the type of the DM and the specific needs of the patients.

Type 1 DM: The treatment of type 1 DM is lifelong insulin replacement. However, alpha glucosidase inhibitors (acarbose, miglitol) can be given to reduce carbohydrate absorption.

Diet modifications, physical exercise and education are also important for the proper control of blood sugar.

Type 2 DM: In type 2 patients, weight reduction should be achieved in obese patients by diet modification and increased physical activity. Metformin is the first line therapy in type 2 diabetes patients. If this is inadequate to achieve or maintain A1c target over 3 months, second oral agent (sulfonylurea, thiazolidinediones, gliptin, SGLT 2 inhibitors) or GLP-1 receptor agonist or insulin are added alone or in combination. If the combination of oral drugs fails to control blood glucose levels, insulin or GLP 1 receptor agonists therapy is instituted. If newly diagnosed type 2 diabetic patient has markedly elevated glucose levels or A1c and/or has severe symptoms, insulin may be considered (alone or with other additional agents) from the outset.

Indications of insulin use in type 2 DM are summarized as below:
- As an initial therapy in patients with severe weight loss
- As add on therapy when other agents fail to achieve the target.
- Patients with hepatic or renal disease where oral agents are contraindicated.
- Patients who are acutely ill (DKA, HHS), and
- During pregnancy.

Recent guidelines for management of type 2 diabetes: Metformin should be started as first line therapy, unless contraindicated, along with lifestyle modifications (Diet, weight management and exercise) at the time type 2 diabetes is diagnosed. Further choice of medication depends on patient characteristics (established atherosclerotic cardiovascular disease (ASCVD) or indicators of high ASCVD risk, heart failure or CKD), weight, safety, risk for hypoglycaemia, tolerability, cost and patient preferences. Additional agent is added afront if patient has established ASCVD or indicators of high ASCVD risk, heart failure or CKD.

- For patients with established ASCVD or indicators of high ASCVD risk (such as patients >55 years of age with coronary, carotid, or lower-extremity artery stenosis > 50% or left ventricular hypertrophy)
SGLT2 inhibitor or GLP-1 RA is added. If A1c remains above target both the drugs (SGLT2 inhibitor and GLP-1 RA) can be combined or other drugs with cardiac safety can be added like thiazolidinediones (Pioglitazone), DPP-4 inhibitor (if not on GLP-1 RA), basal insulin or sulfonylurea may be added.
- For patients with heart failure—SGLT2 inhibitor is preferred.
- For patients with CKD (chronic kidney disease)—SGLT2 inhibitor is added. If it is contraindicated or not tolerated, GLP-1 RA is given.

If patient has no established ASCVD or no indicators of high ASCVD risk, heart failure or CKD and A1c is above target
- DPP-4 inhibitor, GLP-1 RA, SGLT2, Thiazolidinediones (Pioglitazone), or sulfonylurea are used alone or in combination.
b. DPP-4 inhibitor, GLP-1 RA and SGLT2 are preferred if hypoglycemia is a concern.
c. If weight loss is required, GLP-1 RA or SGLT2 inhibitor is preferred.
d. Sulfonylureas and pioglitazone are economical drugs and are preferred usually if cost is a limiting factor.

Basal insulin (human NPH or one of the longacting insulin analogs) is added if A1c is still high after giving combination of 3 drugs. Recent guidelines recommend adding GLP-1 receptor agonists as preferred option to an oral regimen if glucose is not controlled and HbA1c is high. Most GLP-1 RA are injectables drugs, poorly tolerated by some patients and are also costly as compared to insulins. Oral semaglutide is now available.

Metabolic Syndrome

The metabolic syndrome (syndrome X, insulin resistance syndrome) consists of a constellation of metabolic abnormalities that confer increased risk of cardiovascular disease (CVD) and diabetes mellitus (DM). The major features of the metabolic syndrome include central obesity, hypertriglyceridemia, low high-density lipoprotein (HDL) cholesterol, hyperglycemia, and hypertension **(Table 9.21)**. Risk factors include obesity, sedentary lifestyle, aging, diabetes mellitus, coronary heart disease, lipodystrophy and genetic factors. Main pathophysiology behind its development is insulin resistance. Other contributing factors are glucose intolerance, hypertension, dyslipidemia and proinflammatory cytokines. Metabolic syndrome confers a 2 fold increase in the relative risk for atherosclerotic cardiovascular disease and a five-fold increase in the risk of developing diabetes as compared with people without syndrome. Treatment involves diet and lifestyle modifications, increase physical activity and appropriate control of blood glucose, blood pressure and lipids.

Table 9.21: IDF (International Diabetes Federation) criteria for metabolic syndrome*.

- Waist circumference ≥ 90 cm in males, ≥ 80 cm in females
  Plus
- Two or more of the following:
  – Fasting triglycerides >150 mg/dL or specific treatment for this abnormality
  – HDL cholesterol <40 mg/dL in males and <50 mg/dL in females or specific treatment for this abnormality
  – Blood pressure >130 mm systolic or >85 mm diastolic or specific treatment for hypertension
  – Fasting plasma glucose >100 mg/dL or previously diagnosed type 2 diabetes mellitus

*If BMI is 30 kg/m², central obesity is assumed and there is no need to measure waist circumference.

Hypoglycemia

Hypoglycemia means low blood sugar levels, generally <50 mg/dL. However, the threshold may vary widely from patient to patient. This is the most common complication of insulin therapy. Hypoglycemia can also occur due to sulfonylurea therapy. Risk factors for the development of hypoglycemia include skipped meal, delay in the meal, unusual physical exertion, alcohol ingestion and drug overdose. Hypoglycemia can also occur in other conditions such as insulinomas (beta islet tumor), liver disease, adrenal insufficiency and hypopituitarism.

Clinical Presentations

Manifestations of hypoglycemia are commonly due to activation of autonomic nervous system and secondary to glucose deprivation of the brain. Autonomic symptoms are sweating, trembling, palpitation, hunger and anxiety. Neurological manifestations are impaired concentration, irritation, confusion, seizures and coma. Nausea, headache and tiredness are non-specific symptoms.

Diagnosis

The diagnosis is made by the measurement of plasma or capillary blood glucose.

Treatment

The treatment depends upon the severity of hypoglycemia and consciousness level of the patient.
- If the patient is able to swallow, rapidly absorbable carbohydrates can be administered orally (glucose and sugar). Alternatively milk, fruit, candy bars, or biscuits may be given to patients with mild hypoglycemia.
- If the patient is unable to swallow or is in severe hypoglycemia, intravenous glucose (20–50 mL of 50% dextrose) is given initially. This is followed by an infusion of 10% dextrose to maintain blood glucose above 100 mg/dL.
- Glucagon injection (1 mg SC or IM) may be given in severe hypoglycemia if intravenous access can not be established promptly.
- Prevention of hypoglycemia includes proper education regarding causes and symptoms of hypoglycemia and proper adjustment in medication and diet.

IMPLICATIONS ON DENTAL PRACTICE

- Oral conditions seen in diabetic patients include burning mouth, altered wound healing and increased incidence of infections. Xerostomia may result from diabetes *per se* or from medications.
- Diabetes is a risk factor for the prevalence and severity of gingivitis and periodontis. Periodontal infection may adversely affect glycemic control. Proper dental treatment may have favorable effects on glycemic control.
- Diabetes may be associated with the increased incidence of oral candidiasis. Severe diabetes with ketoacidosis may predispose patient to mucormycosis of the paranasal sinuses and nose.
- Blood sugar should be adequately controlled before any surgery.
- The normal pattern of food intake may be disturbed by dental disease or dental treatment. This can interfere with diabetic control.
- Most common emergency in diabetic patients during dental treatment is hypoglycemia. A proper history about the time of meals and anti-diabetic medications must be recorded. Easily absorbable carbohydrates (glucose, sugar, candies, chocolates, and fruit juices) should be available for emergency use.
- Patients with Cushing's syndrome may develop complications following dental procedures. These include excessive bleeding, poor wound healing and increased susceptibility to infections.
- Patients with Cushing's syndrome have higher incidence of candida and other fungal infections.
- Brown or black pigmentation of the oral mucosa is seen in patients with Addison's disease (adrenal insufficiency). This condition must be suspected if there is hypotension, weakness, nausea, anorexia, vomiting, abdominal pain and weight loss.
- In hyperthyroidism, elevated systolic blood pressure may require caution. Longer duration of local pressure is needed to stop bleeding in such cases. Patients may be difficult to deal as they may be anxious and irritable.
- Deposition of subcutaneous mucopolysaccharides in hypothyroidism may lead to impaired ability of small vessels to contract when cut. This may result in excessive bleeding. Hence, local pressure is required for longer period to control bleeding.
- There is also a delayed wound healing and increased risk of infection due to poor healing in hypothyroidism.
- Use of sedatives, opioid analgesics and tranquillizers may precipitate myxedema coma in patients with hypothyroidism.
- Well controlled hyperthyroidism and hypothyroidism do not pose any additional risk for dental procedures.

- Dryness of the mouth may be present in diabetes insipidus.
16. Brown tumor of the jaw should be differentiated from giant cell granuloma of the jaw.
17. Enamel hypoplasia, delayed eruption and chronic mucocutaneous candidiasis may occur in idiopathic congenital hypoparathyroidism.

SELF ASSESSMENT

Multiple Choice Questions

1. Excess of cortisol causes:
   - A. Conn's syndrome
   - B. Cushing's syndrome
   - C. Diabetes insipidus
   - D. Acromegaly
2. Signs of hypoglycemia include the following, *except*:
   - A. Sweating
   - B. Mental confusion
   - C. Tachycardia
   - D. Hyperpyrexia
3. Which of the following is associated with tetany:
   - A. Chvostick's sign
   - B. Kussmaul's sign
   - C. Corrigan sign
   - D. Lock jaw
4. Features not associated with type 2 diabetes mellitus:
   - A. Onset after 30 years
   - B. Obesity
   - C. Ketoacidosis very common
   - D. Insulin resistance
5. Initial drug preferred in type 2 obese diabetics:
   - A. Gliclazide
   - B. Repaglinide
   - C. Metformin
   - D. Acarbose
6. Treatment of choice for type 1 diabetics:
   - A. Metformin
   - B. Insulin
   - C. Acarbose
   - D. Glipizide
7. Earliest feature in diabetic nephropathy is:
   - A. Hematuria
   - B. Raised serum creatinine
   - C. Microalbuminuria
   - D. Overt proteinuria
8. All of the following hormones are secreted by anterior pituitary, *except*:
   - A. ACTH
   - B. TSH
   - C. ADH
   - D. FSH
9. Bone pain, bone cysts, fracture and renal stones are found in:
   - A. Multiple myeloma
   - B. Hyperparathyroidism
   - C. Osteomalacia
   - D. Marfan's syndrome
10. In alkalosis, following is true:
    - A. Normal total serum and normal ionic calcium
    - B. Low total serum and normal ionic calcium
    - C. Normal total serum and low ionic calcium
    - D. Low total serum and low ionic calcium
11. Tetany may occur in:
    - A. Alkalosis
    - B. Hyperparathyroidism
    - C. Myxedema
    - D. Hyperglycemia
12. Following are features of diabetes insipidus, *except*:
    - A. Polyuria
    - B. Polydipsia
    - C. Polyphagia
    - D. High plasma osmolality
13. Most common cause of thyrotoxicosis is:
    - A. Graves' disease
    - B. Multinodular goiter
    - C. TSH secreting pituitary tumor
    - D. Toxic adenoma
14. Pretibial myxedema is seen in:
    - A. Hypothyroidism
    - B. Graves' disease
    - C. Hashimoto's disease
    - D. All of the above
15. Which one of the following is the early feature of hypothyroidism:
    - A. Low T_3
    - B. High TSH
    - C. Low T_4
    - D. Low TSH
16. In hypoalbuminemia, following is true:
    - A. Low total serum calcium
    - B. Low ionized calcium
    - C. Low total serum calcium and low ionized calcium
    - D. Low total serum calcium and normal ionized calcium
17. Following is seen in hypocalcemia:
    - A. Convulsions
    - B. Laryngeal spasm
    - C. Perioral paresthesia
    - D. All of the above
18. The common causes of hypocalcemia include all, *except*:
    - A. Chronic renal failure
    - B. Hypoparathyroidism
    - C. Vitamin D deficiency
    - D. High serum albumin
19. Hypercalcemia associated with malignancy is most often mediated by:
    - A. Parathyroid hormone
    - B. Parathyroid-related protein (PTHrP)
    - C. Interleukin-6
    - D. Calcitonin
20. Hyperthyroidism is treated by:
    - A. Carbimazole
    - B. Radioactive iodine
    - C. Subtotal thyroidectomy
    - D. All of the above
21. Glycated Hb (HbA1) provides measure of glucose control over a period of:
    - A. Within 6 hours
    - B. Within one week
    - C. Within 1–3 weeks
    - D. Within 8–12 weeks
22. Which one is not a feature of hyperglycemic hyper-osmolar state:
    - A. Severe hyperglycemia
    - B. Marked dehydration
    - C. High incidence of thromboembolic complications
    - D. Presence of ketosis
23. Which of the following drug is not a insulin secretogog:
    - A. Glipizide
    - B. Glimperide
    - C. Repaglinide
    - D. Rosiglitazone
24. Hypoglycemia is not a complication of:
    - A. Glipizide
    - B. Glimperide
    - C. Metformin
    - D. Repaglinide
25. Drug which inhibits absorption of glucose from intestine is:
    - A. Gliclazide
    - B. Pioglitazone
    - C. Acarbose
    - D. Natiglinide
26. SGLT2 inhibitors have been approved for use in:
    - A. Diabetes mellitus
    - B. Hypertension
    - C. Angina pectoris
    - D. Bronchial asthma
27. Which of the following is a sodium glucose transport inhibitor (SGLT2):
    - A. Liraglutide
    - B. Colesevelam
    - C. Pramlintide
    - D. Canagliflozin
28. Dapagliflozin inhibits which of the following receptor:
    - A. SGLT 1
    - B. SGLT 2
    - C. SGLT 3
    - D. SGLT 4
29. All of the following are DDP IV inhibitors, *except*:
    - A. Linagliptin
    - B. Monagliptin
    - C. Saxagliptin
    - D. Vildagliptin

30. **Increased risk of pancreatitis has been associated with which of the following drug:**
    A. Canaglifozin
    B. Sitagliptin
    C. Acarbose
    D. Glimepride
31. **The mechanism of action of dapagliflozin is:**
    A. Increased secretion of insulin from pancreas
    B. Decrease hepatic glucose output
    C. Inhibition of reabsorption of glucose from renal tubules
    D. Inhibition of glucose absorption from intestine

Fill in the Blanks

1. Moon face and buffalo hump are seen in _____.
2. Active form of thyroid hormone is called _____.
3. Trousseau's sign is present in _____.
4. Normal level of total serum calcium is _____.
5. Carpopedal spasm (main d'accoucheur) is a feature of _____.
6. Goiter, bruit over thyroid gland, ophthalmopathy and dermopathy is seen in thyrotoxicosis due to _____.
7. Condition when the production of PTH is normal but there is tissue resistance to PTH is _____.
8. Most common cause of primary hyperparathyroidism is _____.
9. Basal ganglion calcification and cataract formation are seen in _____.
10. Fasting plasma glucose more than _____ is diagnostic of diabetes mellitus.
11. Impaired fasting plasma glucose is between _____ and _____ mg/dL.
12. Rapid and deep breathing in diabetic ketoacidosis is known as _____.
13. Microalbuminuria is defined as excretion of _____ to _____ albumin daily.
14. The drug of choice in hypertension with diabetes mellitus is _____.
15. The insulin which can be given intravenously is _____.

CHAPTER 10

Infections

MEASLES (RUBEOLA)

Measles (Rubeola) is an acute paramyxoviral infection. It is a cause of major morbidity and mortality in children worldwide.
- *Mode of transmission:* Measles is a highly infectious disease. It spreads through infected droplets. Patients in pre-eruptive and catarrhal phase are most infectious.
- Incubation period is about 7–14 days.
- Illness confers permanent immunity.

Clinical Features

- Illness starts with high fever, dry cough, sore throat, malaise and redness of conjunctivae. There may be photophobia.
- After about 2 days of fever, tiny white spots surrounded by red margin appear on buccal mucosa. These *'Koplik's spots'* are pathognomonic of measles **(Fig. 10.1)**.
- Rashes appear over the face and behind the ears 4 days after the onset of fever. These *non-pruritic erythematous maculopapular rashes* descend and involve the whole body **(Fig. 10.2)**. The rashes fade in order of appearance.
- Other features include pharyngeal edema, red tongue, generalized lymphadenopathy, and splenomegaly.
- Disease is more severe and prolonged in adults. The clinical features may be atypical.

Complications

- *Neurological:* Such complications are rare. Encephalitis can occur after 3–7 days of the appearance of rashes. Other complications are aseptic meningitis and transverse myelitis. Subacute sclerosing panencephalitis (SSPE) is a very late complication which occurs years after the initial infection.

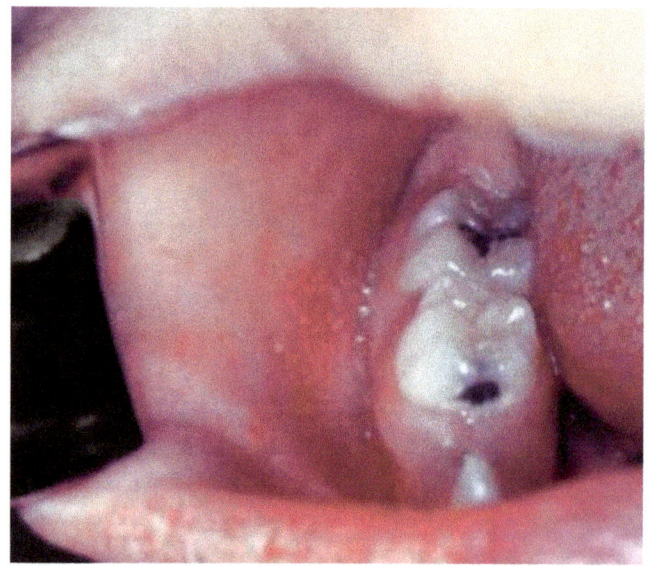

Fig. 10.1: Koplik spot in a case of measles.

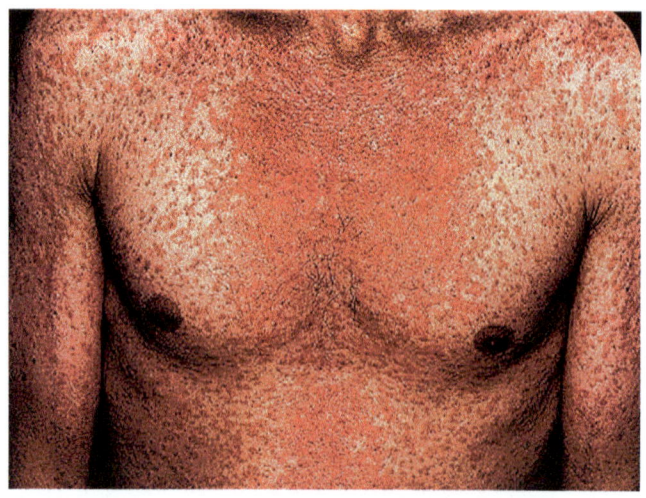

Fig. 10.2: Measles patient.

- *Respiratory:* Pneumonia or bronchopneumonia can occur due to the measles virus or due to secondary bacterial infection. This is the most common complication of measles in adults. Bronchiectasis may occur in children.
- Otitis media is the most common complication in young children.
- Cervical adenitis and pancreatitis are uncommon complications.
- *Gastrointestinal:* Possible complications are gastroenteritis, hepatitis and ileocolitis.

Laboratory Diagnosis

- Blood examination shows leukopenia. Leukocytosis suggests the presence of bacterial infection. Thrombocytopenia is common.
- Specific diagnosis can quickly be made by the immunofluorescence techniques which detect the presence of viral antigens in the respiratory secretion.
- RT-PCR can detect viral RNA.
- Specific IgM antibodies suggest recent infection.

The important differential diagnoses include drug reaction, infectious mononucleosis and mycoplasma infection.

Management

The management of measles is mainly symptomatic and supportive.
- The patients should be isolated for the week following onset of rashes and put on bed rest.
- Antipyretics and fluid therapy may be needed.
- Vitamin A administration has been shown to reduce morbidity in children. The dose is 2,00,000 IU once a day for 2 days in children >1 year of age.
- Antibiotics should not be used routinely and should be given only to treat bacterial complications.
- Antiviral drug ribavirin may be considered for use in immune-compromised patient.
- Zinc supplementation may help in improving immune function.
- SSPE is managed symptomatically.

Preventions

- Live attenuated measles vaccine should be given at the age of 9 months to all children **(Table 10.1)**. However a combined measles, mumps and rubella (MMR) vaccine can be given at the age of 12–15 months. MMR booster is given at 4–12 years of age. This provides life long protection.
- Immunoglobulin if given to immune-competent person within 72 hours of exposure usually prevents infection. It also prevents development of clinical disease in most persons who get infected.
- Post-exposure prophylaxis is indicated for immune-compromised persons within 6 days of contact. A dose of immunoglobulin 0.25 mL/kg is given in adults. This is followed by vaccinations after 3 months. Vaccine and immunoglobulin should not be given concurrently.

	Table 10.1: National immunization schedule.
At birth	BCG (Bacillus Calmette-Guerin vaccine), oral polio, Hepatitis B
At 6 weeks	BCG (if not given at birth), DPT (Diphtheria, Tetanus, Pertussis) and oral polio, Hepatitis B, fIPV (fractional inactivated polio vaccine), Rotavirus, Hib (*Haemophilus influenzae* type b), PCV (Pneumococcal Conjugate Vaccine)*
At 10 weeks	DPT (Diphtheria, Tetanus, Pertussis) and oral polio, Hepatitis B, Rotavirus, Hib (*Haemophilus influenzae* type b)
At 14 weeks	DPT (Diphtheria, Tetanus, Pertussis) and oral polio, Hepatitis B, fIPV(fractional inactivated polio vaccine), Rotavirus, Hib (*Haemophilus influenzae* type b), PCV (Pneumococcal Conjugate Vaccine)
At 9-12 months	Measles/MR (Measles Rubella), PCV (Pneumococcal Conjugate Vaccine), JE (Japanese encephalitis vaccine)**
At 16–24 months	DPT (Diphtheria, Tetanus, Pertussis) and oral polio, measles/MR (Measles Rubella), JE (Japanese encephalitis vaccine)
At 5–6 years	DPT (Diphtheria, Tetanus, Pertussis)
At 10, 16 years	Td vaccine (Tetanus and adult diphtheria)

*PCV is given in selected states/districts
**JE in endemic districts only

MUMPS

Mumps is a systemic viral infection caused by paramyxovirus.
- It spreads through respiratory droplets or saliva.
- Multiplication of the virus in the upper respiratory tract epithelium is followed by a phase of viremia. Subsequently various organs such as salivary glands, pancreas, meninges and gonads are involved.
- Incubation period is 14–21 days.
- Patients become infective one day before the appearance of symptoms and remain so for a week.

Clinical Features

The prodromal symptoms like fever, malaise and myalgia appear first.

This is followed by bilateral tender parotid swelling generally within next 24 hours. Both parotids may not be involved simultaneously in some. Orifice of Stensen's duct may be red and swollen. Other salivary glands (submaxillary, sublingual) are less commonly affected. There can be pain during eating, swallowing or talking. The glandular swelling disappears within a week **(Fig. 10.3)**.

Complications

Common complications are meningitis, orchitis or oophoritis and pancreatitis. Other complications are shown in **Table 10.2**.

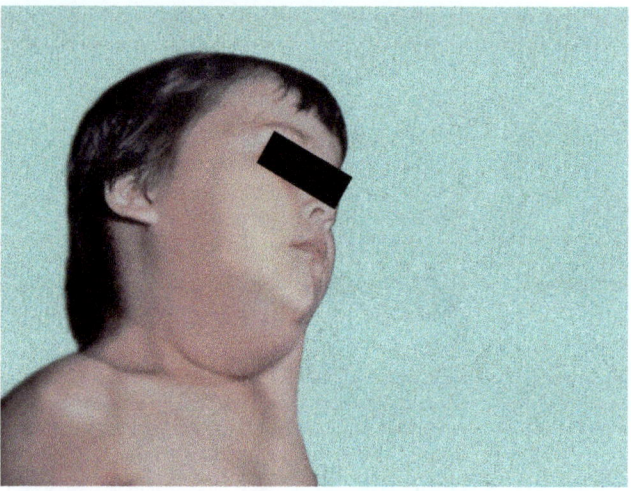

Fig. 10.3: Mumps patient.

Table 10.2: Complications of mumps.

Common
- Aseptic meningitis
- Orchitis/oophoritis
- Pancreatitis

Rare
- Hepatitis
- Myocarditis
- Thyroiditis
- Nephritis
- Arthritis
- Thrombocytopenia
- Encephalitis
- Guillain-Barré syndrome

- Aseptic meningitis may occur in both children and adults. Presence of stiff neck, headache and drowsiness suggests meningitis. Cerebrospinal fluid (CSF) findings show mild pleocytosis (mostly lymphocytes), and raised protein. Unlike other viral meningitis the sugar level in CSF may be low. The meningitis is self-limiting.
- Generally, unilateral orchitis occurs in postpubertal males. This is the most common complication among postpubertal males. There is pain, tenderness and swelling of the testicle. Testicular atrophy may occur but sterility is rare. Lower abdominal pain in females suggests oophoritis.
- Mumps is the leading cause of pancreatitis in children. This presents with upper abdominal pain, nausea and vomiting.

Investigations

- Serum amylase is raised either due to parotitis or pancreatitis.
- There may be relative lymphocytosis in the peripheral blood.
- Diagnosis can be confirmed by isolating the virus or detecting by PCR from saliva, throat, CSF or urine during first few days of illness.

Table 10.3: Causes of parotid swelling.

Unilateral
- Parotid cyst parotid tumor
- Stone in the parotid duct

Bilateral
Infectious
- Viral: Mumps, coxsackie, HIV, influenza, EBV
- Bacterial: *S. aureus,* streptococci, gram-negative bacteria

Non-infectious
- Sarcoidosis
- Sjögren's syndrome
- Diabetes mellitus
- Cirrhosis
- Drugs (propylthiouracil, phenothiazine)

- Demonstration of specific IgM antibody or four-fold rise in IgG antibody titer in acute and convalescent sera also help in the diagnosis.
- There may be mild rise in blood urea and serum creatinine.

Differential Diagnosis

The parotitis in mumps should be differentiated from other causes of parotid swelling. The **Table 10.3** shows other causes of parotid enlargement.

Treatment

- The patient should be isolated until the swelling subsides.
- The patient needs bed rest during the febrile period.
- The treatment of parotitis, meningitis and pancreatitis is purely symptomatic.
- Analgesics and cold or warm compresses are helpful in relieving parotid pain.
- The role of prednisolone in the management of orchitis is not fully established. However, it may reduce the discomfort of orchitis. Interferon alpha has been shown to be helpful in some cases of orchitis.

Prevention

- The infection confers life long immunity.
- The primary prevention of mumps is done by the administration of live attenuated vaccine. MMR vaccine is given during 12–15 month of age **(Table 10.1)**. The vaccine provides life long immunity.
- The vaccine can also be given to susceptible adults who have not had mumps. However, this is contraindicated in pregnant women and immune-compromised individuals.

RUBELLA (GERMAN MEASLES)

Rubella or German measles is a systemic viral infection caused by togavirus.
- Infection spreads through droplets.
- Incubation period is 14–21 days.

- Patients are infective from up to a week before to two weeks after the onset of the rash.
- Skin, joint and placenta are mainly involved.

Clinical Features

The main presenting features are fever, lymphadenopathy and rash. In many, the infection is subclinical.
- Fever is mild and occurs on the first day of the rash.
- There may be coryza and conjunctivitis.
- Rash is maculopapular and nonconfluent which begins on the face and then spreads downwards. Petechial rash may appear on the soft palate (Forchheimer spots).
- Posterior auricular, cervical and suboccipital lymphadenopathy is typically present.
- The most devastating effect of rubella is on the fetus if infection occurs in pregnant women during first trimester and early second trimester.
- Spontaneous abortion may occur.
- *Congenital rubella:* Classical signs of congenital rubella are cataract, heart disease (patent ductus arteriosus, pulmonic stenosis), deafness and other defects such as mental retardation, autism, microcephaly and retinopathy.

Complications

Polyarthritis occurs in about 25% adult female patients. Other complications are bleeding due to thrombocytopenia and vascular damage, encephalitis and hepatitis.

Investigations

The diagnosis is made by the demonstration of virus or specific antibodies. The presence of IgM antibody or fourfold rise in IgG antibodies in paired acute and convalescent sera is diagnostic. The IgM antibody can be false-positive therefore this alone may not be diagnostic of rubella.

Treatment

There is no specific therapy. The fever and joint pain are managed symptomatically.

Prevention

The rubella vaccine (in form of MMR) is given to children at 12–15 months of age **(Table 10.1)**. A second dose is given at 4 years. Immunoglobulin (20 mL) given in pregnant females within 72 hours of exposure to rubella reduces the risk of infection.

CHICKENPOX (VARICELLA) AND HERPES ZOSTER (SHINGLES)

Varicella-zoster virus is a human herpes-virus 3. It causes two important clinical entities in humans: chickenpox (varicella) and herpes zoster (shingles).

Chickenpox

It is a highly contagious disease. The spread of infection is through inhalation of infected droplets (aerosol) or through contact with the skin lesions. Incubation period is 10–21 days.

Clinical Features

Chickenpox is generally a disease of children, although it can also occur in adults. The disease is mild in children and more severe in adults, pregnant women and immunocompromised individuals.
- Initial manifestations are fever and malaise followed by the appearance of rash. Rashes appear first over mucous membrane and then spread in centripetal distribution over skin (more in the trunk, sparse in limbs). Initial lesions are pruritic and maculopapular which eventually evolve into vesicles, pustules and finally crusts **(Figs. 10.4 A and B)**. Successive new crops of lesions appear so that all stages of rashes are seen simultaneously *(pleomorphic rash)*.
- Patient is infective till crusts slough and separate (7–14 days).

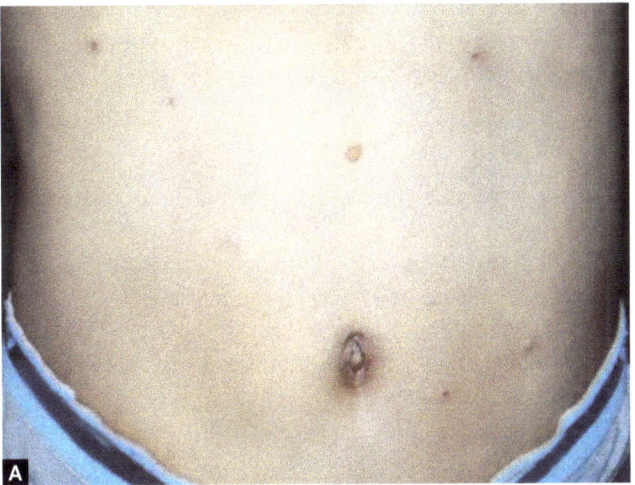
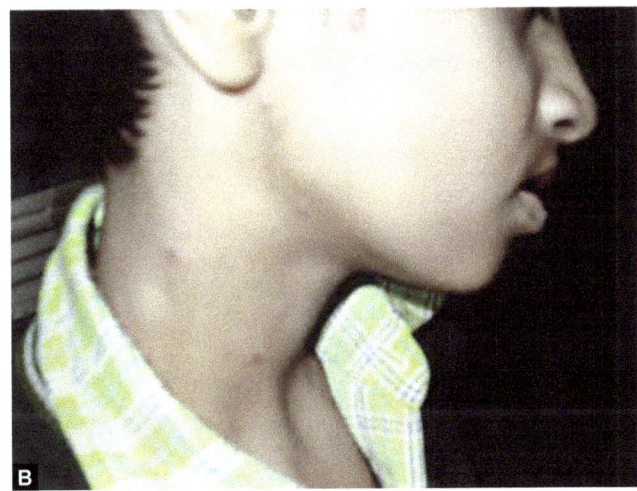

Figs. 10.4A and B: (A) Pleomorphic rash over abdomen in chickenpox; (B) Rash over face.

- Intense itching leads to infection due to scratching of lesions.
- After the primary infection, the virus remains dormant in nervous tissue. Reactivation later in life may lead to herpes zoster, which is more common in elderly.

Complications

- The most common complication of chickenpox is secondary infection of the skin lesions by *Streptococcus pyogenes* or *Staphylococcus aureus* (**Table 10.4**).
- Acute cerebellar ataxia and meningitis may occur after 3 weeks of onset of rash. It is generally self-limiting. Encephalitis and Guillain-Barré syndrome are other rare neurological complications.
- Varicella pneumonia is a serious complication of varicella. It is more common in adults especially pregnant women and immune-compromised patients. It manifests as tachypnea, cough, dyspnea and fever.
- Hepatitis can occur in small number of patients.
- Other complications include myocarditis, nephritis and arthritis.
- Infection in females during first trimester of pregnancy can lead to congenital malformations in fetus *(congenital varicella)*. Mortality rate in neonates is high if they get infection within five days of delivery *(perinatal varicella)*.
- *Reye's syndrome* (fatty liver with encephalopathy) may complicate children with varicella who receive aspirin.

Diagnosis

Diagnosis is usually clinical from the typical appearance of the lesions.
- Confirmation of infection is made by isolation of varicella on tissue culture or by detection of viral DNA by PCR in the vesicular fluid or scrapings.
- Serological diagnosis by the demonstration of rising titers of antibody is also helpful.
- Multinucleated giant cells can be demonstrated by Tzanck smear.
- Leukopenia, thrombocytopenia and raised liver enzymes may be present.

Treatment

- *General:*
  - The patient is isolated till the complete sloughing of crusts.

Table 10.4: Complications of varicella infection.

- Secondary bacterial infection
- Cerebellar ataxia, meningitis, encephalitis, GB syndrome
- Pneumonia
- Hepatitis
- Myocarditis
- Nephritis
- Arthritis
- Reye's syndrome
- Congenital malformation

- Personal hygiene should be maintained to prevent skin infection. Nails should be closely cropped.
- Antipruritic agents, tepid water baths and wet compresses can be used to ease pruritus.
- Aspirin should be avoided in children as it can lead to Reye's syndrome.
- *Antiviral therapy:* Antiviral therapy is not required in immune-competent children and adolescents with uncomplicated varicella disease. However it is useful in adults. Antiviral is of benefit particularly in immune-compromised host and complicated varicella. Acyclovir 800 mg orally five times a day or valacyclovir 1 g orally thrice a day or famciclovir 250 mg orally three times a day for 7 days is given within 24-72 hours of onset of rashes.

Prevention

- Live attenuated varicella vaccine can be given to children >1 year of age who have not had chickenpox. A single dose is adequate. Sero-negative adults should receive two doses 1-2 months apart.
- Varicella-zoster immunoglobulin (VZIg) is given to susceptible individuals (HIV positive, pregnant ladies, premature infants, neonates born to mothers who develop varicella in perinatal period) within 7 days of exposure to an active varicella case.
- Susceptible individuals who are not eligible for VZIg or who have had exposure more than 4 days before should receive acyclovir. Acyclovir is initiated in these patients after seventh day of exposure.

Herpes Zoster

Herpes Zoster is due to reactivation of latent varicella-zoster virus from the dorsal root ganglion. Its incidence is highest in the sixth decade, although it can occur at all ages.

Clinical Features

Severe pain occurs initially and is followed by the appearance of rash after 2-3 days.
- Rashes are initially erythematous maculopapular, which evolve into vesicles and pustules (**Figs. 10.5A and B**). These occur along the distribution of nerve root (dermatome). Thoracic and lumbar roots are more commonly involved (**Fig. 10.6**). The rash usually subsides in 1-2 weeks. However, it may take 4 weeks for the skin to become normal.
- In immunosuppressed patients (such as HIV/AIDS), the rash may be multidermatomal and occur recurrently (**Fig. 10.7**).
- Lesions may appear on the face, mouth, tongue and eye if branches of the trigeminal nerve are involved (**Fig. 10.8**).
- *Ramsay Hunt syndrome:* Ipsilateral facial palsy, loss of taste over the anterior two-third of tongue and painful vesicles in the external auditory canal can occur if geniculate ganglion is involved.

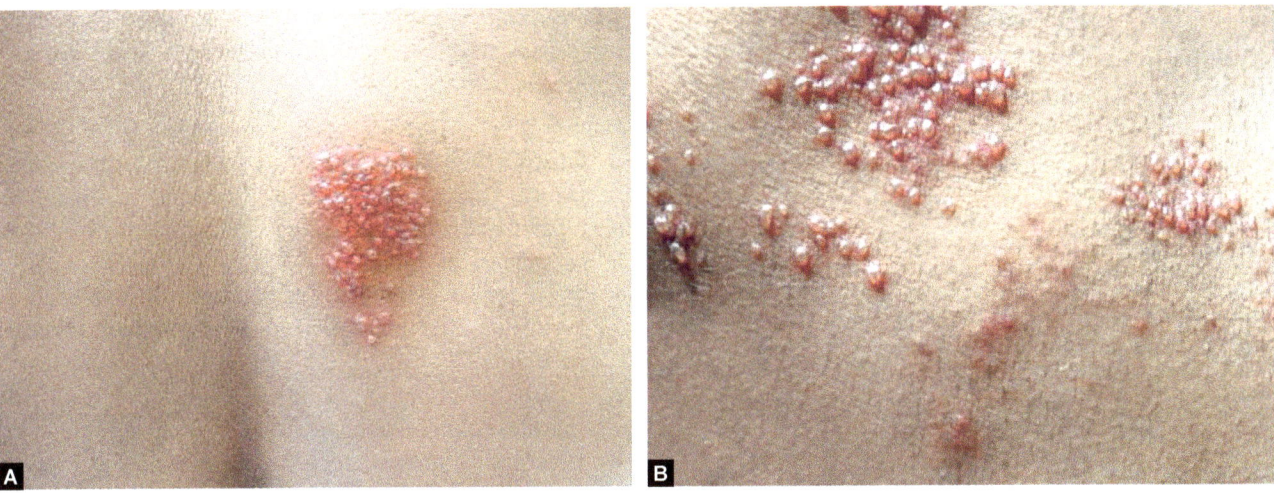

Figs. 10.5A and B: Rash over thoracic dermatomes in herpes zoster.

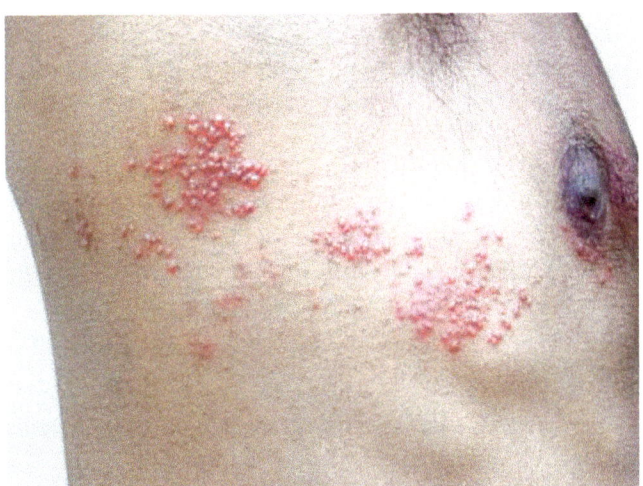

Fig. 10.6: Rashes over dermatomal areas of thoracic and lumbar roots.

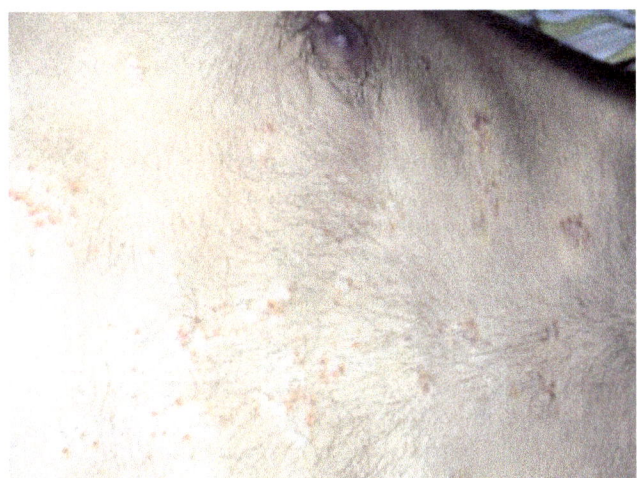

Fig. 10.7: Multidermatomal herpes zoster in a immunocompromised patient.

Complications

- Most common complication is post-herpetic neuralgia; pain persists for 1–6 months or more following healing of the rash. This is more common in elderly and females.
- Superadded bacterial infections
- Herpes zoster ophthalmicus and vision loss if iris is involved.
- Other complications are meningitis, myelitis and encephalitis.

Treatment

Antiviral therapy (acyclovir, valacyclovir, famciclovir) is helpful as it accelerates the healing and reduces the pain during attack. It also reduces the incidence and severity of post-herpetic neuralgia. The dose of acyclovir is 800 mg five times a day for 7–10 days and of valacyclovir is 1000 mg three times a day for 5–7 days. The dose of famciclovir is 500 mg three times a day for 7 days.

Post-herpetic neuralgia is treated with analgesics, amitriptyline, gabapentin, capsaicin cream and lidocaine patches.

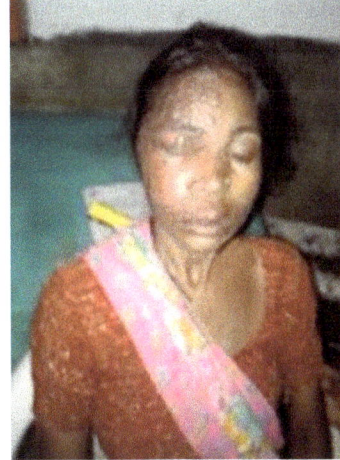

Fig. 10.8: Herpes zoster involving trigeminal dermatome.

HERPES SIMPLEX

Herpes viruses are associated with various human diseases. Eight types of herpes viruses may cause disease in humans (**Table 10.5**). Primary infection with herpes virus may be

Table 10.5: Human herpes viruses.

Virus	Disease

Herpes simplex (HSV)/ Herpesvirus hominis
  HSV type 1
  HSV type 2	

Varicella zoster virus (VZV)- Type 3	Causes chickenpox and shingles (Herpes zoster)
Epstein-Barr virus (EBV)-Type 4	Causes infectious mononucleosis
Cytomegalovirus (CMV)-Type 5	
Human herpes virus (HHV-6)	Causes exanthema subitum
Human herpes virus (HHV-7)	Causes disease in immunocompromised patients
Human herpes virus (HHV-8)	Associated with Kaposi's sarcoma

subclinical and is followed by latent stage. Each type of virus may affect particular organ. Immunodeficiency or impaired immunity later in life is associated with recurrences or relapses due to reactivation of virus.

Herpes Simplex (HSV)/Herpes Virus Hominis

HSV-1 and HSV-2 infections are associated with mucocutaneous lesions. HSV-1 causes mainly oral lesions while HSV-2 causes lesions in genital area predominantly.

Source of Infection

The source of infection is patients suffering from primary infection or recurrences. Asymptomatic shedding of virus occurs after primary infection or shedding may occur during symptomatic recurrences and lead to transmission.

Clinical Presentation

Primary infection may be asymptomatic or may cause gingivostomatitis or pharyngitis. Systemic manifestations are more common during primary infection and patient may present with fever, myalgias, weakness and cervical lymphadenopathy. HSV-1 disease mainly involves mouth and oral cavity **(Fig. 10.9)**. Lesions may occur on gingiva, soft palate, tongue and lips. Lesions in oral area are characterized by vesicles, which occur in groups. Vesicles later ulcerate and epithelize in few weeks.

Recurrence: After primary infection, virus remains in latent stage in ganglion of sensory nerves. Stress, infection, radiotherapy, chemotherapy, sunlight, drugs and impaired immunity may lead to reactivation of virus and recurrences.

- Recurrences usually are associated with milder disease, few lesions and heal more rapidly as compared to primary infection.
- Recurrent herpes labialis is more commonly a manifestation of reactivation.
- Ulcerations on lips, oral mucosa or facial skin may occur due to reactivation of HSV from the trigeminal ganglia.
- Patient may develop oral-labial lesions few days after procedures like *trigeminal root decompression and dental extraction.*
- Ulceration in oral mucosa is difficult to differentiate from aphthous ulcers, traumatic ulcers and drug-induced ulcers.

In immunosuppressed individuals, infection is more severe and extends into deeper tissues. Lesions are characterized by severe pain, inability to eat, bleeding and necrosis. Differential diagnosis includes bacterial infections, fungal infections, drug-induced ulcers and trauma.

Other Manifestations

Bell's palsy: HSV-1 has also been associated with Bell's palsy (infranuclear VII nerve palsy). See Chapter 8.

Genital herpes: HSV infection may also cause vulvovaginitis and cervicitis in females, balanitis in males. Bilateral lesions of external genitalia occur. HSV may also cause rectal infection (proctitis) and perianal infection.

- Primary genital herpes may be associated with systemic manifestations like fever, headache, weakness, myalgia and inguinal adenopathy.
- Lesions occur in form of painful grouped vesicles or pustules in the genital and perianal regions that ulcerate. Discharge (vaginal, urethral), dysuria and itching may occur.
- First episode of HSV-1 and HSV-2 are similar clinically, however, recurrent genital herpes is more common with HSV-2 infection. HSV-2 infection increases the risk of acquiring HIV infection. In HIV infection recurrences of HSV-2 occur more frequently.

Eye involvement: HSV infection can cause keratitis, keratoconjunctivitis and chorioretinitis. Keratitis presents as acute pain, blurred vision, chemosis and dendritic ulcers of cornea. HSV infection of eye can lead to blindness.

Congenital herpes: Transmission of infection occurs during delivery or during intrauterine stage. Disseminated and potentially fatal infection may occur in neonates (congenital herpes). It is characterized by visceral and CNS involvement.

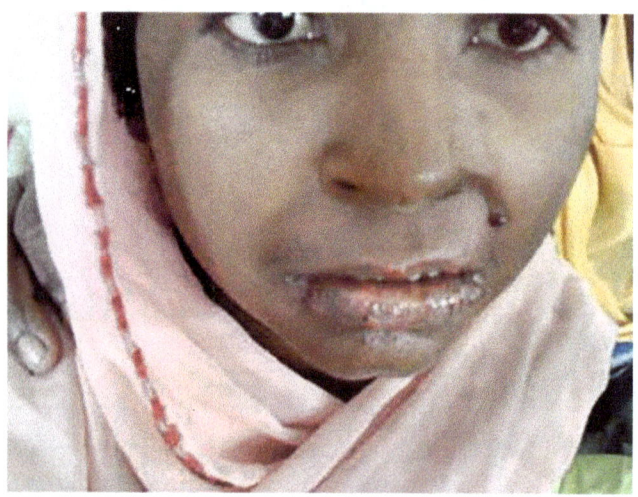

Fig. 10.9: Herpes simplex labialis.

Maternal infection during pregnancy is associated with highest risk of transmission.

Skin: HSV infection in patients with eczema may result in severe infection involving large areas of skin and oral lesions may spread to visceral organs (eczema herpeticum).

Infection of the finger (herpetic whitlow) may occur as a complication of HSV oral or genital infection or through occupational infection. Vesicular or pustular lesion of fingertip occurs with edema, redness and tenderness. Lesion may be difficult to differentiate from pyogenic bacterial infection. Erythema multiforme, Stevens-Johnson syndrome, and toxic epidermal necrolysis can also be the presentation in HSV infection.

Nervous system: HSV infection can cause encephalitis, the most serious complication of herpes simplex infection. Recurrent benign lymphocytic meningitis (Mollaret's meningitis) is another CNS complication of HSV infection.

Diagnosis

Diagnosis is usually clinical but to differentiate from other vesicular eruptions laboratory tests may be needed.

- Multinucleated giant cells or intranuclear inclusion bodies can be demonstrated in scrapings from the lesion and staining with Giemsa's stain (Tzanck preparation) or Papanicolaou's stain. These findings may be present in other viral infection like VZV infection.
- Confirmation of HSV can be done by detection of HSV DNA by PCR, culture from vesicular fluid and direct fluorescent antibody staining of scraped lesions.
- Serology is useful in primary infections.
- CSF-PCR is useful in HSV encephalitis.

Treatment

In immune-competent persons, therapy is usually not required but if initiated early it may ameliorate or shorten the duration of symptoms. Antiviral treatment is effective if started in initial stages (first 48 hours). Severe manifestations require antiviral therapy irrespective of time of presentation.

Serious manifestations (CNS infections, visceral HSV infections, neonatal infection, disseminated infections) require intravenous administration of acyclovir (10 mg/kg 8 hourly for 10 days).

Acyclovir, valacyclovir and famciclovir are used for treatment and these agents inhibit the viral DNA polymerase. Treatment of mucocutaneous herpes is given in **Table 10.6**.

For eye infections, various topical preparations are available (idoxuridine, vidarabine and cidofovir).

Prevention

- Use of barrier contraception during sexual activity (condoms) decreases the rate of transmission of HSV infection.
- Valacyclovir 500 mg once daily reduces chances of transmission of infection between sexual partners.

Table 10.6: Treatment of herpes simplex infection.

Primary HSV	
• Acyclovir	200 mg five times daily for 7–14 days
• Valacyclovir	1 g twice daily for 7–14 days
• Famciclovir	250 mg three times daily for 7–14 days
• Acyclovir	IV 5 mg/kg 8 h for 5 days in severe primary infection
Recurrent HSV	
Orolabial	
• Famciclovir	1500 mg single dose or 750 mg bd for 1 day
• Valacyclovir	2 g single dose or 2 g bd for 1 day
Genital	
• Acyclovir	800 mg tid for 2 days or 200 mg five times for 5 days
• Valacyclovir	500 mg bd for 3 days
• Famciclovir	1500 mg single dose or 750 mg bid for 1 day or 125 mg bd for 5 days
Disease suppression	
• Acyclovir	400 mg bd
• Valacyclovir	500 mg –1 g daily
• Famciclovir	250 mg bd or 500 mg once daily

- Isolation and use of gloves, gowns and hand washing decrease spread of infection from patients with mucocutaneous, genital and disseminated infection to hospital staff and other patients
- There is no approved herpes vaccine.

INFECTIOUS MONONUCLEOSIS

Infectious mononucleosis is mostly caused by Epstein-Barr virus (EBV), a human herpes virus (HHV-4) and is characterized by fever, lymphadenopathy, pharyngeal inflammation, and atypical lymphocytes on peripheral blood smear examination.

EBV is also associated with many tumors including nasopharyngeal carcinoma, Burkitt's lymphoma, Hodgkin's disease and B cell lymphoma in immunosuppressed persons.

Source of Infection

Its mode of transmission is saliva, contact with oral secretions of patients or asymptomatic carriers. About 90% of asymptomatic seropositive persons have virus in their saliva. It is also transmitted through blood transfusion and bone marrow transplantation. The incubation period is generally 4–8 weeks but it may be longer.

Pathogenesis

The virus infects epithelial cells of the oral cavity and salivary glands and is shed in salivary secretions. Lymphocytes in tonsils may be infected directly or B lymphocytes may get infected after contact with epithelial cells. The virus then spreads through bloodstream. Lymphoid tissue is enlarged because of proliferation and expansion of B cells and reactive

T cells. Activated B cells produce antibodies against EBV antigens and host cells. CD4+ T cells decrease in number and CD8+ T cells increase leading to inverse CD4+/CD8+ cells ratio. B cells form the reservoir for EBV in the body.

Clinical Features

Infection may occur at any age.
- In developing countries infection occurs most commonly in early childhood. Infection is usually subclinical and most patients are asymptomatic. By adulthood majority of population has antibodies against EBV.
- In developed countries infection occurs during adolescence and young adults (10–36 years). In this situation many patients have typical infectious mononucleosis (IM).
  - It presents with nonspecific symptoms like fever, myalgia, weakness and malaise.
  - Pharyngitis with or without tonsillitis is usually present.
  - Lymphadenopathy, mainly posterior cervical group of lymph nodes are involved but generalized lymphadenopathy may also be seen. Lymph nodes are tender, mobile and discrete.
  - Splenomegaly may be seen in second or third week of illness. Maculopapular rash is present in 5–15% of cases. If ampicillin is given, most patients (>90%) will develop rash.

Complications

Most cases are self-limiting but complications may be seen in some patients **(Table 10.7)**.
- Complications may be due to CNS involvement (meningitis, encephalitis, cranial nerve palsies mostly VII nerve, transverse myelitis and polyneuritis).

Table 10.7: Complications of Infectious mononucleosis.

Central nervous system complications
- Meningitis
- Encephalitis
- Cranial nerve palsies
- Acute transverse myelitis
- Polyneuritis

Airway obstruction
- Splenic rupture
- Bacterial superinfection

Hematological complications
- Autoimmune hemolytic anemia
- Granulocytopenia
- Thrombocytopenia
- Red cell aplasia
- Pancytopenia

Rare complications
- Hepatitis
- Myocarditis
- Pericarditis
- Interstitial nephritis
- Interstitial pneumonia

- Upper airway obstruction occurs because of enlargement of lymphoid tissue in tonsils and adenoids and is an indication for hospitalization.
- Coombs positive hemolytic anemia may occur because of formation of antibodies against the red cell antigen. Granulocytopenia and thrombocytopenia may also occur.
- Hemophagocytic lymphohistiocytosis may occur in EBV infection.

Laboratory Findings

- After a week of illness, WBC count is elevated with lymphocytosis and atypical lymphocytes. Atypical lymphocytes are larger than normal lymphocytes with plenty of cytoplasm, vacuoles and dark chromatin with indented cell membrane. For diagnosis at least 20% of peripheral lymphocytes must be atypical. Granulocytopenia, thrombocytopenia may be seen.
- Serum levels of aminotransferases and alkaline phosphatase are usually elevated. Bilirubin levels may be raised in some cases.
- Presence of heterophile antibodies in serum is an important test for the diagnosis. Tests for heterophile antibodies are positive in about 40% of patients in first week of illness but they become positive in almost 90% of cases during the third week. Heterophile antibodies when adsorbed in guinea pig kidney, agglutinate erythrocytes of other species, e.g., sheep, horse or cow. Paul-Bunnell test or slide test (Monospot test) is used to demonstrate presence of heterophile antibodies.
- Elevation in other antibodies directed at various EBV antigens may also be useful in diagnosis patients who don't have heterophile antibodies and patients with atypical presentation. These include:
  - IgM and IgG antibodies against viral capsid antigen (anti-VCA)
  - Antibodies to early antigen (anti-EA-D and anti-EA-R)
  - Antibodies to EBV nuclear antigen (anti-EBNA)
- Detection of EBV DNA by polymerase chain reaction is useful in demonstrating virus in EBV-associated malignancies and for diagnosis in immunocompromised individuals when serology is not helpful.

Differential Diagnosis

Most of the cases of IM are due to EBV. Few percentages of cases may be caused by cytomegalovirus (CMV). IM caused by CMV is less severe and heterophile antibody test is negative. Other less common causes of IM are acute toxoplasmosis, acute HIV infection, HHV-6, hepatitis virus and hypersensitivity drug reactions. Exudative pharyngitis and heterophile antibodies are not seen in other causes of IM.

Treatment

Treatment is usually symptomatic as majority of patients will recover.

- Rest and avoidance of excessive exertion are helpful.
- Acetaminophen and other nonsteroidal anti-inflammatory drugs (NSAIDs) are used for symptomatic relief. Warm saline gargles and throat irrigation also provides relief.
- Acyclovir therapy is not effective and is not recommended.
- Glucocorticoids (prednisolone) are used in airway obstruction, autoimmune hemolytic anemia, hemophagocytic lymphohistiocytosis (HLH) and severe thrombocytopenia. Glucocorticoid therapy is not recommended in uncomplicated cases.
- Acyclovir in dosage of 400–800 mg five times a day has been shown to be effective in oral hairy leukoplakia.
- Ampicillin, amoxicillin and other penicillin should be avoided because they can precipitate rash in patients of IM.
- Monoclonal antibodies to CD20 (Rituximab) have been useful in some cases, notably in X-linked lymphoproliferative syndrome.
- Patients should avoid sports activities for few weeks until splenomegaly has resolved because of the danger of splenic rupture.

Other EBV-Associated Diseases (Table 10.8)

- EBV-associated lymphoproliferative disease may occur in immunodeficient patients including AIDS patients, post-transplant patients and patients with severe combined immunodeficiency. In such patients it may cause B cell hyperplasia or B cell lymphoma.
- Duncan's disease is a X-linked recessive lymphoproliferative syndrome seen in young boys who develop fatal lymphoproliferative syndrome after EBV infection.
- *Oral hairy leukoplakia* is seen in HIV infection and is characterized by raised, corrugated lesions on tongue; EBV-DNA can be detected from these lesions **(Fig. 10.10)**.
- It is associated with Burkitt's lymphoma (90% of cases in Africa and about 15% of cases in USA). EBV-DNA can be detected from tumor tissue and these patients have high titer of antibodies to EBV.
- Nasopharyngeal carcinoma is also associated with EBV infection. EBV-DNA levels in plasma correlates with poor prognosis and EBV-DNA levels in such patients are used to monitor patients.
- EBV infection is also associated with Hodgkin's lymphoma (especially mixed cellularity type). Viral antigen and EBV-DNA can be demonstrated in Reed-Sternberg cells in

Table 10.8: Diseases associated with Epstein-Barr virus (EBV).

- Infectious mononucleosis
- Hodgkin's lymphoma
- Non-Hodgkin lymphoma
- CNS lymphoma in AIDS patients
- Burkitt's lymphoma
- Post-transplant lymphoproliferative disease
- Nasopharyngeal carcinoma
- Oral hairy leukoplakia
- X-linked recessive lymphoproliferative syndrome (Duncan's disease)

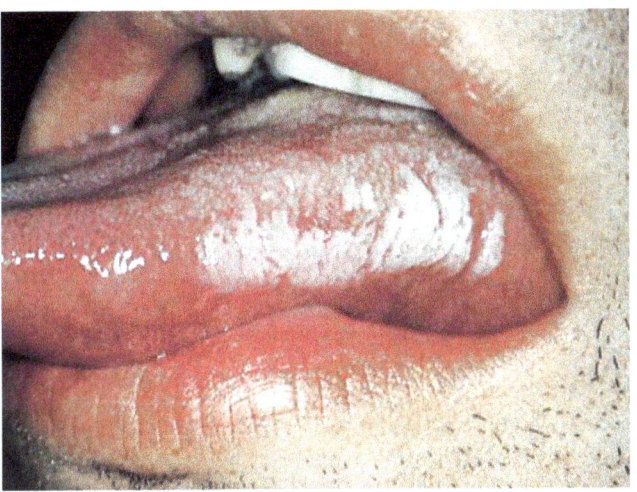

Fig. 10.10: Oral hairy leukoplakia.

such patients and patients have high levels of antibodies to EBV.

DIPHTHERIA

Diphtheria although eradicated from most of the developed world still occurs in developing countries.

- This is caused by aerobic gram-positive bacteria *Corynebacterium diphtheriae*.
- Infection occurs mostly in the upper respiratory tract via droplets which spread from the cases or carriers. Occasionally bacteria may primarily infect conjunctiva, genital tract or skin wounds.
- The organism *does not invade the tissue*. The manifestations occur due to damage of heart muscle and nervous system by the *soluble bacterial exotoxin* absorbed at the site of infection.
- Incubation period is 2–4 days.

Clinical Manifestations

The presentations may be predominantly nasal, laryngeal, pharyngeal or cutaneous.

- Pharyngeal form is the most common one. The initial presentations are usually mild fever, sore throat and membrane formation over tonsils. The membrane is grayish, firm and adherent, surrounded by a zone of inflammation. The membrane often extends beyond the margin of tonsils unlike the exudates in staphylococcal pharyngitis. Swelling in the neck may occur along with tender lymphadenopathy *(bull neck)*.
- Husky voice, high-pitched cough and respiratory obstruction may occur due to laryngeal involvement.
- Patients may have epistaxis and nasal obstruction.
- Death may occur due to acute circulatory failure **(Table 10.9)**.

Complications

The important complications are respiratory obstruction, myocarditis and neurological involvement.

Table 10.9: Clinical manifestations of diphtheria.

- Mild fever, sore throat
- Tachycardia
- "Pseudomembrane" over tonsils, larynx, nasal cavity
- Hoarseness of voice
- Respiratory obstruction
- Acute circulatory failure

Complications
- Myocarditis
- Palatal and laryngeal paralysis
- Peripheral neuropathy

- Manifestations of diphtheric myocarditis include arrhythmia, conduction defects and cardiomyopathy.
- Neurological complications appear 3-5 weeks after the onset of diphtheria and are in the form of palatal palsy, paralysis of accommodation and polyneuritis.

Diagnosis

A definitive diagnosis of diphtheria is made on the basis of typical clinical presentations including 'pseudomembrane' and isolation of *C. diphtheriae* from the lesions. Diphtheric pseudomembrane should be distinguished from other pharyngeal exudates due to staphylococcal infection, infectious mononucleosis and candida.

Treatment

The patient is managed in isolation.
- The most important step is the prompt administration of antitoxin since the antitoxin if given late cannot neutralize the toxin which is already bound to the tissues. The dose of antitoxin is given in **Table 10.10**. A history of previous horse serum administration and any allergic reaction must be sought. A small test dose is given to detect the allergy. Injectable adrenaline must be ready so as to be used in case anaphylaxis occurs.
- Antibiotic (penicillin, amoxicillin or erythromycin for 10-14 days) is given to eliminate *C. diphtheriae* so that the spread of infection to others is prevented. The dose of erythromycin is 500 mg 6 hourly and that of amoxicillin is 500 mg 8 hourly. Clarithromycin and azithromycin are equally effective.
- Treatment with glucocorticoids has not been shown to reduce the risk of myocarditis or polyneuropathy.
- An urgent tracheostomy may be needed in case of respiratory obstruction.
- Following recovery, the patient should be immunized with diphtheria toxoid.
- The patient is isolated till three daily consecutive cultures are negative for the organism.

Table 10.10: Dose of diphtheria antitoxin.

Mild cases	4000–8000 units IM
Moderate cases	16000–40000 units IM
Severe cases	up to 100000 units IV

Prophylaxis

- Active immunization for diphtheria is a part of immunization program in children. A combined vaccine DPT is used **(Table 10.1)**.
- Susceptible contact person should be given booster dose of toxoid and a course of antibiotic such as erythromycin.

ENTERIC FEVER (TYPHOID FEVER)

Enteric fever (typhoid fever) is a systemic disease caused by *Salmonella typhi* and *Salmonella paratyphi A, B,* and *C*. Humans are the only host for *S. typhi* and *S. paratyphi*.
- In most, the infection results from consumption of contaminated food or water.
- Sources of infection are acutely infected patients or chronic carriers.
- Incubation period is generally 5–14 days, but can be longer.

Pathophysiology

Organisms enter the intestinal epithelial cells and subsequently invade and multiply in macrophages in Peyer's patches, mesenteric lymph nodes and the spleen. This is followed by a phase of bacteremia. The organisms may spread to the lungs, gallbladder, kidneys and central nervous system. Finally, bacteria localize mainly in the lymphoid tissues of the distal small intestine. The typical lesion occurs in the Peyer's patches in small intestine which become swollen, ulcerate and heal. Bleeding and perforation may occur.

Clinical Features

The onset is insidious.
- Initially patient presents with prodromal symptoms such as malaise, headache, cough, sore throat, abdominal pain and constipation followed by the appearance of fever. Children may present with diarrhea and vomiting.
- Fever typically rises in stepwise fashion for few days and then attains plateau. It disappears over 7-10 days in uncomplicated cases.
- There may be relative bradycardia.
- Tongue may be coated.
- Spleen becomes palpable in second week.
- Rashes (rose spots) may appear on the back and upper abdomen at the end of first week. These are pink maculopapular rashes that fade on pressure and disappear in 3-4 days.

About 5% of patients with enteric fever become long-term asymptomatic carriers who continue to shed bacteria in stool or urine. Women, patients with gallstones or gastrointestinal malignancies are more likely to become carriers.

Complications

Important complications are intestinal perforation and/or intestinal hemorrhage which occur in untreated cases in

Table 10.11: Complications of enteric fever.
• Intestinal perforation
• Intestinal hemorrhage
Others
• Osteomyelitis
• Arthritis
• Cholecystitis
• Meningitis, neuritis, GB syndrome
• Myocarditis, pericarditis
• Nephritis
• Parotitis
• Psychosis
• Disseminated intravascular coagulation

third and fourth week. Presence of tachycardia, hypotension, abdominal pain and tenderness, dark or fresh blood in stool and leukocytosis suggest these complications. Other complications are shown in **Table 10.11**.

Investigations

- Blood culture is positive for *S. typhi* or *S. paratyphi*. The yield is higher in first week of illness (90% in untreated cases) but decreases to 50% by third week.
  - Culture of bone marrow may be positive when blood cultures are negative.
  - Stool, urine, rose spots and gastrointestinal secretions can also reveal positive culture. Stool culture is positive during the third week of infection.
- White blood cell counts are normal but leukopenia can occur. Leukocytosis may occur in children or when infection is complicated by intestinal perforation or hemorrhage.
- Serological tests are available but these are not reliable because of high false-positive and false-negative rates. Widal test detects antibodies to the causative organisms and is usually positive by the second week. Administration of antibiotics or previous typhoid vaccination may interfere with the interpretation of Widal test.

Treatment

- Treatment includes administration of antibiotics parenterally or orally depending on patient's condition.
- Effective antibiotics are fluoroquinolones, third generation cephalosporins (ceftriaxone, cefotaxime,

cefixime and cefpodoxime) and azithromycin (**Table 10.12**). The treatment is given for either ten days or at least five days after resolution of fever.
- Ampicillin, amoxycillin, chloramphenicol and trimethoprim-sulfamethoxazole (TMP-SMX) are generally not used now because of resistance. Quinolone resistance has also been reported.
- Dexamethasone is indicated in severe cases (altered sensorium or shock) as a single dose of 3 mg/kg followed by 8 doses of 1 mg/kg every 6 hourly.
- Carriers are treated with oral antibiotics (amoxycillin, ciprofloxacin, TMP-SMX) for 6 weeks.
- Eradication of disease may need surgery of anatomical abnormality such as biliary stone.

Prevention

- Immunization is indicated in close household contacts, travellers to endemic area and during epidemics. Multiple dose oral vaccines or single dose parenteral vaccines are available. These provide protection for 5 and 3 years respectively.
- Other preventive measures are proper waste disposal and protection of food and water from contamination.
- Carriers should not work as food handlers.

GONORRHEA

Gonorrhea is caused by *Neisseria gonorrhoeae*, a gram-negative diplococcus. It is transmitted through sexual activity (vaginal, oral, anal sex). Sexually active young population is the most commonly affected one. The incubation period is 2–10 days.

Clinical Features

Infection may be asymptomatic, or they may present as the following:
- In males, urethra is most commonly involved. Dysuria and purulent urethral discharge are initial symptoms. It may progress to involve the prostate, epididymis and periurethral glands. Chronic infection may lead to urethral stricture and prostatitis. In homosexual men, rectal infection may occur which is either asymptomatic or presents with discharge, discomfort or rectal bleeding.
- In females, the infection may be asymptomatic in 50% cases. Urethral infection may present as dysuria, discharge or increased frequency. Vaginitis or cervicitis may occur and present as vaginal discharge. Infection of Bartholin's glands and periurethral glands is also common. Rectum may be involved due to anal sex or spread from urogenital infection. Uterus and fallopian tubes may be involved resulting into salpingitis. Chronic salpingitis may lead to scarring of fallopian tubes and sterility. Pelvic inflammatory disease (PID) refers to mixed infection with gonococci, chlamydia and anerobes. It may present as

Table 10.12: Usual antibiotics for enteric fever.		
Drug	Dose	Duration
Ciprofloxacin	500–750 mg twice daily	10–14 days
Ofloxacin	300–400 mg twice daily	10–14 days
Levofloxacin	500 mg daily	10–14 days
Ceftriaxone	1–2 g IV or IM daily	10–14 days
Cefixime	400 mg twice daily	10–14 days
Azithromycin	1 g once daily	5 days

lower abdominal pain, discharge, pain during coitus and vaginal bleeding.
- Pharyngeal gonorrhea may be asymptomatic or present as sore throat and occurs due to oral sex.
- Eye involvement occurs in the form of conjunctivitis due to direct inoculation of gonococci. The purulent conjunctivitis and edema of eyelids are found in neonates (ophthalmia neonatorum). It may lead to panophthalmitis. Urgent treatment is required to prevent corneal damage and loss of vision.
- Dissemination of gonococci through bloodstream from primary site may cause bacteremia and systemic infection. Intermittent fever, arthritis, tenosynovitis and skin involvement are common. Rash may be maculopapular or hemorrhagic. Endocarditis and meningitis are rare presentations.

Differential Diagnosis

Gonorrhea should be differentiated from non-gonococcal urethritis or vaginitis due to *Chlamydia trachomatis*, trichomoniasis, candidiasis, bacterial vaginosis.

Investigations

- Smear examination of the discharge may show gram-negative diplococci in polymorphonuclear leukocytes.
- Diagnosis is confirmed by culture.
- Ligase chain reaction (LCR) assay may detect both *N. gonorrhoeae* and *Chlamydia trachomatis* in urethral or cervical swab and urine.

Treatment

- Antimicrobial is started as soon as possible. *A single dose is curative in uncomplicated infection* **(Table 10.13)**. Cefixime and ceftriaxone are first line agents because of fluoroquinolones resistance. In view of emerging resistance to cephalosporins, single dose of oral azithromycin (1 g) is generally added to the single dose of ceftriaxone (250–500 mg intramuscular). Spectinomycin should be used if patient is allergic to penicillin. Doxycycline (100 mg twice daily for 7 days) or azithromycin (1 g orally) is generally added to cover other coinfections like chlamydia.

Table 10.13: Drugs used in the treatment of uncomplicated gonorrhea.

Drug	Dose	Route
Cefixime	400 mg	Orally
Ceftriaxone	250 mg	Intramuscularly
Ciprofloxacin	500 mg	Orally
Ofloxacin	400 mg	Orally
Levofloxacin	250 mg	Orally
Spectinomycin	2 g	Intramuscularly
Azithromycin	1 g	Orally
Doxycycline	100 mg BD	Orally

- Complicated infection requires prolonged therapy. PID is treated with antimicrobials effective against gonococci, chlamydia and anerobes. Complicated gonorrhea (Salpingitis, prostatitis, arthritis, bacteremia) is treated by any of the following:
  - Ceftriaxone 1 g intravenously daily followed by oral cefixime 400 mg daily for total 7 days plus azithromycin orally 1 g single dose.
  - Cefoxitine 2 g intravenous 6 hourly or cefotetan 2 g intravenous 12 hourly plus oral doxycycline 100 mg 12 hourly for 7 days.
  - Clindamycin 900 mg intravenous 8 hourly plus gentamycin 80 mg intravenous 8 hourly is also effective.
- All sexual partners and patient should be tested and treated for syphilis and human immunodeficiency virus (HIV).

Prevention

The preventive methods include education, and adoption of mechanical measures like condoms. Sexual partners of the patient should be treated. The patient is advised to abstain from sex until therapy is completed. Effective drugs in therapeutic dosage if taken within 24 hours of exposure may abort an infection.

SYPHILIS

Syphilis is sexually transmitted chronic systemic infection caused by *Treponema pallidum*. It is transmitted during sexual contact through abrasions in skin or mucous membranes. It can be transferred from mother to fetus via placenta (congenital syphilis).

Transmission may also occur by blood transfusion, kissing and percutaneous injury.

Clinical Manifestations

The clinical features of syphilis are broadly classified as early and late syphilis.
a. Early syphilis includes primary syphilis, secondary syphilis and latent syphilis.
b. Late syphilis includes 'Late' latent syphilis and tertiary syphilis (benign tertiary syphilis, cardiovascular and neurosyphilis).

Early Syphilis

Primary Syphilis

Primary syphilis is the first stage in the natural history of the disease.
- Incubation period is 10–90 days (average 2–4 weeks).
- Typical lesion is a chancre, which develops at the site of the inoculation, usually located on the penis in heterosexual males. It begins as a painless papule that ulcerates and becomes indurated.

- Inguinal lymph nodes are enlarged, rubbery, discrete and non-tender. It heals without treatment in 2–6 weeks; a scar may form, particularly if secondary bacterial infection has occurred.
- In homosexual male, lesion can occur in rectum or anal canal. In female patients, cervix and labia are common primary sites. Atypical primary sites of chancre include tongue, tonsils, nipple and fingertips.

The differential diagnosis of primary chancre is chanchroid (painful nonindurated ulcer), lymphogranuloma venereum, genital herpes and neoplasm.

Secondary Syphilis

Secondary stage occurs 6–8 weeks after the development of chancre. The manifestations are due to the dissemination of *Treponema pallidum* to distant sites. Main features are fever, rash and lymphadenopathy.
- Rashes are non-pruritic and symmetrical. The palm and soles are generally involved. Rashes may be in the form of macular, papular, pustular or follicular or a combination of these but not vesicular.
- Mucosal patches and ulcers may occur in the oral cavity, and genitalia. These are highly infectious. In the oral cavity the lips, oral mucosa, tongue, palate and pharynx may be involved. Differential diagnosis of oral ulcers in secondary syphilis is given in **Table 10.14**.
- "Weeping" papules over warm and moist areas like vulva and perianal region are called *candyloma lata*.
- Lymphadenopathy is generalized, non-tender, discrete and rubbery.
- Other features are meningitis, cranial nerve palsies, uveitis, hepatitis, gastritis, periostitis, glomerulonephritis. alopecia (moth-eaten appearance) may also occur.

Latent Syphilis

Latent syphilis is characterized by positive serological tests for syphilis, absence of clinical manifestations and normal CSF.
- The latent phase during first year of infection is known as *early latent syphilis* when the patient is sexually infectious.
- *Late latent syphilis* begins after 1 year of infection in untreated patients. This stage is sexually non-infectious.

However, transmission of infection through blood or placenta may occur in both early and late latent syphilis.

Table 10.14: Differential diagnosis of oral lesions in secondary syphilis.

- Aphthous ulcers
- Ulcerative stomatitis
- Herpes simplex
- Infectious mononucleosis
- Primary HIV infection
- Agranulocytosis
- Stevens-Johnson syndrome
- Behcet syndrome
- Reiter's syndrome

Latent syphilis may persist throughout life or could end in the development of late syphilis (tertiary syphilis) in 30 to 40% cases.

Tertiary Syphilis

Benign Tertiary Syphilis

Benign tertiary syphilis may develop between 3–10 years of infection and can involve skin, mucous membrane, bone, muscle or viscera. Chronic granulomatous lesion (gumma) is the characteristic feature. Gumma can be single or multiple and most commonly involved sites are the skin, bone, mouth, upper respiratory tract, liver and the stomach. Upper respiratory gumma can lead to perforation of the palate or nasal septum. Gummatous tongue may heal to develop leukoplakia which is premalignant.

Other causes of granulomatous lesions such as tuberculosis, sarcoidosis, leprosy and fungal infection must be considered in the differential diagnosis of gumma.

Cardiovascular Syphilis

Cardiovascular Syphilis may present after many years of infection. Aorta, coronary ostia and aortic valve may be affected leading to aortic aneurysm, angina and aortic regurgitation.

Neurosyphilis

Neurosyphilis takes years to develop. Neurosyphilis may be asymptomatic or symptomatic.
- Asymptomatic neurosyphilis is characterized by CSF abnormalities in the absence of clinical signs.
- Symptomatic neurosyphilis may present as:
  - Meningovascular syphilis
  - General paresis of insane
  - Tabes dorsalis.

Some important clinical features are Argyll Robertson pupil and Charcoat's joints. *Argyll Robertson pupil* is small irregular pupil which reacts to accommodation but not to light.

Congenital Syphilis

Transmission of infection from untreated mother to fetus transplacentally can lead to congenital syphilis. Untreated maternal syphilis can lead to stillbirth, premature birth and neonatal death. A child may be born with syphilitic features, same as in secondary syphilis, or may develop manifestations during first few weeks of life.
- Features of early syphilis are rhinitis (snuffles), maculopapular rash, condyloma lata, mucus patches, periostitis, lymphadenopathy, hepatosplenomegaly, anemia and thrombocytopenia. This stage is infectious.
- Some children remain in latent phase and develop features of congenital syphilis or residual stigmata after 2 years. Late congenital syphilis presents as benign tertiary

syphilis, interstitial keratitis, deafness, neurosyphilis, and Clutton's joint (bilateral knee effusion).
- Stigmata include *Hutchinson's teeth, mulberry molars,* frontal bossing, saddle nose, *maxillary hypoplasia,* high arched palate, rhagades and saber tibia.
    - Hutchinson's teeth are widely spaced peg-shaped notched upper central incisors.
    - Mulberry molars are sixth year molars with poorly developed cusps.
    - Rhagades are linear scars at angle of the mouth, nose and anus following secondary bacterial infection of the rashes.

Investigations

T. pallidum cannot be cultured in vitro hence diagnosis depends on (a) Microscopic examination, (b) serological tests and (c) other tests.

a. *Dark-field microscopic* examination may show motile spirochaetes from lesions in infectious syphilis. Fluid from chancre, regional lymph nodes or moist cutaneous lesions in early syphilis or congenital syphilis is used for this purpose. The sensitivity is around 90%. Organism is not found in late syphilis.
   The direct fluorescent antibody *T. pallidum* test (DFA-TP) is also used to detect the pallidum in fixed smears prepared from lesions. PCR test is also used in some centers.
b. *Serological tests:* Tests used in the diagnosis of syphilis are given in **Table 10.15**.
   Non-treponemal antibody tests: Commonly used non-treponemal tests are Venereal Disease Research Laboratory (VDRL) and Rapid Plasma Reagent (RPR) tests. These tests measure the ability of serum to flocculate cardiolipin-lecithin-cholesterol antigen complex. These tests are used for primary screening and are positive 4 weeks after the primary infection, secondary syphilis and at birth in congenital syphilis. False-positive reactions may occur in other diseases and diagnosis must be confirmed by specific treponemal antibody test. The titer correlates with disease activity and can be used to monitor the response to therapy.
   Treponemal antibody tests: Specific tests like Fluorescent treponemal antibody-absorbed test (FTA-ABS), *T. pallidum* hemagglutination test (TPHA), Agglutination assays for antibodies to *T. pallidum* are used to confirm the diagnosis as these are negative in non-treponemal infections. These are positive in primary and secondary syphilis.
   Enzyme immunoassay (EIA) or Chemiluminescence immunoassay (CIA): These tests are based on reactivity to recombinant antigens and are used for screening.
c. *Other tests*: CSF examination is required in late syphilis such as in benign tertiary syphilis, cardiovascular syphilis and neurosyphilis. It should also be examined in seropositive patients with neurological signs. Biopsy may be required to diagnose gumma. Chest X-ray, ECG and echocardiography are done to detect cardiovascular syphilis.

Treatment

Penicillin G is the drug of choice in all stages of syphilis. Alternatively tetracycline, doxycycline, cephalosporin, and azithromycin can be used in penicillin allergic patients **(Table 10.16)**.
- *Treatment of early syphilis (primary, secondary and early latent):* Single dose of benzathine penicillin G is the drug of choice. Alternatively, two weeks course of tetracycline or doxycycline can be given in penicillin sensitive patients. Ceftriaxone (for 8–10 days) or azithromycin (single dose) are also effective.
- *Treatment of late syphilis (late latent, cardiovascular, benign tertiary):* Lumbar puncture is done to examine CSF. If CSF is abnormal, patient is treated for neurosyphilis.
    - Patients with normal CSF are treated with benzathine penicillin weekly for 3 weeks. Alternatively, doxycycline or tetracycline is given for 4 weeks.
    - Neurosyphilis (asymptomatic or symptomatic) is treated with aqueous penicillin G for 10–14 days. Probenecid is added if procaine penicillin G is given. Alternatively intravenous ceftriaxone 2 g daily can be given for 10–14 days.
- Drugs indicated in neurosyphilis are penicillin and ceftriaxone. Patients allergic to penicillin are treated after desensitization.
- Penicillin is the only drug which has documented efficacy in pregnancy.
- *Jarisch Herxheimer reaction:* This is a mild acute febrile reaction, which occurs following initiation of treatment. The features are fever, chills, myalgia, headache, tachycardia and hypotension. The reaction occurs due to release of toxic products after massive destruction of

Table 10.15: Serological tests for syphilis.

Non-treponemal tests
- Venereal disease research laboratory test (VDRL)
- Rapid plasma reagin test (RPR)

Treponemal antibody tests (specific)
- Fluorescent treponemal antibody-absorbed test (FTA-ABS)
- *T. pallidum* hemagglutination test (TPHA)
- Agglutination assays for antibodies to *T. pallidum*.

Table 10.16: Drugs used in syphilis.

Benzathine penicillin G	2.4 million units	IM, single dose
Aqueous penicillin G	18–24 million units daily	IV, divided doses
Procaine penicillin G	2.4 million units daily	IM, divided doses
Probenecid	500 mg qid	Oral
Doxycycline	100 mg bd	Oral
Tetracycline	500 mg qid	Oral
Azithromycin	2 g	Oral single dose
Ceftriaxone	1–2 g daily	IM/IV

spirochetes. Treatment is symptomatic. The symptoms generally resolve within 24 hours.

Prevention

Use of condom is helpful in prevention. Following exposure to infectious syphilis, azithromycin 1 g single dose or procaine penicillin G 2.4 million units IM may be used to prevent infection.

AMEBIASIS

Amebiasis is an infection caused by the intestinal protozoan *Entamoeba histolytica*. The infection is spread by cysts which are present in water and uncooked food contaminated by human feces. About 90% of infections are asymptomatic.

Pathogenesis

- The trophozoites are released from cysts in the intestine and invade the mucous membrane of the large bowel, chiefly the cecum. They can produce flask-shaped ulcers surrounded by healthy mucosa. These ulcers can bleed or lead to perforation.
- Rarely, intestinal infection may lead to formation of mass lesion *(ameboma)*.
- Trophozoites may reach the liver through the portal vein and cause parenchymal destruction leading to the formation of *amebic liver abscess*. The abscess is usually found in right lobe of the liver.
- Other extraintestinal sites such as genitourinary tract, skin and cerebrum may become involved rarely.

Clinical Manifestations

- In endemic areas, around one-third of the population is asymptomatic passers of amebic cysts.
- Usual symptom is frequent loose stools containing mucus with or without blood. The stool has an offensive odor. This is known as *amebic dysentery*. There may also be mild abdominal pain.
- On palpation, the colon particularly cecum is tender. Cecal involvement may mimic acute appendicitis.
- Acute diarrheal presentation with blood in stool mimics bacillary dysentery or ulcerative colitis.
- Presentation may be severe in elderly and in immuno-compromised individuals.

Differential Diagnosis

Intestinal amebiasis should be differentiated from bacterial diarrhea caused by *Shigella, Salmonella, Vibrio, Enteroinvasive E.coli* and *Campylobacter*. Amebic liver abscess can be a cause of prolonged pyrexia without any localizing sign. Hence it must be suspected in a case of pyrexia of unknown origin.

Amebic Liver Abscess

- Symptoms are fever with chills, malaise and pain in right upper abdomen and right shoulder.
- Liver is enlarged and tender. Jaundice is rare.
- Large abscess may rupture through the diaphragm into the lung. The contents of the abscess thus may be coughed out. Occasionally the abscess may rupture into the pleural cavity, peritoneal cavity or pericardial sac.
- Diagnosis is suspected on clinical grounds and confirmed by ultrasonography.

Investigations

- Fresh stool examination reveals the presence of trophozoites or amebic cysts. Trophozoites are diagnostic of acute dysentery. The stool is positive for heme (occult blood).
- Sigmoidoscopy may reveal typical flask-shaped ulcers. Biopsy of the margin of the ulcer may show the presence of trophozoites.
- X-ray chest may reveal raised diaphragm in cases of liver abscess.
- Ultrasonography confirms the diagnosis of liver abscess **(Figs. 10.11 and 10.12)**. Amebic liver abscess is generally solitary. Presence of multiple abscesses indicates pyogenic liver abscess.
- Aspiration of abscess: The aspirated fluid is pink to chocolate brown color *(Anchovy sauce)* and may contain free amebae.
- Immunofluorescence techniques show the presence of antibodies in the serum of about 95% patients with amebic liver abscess and 60% with amebic dysentery.
- Blood tests reveal mild leukocytosis, normal liver transaminases and raised alkaline phosphatase.

Management

- The drug of choice is metronidazole in dosage of 750–800 mg 8 hourly for 5–10 days. The common side effects

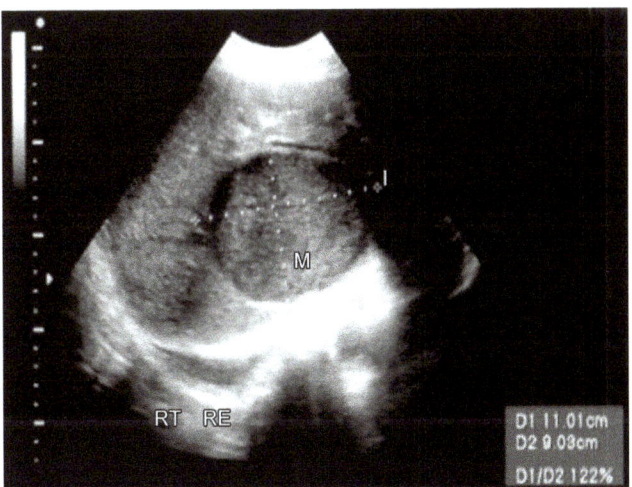

Fig. 10.11: Ultrasound showing solitary abscess (Amebic liver abscess).

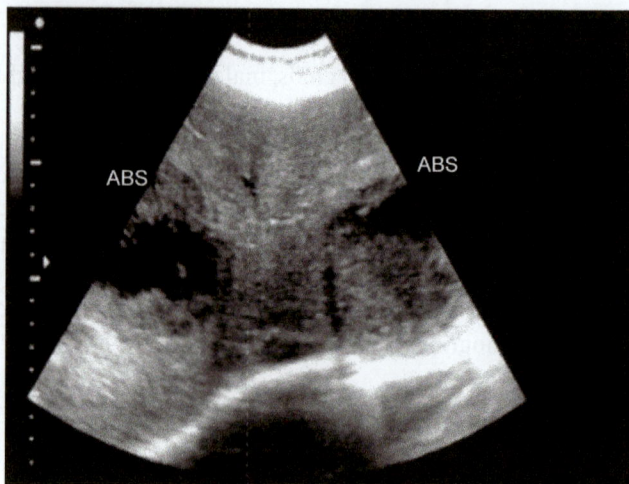

Fig. 10.12: Ultrasound showing multiple abscesses (Pyogenic liver abscess).

of metronidazole are metallic taste and disulfiram like reaction. Longer acting nitroimidazoles (tinidazole, ornidazole) are equally effective. Tinidazole is given as daily single dose of 2 g for 3 days. This is followed by administration of diloxanide furoate 500 mg 8 hourly for 10 days or iodoquinol 650 mg 8 hourly for 21 days to eliminate luminal parasites. Chloroquine and emetine used previously should preferably be avoided because of their significant side effects.

- Asymptomatic cyst passers or carriers can be given luminal agents like diloxanide furoate (500 mg 8 hourly for 10 days) or iodoquinol (650 mg 8 hourly for 21 days).
- Nitazoxanide is a new addition. The dose is 500 mg twice daily for 3 days. It is effective against trophozoites in both tissue and gut lumen.
- The amebic liver abscess is treated with medications as mentioned above. The aspiration of the amebic liver abscess is indicated if it is large and threatens to burst or does not respond promptly (within 72 hours) to drug therapy. Aspiration may also be needed to differentiate it from pyogenic liver abscess especially in case of multiple abscesses.

MALARIA

Malaria is a parasitic infection caused by *Plasmodium vivax, P. falciparum, P. ovale* (*curtisi* and *wallikeri*), *P. malariae* and *P. knowlesi*. Globally around 0.5 million people die each year due to malaria, mostly due to *P. falciparum* infection. Currently malaria is appearing in the areas from where it had disappeared.

Transmission of Malaria

Malaria is transmitted from human to human through bite of infected female Anopheles mosquitoes. There is no animal reservoir for human malaria. Other rare routes of transmission are transplacental and through blood transfusion.

Life Cycle

The mosquito is infected with the sexual form of parasite (gametocyte) when it feeds on human blood. These gametocytes develop into sporozoites in the salivary gland of the mosquito within 7–20 days.

When the infected mosquito bites an uninfected human, inoculated sporozoites travel to the liver within half an hour. In the hepatic cells, the sporozoites transform into merozoites (exoerythrocytic stage). However, in cases of *P. vivax* and *P. ovale* infections, some sporozoites remain in dormant form in liver (hypnozoites) for a period of upto a year or more. Hypnozoites can reactivate later and cause delayed primary infection or relapses. Relapse can also occur if treatment is not given to eradicate hypnozoites.

Merozoites leave the liver and infect erythrocytes. In the erythrocytes, merozoites go through the stages of ring form, trophozoite and schizont **(Fig. 10.13)**. The rupture of schizont causes release of plenty of newly produced merozoites in the blood (asexual erythrocytic stage). This event is accompanied with the febrile episode.

The newly released merozoites invade erythrocytes to repeat the erythrocytic cycle. However, some merozoites develop into gametocytes (sexual form) that can transmit malaria.

Recurrent malaria can occur in all four types of plasmodium infections due to the failure of treatment to eradicate all infected erythrocytes *(recrudescence)*.

Pathogenesis

P. falciparum invades erythrocytes of all ages whereas *P. vivax* and *P. ovale* preferably invade reticulocytes and *P. malariae* normoblasts. Parasitemia is most severe in *P. falciparum* infection; more than 2% of all erythrocytes can be infected. That is why the hemolysis is most severe in *P. falciparum* infection. Erythrocytes infected with *P. falciparum* adhere to capillary endothelium (cytoadherence), agglutinate with other infected erythrocytes and form rosettes with uninfected erythrocytes. This leads to ischemia and dysfunction of various organs such as brain, liver, kidney, lungs and the gut.

Clinical Features

The approximate incubation period is 12 days in case of *P. falciparum*, 14 days for *P. vivax* and *P. ovale* and 30 days for *P. malariae*.

The typical clinical feature is fever with chills and rigors. This may be associated with nonspecific symptoms such as headache, fatigue, myalgia, arthralgia and abdominal symptoms like anorexia, nausea, vomiting, diarrhea and pain. Initially, there is shaking chills for few hours (cold stage) followed by high fever (hot stage) and marked sweating (sweating stage). The fever is intermittent which may occur every other day in *P. vivax* and *P. ovale* infection *(tertian malaria)*, every third day in *P. malariae* (quartan malaria). *P. falciparum* has no specific pattern of fever.

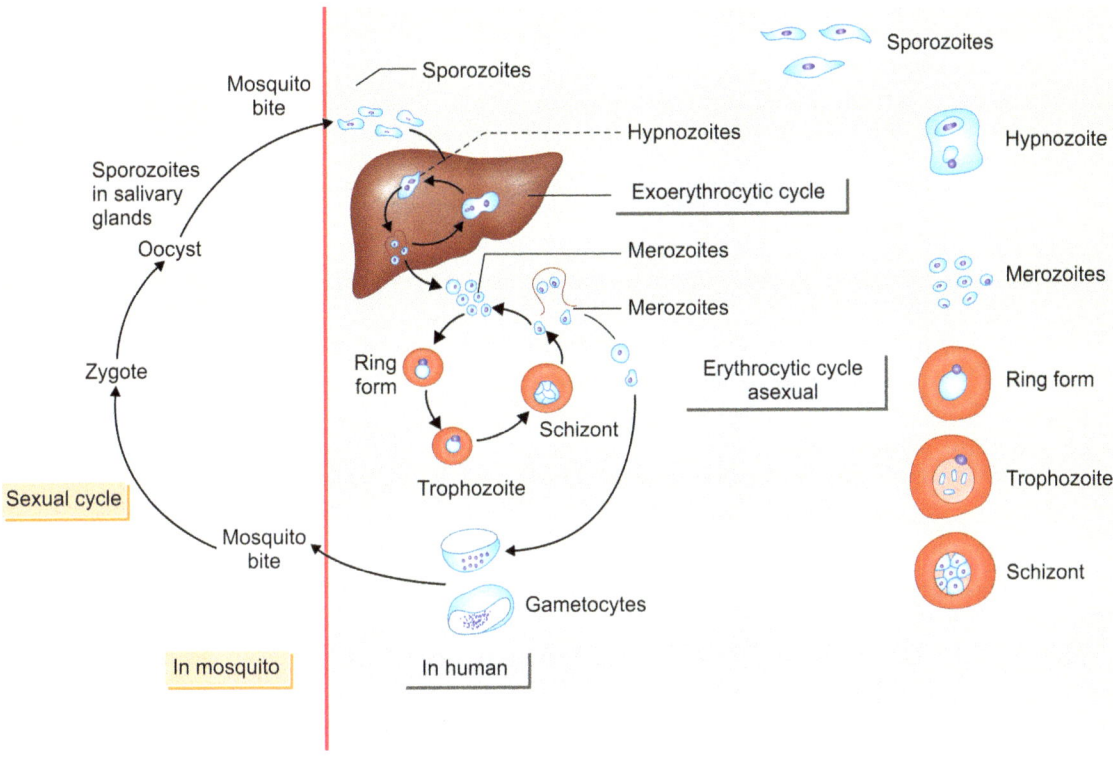

Fig. 10.13: Life cycle of malarial parasite.

The patients may have anemia and mild jaundice due to hemolysis. Splenomegaly is usual while mild hepatomegaly may also occur.

Severe Falciparum Malaria

Severe falciparum malaria is most dangerous form of malaria and is responsible for most of the deaths. Cerebral malaria is the most serious complication. It is characterized by confusion, coma, convulsions and neurological signs. Severe intravascular hemolysis may lead to hemoglobinuria *(black water fever)*. Other complications of falciparum malaria are given in **Table 10.17**. Complications are more frequent in children and pregnant females.

Chronic Complications of Malaria

Tropical splenomegaly (hyperactive malarial splenomegaly): Abnormal immune response to repeated attacks of malaria may result in massive splenomegaly, hepatomegaly and raised titers of IgM and malarial antibodies.

Table 10.17: Complications of falciparum malaria.

- Cerebral malaria
- Acute noncardiogenic pulmonary edema (ARDS)
- Acute tubular necrosis and renal failure
- Hyperpyrexia
- Hypoglycemia
- Severe anemia
- Metabolic acidosis
- Bleeding and disseminated intravascular coagulation (DIC)
- Hypotension and shock
- Convulsions

Nephrotic syndrome: Chronic and repeated infections with *P. malariae* may cause immune-mediated injury to renal glomeruli and cause nephrotic syndrome.

Investigations

- Thick and thin blood films stained with Giemsa and Wright's stain are examined for the presence of sexual and asexual forms of the parasites. The presence of asexual forms is important for the diagnosis of the infection. Sexual forms appear late and may persist even after the treatment of the infection.
- Antibodies are detectable 8–10 days after the onset of symptoms and persist for years. Hence, serological tests are neither helpful in the diagnosis of initial acute attack nor in the differentiation of current or past infections.
- Antigen detection methods (ELISA and dipstick format), polymerase chain reaction and indirect fluorescent antibody tests are commercially available for the diagnosis.
- Normocytic normochromic anemia is usually present. Laboratory findings in severe falciparum malaria include altered hepatic and renal function tests, acidosis and hypoglycemia.

Treatment

Several drugs are available for the treatment of malaria. The drugs are given in **Tables 10.18 to 10.20**. Treatment guidelines are given in **Table 10.21**.

Uncomplicated malaria is defined as malaria without signs of severity or vital organ dysfunction. Uncomplicated malaria can be treated by oral antimalarials. Patients who

Table 10.18: Drugs used in malaria.

Drug	Adult dose and side effects
Chloroquine	1g salt (600 mg base) initially, then 0.5 g (300 mg base) at 12, 24 and 36 hours. Parenteral dose: IV infusion; 10 mg/kg base in 8 hours then 15 mg/kg in next 24 hours **or** seven IM doses of 3.5 mg base/kg every 6 hour. Side effects: Nausea, postural hypotension, distaste, cardiac arrhythmia and severe hypotension if given IV
Quinine	Oral: 10 mg salt/kg thrice a day for 7 days plus Doxycycline 100 mg twice a day for 7 days or tetracycline 500 mg 4 times a day for 7 days **or** clindamycin 900 mg 3 times a day for 7 days.
Mefloquine	Oral: 750 mg followed by 500 mg after 12 hours. Side effects: Convulsion, neuropsychiatric symptoms
Sulfadoxine/pyrimethamine	25/1.25 mg/kg single oral dose (3 tablets of 500/25 mg) Side effects: Hypersensitivity, megaloblastic anemia
Primaquine	15 mg base daily for 14 days Side effects: Hemolysis (in G6PD deficiency patients), nausea, diarrhea, methemoglobinemia
Artesunate	Oral: 4 mg/kg followed by 2 mg/kg per day for 4 days
Artemether	Oral dose same as artesunate
Artemisinin-based combination therapies (ACTs) • Artemether plus lumefantrine • Artesunate plus mefloquine • Artesunate plus amodiaquine • Artesunate plus sulfadoxine-pyrimethamine • Dihydroartemisinin plus piperaquine	

Table 10.19: Artemisinin-based combination therapies (ACTs).

Drugs in combination	Dose in mg /kg	Dose
Artesunate plus sulfadoxine-pyrimethamine (SP)	Artesunate 4 mg/kg over 3 days and SP 25/1.25 mg/kg as single dose on day 1	Artesunate 1 tablet of 200 mg for 3 days and 3 tablets of SP (500/25 mg) on day 1
Artemether plus lumefantrine	Artemether 1.7 mg/kg and lumefantrine 12 mg/kg for 3 days	Artemether 80 mg plus lumefantrine 480 mg tablet twice daily for 3 days
Artesunate plus mefloquine	Artesunate 4 mg/kg over 3 days and mefloquine 25 mg/kg split over 2–3 days	Artesunate 1 tablet of 200 mg for 3 days and mefloquine 1000 mg on day 2 and 500 mg on day 3
Artesunate plus amodiaquine	Artesunate 4 mg/kg and amodiaquine 10 mg/kg once daily for 3 days	Artesunate 1 tablet of 200 mg for 3 days and 612 mg tablets once daily for 3 days
Dihydroartemisinin plus piperaquine	Dihydroartemisinin 2 mg/kg plus piperaquine 18 mg/kg once daily for 3 days	Total dose (6/48 mg/ kg in divided doses) may be given once orally daily for 3 days. Alternatively total dose can be given in divided doses at 0, 8, 24 and 48 hours

Table 10.20: Drugs for severe malaria.

Drug	Dose	Follow-up treatment	Comments
Artesunate	Parenteral: 2.4 mg/kg IV followed by 1.2 mg/kg at 12 and 24 hours then once daily Side effects: Anaphylaxis, urticaria, fever, lowers reticulocyte count	• Artesunate plus SP, or • Artesunate plus amodiaquine or • Artesunate plus clindamycin/doxycycline for 7 days	First choice
Quinine	Parenteral dose: IV infusion 20 mg of salt/kg over 4 hours followed by 10 mg/kg infused over 2–8 hours every 8 hours. Start oral therapy when possible Side effects: Nausea, vomiting, tinnitus, hearing loss (Cinchonism), hypotension if given IV	• Clindamycin for 7days • Doxycycline for 7 days (not in pregnancy and children < 8 yrs)	• Alternative regimen • Quinine is drug of choice in first trimester of pregnancy
Artemether	Parenteral: 3.2 mg/kg IM followed by 1.6 mg/kg daily Side effects: Same as artesunate	Artemether plus lumefantrine	Only used if artesunate and quinine are not available

cannot tolerate oral therapy should be treated by parenteral administration for few days followed by oral therapy when they are able to tolerate oral therapy.

• Chloroquine, quinine, artesunate, pyrimethamine and mefloquine act on blood schizonts and gametocytes of *P. vivax, P. ovale* and *P. malariae.*

Table 10.21: Treatment guidelines.	
Infection	WHO recommendation
Non-falciparum malaria	Chloroquine plus primaquine 0.25 mg base/kg once daily for 14 days
Uncomplicated *P. falciparum* infection	Artemisinin-based combination therapy (ACTs) plus a single dose of primaquine 0.75 mg base/kg; maximum 45 mg
Severe malaria	Artesunate IV first choice, Quinine infusion or artemether IM are alternatives
Malaria in pregnancy	**Uncomplicated malaria** *First trimester*: Quinine plus clindamycin for 7 days (artesunate plus clindamycin for 7 days is alternative) *Second and third trimester*: ACTs (Quinine plus clindamycin is alternative) **Severe malaria** Parenteral artesunate, quinine or artemether

- Only primaquine acts against hypnozoites and prevent relapse in *P. vivax* and *P. ovale (radical cure)*. The gametocytes of *P. falciparum* are killed by primaquine. Primaquine is contraindicated in patients with G6PD deficiency.
- Chloroquine is the drug of choice in uncomplicated malaria except in chloroquine resistant *P. falciparum* infection. Primaquine is added for 14 days in the case of *P. vivax* and *P. ovale* infection to destroy the hypnozoites and to prevent relapse. Single dose of primaquine is recommended in *P. falciparum* infection along with chloroquine.
- In severe attacks, parenteral therapy is started and switched to oral as soon as possible.
- Artemisinin (qinghaosu, Chinese herbal drug) is effective against all erythrocytic stages of human malarial parasite. Artesunate, artemether and dihydroartemisinin are analogs of artemisinin. These drugs have short half life and are recommended to be used in conjunction with a long acting agent for treatment of malaria (artemisinin-based combination therapy, ACT). These are not useful in prophylaxis because of short half life. The ACTs that are most commonly used are:
  – Artemether plus lumefantrine
  – Artesunate plus mefloquine
  – Artesunate plus amodiaquine
  – Artesunate plus sulfadoxine-pyrimethamine
  – Dihydroartemisinin plus piperaquine.

If artemisinin derivatives are used alone as monotherapy or in combination with rapidly eliminated agents (tetracycline or clindamycin) the duration of treatment should be 7 days.

Treatment of Resistant Malaria

- Resistance to chloroquine is usually observed in *P. falciparum* malaria. WHO recommends the use of combination therapy with artemether plus lumifantrine or other ACTs for treatment of uncomplicated resistant falciparum malaria in most regions **(Table 10.19)**.

The alternative treatment is oral quinine sulfate plus doxycycline (200 mg daily), tetracycline (250 mg 6 hourly) or clindamycin (600 mg 12 hourly) for 7 days.
- Patients who cannot take medication orally are given IV artesunate or quinine. Parenteral artemether can be given if artesunate and quinine are not available. Oral treatment is started as soon as possible.

Severe Malaria

Severe malaria should be treated with parenteral antimalarial therapy **(Table 10.20)**. Patients having one or more clinical criteria given in **Table 10.22** are considered having severe malaria.

Cerebral Malaria

Patients are hospitalized promptly. The management includes appropriate parenteral antimalarial chemotherapy, detection and treatment of fluid, electrolyte, acid-base abnormalities and other complications.

Prophylaxis

Chemoprophylaxis should begin one week before entering the malarious area and should be given till 4 weeks after leaving it. The drug of choice for prophylaxis is chloroquine (300 mg base weekly). In regions with chloroquine resistant malaria, proguanil (100 mg once a day) plus atovaquone (250 mg), mefloquine (250 mg weekly), primaquine (30 mg base daily) or doxycycline (100 mg daily) can be used.

Other preventive measures are wearing long sleeve shirts and trouser, using mosquito repellents and nets and using screens in houses.

HUMAN IMMUNODEFICIENCY SYNDROME (HIV)/ACQUIRED IMMUNODEFICIENCY SYNDROME (AIDS)

HIV/AIDS is a global pandemic. It was first detected in USA in 1981 whereas the first case of HIV infection was diagnosed in India in 1986. Now almost all countries of the world have it.

According to a recent estimate around 1.7 million people were newly infected with HIV in the year 2019 and total 38 million people are infected with HIV worldwide (2019).

Table 10.22: Clinical criteria for severe malaria.
- Impaired consciousness/coma - Repeated seizures - Renal failure - Acute respiratory distress syndrome (ARDS) - Hypotension - Disseminated intravascular bleeding (DIC) - Severe anemia - Spontaneous bleeding - Acidosis - Hemoglobinuria - Parasitemia of >5%

In India, there are around 2.34 million HIV positive individuals in India (2019). Highest number of cases was reported in Maharashtra, Andhra Pradesh, Karnataka, Uttar Pradesh and Telangana. Worst affected states (percent wise population infected) were Mizoram, Nagaland, Manipur, Andhra Pradesh and Meghalaya.

Mode of Transmission

- The most common mode of transmission of HIV in India as well as worldwide is heterosexual contact. In India, around 85–90% patients have received infection through unsafe sex with commercial sex workers (CSW), mostly in metropolitan cities. In Mumbai, about half of the CSW are HIV positive.
- Other modes of transmission are through contaminated blood or blood products, contaminated syringes (as in IV drug abusers) and from infected mother to fetus/newborn baby **(Table 10.23)**.
- The transmission of HIV from mother to child occurs mostly during labor although it can happen during any time in pregnancy or after birth, through breastfeed.
- Stool, saliva, sweat, urine have not shown to transmit infection although viral particles have been demonstrated in these fluids.

Causative Organism

Most cases of AIDS (98%) are due to HIV 1 while HIV 2 is responsible in only few cases particularly in Africa. The course of HIV 2 is less aggressive. Human immunodeficiency virus is a retrovirus belonging to lentivirus family **(Fig. 10.14)**. It is a RNA virus. HIV 1 is subdivided into three groups, M (major), O (outlier) and N. The most common group is M, which is further classified into nine subtypes or clades, lettered A, B, C, D, F, G, H, J, and K. Subtype C is prevalent in India whereas subtype B is common in North America and Europe. HIV 2 is of 5 subtypes, A, B, C, D and E.

Pathogenesis

HIV infects CD4 positive immune cells chiefly T helper lymphocytes, but other cells like B lymphocytes, monocytes, dendritic cells and microglial cells are also infected. A glycoprotein gp 120 present on the surface membrane of the virus has high affinity with the CD4 molecule present on the surface of immune cells. Certain coreceptors such as CXCR4 (on lymphocytes) and CCR5 (on monocytes) are also needed for the binding of the virus over cell surface. Following binding with the lymphocytes, HIV enters the cell **(Fig. 10.15)**. Its genomic RNA is released in the cytoplasm and converted into viral DNA by a unique enzyme *reverse transcriptase*. Viral DNA is integrated into the host cell DNA and captures the genetic machinery of the host cell. This leads to the rapid production of viral genome, which attains the shape of full virus with the help of protease enzymes.

Clinical Stages

The course of HIV disease follows various stages **(Table 10.24)**. Clinical stages of HIV disease have also been classified by WHO **(Table 10.25)**.

Acute HIV Syndrome

About half to two-third of the patients infected with HIV develop prodromal symptoms 3–6 weeks after infection. This stage is known as acute HIV syndrome and is characterized by fever, myalgia, arthralgia, rashes, lymphadenopathy, thrombocytopenia and neurological syndromes. In some this phase goes unnoticed. The symptoms spontaneously resolve within 3–4 weeks. The plasma viral load is very high during this stage.

Asymptomatic Stage

Following resolution of the acute HIV syndrome, infected individuals remain asymptomatic (clinical latency) for 2–8 years, although HIV continues to multiply and damage the immune system of the patient. There is a progressive decline in the CD4 count.

Mildly Symptomatic Disease

There is mild immune deficiency leading to manifestations, although these are not AIDS defining illnesses. The manifestations are oral or vaginal candidiasis, hairy cell leukoplakia, herpes zoster, bacillary angiomatosis, pelvic inflammatory disease and idiopathic thrombocytopenic purpura.

Table 10.23: Modes of transmission of HIV.

- Sexual route (heterosexual, homosexual)
- Parenteral route:
  - blood and blood products
  - injection drug users
  - occupational injury
- Mother-to-child transmission

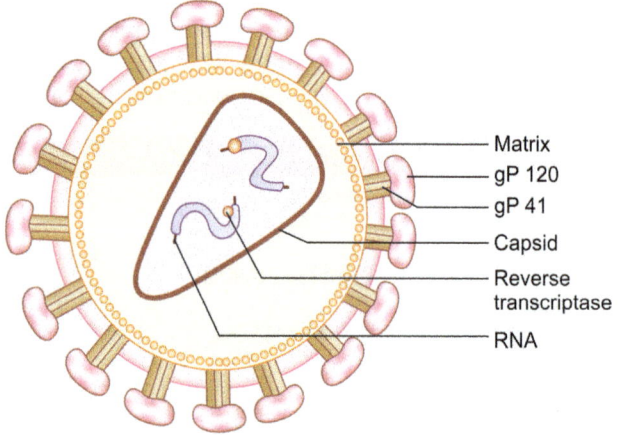

Fig. 10.14: Human immunodeficiency virus.

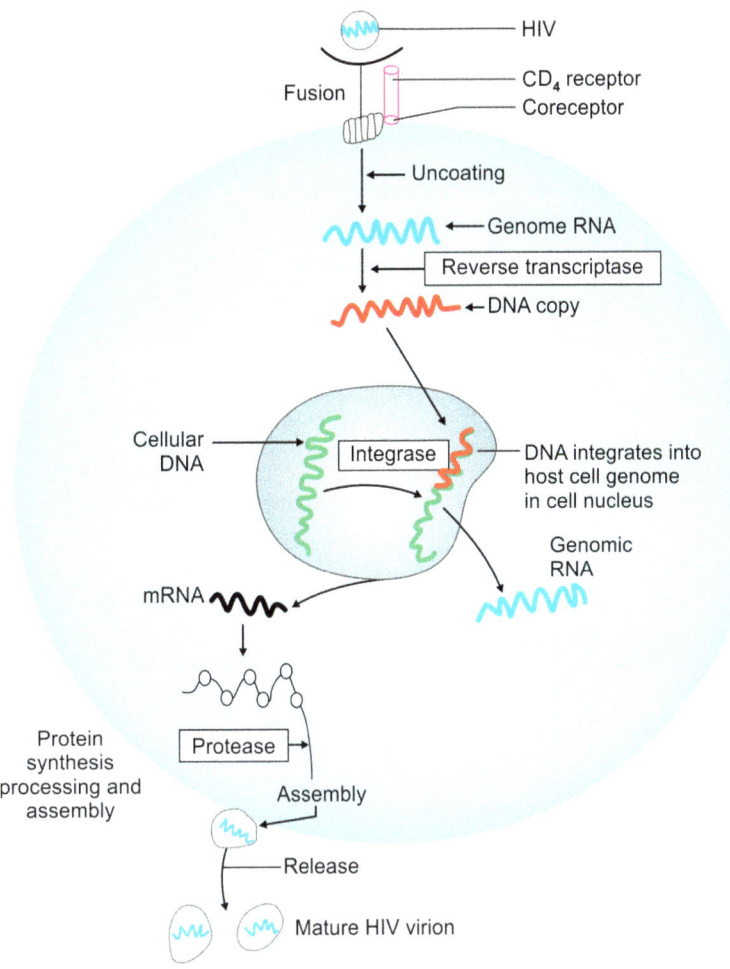

Fig. 10.15: Pathogenesis of HIV disease.

Table 10.24: Clinical stages of HIV disease.
- Acute HIV syndrome
- Asymptomatic stage
- Symptomatic stage
  - Mildly symptomatic disease
  - Advanced disease (AIDS)

Acquired Immunodeficiency Syndrome

As the disease progresses, there is a significant decrease in the CD4 count.
- Constitutional symptoms include unexplained weight loss (>10%), fever (>1 month) and chronic diarrhea. The patient may become severely cachexic **(Fig. 10.16)**. Persistent generalized lymphadenopathy may occur.
- A number of opportunistic infections may occur when CD4 count falls below 200/mm^3.
- Important opportunistic infections are tuberculosis (pulmonary and extrapulmonary), oroesophageal candidiasis **(Fig. 10.17)**, cryptococcal infection, herpes zoster **(Figs. 10.18A and B)**, toxoplasmosis, cytomegalovirus and *Pneumocystis carinii (now known as Pneumocystis jiroveci)* pneumonia.

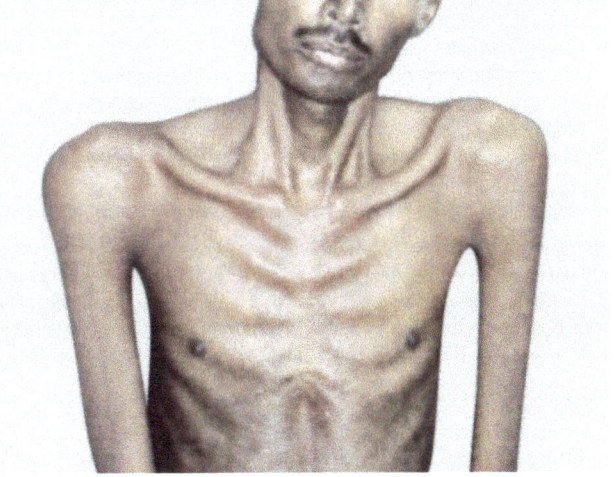

Fig. 10.16: Severely cachexic AIDS patient.

- Tuberculosis is the most common opportunistic infection in HIV patients in India.
- Patients may also have malignancies like Kaposi sarcoma and lymphoma.
- Diffuse skin eruption due to Molluscum contagiosum may be seen in patients with advanced HIV disease **(Fig. 10.19)**.

Table 10.25: WHO clinical staging in adults and adolescents.

Clinical stage 1
- Asymptomatic
- Persistent generalized lymphadenopathy

Clinical stage 2
- Unexplained moderate weight loss (<10% of presumed or measured body weight)[1]
- Recurrent respiratory tract infections (sinusitis, tonsillitis, otitis media, pharyngitis)
- Herpes zoster
- Angular cheilitis
- Recurrent oral ulceration
- Papular pruritic eruptions
- Seborrheic dermatitis
- Fungal nail infections

Clinical stage 3
- Unexplained[2] severe weight loss (>10% of presumed or measured body weight)
- Unexplained chronic diarrhea for longer than one month
- Unexplained persistent fever (above 37.5°C intermittent or constant for longer than one month)
- Persistent oral candidiasis
- Oral hairy leukoplakia
- Pulmonary tuberculosis
- Severe bacterial infections (e.g. pneumonia, empyema, pyomyositis, bone or joint infection, meningitis, bacteremia)
- Acute necrotizing ulcerative stomatitis, gingivitis or periodontitis
- Unexplained anemia (<8 g/dL), neutropenia (<0.5 × 10^9/L) and or chronic thrombocytopenia (<50 × 10^9/L[3])

Clinical stage 4[3]
- HIV wasting syndrome
- Pneumocystis pneumonia
- Recurrent severe bacterial pneumonia
- Chronic herpes simplex infection (orolabial, genital or anorectal of more than one month's duration or visceral at any site)
- Esophageal candidiasis (or candidiasis of trachea, bronchi or lungs)
- Extrapulmonary tuberculosis
- Kaposi sarcoma
- Cytomegalovirus infection (retinitis or infection of other organs)
- Central nervous system toxoplasmosis
- HIV encephalopathy
- Extrapulmonary cryptococcosis including meningitis
- Disseminated nontuberculous mycobacterial infection
- Progressive multifocal leukoencephalopathy
- Chronic cryptosporidiosis
- Chronic isosporiasis
- Disseminated mycosis (extrapulmonary histoplasmosis, coccidiomycosis)
- Recurrent septicemia (including non-typhoidal salmonella)
- Lymphoma (Cerebral or B cell non-Hodgkin)
- Invasive cervical carcinoma
- Atypical disseminated leishmaniasis
- Symptomatic HIV-associated nephropathy or symptomatic HIV-associated cardiomyopathy

[1]Assessment of body weight in pregnant woman needs to consider expected weight gain of pregnancy.
[2]Unexplained refers to where the condition is not explained by other conditions.
[3]Some additional specific conditions can also be included in regional classifications (e.g. reactivation of American Trypanosomiasis (meningoencephalitis and/or myocarditis) in Americas region, Penicilliosis in Asia).

Diagnosis

- Diagnosis of HIV infection is generally based on the detection of antibodies against viral proteins in the serum of the patients. The tests are ELISA and western blot. The former is more sensitive and is used for the screening whereas the later is more specific and is needed to confirm the diagnosis if the ELISA test is inconclusive.
- According to NACO guidelines, two different ELISA in symptomatic and three different ELISA in asymptomatic are required to be positive for the diagnosis of HIV infection.
- ELISA test may be negative during the first 3–6 weeks of infection when detectable amount of antibodies may not have formed. During this *'window period'* tests based on detection of antigens (p24) or viral RNA through RT-PCR (reverse transcriptase-polymerase chain reaction) are recommended.
- The CD4 count, measured by flow cytometry tells about the current immune status of the patient and guides us to start prophylactic therapy and anti-retroviral treatment. Viral RNA load suggests the prognosis of the patient.
- Patients are investigated for the evidence of co-infection with hepatitis B, and hepatitis C and positivity for syphilis (VDRL test).
- Investigations are also performed, if need be, to detect the presence of opportunistic infections.

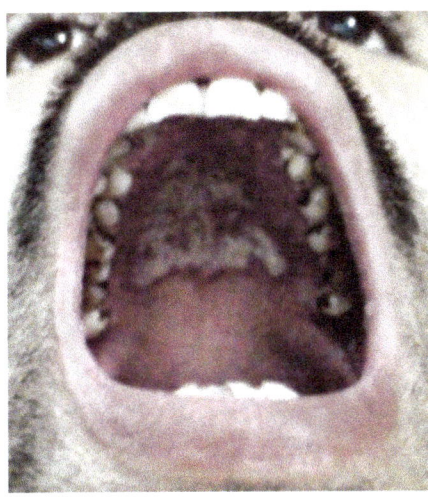

Fig. 10.17: Oral candidiasis.

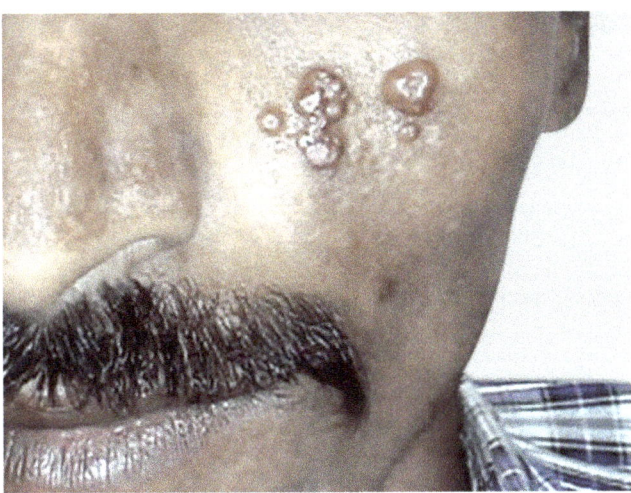

Fig. 10.19: Molluscum contagiosum.

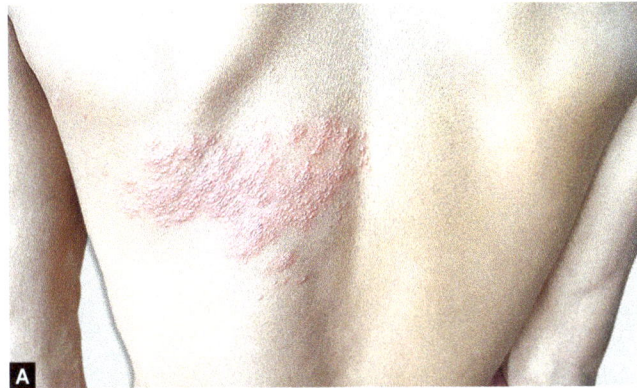

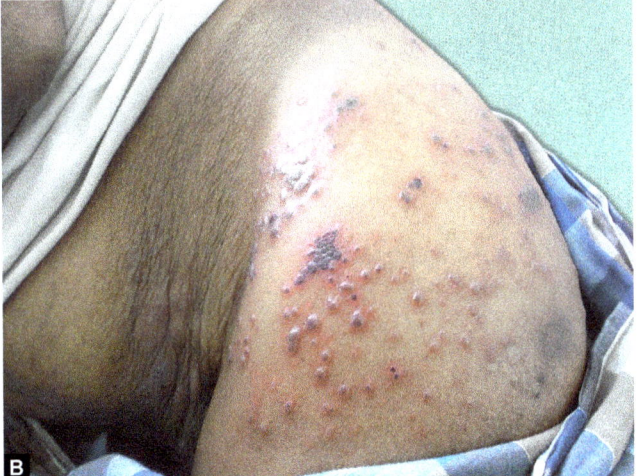

Figs. 10.18A and B: Herpes zoster in: (A) Thoracic region; (B) Left gluteal region.

- Besides these, complete blood count, liver function tests, blood urea, serum amylase, blood sugar and lipid profile are done as the baseline before initiation of anti-retroviral therapy.

Management of HIV Infection

The management of HIV disease starts the day the patient is diagnosed. The initial assessment includes a detailed history, mainly about occupation, mode of infection, fever, weight loss, loose motions, cough, dyspnea, rashes, lymphadenopathy, neurological problems and oral ulcer. The examination must include a detailed general and physical examination. Following are the main components of the management:
- Counseling
- Prevention of spread of infection
- Prophylaxis of opportunistic infections (OI)
- Treatment of opportunistic infections
- Anti-retroviral therapy.

- *Counseling:* Initially patient needs counseling so as to be able to cope up with stress. He is also counseled about the nature of disease and possibilities of the benefits and the risks of the treatment. He should also be convinced as regards regular follow-up visits to the doctor for initial assessment, prophylaxis for opportunistic infections and anti-retroviral therapy.
- *Prevention of spread of infection:* HIV positive individuals should also be advised to refrain from donating blood and unsafe sex so that they may not spread HIV infection to others.
- *The initiation of primary prophylactic therapy:* Prophylaxis of OI depends on the CD4 count. Recent NACO guidelines recommend administration of isoniazid in all patients with HIV who do not have active tuberculosis. This is given along with pyridoxine. A recommended schedule is given in **Table 10.26**.
- *Management of opportunistic infection:* Prompt diagnosis of OI and effective treatment has resulted into improved survival of HIV patients. The control of OI also retards the progression of HIV. Some infections are to be treated life long.

The co-infection of tuberculosis with HIV poses special problem in India and other developing countries. The presence of tuberculosis adversely affects the prognosis of HIV infection and the presence of HIV infection in tuberculosis leads to problem in the diagnosis as the manifestations are more commonly atypical. HIV positive

Table 10.26: Primary prophylaxis of opportunistic infections.

Infections	Indications	Medications
Pneumocystis carinii	CD4 count <350/mm³	Cotrimoxazole, dapsone, pentamidine
Toxoplasmosis	CD4 count <100/mm³	Co-trimoxazole, pyrimethamine plus dapsone
Cytomegalovirus	CD4 count <50/mm³	Gancyclovir
Mycobacterium avium complex (MAC)	CD4 count <50/mm³	Azithromycin, clarithromycin, rifabutin
Tuberculosis	All patients without active TB	Isoniazid

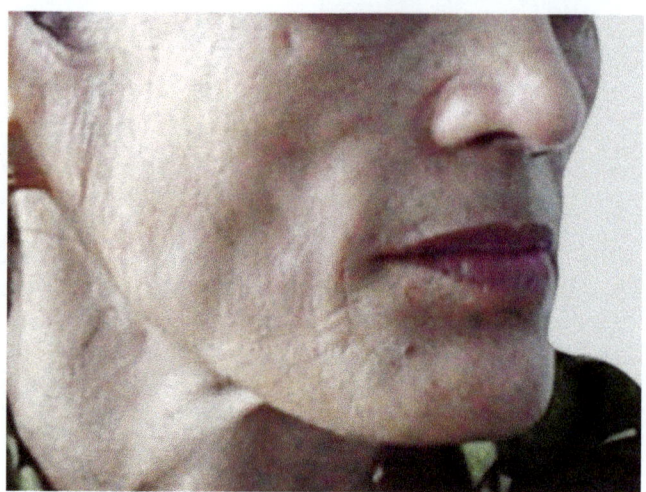

Fig. 10.20: Lipodystrophy.

patients are 15 times more prone to have reactivation of tuberculosis than their HIV negative counterparts.

Treatment of tuberculosis is same in HIV positive individuals as in HIV negatives. However, special precaution should be taken regarding the interaction between rifampicin and anti-retroviral drugs. In such cases, rifabutin is preferred over rifampicin.

- *Anti-retroviral therapy (ART):* The availability of anti-retroviral drugs has transformed the prognosis in HIV patients. Now HIV disease is regarded as chronically manageable disease rather than an essentially fatal disease.
    - The anti-retroviral therapy reduces viral load, improves the immune status of the patients (increases CD4 count) and thus decreases the incidence of opportunistic infections.
    - All persons diagnosed with HIV infection should be given ART regardless of CD4 count or WHO clinical staging.
    - ART should not be started in presence of severe form of active opportunistic infection (OI). OI should be treated and stabilized before commencing ART.

Limitations of ART

- ART is not curative. Only 70–80% patients respond to ART.
- Treatment needs to be given life long.
- There is also the problem of drug resistance.
- Anti-retroviral drugs are not free from toxic effects. These can lead to significant complications like gastrointestinal intolerance, hepatotoxicity, nephrotoxicity, bone marrow failure, pancreatitis, lipodystrophy **(Figs. 10.20 and 10.21)**, myopathy, neuropathy and increased cardiovascular mortality. Anemia is a common side effect of zidovudine (AZT) while neuropathy may occur with stavudine therapy. Side effects of first line ART drugs are given in **Table 10.27**.
- There may be interaction between ART drugs and other concomitant medications. This may require change in the dosage of drugs.

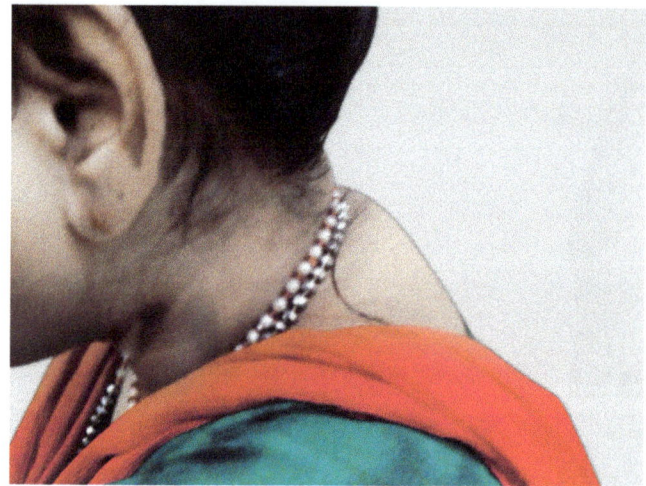

Fig. 10.21: Fat deposition at the back of neck; a toxicity of antiretroviral drugs.

Table 10.27: First line ART drugs and their side effects.

Name	Dose	Side effects
Tenofovir disoproxil fumarate (TDF)	300 mg OD	Renal toxicity, osteomalacia, flare of HBV infection
Tenofovir alafenamide (TAF)	25 mg OD	Nausea, less renal toxicity
Lamivudine	300 mg OD	Flare of HBV infection
Dolutegravir	50 mg OD	Insomnia, allergy, hepatotoxicity, weight gain, fetal neural tube defect
Abacavir	300 mg BD	Hypersensitivity (in HLAB5701 positives), anorexia, nausea

Anti-retroviral Drugs and Regimens

More than 20 drugs are approved for therapy. Most drugs are directed against viral enzymes such as reverse transcriptase and protease. Recent drugs like entry inhibitors and integrase inhibitors are now being used. Anti-retroviral drugs are listed in **Table 10.28**.

Table 10.28: Anti-retroviral drugs.

Reverse transcriptase inhibitors (RTI)
Nucleoside RTI (NRTI)
- Zidovudine
- Stavudine
- Lamivudine
- Didanosine
- Emtricitabine
- Abacavir

Non-nucleoside RTI (NNRTI)
- Nevirapine
- Efavirenz
- Delavirdine
- Rilpivirine
- Etravirine
- Doravirine

Nucleotide RTI
- Tenofovir disoproxil fumarate (TDF)
- Tenofovir alafenamide (TAF)

Protease inhibitors (PI)
- Saquinavir
- Ritonavir
- Indinavir
- Nelfinavir
- Atazanavir
- Lopinavir
- Fosamprenavir
- Darunavir
- Amprenavir
- Tipranavir
- Nelfinavir

Entry inhibitors
- Enfuvirtide (T20) (fusion inhibitor)
- Maraviroc

Integrase inhibitor
- Raltegravir
- Dolutegravir (DTG)
- Elvitegravir
- Bictegravir
- Cabotegravir

Post-attachment inhibitors
- Ibalizumab

Triple drug therapy is the gold standard. Mono or dual drug combination is contraindicated since these are often ineffective and lead to the emergence of resistance.

The combinations are:
- 2 NRTI plus 1 Integrase strand transfer inhibitor (ISTI)
- 2 NRTI plus 1 NNRTI
- 2 NRTI plus 1 PI (boosted with ritonavir).

ART Regimen in ART-naive Adults and Adolescents

- Recent NACO guidelines prescribe the use of dolutegravir as third agent in addition to tenofovir and lamivudine. The reason for choosing dolutegravir over efavirenz are:
  – Effective against HIV 2
  – Rapid viral suppression: Achieves viral suppression sooner than efavirenz
  – Fewer toxicities and side effects: Rash, dizziness and neuropsychiatric events are significantly more common with EFV.
  – More potent regimen: No resistance to DTG has been observed in trials.
  – Minimal drug interactions
  – High genetic barrier.
- As per current NACO guidelines (2020) preferred first line ART regimen for all PLHIV (age >10 years and weight >30 kg) is fixed dose combination (FDC) of Tenofovir (300 mg) + Lamivudine (300 mg) + Dolutegravir (50 mg) – single tablet once daily, this can be given at bedtime or any fixed time everyday as per patient's convenience (TLD regimen).
- Same regimen (TLD) is given to persons infected with HIV1 or HIV2 or both.
- For PLHIV with body weight <30 kg the recommended regimen is Abacavir 600 mg + Lamivudine 300 mg, one tablet plus Dolutegravir (50 mg) once daily.
- In patients with deranged renal functions (increased serum creatinine) the preferred regimen is Abacavir 600 mg OD plus Lamivudine (as per creatinine clearance) with Dolutegravir 50 mg once daily.
- If PLHIV is taking rifampicin containing anti-tubercular treatment, single tablet (FDC) of Tenofovir (300 mg) + Lamivudine (300 mg) + Dolutegravir (50 mg) is given in evening with additional dose of Dolutegravir 50 mg in morning.

TLD and Adult Women and Adolescent Girls of Childbearing Age

- Effective contraception should be offered to adult women and adolescent girls of childbearing age or potential.
- Risks of dolutegravir (DTG) in WCBP include adult morbidity resulting from DTG-associated weight gain and neonatal deaths among the infants of pregnant women with DTG-associated weight gain
- Adult women and adolescent girls of childbearing age or potential who wish to become pregnant should be fully informed of the potential increase in the risk of neural tube defects.
- In case a woman does not want to initiate TLD after adequate counseling, she should be initiated on TLE
- It is safe to initiate DTG-based regimen in pregnant women beyond first trimester.
- If woman is identified to be pregnant after the first trimester, DTG should be initiated or continued for the duration of the pregnancy.

Females in reproductive age group who opt out of TLD
a. Tenofovir + Lamivudine + Efavirenz
b. If Efavirenz is contraindicated (HIV2/HIV1 and 2/prior NNRTI exposure) then Tenofovir + Lamivudine +LPV/r (TL-1OD, LPV/r -2BD).

The response to therapy is monitored clinically, immunologically and by viral load reduction. In patients who respond, there is a rise in CD4 count and decrease in the plasma viral load.

Occupational Exposure and Post-exposure Prophylaxis

There is a minimal but definite risk of infection to the health care worker following exposure to patient's blood and body fluids. To minimize this, certain precautions and steps are to be taken. This is known as post-exposure prophylaxis (PEP).

- The chance of transmission of infection depends on the severity of exposure, the stage of the disease in the patient and measures taken after exposure. The guidelines for PEP are given in **Figure 10.22** (NACO guidelines 2014).
- Majority of occupational infections occur percutaneously through needlesticks and other instruments contaminated with blood. The mucocutaneous transmission of HIV may also occur. Risk of infection following percutaneous exposure to contaminated blood is about 0.3% and after mucous membrane exposure 0.09%.
- Following needlestick injury, the part should be thoroughly washed with soap and water. The injured finger should not be put in the mouth reflexly. Open wounds should be irrigated with saline. Antiseptic agents can be applied but caustic agents are avoided. Mucous membrane is flushed with copious amount of water. Eyes are irrigated with clean water or sterile saline.
- The need for PEP is decided as mentioned below:

For exposure code 1 and HIV source code 1	PEP not recommended
For exposure code 1 and HIV source code 2	PEP given
For exposure code 2 and HIV source code 1–2	PEP given
For exposure code 3 and HIV source code 1 or 2	PEP given
For exposure code 2 or 3 and HIV source code unknown	PEP if high prevalence

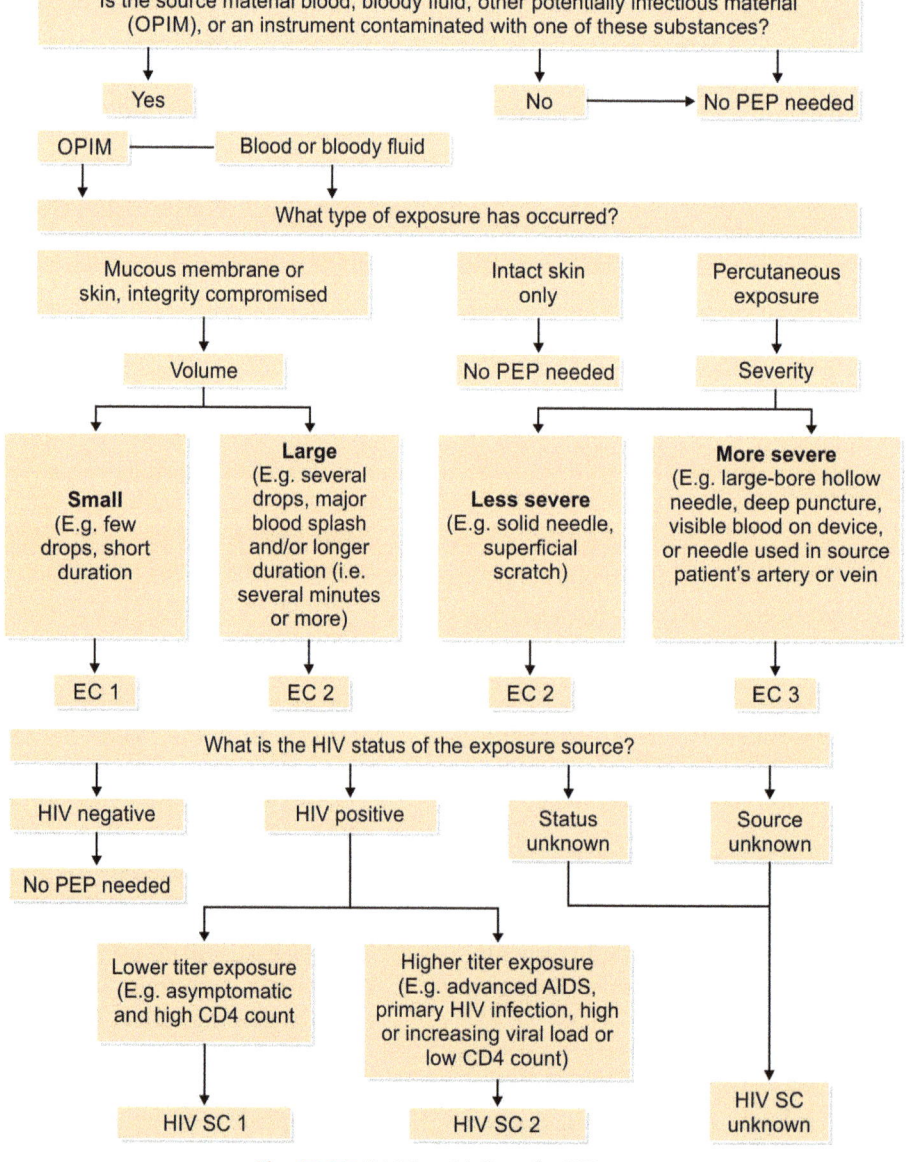

Fig. 10.22: NACO guidelines for PEP.

Table 10.29: Regimen for PEP (NACO 2020).

Tenofovir (TDF) 300 mg *plus*
Lamivudine (3TC) 300 mg *plus*
Dolutegravir (50 mg)
To be taken within 2 hours of exposure and continued for 4 weeks

Recommended PEP regimen for adults
- According to recent NACO guidelines, all individuals who are to receive PEP are given three-drug regimen. It includes one tab (FDC) of **Tenofovir (TDF) 300 mg + Lamivudine (3TC) 300 mg + Dolutegravir (50 mg) given** immediately within 2 hours of exposure followed by one tab once daily next day onwards, to be continued for 4 weeks **(Table 10.29)**.
- Universal precaution must be taken to protect health care worker from HIV patients.

Prevention of HIV Infection

The prevention of HIV infection can be achieved by taking the following measures:
- To practice safe sex: Use of condom can effectively reduce the chance of infection.
- Use of sterilized syringes and needles and instruments for every injection, immunization and surgery.
- Screening of all blood and blood products for HIV infection.

Prevention of Parent to Child Transmission (PPTCT) of HIV Infection

The success story of ART in the prevention of transmission of HIV infection from mother to fetus/newborn has instilled hopes. According to recent NACO guidelines, all HIV positive pregnant and breastfeeding women should be initiated on ART irrespective of their CD4 counts. This consists of a three-drug combination, preferably tenofovir (300 mg), lamivudine (300 mg) and dolutegravir (50 mg) taken orally as single dose. However due to risk of neural tube defect associated with dolutegravir, TLD regimen is avoided during first trimester. Alternative regimen is combination of tenofovir (300 mg), lamivudine (300 mg) and efavirenz (600 mg). Exposed newborn is given nevirapine 2 mg/kg once daily for 6 to 12 weeks.

Oral Manifestations in HIV Disease

Oropharyngeal lesions are common in HIV infection and are mostly due to secondary infections **(Table 10.30)**.
- The presence of *oral candidiasis* (thrush) may be an indicator of underlying HIV disease. Thrush appears as white, cheesy exudates on erythematous mucosa in the posterior oropharynx. Diagnosis is based on the examination of scraping for fungal elements.
- Palatal, glossal or gingival ulcer may also result from *cryptococcal disease or histoplasmosis.*

Table 10.30: Oral manifestations in HIV infection.

Infections
Fungal
- Candidiasis
- Histoplasmosis
- Cryptococcosis

Viral
- Oral hairy leukoplakia (EBV)
- Herpes simplex
- Cytomegalovirus
- Varicella zoster
- Papillomavirus

Bacterial
- Periodontal infections
- Necrotizing ulcerative gingivitis
- Necrotizing stomatitis

Neoplasms
- *Kaposi sarcoma*
- *Lymphoma*

Idiopathic oral aphthous ulcers

HIV salivary gland disease (DILS)*

Cervical lymphadenopathy

*Diffuse infiltrative CD8 lymphocytosis syndrome.

- *Oral hairy leukoplakia* is a white corrugated lesion presumed due to EBV. It occurs mostly on the lateral borders of the tongue but may involve adjacent buccal mucosa. It does not transform into malignancy. The presence of this lesion is highly suggestive of concurrent HIV infection and is more prevalent in advanced disease. Diagnosis is clinical and usually no treatment is required as it does not cause any symptoms.
- *Herpes simplex* may manifest as recurrent single or multiple oral or labial ulcers. Oropharyngeal ulcers can also be due to *Cytomegalovirus* (CMV). *Herpes zoster* can lead to ulcers in the trigeminal nerve distribution.
- *Papilloma virus* infection can present as pink or white single or multiple warts in the oral cavity. These are usually asymptomatic. The treatment is surgery, laser excision, cryotherapy or coagulation.
- Periodontal infections may become rapidly destructive which are difficult to manage. Anaerobic bacteria play a dominant role. Aggressive necrosis and ulceration of free gingival margin *(necrotizing ulcerative gingivitis)* may occur. The dissemination of this process to adjoining oral mucosa and palate leads to *necrotizing stomatitis*. Extension of ulcer can lead to bone destruction, tooth loosening and loss. These lesions are associated with pain, fever, gingival bleeding and foul breath. The treatment includes mouthwashes with povidine-iodine followed by chlorhexidine. Local debridement of necrotic material may be needed. Antibiotics (clindamycin, metronidazole, amoxicillin-clavulanate) are given in severe infection.
- Neoplasms of the oral cavity may occur. The mouth is the common site for *Kaposi's sarcoma*. The lesions are red or violet, flat, raised and nodular found usually over hard palate. Bulky lesions may ulcerate and bleed. They may

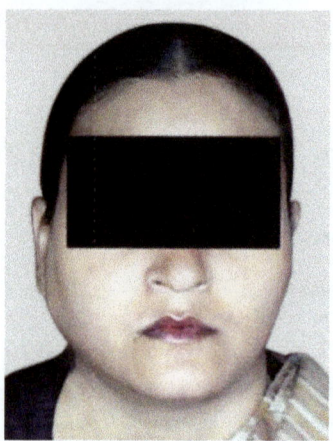

Fig. 10.23: Diffuse infiltrative lymphocytosis syndrome in HIV patient.

cause pain and swallowing problems. Diagnosis is made by biopsy.
- *Lymphoma* may manifest as nodules, ulcers or diffuse swelling in the oral cavity.
- Recurrent painful, single or multiple *aphthous ulcers* may occur in HIV disease. Large destructive ulcers are seen in advanced HIV disease. The treatment includes application of local anesthetic and steroids. In case of larger lesions, biopsy is done to rule out infectious or neoplastic cause. Thalidomide (200 mg/day orally) for 4 weeks is effective treatment for large ulcers. Systemic steroids can also be tried.
- *Diffuse infiltrative CD_8 lymphocytosis syndrome* (DILS) may present as bilateral salivary gland enlargement, usually parotid **(Fig. 10.23)** and xerostomia. Xerophthalmia can also occur. *Sjögren syndrome* and lymphoma may develop in these patients.

COVID-19

Corona virus disease 19 (Covid 19) is a disease caused by severe acute respiratory syndrome corona virus-2 (SARS-CoV-2), a enveloped positive-stranded RNA virus. Other severe outbreaks caused by corona virus are severe acute respiratory syndrome (SARS) in 2002-2004 and Middle East respiratory syndrome (MERS) in 2012.

Covid-19 cases were first reported from Wuhan, a city in the Hubei Province of China on 31st December 2019. In February 2020, WHO has named this as Covid-19. Since then it involved many countries and WHO declared it as a pandemic on 11th March 2020. A total of 239,110,635 cases with 4,874,702 deaths have been reported worldwide.

Highest number of cases (45,313,353) have been reported from USA USA followed by India (33,985,920) as on 12th October 2021. Total number of Covid-19 related deaths reported in India is 450,991 as on 12th October 2021.

Transmission and Incubation Period

It commonly spreads from human to human by droplets and aerosols generated while coughing, sneezing, talking, etc., from 2 days prior to symptoms to 5-7 days after symptoms of Covid-19. The average incubation period is 5-6 days (range 1-14 days). This is the reason why persons who are exposed are advised to stay quarantined for 14 days so that they if infected, do not spread virus to others.

Clinical Features

There are no specific symptoms or signs attributable to Covid-19. However common symptoms are fever, cough, breathlessness, sore throat, myalgia, loss of smell and taste and generalized weakness. Rarely, it may present with diarrhea and vomiting. Pneumonia is most frequent serious manifestation. Some people are more likely to develop severe clinical features **(Table 10.31)**.

Severe disease can lead to organ dysfunction like acute respiratory distress syndrome (ARDS), acute kidney injury (AKI), cardiac injury which may lead to multiorgan failure and death. Pathogenesis of disease, although not fully known yet, is related to cytokine release (e.g. IL-6), TNF-alpha and thromboembolic phenomenon.

Variants of Concern

As in other viruses, mutations also occur in the SARS-CoV-2 genome over time **(Table 10.32)**. Many variants of SARS-CoV-2 have emerged and have caused severe disease and rapid transmission of disease (variants of concern). These variants are also less neutralized by convalescent and post-vaccination sera. Neutralization by monoclonal antibodies is also reduced. Delta variant was first detected in India. Delta variant spreads rapidly and causes more infections than earlier forms.

Table 10.31: Risk factors for severe disease.

- Age > 60 years (mortality 8-15%)
- Cancer
- Solid organ transplant
- Type 2 DM
- Hematopoietic cell transplant
- HIV
- Use of corticosteroids or other immunosuppressing agents
- Comorbid conditions like COPD, chronic kidney disease, cardiac failure
- Obesity (body mass index ≥30)
- Smoking
- Pregnancy

Table 10.32: SARS-CoV-2 variants.

WHO label	Name (Pango lineage)
Alpha	B.1.1.7
Beta	B1.351, B1.351.2, B1.351.3
Gamma	P.1, P.1.1, P.1.2
Delta	B.1.617.2, AY.1, AY.2, AY.3
Epsilon	B.1.427 and B.1.429

Investigation

- *Nucleic acid amplification test:* Samples are taken from throat and nasal cavity by swab and tests are performed by RT-PCR or TrueNat. The sensitivity of these tests is 50–80% and specificity is around 100%. It takes around 8–10 hours and 2 hours by RT-PCR and TruNat respectively.
- *Rapid antigen test:* It is also done from nasal swab. Its sensitivity is around 50% and specificity is close to 100%. Time to perform the test is less than 1 hour. In case of negative result, RT-PCR test is indicated to confirm the diagnosis.
- *Serology:* Serum IgM and IgG are useful in epidemiological studies only.
- *Chest X-ray and CT scan thorax* are required to detect pneumonia and to classify it into mild, moderate and severe disease **(Table 10.33)**. Abnormalities are often bilateral and peripheral and are seen in lower lobes generally. There is ground glass opacification with or without consolidation **(Figs. 10.24 and 10.25)**.
- *Blood investigations:* CBC, KFT, LFT, RBS.
- *Inflammatory markers:* C-reactive protein, D-dimers, Ferritin, LDH, IL-6.

Common laboratory abnormalities in Covid-19 are mentioned below. Presence of these abnormalities are markers of severity.
- Lymphopenia
- Increased neutrophil-lymphocyte ratio (NLR)
- Elevated aminotransaminase level
- Elevated lactate dehydrogenase level
- Elevated inflammatory markers (ferritin, C-reactive protein, ESR, IL-6)
- Raised D-dimer and fibrinogen degradation products (FDP).

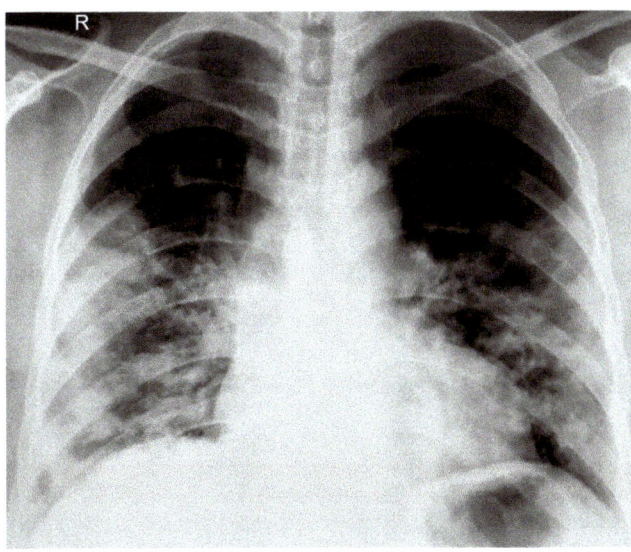

Fig. 10.24: Chest X-ray of Covid-19 positive patient showing B/L pneumonia on lower zone and peripherally located.

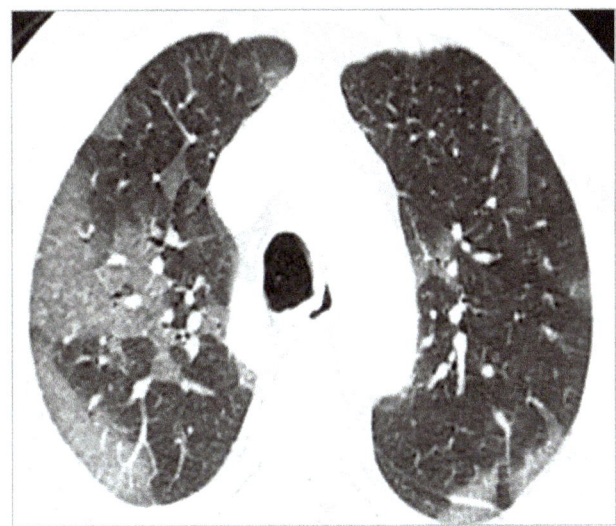

Fig. 10.25: CT scan thorax of Covid-19 positive patient showing B/L patchy ground glass opacities which are peripherally located.

Table 10.33: Clinical catagories of Covid-19.

Category	Clinical features	Radiological involvement
Mild	• No breathlessness • Normal oxygen saturation • RR < 24/Min	**No pneumonia or Lung involvement <25%**
Moderate	Dyspnea and or hypoxia, fever, cough. **Plus** • SpO$_2$ <94% (range 90–94%) on room air • Respiratory rate > 24 per minute	**Pneumonia (Lung involvement 25–50%)**
Severe	Clinical signs of pneumonia **Plus** • Respiratory **rate >30** breaths/min • **SpO$_2$ <90%** on room air	**Severe pneumonia (Lung involvement >50%)**
Critical illness: Multiorgan failure	Complications like ARDS, acute kidney injury, myocarditis, arrhythmias, etc.	

Treatment

Supportive treatment in all categories:
- Tab. Paracetamol 500 mg SOS (for fever)
- Syp. Dextromethorphan 10 mL TDS (for dry cough)
- Tab. Vitamin C 500 mg 1 BD
- Tab. Zinc 50 mg 1 OD
- Tab. Vitamin D$_3$ 60 K Units/week for 1 month
- Saline warm water gargles BD.

Specific treatment: The treatment of Covid-19 according to the Ministry of Health and Family Welfare (MOHFW) guidelines is given below. Drugs generally used in Covid-19 and their contraindications are mentioned in **Tables 10.34 to 10.36**. The knowledge about COVID-19 is evolving. Hence, the indications and choice of drugs may change in light of new evidences.

Table 10.34: Immunomodulators recommended in COVID-19.

- Oral steroids for 10d
- Tab Dexametasone 6 mg od
- Tab Prednisolone 20 mg bd, Tab MPS 16 mg bd
- MDI Budesonide 800 mcg twice daily with spacer × 10d
- Tab Colchicine 0.5 mg twice daily × 10d
- Tab Baricitinib 4 mg od × 10d (Anticoagulation required)
- Tab Tofacitinib 10 mg twice daily × 10d (Anticoagulation required)
- Inj. Tocilizumab 8 mg/kg IV or 324 mg SC (patients on respiratory and/or BP support)
- Inj. Infiximab/adalimumab/Itolizumab/Bevacizumab
- Inj. IVIg (Immunoglobin)

Table 10.35: Dugs used in COVID-19.

Hydroxychloroquine
Azithromycin
Ivermectin
Doxycyclin
Remedesivir
Dexamethasone
Methylprednisolone
Tocilizumab
Anti-coagulants
Convalescent plasma therapy

Table 10.36: Contraindication of drugs.

Hydroxychloroquine	• QT prolongation (> 480 ms) • History of unexplained syncope • Retinopathy • Hypersensitivity to HCQs • Cardiac rhythm disorders • Hypokalemia (K^+ < 3 mmol/L)
LMWH like enoxaparin	• Avoid in patients with high risk of bleeding • Enoxaparin CI in renal failure (Dalteparin is safe) • Platelets count <20,000/cmms
Remdesivir	• AST/ALT > 5 times upper limit of normal (ULN) • Severe renal impairment (i.e., eGFR < 30 mL/min/m² or need for hemodialysis) • Pregnancy or lactating females • Children (<12 years of age)
Tocilizumab	• PLHIV • With active infections (systemic bacterial/fungal) • Tuberculosis • Active hepatitis • ANC < 2,000/mm³ • Platelet count < 100,000/mm³ • Severe hepatic and renal impairment • Age < 18 years, pregnancy and lactation

(PLHIV: people living with HIV/AIDS; ANC: absolute neutrophil count; AST: aspartate aminotransferase; ALT: alanine aminotransferase; eGFR: estimated glomerular filtration rate; HCQ: hydroxychloroquine; LMWH: low molecular weight heparin; CI: contraindicated)

Treatment (As per AIIMS/ICMR-COVID-19 Task Force, May 2021 Guidelines)

- Treatment of mild disease
  - Physical distancing, indoor mask, hand hygiene
  - Hydration, antipyretics (paracetamol), antitussives, multivtamin
  - Monitor temperature and oxygen saturation (SpO_2)
  - Tab Ivermectin 200 mcg/kg once daily × 3d
  - Tab Doxycycline 100 mg bd × 5d
  - Tab HCQS 400 mg BD × 1d fb 400 mg od × 4d
  - Inhalational Budesonide 800 mcg twice daily × 5d (Beyond 5 days of symptoms onset)
  - Immediate medical attention if there is
    » Difficulty in breathing
    » High grade fever/severe cough >5d
    » High risk features
- Treatment of moderate disease
  - Oxygen support (target SpO_2 -92-96%)
  - Non-rebreather face mask (NRFM) preferred
  - Awake proning
  - Anti-inflammatory
  - Inj. Methylprednisolone (MPS) 0.5–1.0 mg/kg in 2 divided doses (equivalent Dexamethasone) × 5–10d
  - Anticoagulation conventional heparin or low molecular weight heparin (LMWH e.g., enoxaparin 0.5 mg/kg subcutaneously OD)
  - Monitor
    » Clinical, work of breathing., oxygen requirement
    » Serial chest X-ray, HRCT if worsening
    » CRP and D-dimer 48–72 h; CBC, LFT and KFT 24–48 h; IL-6 if deterioration
- Treatment of severe disease
  - Admit in ICU, Use non-invasive ventilation (NIV) using Helmet or face mask/Oxygen by HFNC (High flow nasal cannula)
  - Intubation—if high work of breathing/NIV not tolerated
  - Inj Methylprednisolone (MPS) 1–2 mg/kg in 2 divided doses (equivalent Dexamethasone) × 5–10d
  - Anticoagulation conventional heparin or LMWH (enoxaparin 0.5 mg/kg subcutaneously BD)
  - Maintain euvolemia
  - Management of sepsis/septic shock
  - Monitor
    » Clinical, work of breathing., O_2 requirement
    » Serial chest X-ray, HRCT if worsening
    » CRP and D-dimer 48–72 h; CBC, LFT and KFT 24–48 h; IL-6 if deterioration.
- Remdesivir may be given only to patients with moderate to severe disease requiring supplemental oxygen (200 mg IV on day 1 followed by 100 mg IV daily for next 4 days).
- Tocilizumab may be given to patients with severe disease, within 24 to 48 hours of admission, who have no

improvement with steroids and have high inflammatory markers (IL-6, CRP). There should be no active bacterial, tubercular or fungal infection.
- Antibody cocktail drug (Casirivimab and Imdevimab)
  – It is recommended for SARS-CoV-2 positive adults and pediatric patients >12 years (> 40 kg) with mild to moderate symptoms not requiring oxygen, who are at high risk of developing severe COVID-19 and/or hospitalization. Phase 3 trial have shown better results on high risk COVID-19 patients, its use shortened the coronavirus symptoms by 4 days and reduced hospitalization and mortality by 70%.

Prevention

- Frequent hand washing, use of hand sanitizers
- Use of masks
- Respiratory hygiene(Cough etiquettes)
- Avoid touching the face
- Social distancing(6 feet)
- Cleaning and disinfecting objects and surfaces
- Isolate if fever, cough develops

Vaccines

Various types of Covid vaccines are approved for emergency use. There are different types of vaccines, namely:
1. Viral vector
2. Whole inactivated virion
3. RNA vaccine
4. DNA vaccine.

India initially approved two types of vaccines; viral vector (covishield) and whole inactivated virion (Covaxin). Recently Sputnik V (vector), Moderna (mRNA), Johnson & Johnson (vector) and ZyCoV-D (DNA plasmid) vaccines have also been approved. Covishield uses a chimpanzee adenovirus to carry genetic material of the spike protein of SARS-CoV-2 into human cells. Vaccination program was roled out on 16th January 2012 by the Government of India. Generally two doses are administered at interval of 3–12 weeks depending on the type of vaccines and regulatory guidelines.

The effectiveness of vaccine is reported to range from 80–95%. Adverse effects are generally mild in the form of fever, myalgia, headache, dizziness and pain at injection site.

IMPLICATIONS ON DENTAL PRACTICE

- HIV patients are usually able to tolerate all types of dental procedures. No dental modification is needed for patients based on their HIV status. Patients with HIV are not more susceptible to complications after dental treatment regardless of CD4 cell count. Routine use of antibiotic prophylaxis is not recommended in HIV patients. However antibiotics are added in case of neutropenia (count <750/mm^3).
- HIV patients may have xerostomia particularly due to anti-retroviral medications. Xerostomia may also occur due to HIV associated disease of salivary glands. Hence, this should be taken into consideration while planning dental procedures like restorative procedures and fabricating fixed or removable prosthodontics.
- The drug interactions are common with anti-retroviral agents. This should be considered when prescribing any medicine to such patients.
- The practice of universal precaution must be maintained. In case of accidental exposure such as needleprick or injury by sharp instruments, PEP must be immediately followed.
- Patients with HIV disease may present for the first time to dental surgeon with oral manifestations. Most common of these manifestations is oroesophageal candidiasis.
- Gonorrhea may present uncommonly with oral manifestations like inflamed tonsils, lymphadenitis, and painful oral and pharyngeal ulcers.
- Patient with late syphilis may present with leukoplakia which may become malignant.

SELF ASSESSMENT

Multiple Choice Questions

1. **HIV subtype predominantly found in India is:**
   A. Clade E B. Clade C
   C. Clade B D. All
2. **Western blot test for HIV infection is based on the detection of following in the serum of patients:**
   A. Antigen B. Antibody
   C. Viral RNA D. Viral particles
3. **Estimated number of HIV infected people in the world:**
   A. 4 million B. 38 million
   C. 10 billion D. 1 billion
4. **Universal work precaution is needed while caring for:**
   A. Symptomatic AIDS patients
   B. All patients with HIV/AIDS
   C. All patients whether HIV positive or negative
   D. Only during surgery
5. **HIV can infect:**
   A. CD4 T lymphocytes only
   B. CD4 and CD_8 T lymphocytes
   C. All CD4 bearing cells
   D. All cells arising from bone marrow
6. **Most common opportunistic infection in AIDS patients in India is:**
   A. Candidiasis B. Amebiasis
   C. Tuberculosis D. Hepatitis
7. **Mother-to-child transmission of HIV occur mostly:**
   A. During labor
   B. During throughout pregnancy
   C. Through breastfeeding
   D. During last trimester of pregnancy

8. The risk of transmission of HIV through needle injury is:
   A. 2–10%   B. 0.3%
   C. 10–30%   D. 0.09%
9. Following malignancies are increasingly associated with HIV infection, *except*:
   A. Kaposi sarcoma   B. Hodgkin's disease
   C. Carcinoma breast   D. Primary CNS lymphoma
10. Following are at increased risk of getting HIV, *except*:
    A. Truck driver
    B. IV drug abuser
    C. Who frequently donate blood
    D. Those having STD
11. Following are anti-HIV drugs, *except*:
    A. Ritonavir   B. Acyclovir
    C. Saquinavir   D. Efavirenz
12. Following test is used for diagnosis of HIV infection during window period:
    A. Western blot   B. p24
    C. B_2 microglobulin   D. CD4
13. Diagnosis of tuberculosis in HIV positive patients may be difficult because:
    A. Tuberculosis is not common in HIV patients
    B. Presentation of tuberculosis may be atypical
    C. Bacterial strain is different
    D. All the above
14. Following drug is contraindicated in severe anemia:
    A. Efavirenz   B. Stavudine
    C. AZT (Zidovudine)   D. All of the above
15. Following percentage of HIV patients respond to ART:
    A. 10–20%   B. 60–70%
    C. >90%   D. 30–40%
16. Depression is important side effect of:
    A. Lamivudine   B. Efavirenz
    C. AZT (Zidovudine)   D. All of the above
17. Which is true for ART:
    A. ART is least effective
    B. ART is very effective in all patients
    C. ART is accompanied with increased cardiovascular mortality
    D. All of the above
18. Following opportunistic infection may occur even at CD4 count >500/cmm:
    A. CMV
    B. Herpes zoster
    C. *Mycobacterium avium* intracellulare
    D. PCP
19. In resource poor settings, if CD4 facility is not available, following can be used as parameter for starting ART:
    A. Eosinophilia   B. All HIV positive persons
    C. ESR   D. PPD test
20. Following is true during latent period of HIV disease:

	Elisa	p24	Symptoms
A.	+	+++	–
B.	–	–	+
C.	+	+/–	–
D.	–	++	–

21. Following drugs are used in herpes zoster, *except*:
    A. Acyclovir   B. Valacyclovir
    C. Indinavir   D. Famcyclovir
22. Which one of the following is the most common complication of mumps in postpubertal males?
    A. Myocarditis   B. Orchitis
    C. Nephritis   D. Parotid abscess
23. Koplik's spots are seen in:
    A. Mumps   B. Measles
    C. Rubella   D. Chickenpox
24. Following are features of rashes in chickenpox, *except*:
    A. Pleomorphic rash
    B. Rashes are pruritic
    C. First appears in extremities
    D. Rashes are infective till crusts slough
25. Most common complication of chickenpox is:
    A. Encephalitis
    B. Meningitis
    C. Viral pneumonia
    D. Secondary infection of skin lesion
26. Subacute sclerosing panencephalitis (SSPE) is associated with:
    A. Mumps   B. Measles
    C. HIV   D. Japanese encephalitis
27. Following are features of congenital syphilis, *except*:
    A. Mulberry molars   B. Maxillary hyperplasia
    C. High arched palate   D. Rhagades
28. Following drugs are used in syphilis, *except*:
    A. Penicillin   B. Doxycycline
    C. Azithromycin   D. Cotrimoxazole
29. Jarisch Herxheimer reaction can occur following initiation of treatment of:
    A. HIV disease   B. *Plasmodium falciparum*
    C. Syphilis   D. Gonorrhea
30. The longest incubation period is found in which type of malaria:
    A. *P. falciparum*   B. *P. ovale*
    C. *P. vivax*   D. *P. malariae*
31. Primaquin is given for radical cure in:
    A. *P. vivax* and *P. falciparum*
    B. *P. falciparum* and *P. ovale*
    C. *P. vivax* and *P. ovale*
    D. *P. malariae* and *P. ovale*
32. Following agents can be used for chemoprophylaxis of malaria, *except*:
    A. Chloroquine   B. Mefloquine
    C. Doxycycline   D. Quinine
33. Most common site involved in amebiasis is:
    A. Jejunum
    B. Rectum
    C. Cecum
    D. Gastroesophageal junction
34. Most common organ involved in extraintestinal amebiasis is:
    A. Brain   B. Lung
    C. Liver   D. Pancreas
35. Palatal palsy is a complication of:
    A. Mumps   B. Diphtheria
    C. Syphilis   D. Rubella
36. Following may occur through blood transfusion, *except*:
    A. Syphilis   B. HIV
    C. Gonorrhea   D. Malaria

37. **In Covid-19, what does 19 indicates?**
    A. Covid virus identified in 19th centaury
    B. Covid pandemic declared on 19th December 2019.
    C. Panel of 19 doctors discovered this disease
    D. First case of covid disease was identified in year 2019.
38. **Corona virus enters in cell by acting on which receptors?**
    A. ACE receptors
    B. K-Ras receptors
    C. EGFR receptors
    D. None of these
39. **Indication of steroid and heparin in Covid-19 is?**
    A. Patient has hypoxia
    B. Patient has severe pneumonia
    C. IL-6 is increased markedly
    D. All of the above
40. **Following disease are caused by corona virus, except:**
    A. Middle east respiratory syndrome (MERS)
    B. Severe acute respiratory syndrome (SARS)
    C. Covid-19
    D. Swine flu

Fill in the Blanks

1. Forschheimer's spots are seen in _____ infection.
2. Hutchinson's teeth are seen in _____.
3. Gumma occurs in _____ stage of syphilis.
4. Drug of choice in primary syphilis is_____.
5. Syphilis is caused by_____.
6. Cerebral malaria is caused by *Plasmodium*_____.
7. Tropical splenomegaly is associated with_____.
8. Amebiasis is caused by_____.
9. Anchovy sauce pus is a feature of_____.
10. "Bull neck" may occur in _____ infection.
11. Severe Covid-19 disease have oxygen saturation_____ and respiratory rate_____.

CHAPTER 11

Medical Emergencies in Dental Practice

Patients who come for treatment for their problems to dental surgeon may also be suffering from other systemic disorders. Some of these disorders may have direct relevance to the dental illness while others may not. However patients may develop serious life threatening problems during or just after the dental treatment. Emergency situations may arise more commonly when invasive or painful procedures are performed or medically compromised patients are treated. Hence the knowledge of these disorders is necessary in order to avoid or manage emergency situations. A list of important medical emergencies that may occur during dental treatment/procedure is given in the **Table 11.1**. A general guidelines should be followed **(Table 11.2)**.

The dental clinic should be well equipped in order to deal with any emergency. A list of paraphernalia and drugs that must be available in the clinic is given in **Table 11.3**.

History: A quick but discrete history must be taken to know about the past and present illness in the patient and also about the medication he/she is taking. In addition to this, a proper counseling is needed so that the patient understands the nature of treatment he is going to receive and the side effects expected if any. This will allay fear from

Table 11.1: Important medical emergencies in dental practice.

- General: Syncope, postural hypotension
- Cardiovascular: angina, myocardial infarction, cardiac arrest, heart failure, severe hypertension
- Respiratory: Asthmatic attack, hyperventilation, airways obstruction
- Neurological: Seizures, stroke
- Allergic: Anaphylaxis
- Endocrinal: Hypoglycemia, adrenal crisis
- Hematological: Excessive bleeding

Table 11.2: General precautions and guidelines.

- Patient should lay supine while receiving local anesthesia
- Ensure that diabetic patient has taken meal timely
- Always have an assistant
- Assistant should be well versed with techniques such as venepuncture, CPR, monitoring vitals and maintaining airways
- Emergency kit should be readily accessible and periodically checked
- Watch carefully for any change in behavior, breathing pattern, wheeze, sensorium in patient while on procedure
- Have contact phone number of physician/emergency department/ambulance

Table 11.3: List of drugs and equipments to deal with medical emergencies.

Drugs
- Inj. adrenaline (0.5 mL ampules of 1:1000 solution)
- Inj. chlorpheniramine
- Inj. hydrocortisone sodium succinate (100–200 mg)
- Inj. glucagon 1 mg
- Inj. diazepam
- IV dextrose (20%, 50%)
- Glucose powder
- Glyceryl trinitrate 0.3–1 mg
- Aspirin
- Salbutamol solution for nebulizing

Equipments
- Oropharyngeal/nasopharyngeal airway
- Oxygen source
- Suction machine
- Ambu bag
- Tourniquet
- Laryngoscope
- Endotracheal tube
- Sphygmomanometer
- Stethoscope
- IV cannula
- Disposable syringes and needles
- IV drip sets and DNS bottles
- Nebulizer
- Defibrillator

Contact numbers of physician/emergency department/ambulance

Table 11.4: History taking before dental treatment/procedure.
• Any problem during previous dental treatment • Hypertension, angina or any heart disease, diabetes • Seizures, fainting, syncope • Asthma, chronic bronchitis • Bleeding diathesis, anemia, jaundice • Drug allergy • Pregnancy • Risk factors for HIV • Renal disease • Peptic ulcer • Details of present medications

the mind of the patient and build trust and confidence. This will also ensure full cooperation on the part of the patient. Such steps are very helpful in avoiding complications like hypoglycemia, exacerbations of bronchial asthma, vasovagal syncope, surge in blood pressure, intense tachycardia or excessive bleeding. A scheme of history taking is given in **Table 11.4**.

Examination: A quick but thorough clinical examination should be performed before any dental treatment/procedure. This includes general and important systemic examination. Important findings on general physical examination such as blood pressure, anemia, jaundice, must be looked for. Systemic examination should particularly include heart sounds, respiratory sounds, organomegaly, and obvious neurological deficits. A detailed list is given in the **Table 11.5**.

POSTURAL HYPOTENSION (ORTHOSTATIC HYPOTENSION)

Postural hypotension (orthostatic hypotension, OH) is a fall in systemic arterial pressure on assumption of upright posture.

- It is defined as a sustained drop in systolic (>20 mm Hg) or diastolic (>10 mm Hg) blood pressure within 3 minutes of standing.

Table 11.5: Clinical examination.
General • Pallor • Pulse • Blood pressure • Jaundice • Edema • Goiter • Lymphadenopathy • Temperature • Skin **Systemic** • Neurological: higher functions, any deficit • Heart sounds • Lung sounds • Liver • Spleen

Table 11.6: Important causes of postural hypotension.
• Defective postural reflexes: Diabetes, aging, parkinsonism • Drugs: vasodilators, beta blockers, diuretics, antidepressants • Hypovolemia: diarrhea, excessive sweating, hemorrhage, diuretics

- Symptoms of postural hypotension are dimming or loss of vision, light headedness, diaphoresis, nausea, pallor and weakness. Syncope may result if cerebral perfusion is impaired.
- Postural hypotension is generally due to defective postural reflexes, hypovolemia or drugs. A history of medications, previous postural syncope, diabetes and causes precipitating hypovolemia must be obtained before the procedure **(Table 11.6)**.

Management

- Patients who have underlying causes of postural hypotension should be advised to attain upright position slowly. Preferably they may be asked to sit down first for sometimes before standing **(Table 11.7)**.
- Plenty of fluids should be given to prevent hypovolemia.
- These patients should not be made to remain in standing position for long.
- Medications that aggravate the problem should be discontinued and changed.
- Movement of legs prior to rising may facilitate the venous return and help avoid OH.
- Upon development of initial symptoms of OH, patient should immediately be laid supine. He is given water to drink and advised to attain sitting posture slowly as described earlier.
- Advise patient to consult physician for evaluation and treatment of the cause of postural hypotension.

SYNCOPE

Syncope is defined as a transient loss of consciousness due to diminished cerebral perfusion. Syncope is characterized by loss of postural control and spontaneous recovery (for details, see Chapter 5).

It may be preceded by symptoms of 'presyncope' such as lightheadedness, visual blurring, dizziness, sweating and nausea.

Vasovagal Syncope

- This is the most common cause of "common faint" in normal persons.

Table 11.7: Measures to avoid postural hypotension.
• Avoid prolonged standing • Avoid sudden change in posture from lying down position to sitting or standing • Movement of legs prior to standing • Plenty of fluids and salt intake prior to the procedure

- Precipitating factors are hot or crowded environment, severe pain, extreme fatigue, prolonged standing, hunger and emotional situations.
- Vasovagal syncope occurs generally in the sitting and standing posture. Hence, it is essential that the patient is immediately made to lie down (recumbent position) at the earliest.

Treatment

The treatment depends upon the underlying cause. However, certain precautions are to be taken regardless of the cause.

Immediate Actions to be Taken During Syncope

- Patient should be placed in supine position with head tilted to the side to maximize cerebral blood flow and to avoid aspiration.
- Peripheral stimulation like sprinkling cold water over the face may help.
- Clothing should be loosened.
- Patient should not be allowed to rise again till weakness persists.

Instructions to the Patient

- Patient is advised to avoid situations that have caused the syncope.
- He should try to assume a recumbent position as soon as they feel premonitory symptoms.
- Patient who has recurrent syncope should avoid climbing ladders, swimming alone, driving or operating machines.
- Patient is advised to consult physician.

HYPERTENSIVE CRISIS

A sudden rise in blood pressure may occur during the treatment at dental clinic. This may happen due to skipping in the dose of antihypertensive medication or due to fear and anxiety.

History should be taken about the hypertension and its medications and whether the patient has taken the dose timely. The patient is counseled about the nature of treatment/procedure in order to allay fear and anxiety. Blood pressure is measured before the procedure.

Hypertensive crisis includes hypertensive urgencies and emergencies.

Hypertensive urgencies is defined as substantial increases in blood pressure usually with systolic >220 mm Hg or diastolic >120–130 mm Hg. It also includes hypertension with disk edema, progressive end organ complications rather than damage and severe perioperative hypertension. In this situation, BP must be reduced in several hours. Parenteral therapy is usually not needed.

Hypertensive emergencies include hypertensive encephalopathy, hypertensive nephropathy, intracranial hemorrhage, unstable angina, myocardial infarction, acute left ventricular failure with pulmonary edema, aortic dissection and eclampsia. Malignant hypertension is characterized by nephropathy or encephalopathy with accompanying papilledema. Parenteral therapy is generally required (for more details, see Chapter 5).

Management

- Excessive and rapid decline in the BP should be avoided as it may lead to cerebral hypoperfusion and coronary insufficiency.
- In patients with malignant hypertension without encephalopathy, it is advisable to bring down BP over hours. This is done with frequent oral dosing with labetalol or clonidine.
- The parenteral drugs used are nitroprusside, nitroglycerine, dizoxide, esmolol, labetalol, enalaprilat and hydralazine. Intravenous frusemide is given as an adjunct. Parenteral labetalol and nicardipine are effective agents for lowering down the blood pressure in patients with hypertensive encephalopathy.
- Sublingual nifedipine should be avoided in the acute management because it is associated with adverse cardiac events.

ACUTE PULMONARY EDEMA

The symptoms of acute pulmonary edema are rapid onset dyspnea, cough, anxiety and restlessness. Patient cannot remain supine and prefers to sit upright for some relief. The sputum may be profuse, pink and frothy or blood stained. Patient has cold extremities, cyanosis, excessive sweating, tachypnea and tachycardia. Lungs are full with crackles and wheezes.

Precipitating factors for acute pulmonary edema are stress and exertion in a cardiac patient, arrhythmia, myocardial ischemia or hypertensive crisis.

An adequate medical history about the presence of cardiac disease should be taken. One should make sure that patient is regularly taking medications as prescribed for his ailment. The patient should be properly counseled prior to the procedure. The procedure is done in cordial and comfortable environment. The management is summarized in **Table 11.8**.

Table 11.8: Management of acute pulmonary edema.

- Patient is put in sitting posture
- Stoppage of dental procedure
- Reassurance
- Oxygen is administered to improve hypoxia
- IV frusemide (20–80 mg) gives rapid relief
- Call for medical help
- Monitor vital signs
- IV morphine (2–4 mg) can be given
- If no relief, shift the patient to medical emergency

Management of Cardiogenic Pulmonary Edema

Acute pulmonary edema is a life-threatening condition and needs prompt management. An emergency call should be sent to physician/cardiologist.

Initial Supports

- Oxygen is administered to improve hypoxia. In severe cases, positive pressure ventilation may be needed.
- Patient is placed in sitting posture.

Drug Therapy

- *Intravenous morphine* (2–4 mg) is given to relieve anxiety. It also reduces preload through venodilation and thus reduces dyspnea. This can be repeated if needed.
- *Frusemide* (20–80 mg IV) offers rapid improvement in dyspnea by decreasing pulmonary congestion through its venodilator effect prior to causing diuresis. Hence, it is the diuretic of choice in acute pulmonary edema.
- *Intravenous nitroglycerine* is also helpful, particularly in cases of ischemic heart disease. Nitroglycerine decreases preload to heart as it is a venodilator. It is contraindicated if there is hypotension. Nitroprusside infusion is indicated in cases of acute pulmonary edema associated with hypertension.
- *Ionotropic agents* (dopamine, dobutamine) and phosphodiesterase inhibitors (amrinone, milrinone) stimulate myocardial contractility and are useful in patients with hypotension or shock.
- Intravenous recombinant *BNP* (nesiritide) is a potent vasodilator with diuretic properties. It is also effective in acute pulmonary edema.
- *Hemodialysis* may be needed in patients with severe renal failure.

Correction of Precipitating Factors

The precipitating factors of acute pulmonary edema such as severe hypertension, IHD, arrhythmias, volume overload should be adequately managed

CHEST PAIN

Patients with ischemic heart disease may develop retrosternal chest pain due to angina. Occasionally it may develop for the first time during procedure in patient not previously known to be a cardiac patient. Hence, a history should be taken for the presence of heart disease in all patients and also about the medications. The immediate management is done as shown in the **Table 11.9**.

Initial Management of Myocardial Infarction

- *Relief of pain*: Sublingual nitroglycerine (0.4 mg) is given for pain relief. This may be given at interval of 5 minutes. Intravenous nitroglycerine is started if pain reoccurs or

Table 11.9: Management of chest pain (acute coronary syndrome).

- Reassure the patient
- Defer further dental treatment
- Glyceryl trinitrate 0.5 mg sublingual
- Give aspirin 160–325 mg stat
- If pain persists for more than 30 minutes, give clopidogrel 300 mg loading dose and atorvastatin 80 mg
- Summon assistance

there is associated hypertension. Nitrates should not be given if systolic blood pressure is < 90 mm Hg.
- *Antiplatelet agents*: Aspirin (nonenteric coated) in the dosage of 160–325 mg should be given to the patient to chew. Clopidogrel (300 mg loading dose followed by 75 mg/day) should be given to all MI (myocardial infarction) patients as soon as possible in addition to aspirin. Atorvastatin 80 mg should also be given.
- *Oxygen therapy*: Oxygen is administered for initial few hours and continued if hypoxemia is present.
- *Hospitalization*: Patient should be referred for hospitalization in coronary care unit (CCU) with facilities of continuous ECG monitoring and defibrillator as promptly as possible since many patients die within the first 24 hours of onset of symptoms of MI and over half occurs within first hour due to ventricular fibrillation. Patient should be confined to bed rest. The goal is a door-to-needle (thrombolysis) time of <30 min and door-to-balloon [percutaneous coronary intervention (PCI)] time of <90 min.

ASTHMATIC ATTACK

The asthmatic attack may get precipitated before, during or after dental procedure. Important precipitating factors are anxiety, infection, allergy or drugs. The symptoms are acute dyspnea, wheeze, dry cough, tightness in the chest, anxiety, diaphoresis, cyanosis and confusion. Chest examination reveals bilateral rhonchi (see also in Chapter 6). In case the patient is a known case of bronchial asthma, one should make sure that he has properly taken medications as prescribed. In order to avoid the precipitation of acute attack in asthmatic patient, one should:

- Avoid using materials/drugs with allergic potentials
- Assure and calm the patient
- Ensure that patient has taken medicines for asthma as prescribed
- Avoid numerous dental products, which may exacerbate asthma such as some toothpastes, tooth enamel dust and methyl methacrylate.

The patient is urgently managed as discussed below and in the **Table 11.10**. However, if recovery does not occur, he should be shifted to medical emergency department.

Management of Acute Severe Asthma

- *Hospitalization and oxygen therapy:* The patient should be hospitalized for urgent management. Arterial blood

Table 11.10: Management of acute asthmatic attack.
• Stop the procedure
• All dental materials removed from patient's mouth
• Reassure the patient
• Do not lay patient supine, place in comfortable posture
• Administer oxygen
• Nebulize with salbutamol (2.5–5 mg)
• Inject hydrocortisone IV 200 mg
• Call an ambulance in case the condition does not settle

gas analysis, chest X-ray and ECG should be done to assess severity and to rule out other causes. A high concentration oxygen inhalation is given to maintain PaO_2 >60 mm Hg.

- Repeated dosage of short-acting adrenergic drugs (salbutamol 2.5–5 mg or terbutaline 5–10 mg) is given through a nebulizer at an interval of 20–30 minutes. The PEFR should be recorded frequently to assess the response. Metered dose inhaler with a spacer device can alternatively be used. Ipratropium bromide can be added to get additional bronchodilator effect.
- *Systemic steroids:* This is essentially needed in all cases of severe asthma. Inj. hydrocortisone 200 mg or methylprednisolone 125 mg is given intravenously followed by oral therapy with prednisolone (30–60 mg daily).
- Others:
    - Mechanical ventilation is needed in patients with coma, respiratory arrest, exhaustion and deteriorating blood gases despite adequate treatment.
    - IV fluid is administered to prevent dehydration.
    - Antibiotics are not used routinely. These are only given if infection is present.
    - Opiates, sedatives or tranquillizers are contraindicated.

Patient Education and Monitoring of Therapy

- Patients are educated about the nature of disease and its treatment.
- They should also be trained to recognize the severity of their disease and monitor the response to therapy with the use of peak flow meter.

AIRWAYS OBSTRUCTION

During dental procedures, objects such as fragments of tooth, filling materials or segments of bone may find their way into the posterior part of the oral cavity, pharynx and larynx. In conscious patient, airway obstruction is less common due to cough reflex. The symptoms are violent respiratory efforts; feel of choking and deepening cyanosis. Preventive measures should be taken to avoid such events **(Table 11.11)**.

Table 11.11: Prevention of airways obstruction.
• Use of rubber dams wherever possible
• Adequate use of oral packings
• Proper positioning of patient
• Effective uses of dental assistance and suction

If the foreign body is swallowed, its location should be confirmed with the help of radiologists. Tips of broken instruments, burs or dental restorations may have pointed or jagged edges that might injure the gut mucosa. The patient is advised to eat soft bulk diet and to keep watch for evacuation of foreign body. A follow-up X-ray must be done to ensure its elimination.

If the foreign body has been aspirated, certain maneuvers are performed and patient is referred to thoracic surgeon. Different maneuvers are:
- Make patient stand up and use abdominal thrusts until foreign body is expelled (Heimlich maneuver).
- A Trendelenburg position (legs raised) can allow the gravity to move the object close to the oral cavity wherefrom it can be easily removed.
- Use laryngoscope and pharyngeal suction.
- If obstruction persists, insert a cannula of 10–12 IV size through cricothyroid ligament (cricothyrotomy).
- Arrange transfer to hospital for specialized care.

HYPERVENTILATION

Patient may develop hyperventilation (rapid breathing) during dental procedure. This is commonly due to pain, fear and anxiety **(Table 11.12)**. Hyperventilation may result into hypocarbia (low $PaCO_2$) and alkalosis. Symptoms due to hyperventilation are tingling sensation around mouth, fingers and toes, muscle tremors, tetanic spasms of fingers and hand, light headedness and altered sensorium. The problem is self-limiting and does not generally require specific treatment **(Table 11.13)**.

SEIZURES

Seizure is a transient clinical event in the form of motor, sensory, autonomic or psychic manifestations due to abnormal excessive paroxysmal discharges from a group of central nervous system neurons. Precipitating factors for seizures are given in **Table 11.14** (see also in Chapter 8).

Proper history of any seizure disorder must be asked from the patient. If patient has seizure disorder, one should

Table 11.12: Causes of hyperventilation.
• Psychogenic or anxiety
• Fever, pain, sepsis
• Pulmonary diseases (pneumonia, asthma, embolism)
• Cardiac diseases (CHF, hypotension)
• Metabolic acidosis (diabetic, renal, lactic)
• Drug induced (salicylates, methylxanthines)

Table 11.13: Management of hyperventilation.
• Stop the procedure
• Assure the patient
• Put the patient in comfortable position
• Patients may be asked to breathe in a paper bag
• May give mild sedative in case of intense anxiety
• Exclude other causes of hyperventilation

Table 11.14: Precipitating factors for seizures.

- Fatigue
- Skipped meal
- Flashes of light (TV, monitor)
- Loud music/sound
- Sleep deprivation
- Alcohol use or withdrawal
- Physical and emotional stress
- Missing the dose of medication

Table 11.15: Emergency management of seizures.

- Patient is put semi-prone
- Airways patency ensured
- Nothing oral till full recovery
- Protect from injury
- If seizure does not terminate spontaneously, give IV diazepam 10–20 mg or IV lorazepam 4 mg slowly and may repeat if no recovery in 5 minutes
- Shift to medical emergency department

make sure he is taking the medication regularly. Precipitating factors for seizures must be avoided. Emergency management of seizures is summarized in **Table 11.15**.

Management

Immediate Care

- Patient is shifted to a safer place, away from danger (water, fire and machine).
- Patient is turned to the semi-prone position to prevent aspiration.
- Patient should not be left alone until full recovery from seizures as there may be drowsiness and confusion in the postictal stage or the seizures may reoccur.
- Nothing should be given by mouth until the patient has fully recovered.
- If convulsions continue for a prolonged duration (>5 minutes) or reoccur without the patient regaining consciousness, hospitalization is a must.

Oral cavity and airways are cleaned and cleared preferably with a piece of gauze. Finger should not be inserted into mouth to avoid bite injury.

Status Epilepticus

Convulsive status epilepticus refers to continuous seizure activity or intermittent seizures with impaired consciousness in interictal period. Practically seizure activity lasting for more than 5 minutes should be managed as status epilepticus.

Nonconvulsive status epilepticus is defined as impairment or loss of consciousness with electrographic (EEG) seizure activity and clinically absent or subtle motor activity. These patients do not present with convulsions, but with a fluctuating abnormal mental status, confusion and impaired responsiveness. The treatment approach is same as convulsive status epilepticus.

Status epilepticus should be treated as emergency. The patient should be hospitalized.

- Airway is maintained and oxygen is administered.
- Intravenous line is started, a blood sample is withdrawn for laboratory analysis and intravenous dextrose (50% dextrose 25–50 mL) is promptly given. The initial laboratory tests include glucose, electrolytes, calcium, urea, creatinine, liver transaminases and complete blood count.
- Intravenous diazepam (10 mg) or lorazepam (4 mg) is given slowly in 2 minutes. This can be repeated once after 15 minutes if seizures are not controlled. Midazolam 0.2 mg/kg or clonazepam 0.015 mg/kg can also be used.
- If seizures continue beyond 30 minutes, a) intravenous phenytoin (20 mg/kg) at a rate not more than 50 mg/min is given. Alternatively, fosphenytoin can be given in a doses of 20 mg/kg PE (phenytoin equivalents) IV. One should monitor for cardiac arrhythmia and hypotension, b) lacosamide 400 mg IV or levetiracetam 20–30 mg/kg IV may also be given, c) in patients taking valproate and who may be having subtherapeutic levels, valproate 25 mg/kg can be given intravenously.
- If seizures continue the patient is in refractory status epilepticus. An additional dosage of 5–10 mg/kg of phenytoin or 10 mg/kg PE of fosphenytoin may be repeated. Alternatively valproate 30 mg/kg IV may be given over 15 minutes.
- If there is no access to intensive care unit (ICU), phenobarbitone (IV 20 mg/kg) at a rate not more than 50 mg/min is given if seizures are still uncontrolled. An additional dose of 5–10 mg/kg may be repeated if needed. Respiratory depression and hypotension are important adverse events.
- Uncontrolled seizures are finally managed by admission in ICU and general anesthesia and neuromuscular blockade along with ventilatory support. Anesthetic agents used are midazolam, propofol and pentobarbitone.
- Once the status is controlled, long-term anti-epileptic medications are started.
- The underlying cause is identified if any and treated accordingly.

STROKE (CEREBROVASCULAR ACCIDENT)

Stroke means sudden neurological deficit due to focal vascular cause. The incidence of stroke increases with age. The causes and risk factors for stroke are described in Chapter 8. Important risk factors are hypertension, heart disease, diabetes mellitus, old age, smoking and previous vascular events. Patient develops sudden loss of consciousness with paralysis, generally hemiplegia and facial paralysis. The initial management is done in the dental clinic before shifting the patient to the emergency room.

Initial Management

- Stop dental procedure
- Lay the patient supine with head turned to one side
- Do not give anything orally
- Ensure patent airways
- Monitor vitals
- Give oxygen
- Inject 20–50 mL 50% dextrose (in case there is hypoglycemia)
- Arrange for shifting to emergency room

ANAPHYLAXIS

Anaphylaxis is acute type 1 hypersensitive reaction presenting as sudden hypotension, bronchospasm and urticarial skin reaction. Patient may develop respiratory arrest, cardiac arrhythmia and cardiac arrest. Thorough history about any such reaction in the past must be asked (for details, see Chapter 13).

In order to avoid this complication, intradermal sensitivity test should be performed, particularly in case of xylocaine, penicillin, streptomycin, anti-serum and radiographic contrast media. Fainting due to fear or anxiety during or after injection can be confused with anaphylaxis. The management is summarized in **Table 11.16**.

Treatment

Prompt recognition and management of anaphylactic reaction is a must as death may occur within minutes. Upon any suspicion of anaphylaxis, airway, breathing and circulation are assessed.

- *The drug of choice is adrenaline (epinephrine).* This is given in a dose of 0.3–0.5 mg (0.3–0.5 mL of 1:1000 solution) intramuscularly or subcutaneously. Repeated injections can be given at 20 minutes intervals if necessary. Patients who are already being treated with beta adrenergic blocker drugs are refractory to epinephrine. A higher dose of adrenaline is required for the desired effect. Glucagon is also beneficial in such patients. Epinephrine causes bronchodilatation and vasoconstriction and prevents further mast cell degradation. This can also be given sublingually, intravenously or via an endotracheal tube in patients with hypotension and airway compromise.
- Airway management should be a priority. Hundred percent oxygen should be administered. Endotracheal intubation may be necessary. If laryngeal edema does not respond to epinephrine, tracheostomy may be required. Inhalation of β_2 adrenergic agonist (terbutaline, salbutamol) and intravenous aminophylline are helpful in bronchospasm.
- Intravenous fluids are given to maintain intravascular volume. The amount of fluid to be given is adjusted according to the blood pressure and urine output. Vasopressor drugs (Dopamine, norepinephrine) are used if the patient remains hypotensive.
- H_1 receptor antagonists (chlorpheniramine, diphenhydramine, promethazine) are useful in relieving skin symptoms (pruritus, urticaria and angioedema) and abdominal cramps. Addition of H_2 receptor antagonists (ranitidine) may provide better effects.
- Glucocorticoids have no immediate significant effect but may reduce prolonged reactions or relapses. Hydrocortisone (200 mg) or methylprednisolone (125 mg) can be given intravenously.

The patient is observed for 24 hours as the late phase reactions can cause reappearance of symptoms.

HYPOGLYCEMIA

Manifestations of hypoglycemia occurs when blood glucose level falls below 60 mg/dL and neurogenic symptoms appear at around 50 mg/dL (see also Chapter 9). However, the levels of blood sugar at which patients develop symptoms greatly vary. It is one of the most common emergencies in diabetic patients during dental treatment. Important symptoms of hypoglycemia are hunger, sweating and tiredness. Other manifestations are listed in **Table 11.17**.

Hypoglycemia is a complication of insulin or oral hypoglycemic therapy. Risk factors for the development of hypoglycemia include overdose of anti-diabetic medication, skipped meal and delay in the meal, unusual physical exertion and alcohol ingestion. Hypoglycemia can also complicate liver disease, adrenal insufficiency and hypopituitarism.

History prior to the dental treatment/procedure must include whether patient has diabetes. The timing of the intake of the anti-diabetic medication and the meal last taken should be asked. Patient should also be inquired for the presence of any symptoms suggestive of hypoglycemia. In case of any such symptoms, patient is given sugar, glucose or candy to eat. Blood may preferably be drawn before the administration of glucose to allow documentation of low plasma glucose.

Table 11.16: Management of anaphylaxis.

- Patient is laid supine with legs raised
- Give 0.5 ml of 1:1000 adrenaline intramuscularly, may be repeated at every 10 min.
- Inject 10–20 mg chlorpheniramine IV
- Inject 100–200 mg hydrocortisone hemisuccinate IV
- Ventilate with oxygen
- Rapid IV saline infusion
- Be prepared for CPR
- Call ambulance, hospitalize the patient

Table 11.17: Symptoms of hypoglycemia.

- Hunger, sweating, anxiety, irritation
- Palpitation, trembling, nausea, headache
- Confusion, lack of concentration
- Seizures, coma

Diagnosis

The diagnosis is made by the measurement of plasma or capillary blood glucose, which is low.

Treatment

The treatment depends upon the severity of hypoglycemia and consciousness level of the patient.
- If the patient is able to swallow, rapidly absorbable carbohydrates can be administered orally (glucose and sugar). Alternatively milk, fruit, candy bars, or biscuits may be given to patients with mild hypoglycemia.
- If the patient is unable to swallow or is in severe hypoglycemia, intravenous glucose (20–50 mL of 50% dextrose) is given initially. This is followed by an infusion of 10% dextrose to maintain blood glucose above 100 mg/dL.
- Glucagon injection (1 mg SC or IM) may be given in severe hypoglycemia if intravenous access can not be established promptly.
- Prevention of hypoglycemia includes proper education regarding causes and symptoms of hypoglycemia and proper adjustment in medication and diet.

ADRENAL CRISIS

Adrenal crisis is acute adrenal insufficiency. This should be suspected if patient collapses, becomes pale, develops hypotension and there is history of prolonged uses of corticosteroid with a period of withdrawal. The adrenal crisis is precipitated in certain situations **(Table 11.18)**. The patient should be put supine with legs raised and injection hydrocortisone hemisuccinate 200 mg IV is immediately given. Medical specialist/endocrinologist is consulted.

EXCESSIVE BLEEDING

Excessive bleeding during dental procedures is not uncommon. In most cases, it may be related to the procedure itself or as a consequence of anxiety. However, in some cases, when it is due to underlying hemostatic disorders, it may be life threatening. Hemostatic disorders commonly seen in practice are listed in the **Table 11.19**. A proper history of undue bleeding, purpura, ecchymosis, hemarthrosis and intake of antiplatelet or anticoagulants must be taken before the dental procedure.

If patient is a known case of hemostatic disorder, proper management must be done before the procedure (See Chapter 4).
- Stop aspirin/antiplatelet drugs 4–7 days before the procedure
- Maintain platelet count (50,000–1,00,000/cmm) in thrombocytopenic patients
- Avoid NSAIDs in thrombocytopenic patient

Table 11.18: Precipitating factors for adrenal crisis.
- Infections
- Trauma
- General anesthesia
- Steroid withdrawal

Table 11.19: Common hemostatic disorders.
- Hemophilia A
- Hemophilia B
- Idiopathic (autoimmune) thrombocytopenic purpura
- Von Willebrand disease
- Drugs (antiplatelets, anticoagulants)
- Liver disease

- Administer Vitamin K and/or fresh frozen plasma (FFP) in patient with liver disease if prothrombin time is highly raised
- Maintain adequate factor activity in hemophilic patients with administration of factors (factor VIII or IX) an hour before the procedure
- In case of mild hemophilia or von-Willebrand disease (vWD), tranexamic acid or DDAVP may be used.

In case the patient bleeds excessively and prior diagnosis is not known, appropriate blood samples for the investigations must be drawn before administration of any drug/factors. Initial investigations in patients with increased risk of bleeding are given below. Other tests can be done later.
- Complete blood count (including platelet count)
- Prothrombin time (PT)
- Activated partial thromboplastin time (APTT)
- Bleeding time.

For detailed description of hemostatic disorders, readers are advised to see Chapter 4.

DENTAL PROCEDURES IN PREGNANT WOMEN

Elective procedures may be deferred during pregnancy; however, acute and emergent dental problems do arise and should be treated. It is advisable to consult the obstetrician before any intervention. Following points should be kept in mind:
- Local anesthesia is preferred over general anesthesia.
- Prolonged procedures may preferably be avoided.
- Pregnant patients may have gingival hyperplasia which does not need any treatment. The gum swelling resolves after the delivery.
- Pre-eclampsia (hypertension, edema, proteinuria) should be excluded before any procedure.
- Only drugs safe in pregnancy should be prescribed.

CARDIOPULMONARY RESUSCITATION

All health care providers must know the procedures of basic life support (BLS) and advanced cardiac life support (ACLS). When cardiac arrest occurs, BLS must be started immediately.

The goal of resuscitation is to maintain cerebral perfusion until cardiopulmonary function is restored. The longer the period of cardiopulmonary arrest, the lower is the chance of restoring healthy life. Irreversible cerebral damage may occur after 3 minutes of anoxia. Ventricular arrhythmias are responsible for majority of cardiac arrests; hence defibrillation facilities should be available.

Following sequence should be followed during adult resuscitation:

1. Assessment of unresponsiveness
2. Activation of emergency medical services
3. BLS until defibrillation is available
4. Defibrillation if indicated
5. Intubation
6. Administration of appropriate medications (For details, see Chapter 12).

SELF ASSESSMENT

Multiple Choice Questions

1. Which of the following is used in treatment of acute pulmonary edema:
   A. Furosemide
   B. Thiazide
   C. Indapamide
   D. Spironolactone

2. Which of the following is the preferred therapy during acute asthmatic attack:
   A. IV aminophylline
   B. Nebulization with beta 2 agonists
   C. Oral deriphyllin
   D. Inhaled anticholinergics

3. First drug to be given during status epilepticus:
   A. Lorazepam or diazepam
   B. Phenytoin
   C. Phenobarbitone
   D. Levetiracetam

4. Which of the following is drug of choice for acute anaphylaxis:
   A. Antihistamine
   B. Corticosteroids
   C. Adrenaline
   D. Dopamine

5. All of the following are features of hypoglycemia, *except*:
   A. Sweating
   B. Bradycardia
   C. Confusion
   D. Seizures

6. Patient can have spontaneous intracranial bleeding if platelet count is less than--------- cu/mm.
   A. 50000
   B. 30000
   C. 1 lac
   D. 10000

7. Patients with chronic liver disease and deranged international normalized ratio (INR) should be given following agent before surgical procedure
   A. Whole blood transfusion
   B. Factor VIII
   C. Fresh frozen plasma
   D. Platelet transfusion

8. Tranexamic acid is:
   A. Antiplatelet agent
   B. Anticoagulant
   C. Antifibrinolytic agent
   D. Antithrombotic agent

9. Which of the following drug is helpful in stabilizing the blood clot and reduce bleeding:
   A. Vitamin C
   B. Tranexamic acid
   C. Streptokinase
   D. Clopidogrel

CHAPTER 12

Critical Care

SHOCK

Shock is the clinical syndrome when the oxygen delivery fails to meet the metabolic requirements of the tissues. It is due to reduced tissue perfusion leading to decreased delivery of oxygen and metabolic substrates to the tissues.

Cellular dysfunction caused by reduced perfusion leads to release of inflammatory mediators, which further cause changes in the microvasculature leading to more reduced perfusion and ultimately multiple organ failure and death if not treated.

Shock is usually accompanied by low blood pressure (hypotension) and circulatory failure. Mean arterial pressure (diastolic blood pressure plus one-third of pulse pressure) is usually less than 60 mm Hg.

Classification

Classification of shock is given in **Table 12.1**. Hypovolemic shock is the most common form of shock.

Hypovolemic Shock

Hypovolemic shock is caused by any condition causing reduction in blood volume **(Table 12.2)**. Hypovolemic shock is characterized by low cardiac output, low central venous pressure, low Jugular venous pressure (JVP), narrow pulse pressure, cool extremities and sympathetically mediated increased systemic vascular resistance.

It may be caused by:
- Hemorrhage (external or internal)
- Loss of fluid from gastrointestinal tract
- Urinary loss or insensible loss (skin, etc.)
- Sequestration of fluid.

Mild hypovolemia (loss of <20% blood volume) is characterized by few clinical signs like anxiety and tachycardia.

Moderate hypovolemia is characterized by loss of 20-40% of blood volume.

- There are tachycardia, tachypnea, and postural hypotension.
- Blood pressure may be normal in supine position but when patient is made to stand for few minutes, blood pressure may fall and patient may complain of dizziness, light headedness and syncope in standing position.
- Postural hypotension (orthostatic hypotension) is defined as > 20 mm Hg fall in systolic blood pressure and >10% fall in diastolic blood pressure within 3 minutes of standing.

Table 12.1: Classification of shock.

- Hypovolemic
- Cardiogenic
- Obstructive
- Distributive
  Septic
  SIRS (Systemic inflammatory response syndrome)
  Anaphylactic
  Neurogenic
  Drug-induced vasodilatation
  Hypoadrenal

Table 12.2: Causes of hypovolemic shock.

Loss of Blood (Hemorrhagic)
- Trauma
- Gastrointestinal bleed
- Hemothorax
- Hemoperitoneum
- Fracture long bones/pelvis
- Rupture of aortic aneurysm
- Ectopic pregnancy rupture

Loss of Volume (Non-hemorrhagic)
- Diarrhea
- Vomiting
- Burns
- Pancreatitis
- Hyperosmolar states

Severe hypovolemia is defined as loss of >40% blood volume. Clinical features of severe hypovolemia are:
- Hypotension: Systolic blood pressure <90 mm Hg or mean arterial pressure of <60 mm Hg
- Tachycardia: Heart rate >100/min
- Tachypnea: Increased respiratory rate
- Oliguria: Decreased urinary output of <30 mL/hr
- Signs of reduced cerebral perfusion: Agitation, confusion, drowsiness and coma
- Cold and clammy extremities
- Reduced central venous pressure
- Multiple organ failure: Acute lung injury and adult respiratory distress syndrome (ARDS), acute renal failure, liver dysfunction, reduced cerebral perfusion (coma), disseminated intravascular coagulation (DIC).

Diagnosis

Diagnosis is made by history of blood loss or fluid loss and signs of hypovolemic shock mentioned above. Occult blood loss, mainly in gastrointestinal tract and internal hemorrhage, should be ruled out when patient is having postural hypotension and other features of hypovolemic shock but there is no history of blood or volume loss.

Measurement of hemoglobin and hematocrit is misleading, as these values may be normal in acute blood loss despite significant blood loss.

Management

- Patient with shock should be admitted in intensive care unit (ICU).
- Assessment of airway, breathing and circulation is done.
- Blood pressure, pulse rate, respiratory rate, urinary output, arterial oxygen saturation and mental status are continuously monitored.
- Aim is to restore tissue perfusion, maintain cardiac output and oxygen saturation so that there is adequate delivery of oxygen and substrates to the tissues.
- Volume resuscitation to maintain intravascular blood volume and measures to control ongoing losses.
  - Isotonic saline or Ringer's lactate are given through rapid intravenous infusion.
  - Blood transfusion or packed cell transfusion may be required when there is continuing blood loss and hemoglobin is lower than 10 g/dL.
  - Infusion of inotropic agents such as dopamine, dobutamine or vasopressin may be required to maintain adequate cardiac output.
  - Goal is to maintain mean arterial pressure of 60–65 mm Hg.
- Supplemental oxygen is also required to maintain respiratory function. If arterial oxygen saturation is not improving, endotracheal intubation may be required.

Obstructive Shock

This is characterized by acute reduction in cardiac output and development of shock. Important causes of obstructive shock are given in **Table 12.3**.

In cardiac tamponade there is inadequate diastolic filling because of compression of heart which becomes less compliant. Tension pneumothorax, diaphragmatic hernia and positive pressure ventilation causes increase in intrathoracic pressure which causes compression and decreased venous return.

Diagnosis depends on clinical features, X-ray chest and echocardiography.

Management depends on prompt recognition of cause and its treatment (**Table 12.4**).

Septic Shock

Septic shock and anaphylactic shock are classified under distributive shock. Sepsis is the most common cause of distributive shock and carries high mortality.

Sepsis is defined as life threatening organ dysfunction caused by dysregulation of host response to an infection (**Table 12.5**). Sequential organ failure assessment (SOFA) score is used to identify organ dysfunction in sepsis. A score

Table 12.3: Causes of obstructive shock.
- Cardiac tamponade (Pericardial effusion, constrictive pericarditis)
- Tension pneumothorax (Air in pleural space)
- Massive pulmonary embolism
- Diaphragmatic hernia (Herniation of abdominal viscera in thoracic cavity)
- Mechanical ventilation (Excessive positive pressure ventilation)

Table 12.4: Treatment of obstructive shock.

Cardiac tamponade	Pericardiocentesis
Tension pneumothorax	Chest tube placement
Massive pulmonary embolism	Thrombolytic therapy, surgical embolectomy.

Table 12.5: Causes of septic shock/SIRS.

Septic Shock
Infections
- Gram-negative bacteria
  - *E. coli*
  - *Klebsiella*
  - *Proteus*
  - *Pseudomonas*
- Gram-positive cocci
- Gram-negative anerobes
  - *Bacteroides*

SIRS (Systemic Inflammatory Response Syndrome)
- Pancreatitis
- Crush injuries
- Air embolism
- Burns
- Amniotic fluid embolism
- Drugs (Salicylates)

Table 12.6: Quick SOFA (qSOFA) scoring system.

Parameter	Point
Systolic blood pressure <100 mm Hg	1
Altered mental status	1
Respiratory rate >22/minute	1

Score of 2 or more identifies serious patients.

of 2 or more along with the infection is diagnostic of sepsis. SOFA scoring measures dysfunction of 6 organ systems: renal, cardiac, pulmonary, neurological, hepatic and hematological. Quick SOFA (qSOFA) scoring system **(Table 12. 6)** is another way to identify serious patients with suspected infection who need intensive care.

Septic shock is characterized by:
- Presence of sepsis
- Persistent hypotension after adequate volume replacement
- Need for vasopressor to maintain mean arterial pressure > 65 mm Hg.
- Serum lactate level > 2 mmol/L.

Clinical Presentation

Patients present with fever, chills, hypotension, altered mental status and features of end organ failure due to hypoperfusion. In some patients clinical features may point toward specific etiology. Generalized erythroderma may be present in toxic shock syndrome, *Staph. aureus* or *Strep. pyogenes* infection. *N. meningitidis* infection causes hemorrhagic or petechial rashes over skin.

Septic shock is also characterized by hypoperfusion of organs and may lead to dysfunction or failure of many organs if not treated promptly.
- Restlessness, confusion, delirium and coma may result from encephalopathy as a result of hypoperfusion of the brain.
- ARDS may result from increased permeability of pulmonary capillaries and pulmonary edema.
- Acute renal failure may occur due to renal hypoperfusion. Prolonged hypoperfusion or toxic injury may cause acute tubular necrosis.
- Increased levels of serum bilirubin and hepatic enzymes (AST, ALT) suggest hepatic dysfunction.
- DIC is frequently present in severe septicemia.

Investigations

- Blood culture may reveal causative organism.
- Culture of material from local infected foci should also be performed to know causative organism and antibiotic sensitivity.
- TLC reveals increased WBC count and DLC reveals polymorphonuclear leukocytosis.
  Procalcitonin (PCT) is a biomarker that helps in diagnosing sepsis, assessing the response and determining the duration of antibiotic therapy. A value > 0.5 ng/mL is suggestive of bacterial infection while <0.1 ng/mL makes bacterial infection less likely.
- Increased levels of serum urea and creatinine suggest renal dysfunction.
- Increased bilirubin levels and hepatic enzymes (AST, ALT) are usually found.
- Low platelet count, increased prothrombin time (PT) and partial thromboplastin time (aPTT) suggest DIC.
- Arterial blood gas analysis may show hypoxia and metabolic acidosis **(Fig. 12.1)**
- Chest X-ray may show features of ARDS.

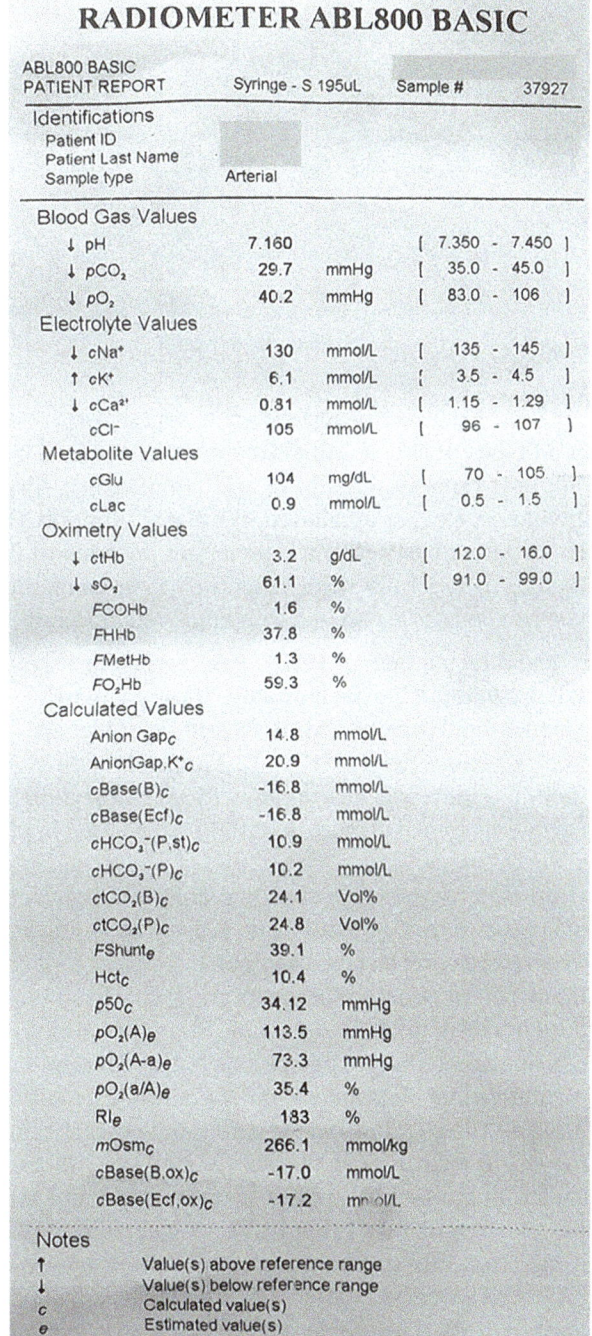

Fig. 12.1: Arterial blood gas (ABG) analysis report showing metabolic acidosis (Low pH, Low HCO_3, Low pCO_2).

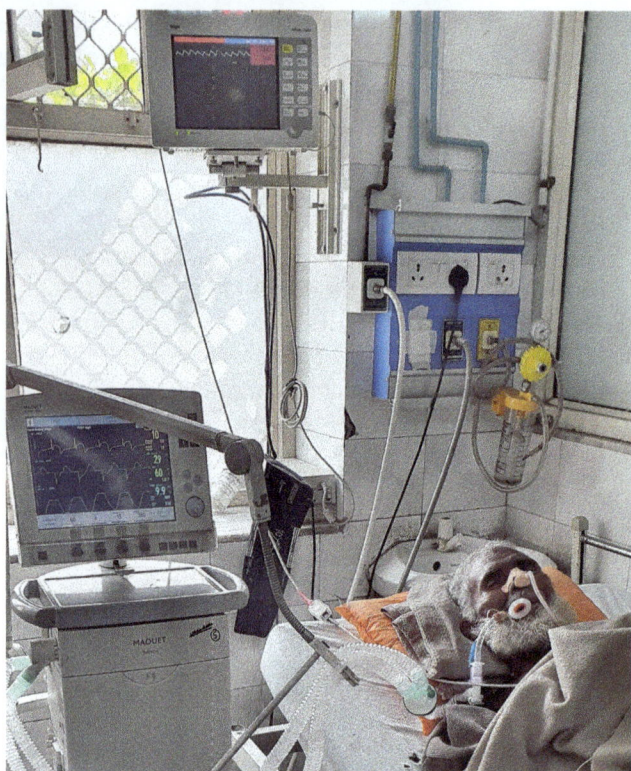

Fig. 12.2: Patient on ventilator.

Management

As in all types of shock, initial treatment consists of basic life support (airway, breathing and circulation): Airway maintenance, oxygen inhalation, ventilatory support **(Fig. 12.2)**. Lactate measurement, intravenous access and fluid resuscitation are important measures in management. Lactate clearance is associated with improved mortality.

Early goal directed therapy (EGDT): Achievement of certain goals helps in reducing the mortality. These goals are:
- Mean arterial pressure (MAP) 65 mm Hg or higher
- Central venous pressure (CVP) 8-12 mm Hg
- Central venous oxygen saturation (ScvO) more than 70%
- Lactate clearance of more than 10% (can be used in place of ScvO.
- Fluid administration is usually required for correction of hypotension. Crystalloid fluid is given at 30 mL/kg for hypotension or if lactate > 4 mmol/L.
- Ionotropic or vasopressor agents are given if hypotension does not respond to fluid therapy. Norepinephrine is the first line agent whereas vasopressin is used as second line.
- Antimicrobial therapy should be started as soon as possible after sending blood sample and other specimen for culture. Empirical therapy is started with broad spectrum antibiotics to cover gram-negative and gram-positive organisms **(Table 12.7)**. Vancomycin is added if infection due to methicillin resistant *Staph. aureus* (MRSA) is suspected. Antibiotics are changed, if required, after culture and sensitivity reports are available. Maximum recommended dose of antimicrobial agents are given intravenously.

Table 12.7: Antibacterial drugs used in septic shock.

Piperacillin-tazobactum	3.375 -4.5 g	q 4-6 h
Imepenem-cilastatin	0.5 g	q 6 h
Meropenem	1 g	q 8 h
Cefipime	2 g	q 12 h
Doripenem	0.5 g	q 8 h
Tobramycin	5-7 mg/kg	q 24 h
Ciprofloxacin	400 mg	q 12h
Levofloxacin	500-750 mg	q 12 h
Aztreonam	2 g	q 8h
Vancomycin	15 mg/kg	q 12 h

- In immunocompetent adult the acceptable regimen include piperacillin-tazobactam or imipenem-cilastatin or meropenem or cefepime. If the patient is allergic to β-lactam agents, ciprofloxacin or levofloxacin or aztreonam is used. Vancomycin should be added to each of the above regimens. In neutropenic patient (< 500 neutrophils/μL) regimens include: (1) imipenem-cilastatin or meropenem or doripenem or cefepime or piperacillin-tazobactam. Vancomycin should be added if staphylococci suspected. In addition, in severe sepsis tobramycin and empirical antifungal therapy with an echinocandin (caspofungin), voriconazole or a lipid formulation of amphotericin B should be added.

Septic shock may be associated with relative adrenal insufficiency. Use of corticosteroids like (hydrocortisone 50 mg 6 h for 5–7 days) is associated with improved survival.

Systemic Inflammatory Response Syndrome

It is characterized by hypotension due to decreased vascular tone (reduced systemic vascular resistance), inadequate cardiac output and normal circulatory volume.

SIRS (systemic inflammatory response syndrome) may be due to infectious or noninfectious etiology and is characterized by fever or hypothermia, leukocytosis or leucopenia, tachypnea and tachycardia.

SIRS is caused by inflammation due to non-infectious causes like pancreatitis, autoimmune disorders, burns, air or amniotic fluid embolism, crush injuries and drugs (salicylates) may also lead to shock.

Cardiogenic Shock

Shock as a result of impaired cardiac function leading to tissue hypoxia in presence of adequate intravascular volume is known as cardiogenic shock (CS). It is most commonly seen after acute myocardial infarction causing pump failure. Other causes of cardiogenic shock are given in **Table 12.8**.

CS secondary to acute myocardial infarction is characterized by:
- Hypotension (Systolic blood pressure < 90 mm Hg, mean arterial pressure <60 mm Hg)
- Decreased cardiac index

Table 12.8: Causes of cardiogenic shock.

- Pump failure
  - Acute myocardial infarction
  - Cardiomyopathy
- Acute myocarditis
- Arrhythmias
- Valvular lesions
  - Acute severe aortic or mitral regurgitation
  - Critical mitral or aortic stenosis
- Rupture of ventricular septum or free ventricular wall
- Pericardial tamponade
- Right ventricular failure due to pulmonary embolism

- Elevated intracardiac pressure (Pulmonary capillary wedge pressure >18 mm Hg), and
- Increased peripheral vascular resistance.

In cardiogenic shock, CVP is usually raised (it is low in hypovolemic shock). Depressed myocardial contractility, usually due to ischemia, results in low cardiac output and hypotension. A vicious cycle is formed as hypotension results in hypoperfusion and ischemia of myocardium and further depression of myocardial contractility. Compensatory reflux arteriolar vasoconstriction leads to reduced blood flow to kidneys, muscle, abdominal viscera and skin while vasodilatation of cerebral and coronary arteries occurs in order to maintain circulation in these territories. Vasoconstriction not only helps in elevating blood pressure but also causes tissue hypoxia and acidosis.

Clinical Features

Shock (Acute circulatory failure, low output state) is a clinical syndrome characterized by:
- Arterial hypotension (Systolic blood pressure <90 mm Hg, mean arterial pressure <60 mm Hg)
- Weak and rapid pulse
- Cold extremities and cyanosis
- Oliguria (low urine output <30 mL/h) and
- Features of altered mentation (agitation, confusion, drowsiness and coma).

In addition, features of underlying cardiac disease are present.

Most patients with acute myocardial infarction present with severe chest pain, dyspnea, anxiety and sweating. Cardiac findings include S3 gallop (third heart sound) and systolic murmurs. Raised jugular venous pressure (JVP) and pulmonary rales are audible in patients with left ventricular failure and cardiogenic shock.

Investigations

Chest X-ray, electrocardiogram and echocardiography are investigations which help in diagnosis. Echocardiogram should be done to find etiology of CS. Pulmonary artery catheterization helps in measurement of filling pressures and cardiac output and helps in diagnosis and proper management (volume replacement and use of pressor agents).

Management

- The aim of therapy is to increase blood pressure sufficient to maintain systemic and coronary perfusion and maintain volume status to ensure proper ventricular function and preventing volume overload.
- Oxygen inhalation is given to maintain PaO_2 of >60 mm Hg. Endotracheal intubation and mechanical ventilation may be required. It reduces work of breathing and increases cardiac pressure which may improve cardiac output.
- Hematocrit is maintained >30%, fluid replacement is done to maintain adequate preload and ventricular function. Excessive fluids may cause pulmonary edema.
- Pressors are administered only after adequate fluid resuscitation.
- Drugs are used to increase blood pressure and cardiac output in patients of CS. The dose is titrated to maintain blood pressure of >90 mm Hg or mean arterial pressure of >60 mm Hg.
  - Dopamine is usually used in CS. It has variable effects according to dosage. At low dose (2 mcg/kg/min) it dilates renal vascular bed and increases glomerular filtration rate because of dopaminergic effects. At moderate dosage (2–10 mcg/kg/min) it stimulates beta adrenergic receptors and increases myocardial contractility (positive ionotropic effect) and heart rate (positive chronotropic effect). At higher dosage (10 mcg/kg/min) it produces vasoconstriction because of alpha adrenergic stimulation.
  - Dobutamine produces greater ionotropic effects as compared to dopamine. It is a synthetic sympathomimetic amine and is given in dosage of 2–20 mcg/kg/min. It also reduces afterload because of its vasodilating effects. Amrinone or milrinone is given with dobutamine.
  - Norepinephrine is a potent vasoconstrictor and ionotropic agent and is given in dosage of 2–10 mcg/min. It is reserved for patients with CS and refractory hypotension. It is also useful in distributive or neurogenic shock.
- Aortic counterpulsation: Intraaortic balloon pumping, a mechanical circulatory assist device, augments arterial diastolic pressure and cardiac output. It is used in patients not responding to medical treatment or in acute valvular insufficiency/VSD. It is inserted percutaneously and the balloon inflates during diastole and deflates during systole, reducing afterload and improving cardiac output. It also increases coronary blood flow during diastole.
- Definitive treatment is directed toward underlying cause. This can be in form of angioplasty, coronary artery bypass grafting, valvular replacement or cardiac transplantation. The rapid establishment of blood flow in infarct-related artery is essential in acute myocardial infarction.

Neurogenic Shock

Neurogenic shock is caused by traumatic high spinal cord injury, effects of spinal anesthesia or head injury.
- It is due to loss of sympathetic tone which results in impaired vasomotor tone causing dilatation of arterioles and veins. Dilatation of vessels leads to venous pooling causing decreased venous return and cardiac output.
- Peripheral examination reveals warm extremities because of venodilation (extremities are cold in hypovolemic and cardiogenic shock due to vasoconstriction) and other features of shock.
- Vagal stimulation which causes increase in parasympathetic tone may result in hypotension, bradycardia and syncope (shock like features). It may mimic neurogenic shock. Pain due to any cause, fright or gastric dilatation may cause reflux vagal stimulation.

Management

Treatment of neurogenic shock includes correction of hypovolemia and drugs such as norepinephrine, phenylephrine which increase sympathetic tone and cause increase in blood pressure.

Hypoadrenal Shock (See also Chapter 9)

There is increased secretion of cortisol from adrenal glands in stress due to any cause like illness, trauma and major surgery. This response is impaired in certain clinical settings leading to decreased secretion of cortisol from adrenal gland and impaired host response to stress. Causes of adrenal insufficiency are given in **Table 12.9**.

Shock due to hypoadrenal state is characterized by hypovolemia, decreased systemic vascular resistance and reduced cardiac output.

Diagnosis

Adrenal insufficiency can be diagnosed by ACTH stimulation test.

Treatment

Hydrocortisone (100 mg every 4-6 h) or dexamethasone (4 mg) is given intravenously, along with volume replacement and intravenous vasopressors.

ACUTE RESPIRATORY DISTRESS SYNDROME

Acute respiratory distress syndrome (ARDS) is most severe form of acute lung injury (ALI) characterized by acute hypoxemic respiratory failure following systemic or pulmonary insult without heart failure. ARDS is a physiological and radiographic syndrome rather than a specific disease.

Table 12.9: Causes of adrenocortical insufficiency.
- Steroid therapy (chronic administration of high dose steroids)
- Atrophy of adrenal glands
- Pituitary injury
- Tuberculosis, amyloidosis, metastatic disease of adrenal glands
- Bilateral hemorrhage in adrenal glands

Table 12.10: Causes of ARDS.

Systemic insult (Indirect lung injury)
- Sepsis
- Multiple blood transfusions
- Severe trauma
- Burns
- Pancreatitis

Pulmonary insult (Direct lung injury)
- Pneumonia
- Aspiration of gastric contents
- Miliary tuberculosis
- Oxygen toxicity
- Pulmonary contusion
- Near drowning
- Toxic inhalation
- High altitude

Causes

Various causes which lead to direct or indirect lung injury cause ARDS. The causes are given in **Table 12.10**.

Pathophysiology

The mechanism of lung injury varies with the etiology, however, the proinflammatory cytokines play a central role in the pathogenesis of lung injury. Damage occurs in the alveolar epithelial cells as well as capillary endothelial cells. This causes increased vascular permeability and decreased production of surfactant. There is accumulation of protein rich fluid and inflammatory cells in the alveoli and interstitium leading to pulmonary edema, alveolar collapse and hypoxemia.

Clinical Features

The usual symptom is rapid onset dyspnea which follows the underlying causative event within 12-48 hours. Examination reveals tachypnea, labored breathing and intercostal retraction. Auscultation of lungs shows bilateral crackles (crepts). Most patients with ARDS have multiorgan failure involving kidneys, liver, gut, CNS and cardiovascular system.

Diagnosis

Diagnosis of ARDS is based on the following criteria:
The Berlin (2012) definition of acute respiratory distress syndrome
- **Timing:** Within 1 week of a known clinical insult or new or worsening respiratory symptoms.
- **Chest imaging:** Bilateral opacities—not fully explained by effusions, lobar/lung collapse, or nodules **(Figs. 12.3A and B)**.

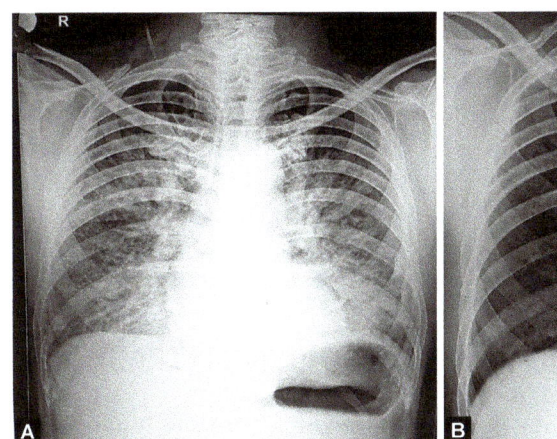
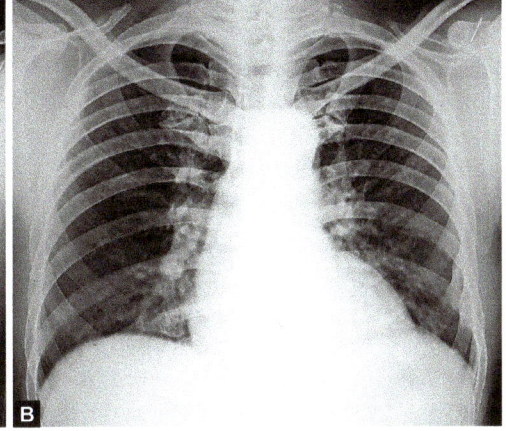

Figs. 12.3A and B: (A) Chest X-ray showing bilateral opacities; (B) Chest X-ray after treatment.

- **Origin of edema:** Respiratory failure not fully explained by cardiac failure or fluid overload. Need objective assessment (e.g., echocardiography) to exclude hydrostatic edema if no risk factor present.
- **Impaired oxygenation:**
  - **Mild:** Partial pressure of arterial oxygen (PaO_2)/Fraction of inspired oxygen (FIO_2) 200–300 mm Hg with positive end-expiratory pressure (PEEP) or continuous positive airway pressure (CPAP) ≥5 cm H_2O
  - **Moderate:** PaO_2/FIO_2 100–200 mm Hg with PEEP ≥5 cm H_2O
  - **Severe:** PaO_2/FIO_2 ≤100 mm Hg with PEEP ≥5 cm.

Differential Diagnosis

Cardiogenic pulmonary edema must be excluded (See Chapter 5).

Investigations

Important investigations include:
- X-ray chest PA view
- Arterial blood gases
- Hemogram
- Blood sugar
- Blood urea/Serum creatinine
- Liver function tests, serum amylase/lipase.

Treatment

General measures include:
- Recognition and treatment of underlying cause
- Minimizing invasive procedures
- Prophylaxis for venous thromboembolism
- Management of nosocomial infection.

Mechanical Ventilation

Goal of protective lung ventilation is that patients should receive a lower tidal volume (Vt) [4-6 mL/ kg predicted body weight (PBW)] to maintenance of plateau pressure (pressure in alveoli) between 25 and 30 cm H_2O. PEEP is adjusted to minimize FiO_2 and provide adequate PaO_2 while avoiding alveolar over distension.

Non-conventional Therapies in Severe ARDS

Prone positioning and extracorporeal membrane oxygenation (ECMO) are non-conventional therapies for life-threatening refractory hypoxemia in severe ARDS patients. In case of ARDS, there is ventilation–perfusion mismatch due to more involvement of dorsal lung alveoli in comparison to ventral. The prone positioning improves ventilation perfusion mismatching due to effect of gravity and heart repositioning. In patients with severe hypoxemic and/or hypercapnic respiratory failure, extracorporeal lung support (ECLS) techniques, including extracorporeal membrane oxygenation (ECMO), is a salvage option. The aim of this strategy is to overcome severe hypoxemia and respiratory acidosis while keeping the lung completely at rest.

In patients with moderate to severe ARDS, use of non-depolarizing neuromuscular blocking agent (NMBA, e.g., cisatracurium) for 48 hours has been shown to improve oxygenation and survival.

Fluid restriction and use of diuretics can reduce left atrial filling pressure leading to reduction in pulmonary edema and improved lung compliance. However hypotension should be avoided.

Currently, use of corticosteroids is not recommended as no mortality benefit has been demonstrated with steroids. Surfactants and inhaled nitric oxide have also been tried.

Prognosis

Mortality is 40–60% on treatment. It is around 90% if ARDS is accompanied by sepsis.

CARDIOVASCULAR COLLAPSE

Cardiovascular collapse is defined as a loss of effective blood flow due to acute dysfunction of heart or peripheral vasculature. Cardiovascular collapse may be caused by:

- Cardiac arrest: Which requires intervention to prevent death.
- Other causes which are transient and non-life-threatening with spontaneous return of consciousness. These include vasovagal syncope postural hypotension, neurocardiogenic syncope or a transient severe bradycardia.

CARDIAC ARREST

Cardiac arrest is defined as abrupt cessation of cardiac pump function. This may be reversible by prompt intervention or can lead to death if no intervention is done. There is aberration in the underlying electrical activity leading to following conditions. Any of these conditions may be responsible for cardiac arrest.
- Ventricular fibrillation (VF)—responsible for 50–80% of arrests
- Asystole
- Persistent bradyarrhythmias
- Pulseless electrical activity (PEA)
- Pulseless sustained ventricular tachycardia (VT).

Sudden Cardiac Death

Sudden cardiac death (SCD) is defined as unexpected nontraumatic death in clinically well or stable patient who dies within 1 hour of onset of symptoms. The causative rhythm in most cases is VF.

Causes of cardiac arrest are given in **Table 12.11**.

Table 12.11: Causes of sudden cardiac death/cardiac arrest.
• Coronary artery disease • Hypertrophic cardiomyopathy • Aortic stenosis and pulmonary stenosis • Cyanotic congenital heart disease • Atrial myxoma • WPW syndrome • Electrolyte abnormalities • Hypoxia • Acidosis • Prolonged QT interval • Brugada syndrome

Management of Cardiac Arrest

Following are important steps in the management of cardiac arrest (see cardiopulmonary resuscitation below).
a. The initial response and basic life support
b. Defibrillation
c. Advanced life support
d. Postresuscitation care
e. Long-term management.

CARDIOPULMONARY RESUSCITATION

All health care providers must know the procedures of basic life support (BLS) and advanced cardiac life support (ACLS). When cardiac arrest occurs, BLS must be started immediately. The goal of resuscitation is to maintain cerebral perfusion until cardiopulmonary function is restored. The longer the period of cardiopulmonary arrest, the lower is the chance of restoring healthy life. Irreversible cerebral damage may occur after 3 minutes of anoxia. Ventricular arrhythmias are responsible for majority of cardiac arrests; hence defibrillation facilities should be available (**Figs. 12.4A and B**).

Following sequence should be followed during adult resuscitation:
1. Assessment of unresponsiveness
2. Activation of emergency medical services
3. BLS until defibrillation is available
4. Defibrillation if indicated
5. Intubation
6. Administration of appropriate medications.

Basic Life Support (BLS)

Airway, breathing and circulation (ABC) are the essentials of BLS. In an unconscious patient, the following is recommended:
- Determine the responsiveness by gently shaking the patient and shouting into ear. Shaking of patient's head and neck should be avoided if trauma to these areas is suspected.

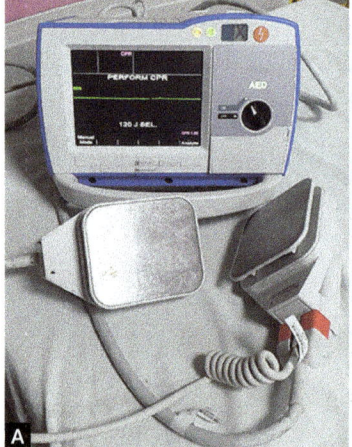
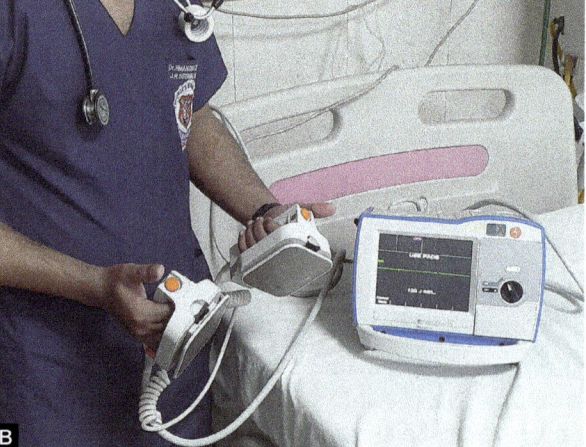

Figs. 12.4A and B: (A) Automatic external defibrillator (AED); (B) Paddles to be applied to chest for DC shock.

- If no response is obtained, activate the emergency medical services system. If breathing problem is the likely cause of unconsciousness (drowning, choking, alcohol intoxication, trauma), resuscitation should be performed before going for help.
- Patient should be laid on firm, flat surface. If the patient is moved, he should be moved as a single unit so that head, neck and body moves simultaneously.
- *Airway:* The patient's mouth should be opened, debris (e.g. mucus and blood) should be removed and dentures should be left in place. Loose or ill-fitting dentures should be removed. Open the patient's airway by flexing the neck and extending the head. The head tilt-chin lift should be performed if neck injury is not suspected. If a cervical injury is suspected, use the jaw thrust manoeuvre to limit the potential for spinal cord injury.
- *Breathing:* Assess for the presence of respiration once the airway is open by the look, listen and feel method. An open airway may be all that is necessary for spontaneous respiration to resume and continue. One should try to feel and hear breath sounds by placing an ear or cheek near to the victim's mouth. Breathing can also be assessed by observing chest and abdominal movements (rise and fall). If the spontaneous breathing is not present, give two slow breaths (1.5 to 2 seconds per breath), taking a breath after each ventilation. Each ventilation should be performed with sufficient volume to make the patient's chest rise. Rapid or high pressure breath may result in gastric distention. If the chest does not rise, the patients head should be repositioned and ventilation attempted again.
- *Circulation:* Cardiac arrest is accompanied by circulatory collapse. Assess circulation by palpating for pulses and checking for signs of perfusion including swallowing or breathing for more than occasional gasps. Absence of carotid pulse for 10 seconds confirms circulatory collapse.
    - External chest compressions should be initiated at a rate of 100-120 per minute in the absence of carotid pulse.
    - The patients should be lying on firm surface.
    - The heel of one hand is placed over the lower half of the victim's sternum and the heel of the second hand is placed over the first with fingers interlocked. Chest compressions are performed with the heel of one hand on the back of the other hand. Hand position should be one inch cephalad to the patient's xiphoid process. With shoulder directly above the hands and elbows in locked position, the patient's sternum should be compressed below to 2.0 to 2.4 inches (5-6 cm).
    - The adequacy of compressions should be assessed periodically by having another rescuer palpate the carotid pulse.
    - Respiratory and circulatory support is continued by providing two effective breaths for every 30 cardiac compressions. Thirty chest compressions should be performed followed by two ventilations. Once the patient is intubated, ventilation can be performed at a rate of 12 per minute without pausing for compressions.
    - Monitor quality of CPR **(Table 12.12)**.

Table 12.12: High quality Cardio-pulmonary resuscitation (CPR).

- Push hard (2 to 2.4 inches or 5-6 cm) and fast (100-120/minute)
- Allow complete chest recoil
- Minimise interruptions in compressions
- Avoid excessive ventilation
- Rotate compressor every 2 minutes
- If no advanced airway, maintain 30:2 compression/ventilation ratio

- Stop BLS for five seconds at the end of first minute and every 1-2 minutes thereafter to determine whether patient has resumed spontaneous breathing or circulation. If spontaneous pulse has returned check the BP and continue ventilation as needed. BLS should not be withheld for more than five seconds except to intubate or defibrillate the patient. Attempts at intubation should not exceed 30 seconds before CPR is resumed.
- If a patient is unconscious and two attempts to ventilate the patient have failed after positioning the head and chin properly, patient should be intubated. if laryngoscope is unavailable, 6 to 10 abdominal thrusts should be performed to remove the airway obstruction. Hands should be positioned properly to avoid damage to the internal organs. After abdominal thrusts, debris should be cleaned from the patient's mouth with a finger and then one should attempt to ventilate the patient. Cricothyrotomy and transtracheal ventilation are rarely necessary for ventilating the patient.

Advanced Cardiac Life Support (ACLS)

ACLS is an extension of BLS and is implemented by a team. Early designation of a team leader facilitates coordination of the efforts. The team leader is responsible for ensuring proper implementation of ACLS. The leader should ascertain that BLS is being properly performed and that defibrillation occurs early when indicated. After this, the leader should ensure the following:

- Proper endotracheal intubation and ventilation
- Placement of functioning IV catheter
- Administration of appropriate cardiovascular medicines
- Diagnosis and treatment of the cause of the arrest

The team leader should examine the patient and determine the events preceding the arrest, obtain a relevant history including current medications and treatments, and obtain appropriate tests (electrolytes, hematocrit, arterial blood gas analysis, ECG, radiographs, etc.) to determine and treat the cause of the arrest. The patient's rhythm and pulse should be assessed after every intervention. The team leader also should determine when termination of resuscitative efforts is warranted.

- ACLS consists of ECG monitoring, endotracheal intubation and setting up an intravenous line in a large peripheral vein or central vein.

- Immediate therapy includes defibrillation, oxygen and administration of cardioactive drugs.
- As soon as possible the cardiac rhythm should be established. If the ECG reveals ventricular arrhythmia or there is doubt to the nature of the rhythm (e.g. Fine VF may be confused with asystole) immediate defibrillation is performed.
- If initial defibrillation attempts are unsuccessful, victim is intubated and setting of intravenous line is performed while the circulation is supported by external chest compressions. If there is any difficulty in intubating the patient, ventilation should be continued by means of an airway, a ventilating bag and oxygen.
- Intravenous epinephrine results in vasoconstriction and increases the proportion of cardiac output delivered to brain.

Sudden unexpected cardiac arrest **(Table 12.13)** occurs due to:
- Ventricular fibrillation (VF)/ventricular tachycardia (VT).
- Asystole and pulseless electrical activity also known as electromechanical dissociation (non-VF/VT).

Majority of deaths are due to VF and rapid VT. Small proportion of deaths occurs due to pulseless electrical activity and remainders are due to asystole.

- VF and pulseless VT is treated with immediate defibrillation, CPR and drugs. Intravenous amiodarone is the first line drug in the refractory VF/pulseless VT.
- Asystole is more difficult to treat but the heart may respond to atropine or epinephrine (adrenaline). Recently vasopressin has been shown to be successful. If there is any sign of slow electromechanical activity (e.g. bradycardia with a weak pulse), emergency pacing should be done.
- Pulseless electrical activity may be due to several potential reversible causes **(Table 12.14)**. It carries a very poor prognosis. Effective treatment involves addressing the underlying cause.

Table 12.13: Causes of unexpected cardiac arrest.
- Cardiac arrhythmias (e.g. ventricular fibrillation)
- Sudden pump failure (e.g. acute myocardial infarction)
- Acute circulatory obstruction (e.g. acute pulmonary embolism)
- Cardiovascular rupture (e.g. myocardial rupture, aortic dissection)
- Vasomotor collapse (e.g. pulmonary hypertension)

Table 12.14: Most frequent causes of pulseless electrical activity.
- Hypovolemia
- Hypoxemia
- Hypokalemia/hyperkalemia
- Hypothermia
- Metabolic acidosis
- Cardiac tamponade
- Tension pneumothorax
- Pulmonary thromboembolism
- Acute coronary syndrome (coronary thrombosis)
- Toxins

SELF ASSESSMENT

Multiple Choice Questions

1. Severe hypovolemia is defined as loss of _____ % of blood volume:
   A. 10 B. 20
   C. 30 D. 40
2. Which of the following is not a characteristic feature of systemic inflammatory response syndrome (SIRS):
   A. Hypothermia B. Leukopenia
   C. Oliguria D. Tachycardia
3. Warm extremities is a feature of:
   A. Hypovolemic shock B. Obstructive shock
   C. Neurogenic shock D. Cardiogenic shock
4. Hypoadrenal shock is characterized by all of the following, *except*:
   A. Decreased secretion of cortisol
   B. Hypovolemia
   C. Increased systemic vascular resistance
   D. Reduced cardiac output
5. All of the following are causes of obstructive shock, *except*:
   A. Massive pulmonary embolism
   B. Tension pneumothorax
   C. Intestinal obstruction
   D. Diaphragmatic hernia
6. All are true about dopamine infusion:
   A. Dilates renal vascular bed
   B. Positive ionotropic effect
   C. Negative chronotropic effect
   D. Causes vasoconstriction
7. During cardiopulmonary resuscitation the chest compression rate should be at least:
   A. 60–70/min B. 80–90/min
   C. 90–100/min D. 100–120/min
8. During cardiopulmonary resuscitation the patients sternum should be compressed to at least:
   A. 1–2 cm B. 2–2.5 cm
   C. 3–4 cm D. 5–6 cm
9. In BLS with no advance airway, compression ventilation ratio should be:
   A. 15:1 B. 20:2
   C. 30:2 D. 25:3
10. Most frequent causes of pulseless electrical activity are all, *except*:
    A. Hypovolemia B. Hypothermia
    C. Hyponatremia D. Hpokalemia

Fill in the Blanks

1. Mild hypovolemia is characterized by loss of _____ blood volume.
2. SIRS (systemic inflammatory response syndrome) is characterized by fever or hypothermia, _____ or _____, tachypnea and tachycardia.
3. Cardiogenic shock (CS) is most commonly seen after____.
4. Cardiogenic shock (CS) is charaterized by mean arterial pressure of _____ mm Hg.
5. In cardiopulmonary resuscitation (CPR) compressor should be rotated every_____.

CHAPTER 13

Anaphylaxis and Drug Allergy

ANAPHYLAXIS

Anaphylaxis is a type I IgE mediated rapidly developing systemic allergic reaction. Exposure to an antigen results in the formation of specific IgE which binds with the mast cells. Once IgE is bound to the surface of mast cells, the individual is primed to develop type I hypersensitivity reaction. Repeat exposure to same antigen in the sensitized individual can lead to the activation of IgE bound mast cells and release of a number of mediators such as histamine, serotonin, leukotrienes and prostaglandins **(Fig. 13.1)**. These mediators cause bronchoconstriction, vasodilatation, fluid exudation and smooth muscle contraction which are responsible for clinical features of the anaphylactic reaction **(Table 13.1)**.

Anaphylactoid reaction: Certain substances can cause activation of mast cells directly (non-IgE mediated) and lead to similar clinical picture. This is known as *anaphylactoid reaction*. Radiocontrast media are the most common cause of anaphylactoid reaction.

Causes

Important causes of anaphylactic reaction are drugs, foodstuffs and insect venoms. These are listed in **Table 13.2**.

Clinical Manifestations

The manifestation may be mild, very severe or life threatening. Type I reaction can occur as systemic disorder (anaphylaxis) or local reaction (urticaria and/or angioedema). Serious

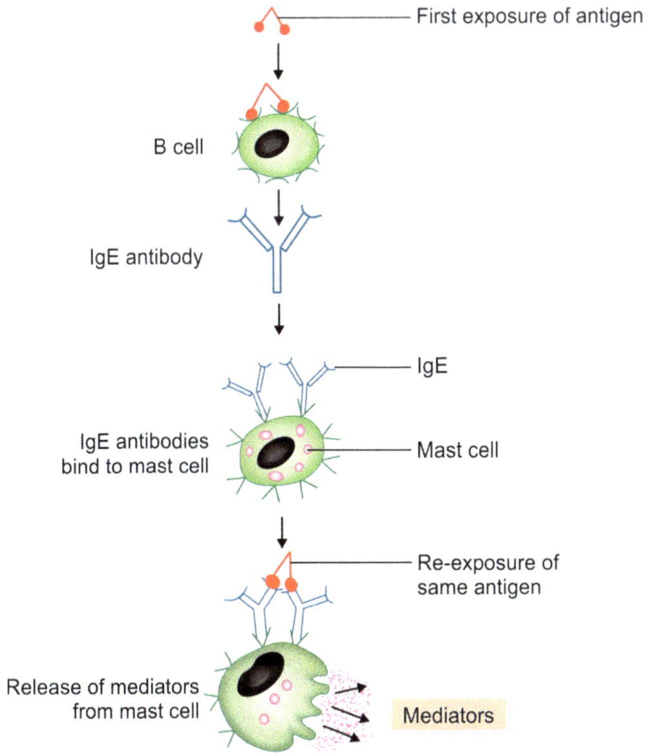

Fig. 13.1: Mechanism of anaphylaxis.

Table 13.1: Mediators and their actions in anaphylaxis.	
Primary mediators	
Histamine	Vasodilatation, increased vascular permeability, bronchospasm, increased mucus secretions
Chemotactic factors (ECF-A, NCF-A)	Chemotaxis of eosinophils and neutrophils
Proteases	Generate other inflammatory mediators
Secondary mediators	
Leukotrienes (LT)	
LTC_4 and LTD_4	Vasoactive and spasmogenic
LTB_4	Chemotaxis of neutrophils, eosinophils and monocytes
Prostaglandins (PGD_2)	Bronchospasm and increased mucus productions
Platelet activating factor (PAF)	Platelet aggregation, histamine release

Table 13.2: Causes of anaphylactic reaction.

Drugs
- Antibiotics: Penicillins, cephalosporins, nitrofurantoin, quinolones
- Amphotericin B
- Local anesthetics: Procaine, lidocaine
- Muscle relaxants: Gallamine, suxamethonium, pancuronium
- Vitamins: Thiamine, folic acid
- Diagnostic agents: Contrast media
- Horse serum: Antithymocyte globulin, antidiphtheric serum
- Enzymes: Streptokinase, chymotrypsin, L-asparaginase

Foods
Milk, eggs, sea food, nuts, grains, beans, gelatin in capsules

Pollen extracts

Non-pollen extracts: Dust mites, animal danders

Insect bites: Honeybee, wasps, Hymenoptera

Latex rubber products

Vaccine preservative: Thimerosal

Table 13.3: Clinical features of anaphylaxis.

Skin	Pruritus, urticaria, angioedema, flushing
Respiratory	Nasal blockade, rhinorrhea, cough, laryngeal edema, breathlessness, hoarseness, stridor, wheezing, cyanosis
Cardiovascular	Tachycardia, palpitation, hypotension, shock, arrhythmia, cardiac arrest
Gastrointestinal	Abdominal pain, nausea, vomiting, diarrhea

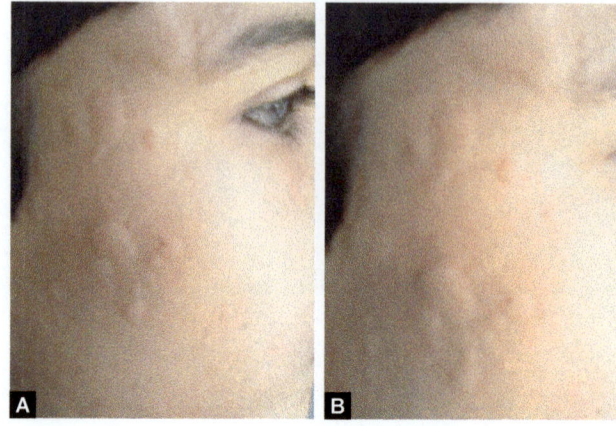

Figs. 13.2A and B: Urticaria.

manifestations occur within seconds to minutes after exposure to antigen. Sometimes, the reaction is delayed by few hours. Important clinical features are given in **Table 13.3**. Respiratory involvement is the most common cause of death.
- Skin lesions in the form of urticaria or angioedema may occur. In mild cases, this could be the only manifestation.
  - Urticaria is a raised flat-topped well-demarcated skin lesion with surrounding erythema **(Figs. 13.2A and B)**. Individual lesions usually last from minutes to hours. They are localized or disseminated and are pruritic.
  - Angioedema is a deeper cutaneous process causing areas of localized nonpitting swelling. It most often involves lips, tongue and eyelids **(Figs. 13.3A and B)**.
- Respiratory distress may occur due to laryngeal edema, laryngospasm or bronchospasm. Patient may have a feeling of tightness of chest, stridor and wheezing.
- Hypotension and shock can occur. Patients have cold extremities, decreased urinary output, peripheral cyanosis and altered sensorium.
- Gastrointestinal manifestations include abdominal cramps, nausea, vomiting and diarrhea.

Diagnosis

The diagnosis of anaphylactic reaction is clinical, based on the history of exposure to the triggering agent and appearance of symptoms and signs within minutes of exposure. An elevated serum tryptase during an episode confirms the diagnosis of anaphylactic reaction.

Treatment

Prompt recognition and management of anaphylactic reactions is a must as death may occur within minutes. Upon any suspicion of anaphylaxis, airway, breathing and circulation are assessed.

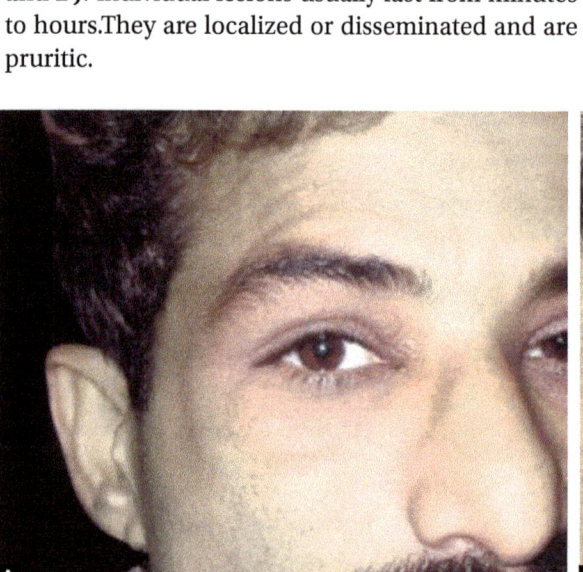
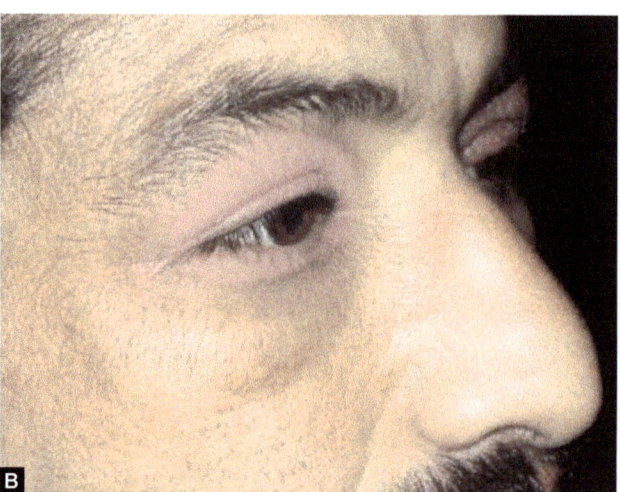

Figs. 13.3A and B: Angioedema.

- *The drug of choice is adrenaline (epinephrine).* This is given in a dose of 0.3-0.5 mg (0.3-0.5 mL of 1:1000 solution) intramuscularly or subcutaneously. Repeated injections can be given at 20 minutes intervals if necessary. Patients who are already being treated with beta adrenergic blocker drugs are refractory to epinephrine. A higher dose of adrenaline is required for the desired effect. Glucagon is also beneficial in such patients. Epinephrine causes bronchodilatation and vasoconstriction and prevents further mast cell degradation. This can also be given sublingually, intravenously or via an endotracheal tube in patients with hypotension and airway compromise.
- Airway management should be a priority. Hundred percent oxygen should be administered. Endotracheal intubation may be necessary. If laryngeal edema does not respond to epinephrine, tracheostomy may be required. Inhalation of β_2 adrenergic agonist (terbutaline, salbutamol) and intravenous aminophylline are helpful in bronchospasm.
- Intravenous fluids are given to maintain intravascular volume. The amount of fluid to be given is adjusted according to the blood pressure and urine output. Vasopressor drugs (dopamine, norepinephrine) are used if the patient remains hypotensive.
- H_2 receptor antagonists (diphenhydramine, promethazine) are useful in relieving skin symptoms (pruritus, urticaria and angioedema) and abdominal cramps. Addition of H_2 receptor antagonists (ranitidine) may provide better effects.
- Glucocorticoids have no immediate significant effect but may reduce prolonged reactions or relapses. Hydrocortisone (200 mg) or methylprednisolone (125 mg) can be given intravenously.

The patient is observed for 24 hours as the late phase reactions can cause reappearance of symptoms.

Prevention of Recurrent Anaphylaxis

- Identification and avoidance of the offending agent is crucial for the prevention of anaphylactic reaction.
- Self-administered epinephrine therapy is advocated for those who develop recurrent anaphylaxis to a food or Hymenoptera sting.
- Venom immunotherapy is tried in patients with anaphylaxis to Hymenoptera sting.

Treatment of Urticaria and Angioedema

These represent mild type I hypersensitivity reactions.
- Ideal treatment is identification and avoidance of specific cause, such as medications, cosmetics, foods.
- Antihistamines (H_1 blocking agents) are given for the control of symptoms. Second generation antihistamines like fexofenadine, cetirizine, levocetirizine, rupatadine, loratidine and desloratidine are used as first line agents. Classic antihistamines such as hydroxyzine is added as an evening dose for better control of the lesions or in refractory cases. H_2 blocking agents (ranitidine) may be added in refractory cases.
- Oral corticosteroids are given to patients with severe symptoms who have not responded to antihistamines.
- Use of ACE inhibitors and ARBs can be associated with the onset of angioedema. They should be discontinued if angioedema develops.

DRUG ALLERGY

Drug reactions are a common medical problem. The basis of drug reaction is idiosyncratic, toxic or immunological.

Immunological reactions can be of various types and occur with relatively low dose. These occur usually after re-exposure to the drug in an individual who has already been sensitized by the previous exposure. Various types of immunological drug reactions are given in **Table 13.4**.

Skin test predicts immediate hypersensitivity reaction. If the test is negative, immediate hypersensitivity reaction will not develop, but delayed non-IgE-mediated reaction may still develop in these cases.

The allergic reactions to drugs can manifest through organ specific syndromes. Important syndromes are as follows:

Cutaneous Reactions

Cutaneous reactions are most common manifestations of drug allergy **(Table 13.5)**.

Table 13.4: Drug reactions (Immune-mediated).

Type of reaction	Mechanism	Features
Anaphylactic	IgE-mediated activation of mast cells and release of mediators	Anaphylaxis, Urticaria, Angioedema
Cytotoxic	IgG and IgM antibodies against cell antigens and complement activation	Autoimmune hemolytic anemia, Drug-induced thrombocytopenia, Interstitial nephritis
Immune complex	Immune complex deposition and complement activation	Serum sickness*, Vasculitis
Cell mediated	T cell activation against cell surface antigen	Photosensitivity, Contact dermatitis

*Rash, fever, arthralgia, lymphadenopathy

Table 13.5: Cutaneous drug reactions.

Common immune-mediated reactions	Severe immune-mediated reactions
- Maculopapular eruptions - Urticaria - Angioedema - Pruritus - Anaphylaxis - Anaphylactoid reaction - Fixed drug eruptions - Allergic contact dermatitis (topical medications)	- Stevens-Johnson syndrome (SJS) - Toxic epidermal necrolysis (TEN) - Drug-induced hypersensitivity syndrome (DIHS)/drug reaction with eosinophilia and systemic symptoms (DRESS) - Serum sickness - Vasculitis - Acute generalized exanthematous pustulosis (AGEP)

- **Urticaria:** It is commonly seen with penicillin, cephalosporin and sulfonamides.
- **Fixed drug eruptions:** These are discrete macular or bullous non-pruritic lesions which occur at the same place each time the drug is administered. Drugs commonly implicated are tetracycline, sulfonamide and penicillin.
- **Photodermatitis:** There are bright erythematous eruption or eczematoid lesions in area exposed to ultraviolet light (sun exposure). Doxycycline, coal tar derivatives and psoralens are important drugs causing photodermatitis.
- **Contact dermatitis:** Local application of neomycin and PABA can lead to dermatitis.
- **Febrile mucocutaneous syndromes:**
  - Common drugs implicated are rifampicin, phenobarbitone, phenytoin, trimethoprim-sulfamethoxazole
  - These are erythema multiforme, Stevens-Johnson syndrome (SJ syndrome), and toxic epidermal necrolysis (TEN or Lyell syndrome)
  - Erythema multiforme is characterized by target lesion on skin
  - SJ syndrome is a severe form of erythema multiforme and presents as popular, urticarial, vesicular or purpuric lesions involving two or more mucosal surfaces **(Fig. 13.4)**. Lyell syndrome (TEN) presents as epithelial bullae and subsequent desquamation **(Fig. 13.5)**.
  - Sloughing of the dermis and mucous membrane occurs in SJS (<10% of total body surface area involved) and TEN (if >30% body surface is involved). Involvement of 10-30% of the body surface area is known as SJS-TEN overlap.
  - The offending drug which has resulted in the above reactions should not be given again.
  - Future skin testing with the offending drug is absolutely contraindicated.

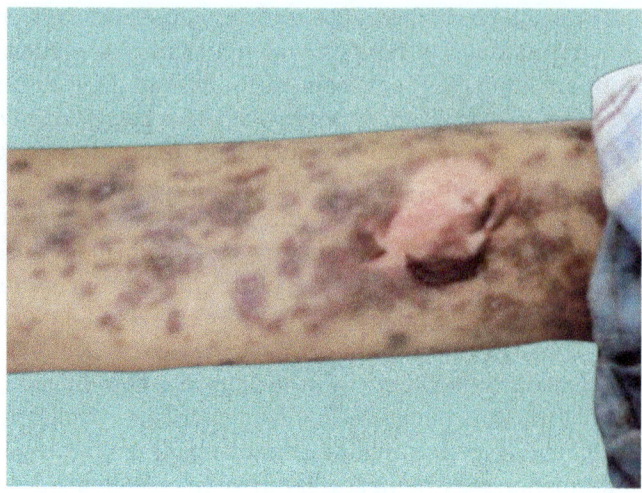

Fig. 13.5: Toxic epidermal necrolysis.

  - Treatment includes:
    » Prompt identification
    » Cessation of culprit drug
    » Supportive care (Fluid management, infection prevention, wound care)
    » Corticosteroid may be useful.
- **Drug-induced hypersensitivity syndrome (DIHS):**
  - It is systemic type of reaction often severe.
  - It occurs 2 to 8 weeks after the drug intake.
  - When associated with eosinophilia, it is known as drug reaction with eosinophilia and systemic symptoms (DRESS)
  - Important complaints are fever, bodyache, morbilliform rash, swelling over face and other body parts.
  - Systemic manifestations are lymphadenopathy, hepatitis, nephritis, pneumonitis, myositis, thyroiditis, myocarditis and gastroenteritis.
  - Blood examination may reveal leukocytosis with or without eosinophilia.
  - It can be accompanied with viral reactivation (EBV, CMV, herpes)
  - Treatment includes:
    » Cessation of offending drug
    » Glucocorticoid
    » Immunosuppressive drugs like mycophenolate mofetil.

Hepatic Syndromes

Hepatic syndromes can present as hepatocellular damage (phenytoin, halothane) and cholestatic jaundice (phenothiazine, erythromycin and azathioprine).

Renal Syndromes

Renal syndromes may present as interstitial nephritis (fever, pyuria, hematuria, proteinuria, rash and eosinophilia). Drugs implicated are methicillin, sulfonamides, and cephalosporins.

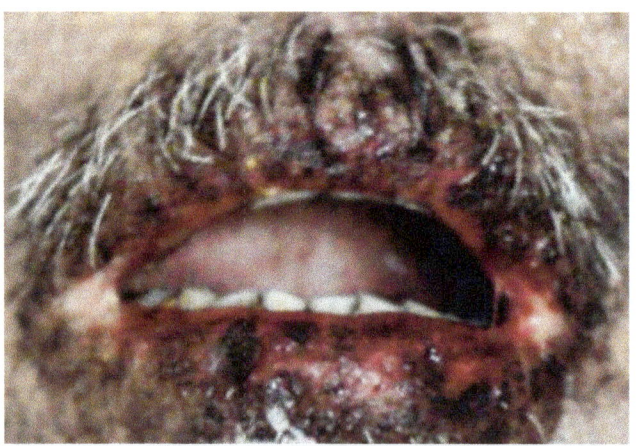

Fig. 13.4: Stevens-Johnson syndrome.

Pulmonary Syndromes

Pulmonary syndromes presents as pulmonary infiltration (nitrofurantoin, gold) and bronchospasm (aspirin, NSAIDs).

Management of Drug Allergy

A careful history is taken for any drug allergy. In case of history of drug reaction, the name of the offending drug and the date of the reaction should be noted. Patients may lose their sensitivity to a drug over time. Prompt appearance of symptoms of drug reaction suggests IgE-mediated anaphylactic reaction. In other types of immune-mediated reactions, symptoms may develop several days after the completion of course of therapy.

Drugs which have caused anaphylaxis should be avoided. However, if no alternative drug is available, skin testing is performed. In case skin test is positive, desensitization is performed. There may be cross reactivity within the same group of antibiotics. A high degree of cross reactivity exists between penicillin, carbapenem and imipenem. Cross reactivity between penicillin and cephalosporin is uncertain, however, latter is avoided if anaphylaxis had occurred due to penicillin.

Treatment

- Discontinuation of suspected drugs.
- If the reaction is mild (skin rash) and the offending drug needs to be given essentially, the drug may not be discontinued. The reaction is treated symptomatically.
- Treatment of anaphylaxis, urticaria and angioedema.

IMPLICATIONS ON DENTAL PRACTICE

- Swelling of the lips and floor of the mouth may occur in angioedema.
- Dry mouth and drowsiness may occur in patients taking antihistamines.
- Emergency kit should always be available in order to deal with any allergic reactions during dental procedures.
- Latex and rubber products can cause allergic reactions. These are now increasingly seen as the use of gloves has become more common with the advent of HIV/AIDS.
- Patients should be in supine position when injections are given. Fainting after injection is common and can be confused with anaphylaxis.

SELF ASSESSMENT

Multiple Choice Questions

1. The drug of choice in a patient with an acute allergic reaction involving bronchospasm and hypotension is:
   A. Aminophylline B. Epinephrine
   C. Dexamethasone D. Chlorpheniramine maleate
2. The blood cell, responsible for humoral immunity are:
   A. T-cells B. B-cells
   C. Both T and B cells D. No cells only antibodies
3. Type I hypersensitivity is mediated by which of the following immunoglobulins:
   A. IgA B. IgM
   C. IgD D. IgE
4. The first drug of choice to be administered in anaphylaxis is:
   A. Atropine B. Adrenaline
   C. Hydrocortisone D. Cetirizine
5. A positive tuberculin test is an example of which hypersensitivity reaction:
   A. Type I B. Type II
   C. Type III D. Type IV
6. Most abundant immunoglobulin is:
   A. IgG B. IgM
   C. IgD D. IgA
7. Which of the following is not true about urticaria:
   A. Skin lesions B. Raised flat-topped lesions
   C. Pruritus is present D. No response to antihistamines
8. Angioedema is commonly seen with the use of:
   A. ACE-inhibitors B. Calcium channel blockers
   C. Beta blockers D. Diuretics
9. Anaphylactoid reaction is:
   A. IgE mediated B. IgG mediated
   C. Non-immunoglobulin-mediated release of mast cells mediators
   D. None of the above
10. Treatment of urticaria includes following, *except*:
    A. Ranitidine B. Amantadine
    C. Fexofenadine D. Hydroxyzine

Fill in the Blanks

1. Anaphylaxis is a type I _____ mediated rapidly developing systemic allergic reaction.
2. Non-IgE mediated activation of mast cells directly occurs in _____.
3. _____ is drug of choice for Anaphylaxis.
4. In toxic epidermal necrolysis (TEN or Lyell syndrome) _____ body surface is involved.
5. Bronchospasm in anaphylactic reaction is mediated by _____ and _____.

CHAPTER 14

Nutrition

DIET AND NUTRITION

Around 40 to 50 nutrients are required by human body which are supplied through the food we eat. These are broadly divided into macronutrients and micronutrients. Macronutrients consist of proteins, fats and carbohydrates. They form the main bulk of food. Micronutrients are vitamins and minerals. They are required in a very small amount.

Energy

Body requires energy for normal function, growth and repair. This is provided by the oxidation of proteins, fats and carbohydrates. Oxidation of one gram of protein or carbohydrates provide 4 kcal (kilocalories) and one gram of fat provides 9 kcal.

The energy requirement mainly depends upon basal energy expenditure (BEE) and physical activity. It also depends upon the energy requirement for metabolizing food (thermic effect of food). Average energy requirement varies according to the age, sex, body composition and physical activity of the individual. An adult male requires 2800-3800 kcal per day and an adult female requires 1800-2900 kcal per day depending upon the type of work (light, moderate or heavy). Requirement increases in pregnancy (+300 kcal) and lactation (+500 kcal).

Protein

Protein is needed for growth and for maintenance of body structure and functions. About 10–15% of the total calories should be provided by the proteins in a healthy diet. Essential amino acids cannot be synthesized in the body and thus should be supplied through food. There are nine essential amino acids namely histidine, isoleucine, leucine, lysine, methionine, phenylalanine, threonine, tryptophan and valine. Usual protein requirement in adults is 1 g/kg per day. The protein requirement increases during growth, pregnancy, lactation and convalescence. The biological value of animal proteins is higher than that of proteins from vegetable sources.

Fat

Fats are concentrated sources of energy. It should provide 30% of the total calorie demand. Dietary fats are chiefly composed of fatty acids and cholesterol. Fatty acids are either saturated or unsaturated. Unsaturated fatty acids are further classified into monounsaturated fatty acids (MUFAs) and polyunsaturated fatty acids (PUFAs). Saturated fats are derived from animal foods and are solid at room temperature. Unsaturated fats are found in vegetable oils. Essential fatty acids, mainly linoleic acid cannot be synthesized in the body and thus is needed in the diet. Linoleic acid is required for the synthesis of other essential fatty acids, linolenic acid and arachidonic acid.

Deficiency of essential fatty acids leads to rough and dry skin (phrenoderma), hair loss and poor wound healing.

Carbohydrate

Dietary carbohydrates mainly consist of simple sugars, complex carbohydrates (starches) and indigestible carbohydrates (dietary fibers). At least 55% of the total calories should come from carbohydrates. Diets high in fibers are associated with lower incidence of digestive and cardiovascular diseases.

Vitamins

Vitamins are organic compounds required by the body for variety of essential metabolic functions. These are grouped as water soluble and fat soluble vitamins. Fat soluble vitamins are vitamin A, D, E and K. Water soluble vitamins are thiamin

Balanced Diet

A balanced diet is defined as a diet which provides adequate amount of energy, amino acids, carbohydrates, fats, vitamins and minerals to maintain health and general wellbeing. The diet should also provide extra amount of nutrients to meet the demands during short periods of deficiency.

Recommended Dietary Allowance (RDA)

Nutritional requirements are generally expressed in the form of RDA. This is the average daily dietary intake that meets the nutrient requirements in healthy persons of a specific sex, age and physiological conditions (pregnancy, lactation).

PROTEIN ENERGY MALNUTRITION

Protein energy malnutrition (PEM) is still a major health problem in the developing countries including India. It occurs mainly in childhood and is an important cause of morbidity and mortality.

PEM occurs due to absolute or relative deficiency of energy and protein. It may be due to inadequate food intake or secondary to illnesses such as diarrhea, respiratory infections, measles and intestinal worms. Factor contributing to PEM are poverty, poor environmental conditions, large family size, poor maternal health, failure of lactation, premature termination of breastfeeding and adverse customs.

Classification

PEM is classified in various ways depending on weight, height, severity and relative contribution of energy or protein deficit. The commonly used classification is Wellcome Trust Classification which is given in **Table 14.3**. Another classification (WHO classification) describes PEM under different nomenclature normal, stunting and wasting.

Clinical Manifestations

The clinical manifestations of PEM range from mild growth retardation and weight loss to distinct clinical forms like kwashiorkor and marasmus (**Figs. 14.1A and B**). The weight to height ratio is low. There is loss of subcutaneous fat, wasting of muscles and edema. Features of specific vitamin deficiency may also be found. Oral manifestations of malnutrition are given in **Table 14.4**.

Kwashiorkor occurs due to protein deficiency while the energy intake is adequate. The child develops dependent

Table 14.1: Recommended dietary allowances (RDA) of vitamins.

Vitamin	Adult male	Adult female	Pregnancy	Lactation
Vitamin A (mcg/d)	900	700	750	1200
Vitamin C (mg/d)	90	75	85	120
Vitamin D (mcg/d)*	15	15	15	15
Vitamin E (mg/d)	15	15	15	19
Vitamin K (mcg/d)	120	90	90	90
Thiamine (mg/d)	1.2	1.1	1.4	1.4
Riboflavin (mg/d)	1.3	1.1	1.4	1.6
Niacin (mg/d)	16	14	18	17
Vitamin B_6 (mg/d)	1.7	1.5	1.9	2.0
Folate (mcg/d)	400	400	600	500
Vitamin B_{12} (mcg/d)	2.4	2.4	2.6	2.8
Pantothenic acid (mg/d)	5	5	6	7
Biotin (mcg/d)	30	30	30	35
Choline (mg/d)	550	425	450	550

*as calciferol (1 mcg is equal to 40 IU)

(B_1), riboflavin (B_2), niacin (B_3), pyridoxine (B_6), cobalamin (B_{12}), folate, pantothenic acid, biotin and L-ascorbic acid (vitamin C). Recommended dietary allowances (RDA) of vitamins are given in **Table 14.1**.

Minerals

Body requires major minerals, electrolytes and trace elements. These are needed for growth, repair and vital body functions. Major minerals are calcium, magnesium and phosphorus. Electrolytes include sodium, potassium and chloride. Trace elements are iron, zinc, copper, manganese, molybdenum, fluoride, iodide, cobalt, chromium and selenium (**Table 14.2**).

Table 14.2: Recommended dietary allowances (RDA) of elements.

Elements	Adult male	Adult female	Pregnancy	Lactation
Iron (mg/d)	8	15	27	10
Calcium (mg/d)	1000	1200	1000	1000
Iodine (mcg/d)	150	150	220	290
Magnesium (mg/d)	400	310	350	310
Phosphorus (mg/d)	700	700	700	700
Chromium (mcg/d)	35	25	30	45
Copper (mcg/d)	900	900	1000	1300
Fluoride (mg/d)	4	3	3	3
Selenium (mcg/d)	55	55	60	70
Zinc (mg/d)	11	8	11	12
Potassium (g/d)	4.7	4.7	4.7	5.1
Sodium (g/d)	1.5	1.5	1.5	1.5
Chloride (g/d)	2.3	2.3	2.3	2.3

Table 14.3: Classification of PEM.

Kwashiorkor	60–80% of expected weight with edema
Under nutrition	60–80% of expected weight without edema
Marasmus	Less than 60% of expected weight without edema
Marasmic kwashiorkor	Less than 60% of expected weight with edema

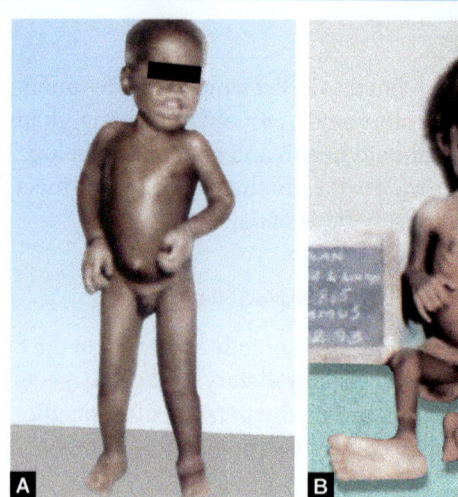

Figs. 14.1A and B: Patients of: (A) Kwashiorkor; (B) Marasmus.

Table 14.4: Oral manifestations in malnutrition.	
Findings	Deficiency of nutrients
Glossitis	Niacin, riboflavin, vitamin B_{12}, folate, pyridoxine
Bleeding gums	Vitamin C, riboflavin
Cheilosis and angular stomatitis	Riboflavin, niacin
Atrophic lingual papillae	Niacin, riboflavin, iron, folate, vitamin B_{12}
Hypogeusia	Vitamin A, zinc
Tongue fissuring	Niacin

edema, ascites, anasarca, 'flaky paint' dermatosis and fatty liver. *Marasmus* is caused by the deficiency of both, energy and proteins. Patient typically develops weight loss, wasting and cachexia. Body fat stores are depleted and muscle mass decreases. There may be intermediate clinical forms having features of both kwashiorkor and marasmus.

Kwashiorkor like PEM may develop in adults following trauma, burn and sepsis. Marasmus like PEM may result from chronic obstructive pulmonary disease, congestive heart failure, cancer and AIDS.

Laboratory Assessments

- Laboratory assessment includes anthropometric measurements for subcutaneous fat and skeletal muscles (mid-arm circumference and thickness of the triceps skin fold of the posterior mid-upper arm).
- Serum levels of protein, minerals, vitamins and assessment of immune functions are important laboratory tests.

Treatment

Treatment of PEM is a slow process. Patients fed rapidly may develop complications like hypokalemia, hypophosphatemia and congestive heart failure due to volume overload.
- Fluid and electrolyte abnormalities and infections are controlled.
- Treatment is directed toward repletion of protein, energy, vitamins and micronutrients.
- Supplementation can be done orally or parenterally.

OBESITY

Obesity is a chronic disease characterized by excessive accumulation of visceral and subcutaneous fat. It is a cause of significant morbidity and mortality. Obesity can be measured by following three methods;

1. **Body mass index:** The most widely used method to measure obesity is body mass index (BMI). BMI is calculated as weight in kilograms (Kg) divided by square of height in meter (kg/m^2). According to Indian consensus guidelines, BMI of 18.5 to 22.9 is normal, 23 to 24.9 is over weight whereas more than 25 is obesity.
2. **Waist to hip circumference ratio:** Accumulation of visceral fat is more dangerous for health than the subcutaneous fat. Abdominal obesity is defined as increased waist/hip ratio more than 0.9 in females and more than 1.0 in males.
3. **Waist circumference:** Waist circumference of more than 90 cm in male and more than 80 cm in females is suggestive of abdominal obesity in Asian Indians.

Etiology

Important factors for the development of obesity are genetic, environmental and behavioral. There are some known selected obesity genes such as *Lep (ob)*, *POMC (proopiomelanocortin)*, and *LepR(db)*. They encode gene products leptin, proopiomelanocortin, and leptin receptor respectively.

Cultural factors like diet composition and physical activity are important in causation of obesity. Sleep deprivation may also cause obesity. Changes in gut microbiome have been linked with obesity. High fat diet with simple rapidly absorbed carbohydrates increase obesity.

Specific causal and treatable factors for obesity are endocrine disorders and drugs **(Table 14.5)**.

Complications of Obesity

Obesity may predispose persons to develop coronary heart disease which is major cause of death. Incidence of cancers

Table 14.5: Specific treatable causes of obesity.
Endocrinal
• Cushing syndrome
• Hypothyroidism
• Insulinoma
• Hypothalamic disorders (tumor, trauma, inflammation)
Drugs
• Antipsychotics, antidepressants
• Corticosteroids
• Insulin, pioglitazone, sulphonylureas
• Sodium valproate, Gabapentin, pregabalin
• Beta blockers

Table 14.6: Complications and associated comorbid conditions of obesity.
Cardiovascualar
• Hypertension
• Dyslipidemia
• Coronary artery disease
• Cor pulmonale
• Varicose veins
• Pulmonary embolism
Endocrine
• Type 2 diabetes
• Metabolic syndrome
• Polycystic ovary syndrome
Cancers
• Breast cancer
• Colon cancer, gallbladder cancer
• Uterine, cervix and endometrial cancer
Musculoskeletal
• Osteoarthritis
• Backache
• Carpal tunnel syndrome
• Gout
Psychological
• Depression
• Low self esteem
• Social stigmatization
Respiratory
• Obstructive sleep apnea
• Asthma
Gastrointestinal
• Gallstones
• Gastroesophageal reflux
• Nonalcoholic fatty liver disease (NAFLD)
Other
• Pseudotumor cerebri
• Urinary stress incontinence
• Glomerulosclerosis

of colorectum in males and breast, endometrium, cervix. Gallbladder and biliary tract in females is higher in obese individuals. Obesity predisposes to type 2 disbetes and knee osteoarthritis. Other complications and associated comorbid conditions are given in **Table 14.6**.

Management

The goal of therapy is to improve obesity related complication and their prevention. Key points are:
1. **Lifestyle modifications:** It includes weight loss diets, increased exercise and eating behavior modification.
2. **Drugs:** Various drugs used are phentermine, orlistat, phentermine plus topiramate, lorcaserin, naltrexone plus bupropion, and GLP-1 receptor agonist liraglutide.
3. **Bariotic surgery:** It is indicated when BMI is more than 37.5 without presence of any obesity-related comorbidities and/or BMI more than 32.5 with the presence of type 2 diabetes or any obesity-related comorbidity. Various procedures are gastric banding, sleeve gastrectomy, roux-en-Y gastric bypass and duodenal switch.

Table 14.7: Criteria for metabolic syndrome.
• Central obesity (waist circumference >90 cm in males/>80 cm in females) Plus
• Any two of the following:
– Triglyceride level >150 mg/dL or specific medication
– HDL cholesterol < 40 mg/dL in males and <50 mg/dL in females or specific medications
– Hypertension BP > 130/85 mm Hg or specific medication
– Fasting plasma glucose > 100 mg/dL or previously diagnosed type 2 diabetes

4. **Treatment of additional risk factors:** It includes cessation of smoking, reduction in alcohol consumption and management of diabetes mellitus, hypertension, hyperlipidemia and obstructive sleep apnea.

Metabolic Syndrome

Metabolic syndrome is constellation of metabolic abnormalities which include increased waist circumference, hypertriglyceridemia, low HDK cholesterol, hypertension and impaired fasting glucose/impaired glucose tolerance/diabetes mellitus. There is increased risk of atherosclerotic and prothrombotic complications. IDF (International Diabetes Federation) criteria of metabolic syndrome are given in **Table 14.7**.

VITAMINS

Vitamins are organic compounds required by the body for variety of essential metabolic functions. These are grouped as water soluble and fat soluble vitamins. **Fat soluble** vitamins are vitamin A, D, E and K. **Water soluble** vitamins are thiamin (B_1), riboflavin (B_2), niacin (B_3), pyridoxine (B_6), cobalamin (B_{12}), folate, pantothenic acid, biotin and L-ascorbic acid (vitamin C).

Vitamins are not synthesized at all or are inadequately synthesized in the body; hence they are required in the diet. They are generally needed in very small quantities for essential functions. Multiple vitamin deficiency is more common than single vitamin deficiency. Body stores for vitamins B_{12} and vitamin A are large and persist for more than a year after being on a deficient diet while folate and thiamine stores are short lived and deplete within weeks. Daily requirement of vitamins are given in **Table 14.1**.

Most deficiencies are associated with malnutrition, malabsorption, alcoholism, medications, total parenteral nutrition, hemodialysis, food faddism or inborn errors of metabolism.

Vitamin deficiency develops gradually and the symptoms are nonspecific in the early stages. The physical findings appear late. Subclinical deficiency of vitamins is common particularly in the geriatric age group and can be recognized by laboratory testing. Excess vitamins can also cause disease **(Table 14.8)**.

Table 14.8: Vitamin deficiency and toxicity.

Vitamin	Physiological role	Deficiency	Excess
Vitamin A	Normal vision, growth, cell differentiation, iron metabolism, immunity	Night blindness, conjunctival xerosis, Bitot's spots, corneal xerosis, keratomalacia, extraocular manifestations- hyperkeratotic skin lesions, growth retardation.	Acute toxicity- increased intracranial pressure, exfoliative dermatitis. Chronic toxicity-cheilosis, glossitis, alopecia, hypercalcemia
Vitamin D	Calcium and phosphate absorption, bone mineralization	Rickets in children, osteomalacia in adults	Hypercalcemia, polyurea, cardiac arrhythmias, renal failure
Vitamin E	Potent antioxidant	Hemolytic anemia, areflexia, ophthalmoplegia, myopathy, retinopathy	Nausea, flatulence, diarrhea, bleeding in patients on oral anticoagulants due to increased requirement of vitamin K
Vitamin K	Important role in the coagulation process	Bleeding from any site	Hemolysis, hyperbilirubinemia
Vitamin B_1	Energy production, peripheral nerve conduction, coenzyme alcohol dehydrogenase	Beri beri, central nervous system manifestations- Wernicke's and Korsakoff's syndrome	
Vitamin B_2	Oxidation-reduction reactions, energy metabolism	Mucocutaneous lesions of the mouth and skin, corneal vascularization, anemia	
Vitamin B_3	Oxidation-reduction reactions	Pellagra (dermatitis, diarrhea and dementia), *bright red glossitis*, stomatitis	Flushing, skin dryness, hepatotoxicity, gout
Vitamin B_6	Amino acid, fat, carbohydrate metabolism and heme synthesis	Glossitis, cheilosis, peripheral neuropathy, personality changes	Sensory neuropathy and dermatitis
Vitamin C	Oxidation-reduction reactions, synthesis of collagen, conversion of dopamine to norepinephrine, iron absorption	Scurvy, impairment of bone growth in children	Gastric irritation, diarrhea, hyperuricemia, raised levels ALT and LDH, hemolysis in cases with G6PD deficiency

Some vitamins are also used as drugs, e.g., niacin for hyperlipidemia and vitamin A for cystic acne and skin wrinkles.

Thiamine (Vitamin B_1)

Functions

- Thiamine pyrophosphate (TPP) acts as a coenzyme in the decarboxylation of alpha-ketoacids and branched-chain amino acids and thus it helps in energy production.
- It acts as a coenzyme for a transketolase reaction that mediates conversion of hexose and pentose phosphates.
- It plays a role in peripheral nerve conduction.
- It is a coenzyme for the enzyme alcohol dehydrogenase.

Sources

Important sources of thiamine are yeast, pork, legumes, beef, whole grains and nuts. Milled and polished rice is a poor source of vitamin B_1. Hence, deficiency of vitamin B_1 is more commonly seen in those with polished rice based diet. Tea and coffee contain thiaminases that destroy the thiamine.

Deficiency

The deficiency of thiamine most commonly occurs in alcoholics. The deficiency presents with nonspecific symptoms in the early stages such as anorexia and irritability. Prolonged deficiency of thiamine causes beriberi. Beriberi may be wet or dry.

- Wet beriberi is characterized by the presence of cardiomegaly, tachycardia, congestive heart failure and peripheral edema.
- Dry beriberi presents with symmetrical sensorimotor neuropathy.

Alcoholics with chronic thiamine deficiency may also have central nervous system manifestations. These include Wernicke's encephalopathy (nystagmus, ophthalmoplegia, cerebellar ataxia and mental impairment) and Korsakoff's syndrome (amnesia, confabulation and impaired learning).

Diagnosis

In most cases, the clinical response to thiamine therapy supports the diagnosis. However, biochemical tests can also be performed to confirm the deficiency. These include an assay of transketolase activity before and after addition of thiamine pyrophosphate and measurement of thiamine levels in blood and serum.

Treatment

Thiamine in a dose of 100 mg/day parenterally is given for 7 days in acute cases. This is followed by 10 mg/day orally till complete recovery. Anaphylaxis has been reported with the parenteral use of thiamine.

Benfotiamine is a newer derivative of thiamine. It is lipid soluble and hence is absorbed much better than water soluble thiamine hydrochloride. It activates the enzyme transketolase ten times more than thiamine.

Riboflavin (Vitamin B$_2$)

Functions

Riboflavin plays an important role in the oxidation-reduction reactions and is a cofactor in a number of enzymes involved in energy metabolism.

Sources

Milk and other dairy products, eggs and green leafy vegetables are important sources. Other sources are cereals, legumes, broccoli and fish.

Deficiency

Riboflavin deficiency is usually due to poor dietary intake and is commonly associated with multiple vitamin deficiencies. People who consume rice as staple diet are more prone to riboflavin deficiency. The clinical manifestations are mucocutaneous lesions of the mouth and skin such as chelosis, angular stomatitis, magenta tongue and seborrheic dermatitis. Corneal vascularization and anemia may also occur.

Diagnosis

The treatment is usually started empirically. However, the diagnosis can be confirmed by measurement of red blood cell and urinary riboflavin concentrations or red blood cell glutathione reductase activity.

Treatment

Riboflavin deficiency is easily treated with oral preparations of the vitamin with the dosage of 5–15 mg/day. It is given till the clinical findings are resolved.

Niacin (Vitamin B$_3$)

Functions

Niacin refers to nicotinic acid, nicotinamide and their derivatives. It serves as a precursor of nicotinamide adenine dinucleotide (NAD) and nicotinamide adenine dinucleotide phosphate (NADP) which are involved in many oxidation-reduction reactions. Unlike other vitamins, niacin is synthesized in the body from the amino acid tryptophan, but to a very small extent.

Sources

Important sources of niacin are milk, eggs, beans and meat. The bioavailability of niacin from cereals especially maize is low.

Deficiency

The deficiency of niacin leads to pellagra (**Fig. 14.2**). This is more common in people who eat corn-based diet. Pellagra can also occur in alcoholics and in inborn errors of tryptophan metabolism (Hartnup's disease).

Pellagra is characterized by dermatitis, diarrhea and dementia. There are dark, dry and scaly lesions in sun exposed areas such as back of the hands, lower legs, face and neck (Casal's necklace). Other features are anorexia, irritability, *bright red glossitis*, stomatitis and weight loss (**Fig. 14.3**). Depression, seizures and psychosis may also occur. Advanced pellagra can result in death.

Diagnosis

Pellagra is generally diagnosed clinically. However, measurement of niacin metabolites in the urine can be performed to confirm the diagnosis.

Treatment

Oral nicotinamide or nicotinic acid (10–150 mg daily) effectively treats pellagra.

Toxicity

Toxicity may occur at high dosage of nicotinic acid used to treat hyperlipidemia. Symptoms include flushing, skin dryness and itching. Others are gastric irritation, hepatotoxicity, hyperglycemia, gout and macular edema.

Vitamin B$_6$ (Pyridoxine)

Functions

Vitamin B$_6$ refers to a group of closely associated substances including pyridoxine, pyridoxal, pyridoxamine and their 5-phosphate esters. Pyridoxal-5-phosphate is a cofactor for a number of enzymes involved in amino acid metabolism. Vitamin B$_6$ is also involved in the metabolism of fat, carbohydrates and several vitamins including the conversion of tryptophan to niacin. It is also involved in heme synthesis.

Sources

Milk, liver, meat, legumes, whole grain cereals, nuts and vegetables are good sources of B$_6$.

Deficiency

Deficiency of vitamin B$_6$ may occur in association with various drugs (isoniazid, cycloserine, oral contraceptives) or alcoholism. Glossitis, cheilosis, weakness are usual features of the vitamin B$_6$ deficiency. Severe deficiency results in the peripheral neuropathy and personality changes including depression and irritability. Microcytic hypochromic anemia and seizures may also occur.

Diagnosis

A low level of pyridoxal phosphate in blood is diagnostic of vitamin B$_6$ deficiency.

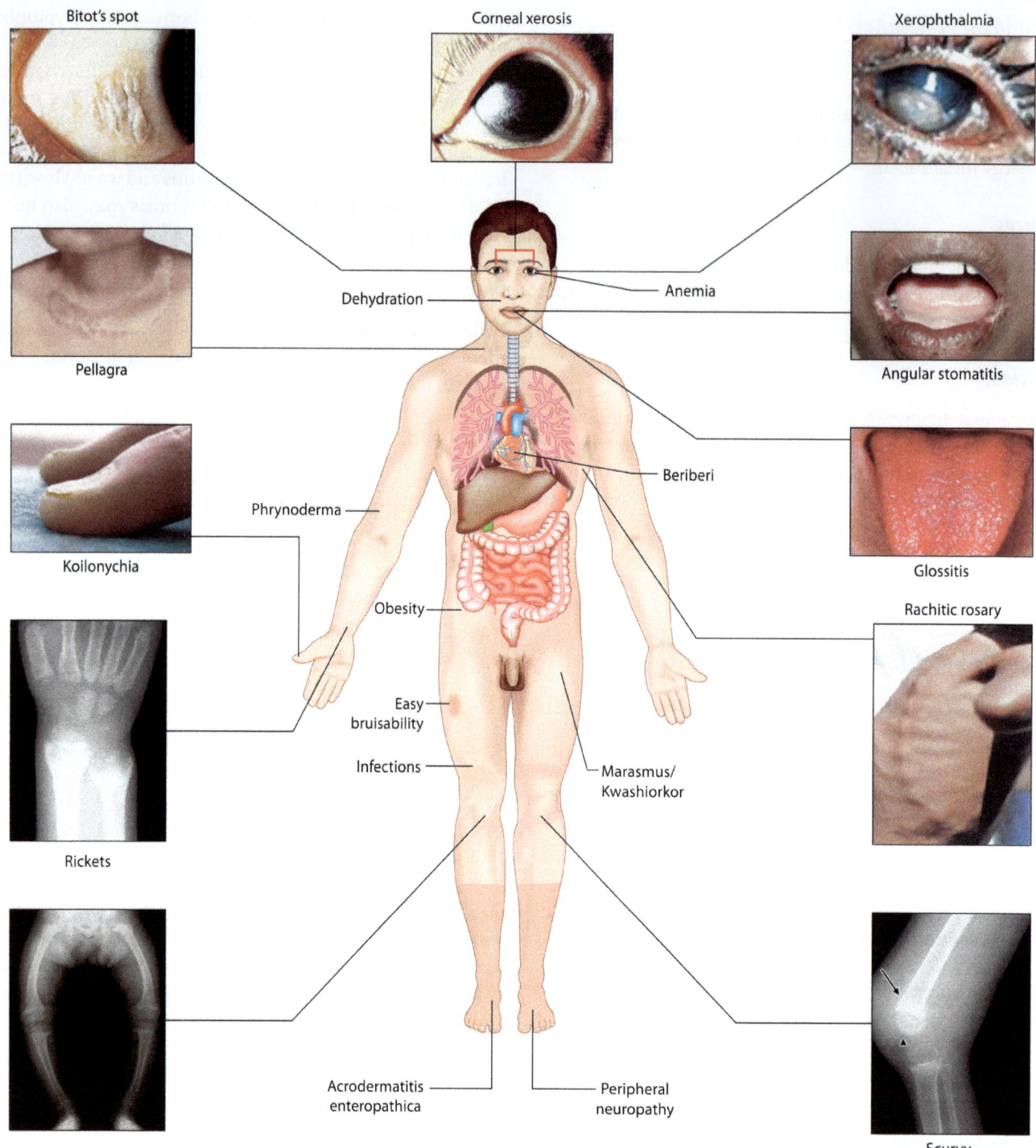

Fig. 14.2: Different manifestations of vitamin deficiencies.

Treatment

Vitamin B_6 is given orally in a dosage of 10–20 mg/day. However, higher doses (100–200 mg/day) are needed in cases with medication-related vitamin deficiency. It is also indicated in the prevention of isoniazid-induced neuropathy.

Toxicity

High doses of vitamin B_6 can cause sensory neuropathy and dermatitis.

Folate and Vitamin B_{12}

These vitamins are discussed in Chapter 4.

Biotin

This is a water soluble vitamin which plays a role in gluconeogenesis and fatty acid synthesis. Dietary sources of biotin are liver, beans, yeast and egg yolk. Significant amounts are also formed by the bacteria of the gut. In adults, the deficiency of biotin results into depression, hallucination,

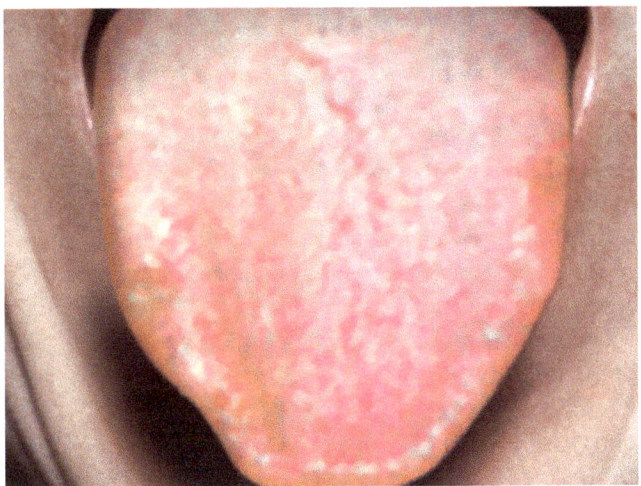

Fig. 14.3: Glossitis.

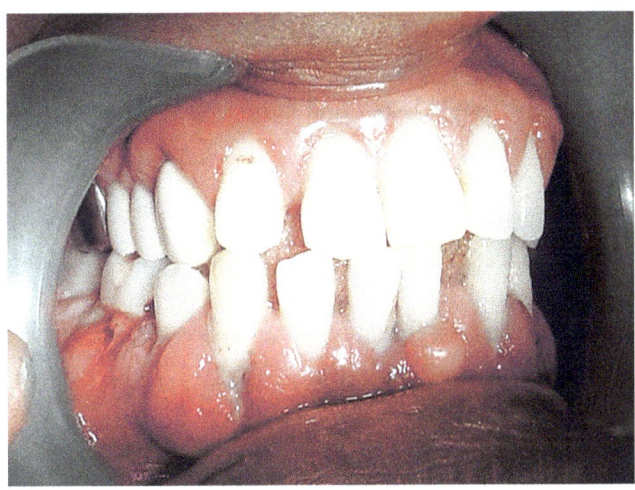

Fig. 14.4: Bleeding gums in scurvy.

paresthesia and anorexia. Seborrheic rash may occur over face. The deficiency of biotin in infants can lead to lethargy, hypotonia and alopecia. Treatment is supplementation of biotin 10 mg/day.

Pantothenic Acid

Dietary sources of pantothenic acid are liver, yeast, egg yolk and vegetables. It plays a role in fatty acid metabolism and in the synthesis of cholesterol and steroid hormones. Deficiency symptoms are nonspecific and are in the form of muscle cramps, paresthesia (burning feet syndrome) and depression.

Choline

Choline is a precursor of acetylcholine, phospholipids and betaine. It is also necessary for the integrity of cell membrane. Deficiency can lead to fatty liver and elevated transaminases levels.

Vitamin C (L-ascorbic Acid)

Functions

Vitamin C is a potent antioxidant which is involved in many oxidation-reduction reactions. It is also required for the synthesis of collagen and conversion of dopamine to norepinephrine. Vitamin C promotes iron absorption because it reduces ferric iron in diet to ferrous form which is better absorbed. It is also involved in drug metabolism, wound healing and carnitine biosynthesis.

Sources

Amla, citrus fruits, guava, green vegetables, potatoes and tomatoes are good sources of vitamin C. The requirement for vitamin C increases under stress, smoking and in those on hemodialysis.

Deficiency

Deficiency may occur in poor, elderly and chronic alcoholics. Vitamin C deficiency causes scurvy in which there is impaired formation of mature connective tissue. The patients may have petechiae, ecchymosis, swollen and bleeding gums (**Fig. 14.4**), hemarthrosis, anemia and poor wound healing. In children bone growth is impaired. *Periodontal signs do not develop in edentulous patients.*

Diagnosis

Diagnosis is made clinically and confirmed by the low level of ascorbic acid in plasma and leukocytes.

Treatment

The usual dose of vitamin C is 200-500 mg/day orally. Studies have reported that high intake of vitamin C may protect against certain cancers. Vitamin C in the dosage of 1–2 g/day may decrease the duration and symptoms of upper respiratory infection.

Toxicity

More than 2 g/day can cause gastric irritation and diarrhea. Higher doses can lead to hyperuricemia and raised levels of alanine amino transferase (ALT) and lactate dehydrogenase (LDH). It can also lead to false-negative test for fecal occult blood and disturbs the urinary glucose estimation.

Vitamin E

Functions

Vitamin E is a collective name for naturally occurring tocopherols. α-tocopherol is the most potent of all tocopherols. It is a powerful antioxidant. Vitamin C, glutathione and various enzymes maintain vitamin E in the reduced state.

Sources

Rich sources of vitamin E are sunflower oil, safflower oil and wheat germ oil. It is also found in meat, nuts, cereals, fruits and vegetables.

Deficiency

Dietary deficiency of vitamin E is rare. Deficiency can occur in chronic and severe malabsorption, abetalipoproteinemia, and in children with chronic cholestatic liver disease or cystic fibrosis.

Manifestations of vitamin E deficiency include hemolytic anemia, areflexia, gait disturbances, decreased vibration and position sense and ophthalmoplegia. Myopathy and retinopathy may also occur. It also causes posterior column and spinocerebellar symptoms.

Diagnosis

Low blood levels of α-tocopherol is diagnostic of vitamin E deficiency.

Treatment

Symptomatic vitamin E deficiency is treated with 800–1200 mg of α-tocopherol daily. Higher doses are required in abetalipoproteinemia. In higher doses, vitamin E protects from intraventricular hemorrhage of prematurity and oxygen-induced retrolental fibroplasias and bronchopulmonary dysplasia.

Toxicity

High dose of vitamin E (>800 mg/day) may interfere with vitamin K metabolism, hence it should not be given to patients taking warfarin. Higher doses can also cause nausea, flatulence and diarrhea.

Vitamin A

Vitamin A (retinol) is a high molecular weight alcohol, synthesized from plant carotenoids. The oxidized metabolites of retinol, retinaldehyde and retinoic acid are also biologically active compounds. Retinaldehyde is required for normal vision and retinoic acid is necessary for growth and cell differentiation. Vitamin A also plays a role in iron metabolism and humoral and cellular immunity.

Sources

Liver and fish have preformed vitamin A. Green leafy vegetable, green and yellow fruits (papaya, mango, pumpkin) and carrots are good sources of β-carotene also known as provitamin A. Milk is a poor source of vitamin A. Fortified food (vanaspati and milk) are also sources of vitamin A.

Deficiency

Vitamin A deficiency is one of the most common vitamin deficiency syndromes and is a common cause of blindness.

Night blindness is the earliest symptom. Conjunctival xerosis, Bitot's spots, corneal xerosis and keratomalacia are other ocular signs of vitamin A deficiency **(Fig. 14.5)**. Xerophthalmia refers to all ocular manifestations of vitamin A deficiency. Keratomalacia is ulceration and necrosis of cornea which may perforate.

Extraocular manifestations include hyperkeratotic skin lesions, anorexia and growth retardation.

Diagnosis

Measurement of serum retinol is diagnostic. Abnormalities of dark adaptation are strongly suggestive of vitamin A deficiency.

Treatment

Ocular changes are treated with 30 mg (100,000 IU) vitamin A intramuscularly or 60 mg (200,000 IU) orally. The dose is repeated every six months in endemic areas.

Toxicity

Acute toxicity has been reported after excess consumption of polar bear liver or intake of more than 150 mg vitamin A. Presentations include increased intracranial pressure, vertigo, diplopia, seizures and exfoliative dermatitis.

Chronic toxicity (ingestion of 15 mg/day for several months) manifests as dry skin, cheilosis, glossitis, alopecia, bone pain, hypercalcemia and increased intracranial pressure.

High dose of carotenoids may cause yellowing of skin (palm and soles) but not the sclera.

Vitamin K

Vitamin K exists in two natural forms, vitamin K1 (phylloquinone) and vitamin K2 (menaquinone). Vitamin K2

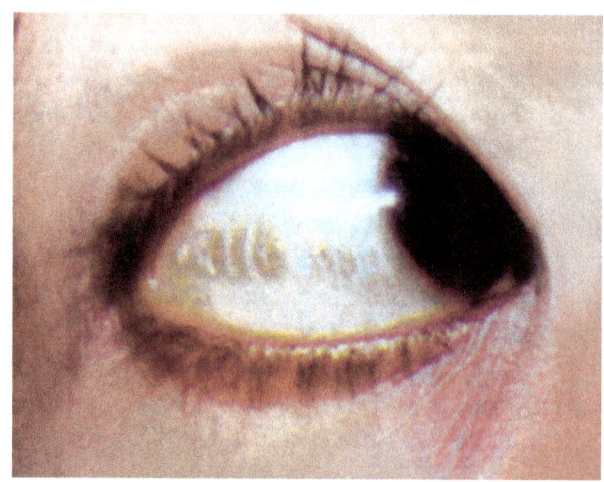

Fig. 14.5: Bitot spots and keratomalacia.

is synthesized by intestinal bacteria and vitamin KI is found in animal and plant sources. Menadione (K3) is a synthetic provitamin which is converted to vitamin K2 by the liver.

Vitamin K plays an important role in the coagulation process by acting as a cofactor for the post-translational gamma carboxylation of factor II, VII, IX and X, protein C and S. These modified proteins are able to bind with platelets in a calcium dependent reaction and participate in the coagulation process more efficiently. Without gamma carboxylation, these factors do not function efficiently. Warfarin type drugs prevent the conversion of vitamin K to its active hydroquinone form.

Sources

Dietary source of vitamin K are green leafy vegetables, fruits, milk, butter, liver and coffee. It is also present in olive oil and soybean oil. Vitamin K2 is endogenously produced by gut bacteria.

Deficiency

Deficiency of vitamin K occurs because of poor diet, malabsorption and broad spectrum antibiotics which suppress colonic flora. Body stores of vitamin K are small, hence deficiency can occur in as little as one week. Newborns are particularly susceptible to vitamin K deficiency because of low stores, low levels of vitamin K in the breast milk, lack of intestinal flora and liver immaturity.

Deficiency of vitamin K may present as bleeding from any site.

Diagnosis

Prothrombin time (PT) is prolonged in mild deficiency. PT and APTT both are elevated in advanced cases; however, PT is elevated to a greater extent. The vitamin K level can be measured by chromatography.

Treatment

The deficiency is treated with 10 mg vitamin K parenterally. Patients with chronic malabsorption should receive 1–2 mg parenterally every week. Newborns are given 1 mg vitamin K intramuscularly at the time of birth as a prophylaxis.

Toxicity

Toxic effects of vitamin K are hemolysis and hyperbilirubinemia which are reported after parenteral use of menadione.

Vitamin D

Vitamin D exists in two forms: ergocalciferol (vitamin D_2) and cholecalciferol (vitamin D_3). Ergocalciferol is derived from plants (the ergot fungus found especially on rye) and cholecalciferol is synthesized in the skin from 7-dehydrocholesterol under the influence of ultraviolet rays present in sunlight or is synthetically produced. Vitamin D is stored largely in fat depots. Cholecalciferol is converted to active forms by hydroxylation in the liver and subsequently in kidneys. In the liver, it is converted to 25-hydroxycholecalciferol (25[OH] D3) and in kidney, to most potent metabolite 1,25-dihydroxycholecalciferol (1,25[OH]$_2$ D_3) or calcitriol.

The main function of vitamin D is to increase absorption of calcium and phosphate from the intestine. It also increases the renal tubular reabsorption of phosphate. Vitamin D promotes bone mineralization. It may also have other systemic effects since vitamin D receptors are found in many body tissues.

Vitamin D is actually a hormone and if sufficient exposure of sunlight is given to the skin it is not required in the diet. It was classified as vitamins when much was not known about it.

Sources

Vitamin D is derived from both sunlight and food. Liver, butter, cheese, egg and fish are important sources of vitamin D. Fish liver oil is the richest source of vitamin D. Other sources are food artificially fortified with vitamin D such as vanaspati and milk (milk as such is a poor source).

Deficiency

Deficiency can occur due to inadequate exposure to sunlight, lack of dietary intake, malabsorption, impaired vitamin D activation (in renal disorders) and resistance to the effects of vitamin D (defective receptors). Drugs such as phenytoin, rifampicin and barbiturates can lead to increased metabolism of vitamin D in liver, thus they can cause vitamin D deficiency.

Vitamin D deficiency leads to rickets in children and osteomalacia in adults. *Rickets* is characterized by growth failure, bony deformities, muscular hypotonia, tetany and convulsion **(Fig. 14.6)**. Bony deformities include curved legs, pigeon chest, Harrison sulcus, rickety rosary,

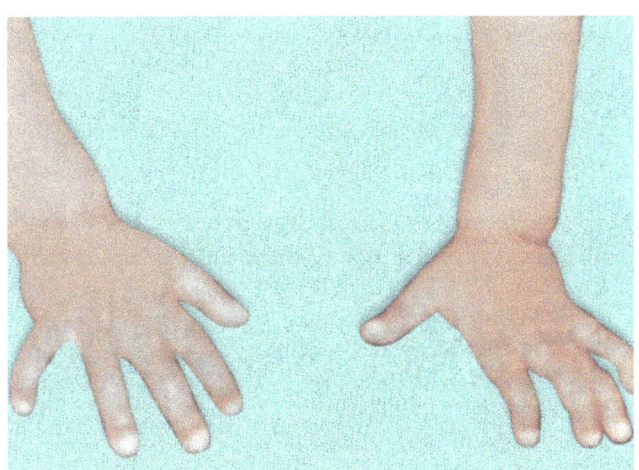

Fig. 14.6: Rickets.

kyphoscoliosis and deformed pelvis. Defective skeleton mineralization, bone fractures and proximal myopathy are found in *osteomalacia*.

Diagnosis

Serum calcium and phosphate levels are low. There is a compensatory increase in PTH level. Serum concentration of vitamin D is low.

Treatment

Treatment involves replacement of vitamin D and calcium. Vitamin D can be replaced in various forms like ergocalciferol, 1-α-hydroxy vitamin D_3 (α-calcidol) and 1,25-dihydroxy vitamin D_3 (calcitriol). The dose of calcitriol is 0.25 to 0.5 µg daily.

Toxicity

Excessive intake of vitamin D may cause hypercalcemia which present as anorexia, nausea, vomiting, thirst, polyurea and drowsiness. Cardiac arrhythmias, renal failure and coma may occur.

IMPLICATIONS ON DENTAL PRACTICE

- Burning mouth syndrome, mouth ulcers, glossitis, gum bleeding and angular stomatitis may be the first presentation of nutritional deficiency.
- Undernutrition in children can result in retarded tooth eruption.
- Undernutrition can lead to immunodeficiency which predisposes to the development of oral ulcerations, necrotizing gingivitis and gangrenous stomatitis.
- Dysphagia may be a manifestation of iron deficiency.

SELF ASSESSMENT

Multiple Choice Questions

1. Alcoholics are prone to develop deficiency of:
   A. Vitamin D B. Vitamin B_1
   C. Vitamin C D. Vitamin E
2. Vitamin B_{12} deficiency can give rise to all of the following, *except*:
   A. Myelopathy B. Optic atrophy
   C. Peripheral neuropathy D. Myopathy
3. All of the following are true about manifestations of vitamin E deficiency, *except*:
   A. Hemolytic anemia
   B. Posterior column abnormalities
   C. Cerebellar ataxia
   D. Autonomic dysfunction
4. Following is true about Vitamin A:
   A. Water soluble
   B. Deficiency causes impaired vision
   C. Maintains normal plasma calcium levels
   D. Is required for formation of plasma clotting factors
5. The final metabolically active form of vitamin D is synthesized in:
   A. Kidney B. Liver
   C. Bone D. Skin
6. Glossitis and angular stomatitis are features of all the vitamins, *except*:
   A. Niacin B. Pyridoxine
   C. Riboflavin D. Ascorbic acid
7. All the following are causes of bleeding gums, *except*:
   A. Acute myeloblastic leukemia
   B. Phenytoin therapy
   C. Scurvy D. Candidiasis
8. Deficiency of vitamin D can lead to:
   A. Hypercalcemia
   B. Decreased absorption of calcium from intestine
   C. Decreased renal excretion of calcium
   D. Increased renal calcium excretion
9. The syndrome of angular oral fissure, corneal vascularization and glossitis is due to:
   A. Pyridoxine deficiency
   B. Niacin deficiency
   C. Riboflavin deficiency
   D. Xerophthalmia (vitamin A deficiency)
10. Sensory neuropathy can occur with high doses of which of the following vitamin:
    A. Thiamine B. Pyridoxine
    C. Niacin D. Vitamin B_{12}
11. Which of the following is used to treat hyperlipidemia:
    A. Vitamin A B. Vitamin D
    C. Niacin D. Vitamin E
12. Increased intracranial pressure can occur with excess doses of:
    A. Vitamin A B. Vitamin K
    C. Vitamin E D. All of the above
13. Consumption of polar bear liver can cause acute toxicity of:
    A. Vitamin A B. Vitamin C
    C. Vitamin K D. Folic acid
14. Following is used in hyperhomocysteinemia:
    A. Folic acid B. Pyridoxine
    C. Riboflavin D. Ascorbic acid
15. Which of the following is a cardiac risk factor?
    A. Hyperhomocysteinemia
    B. Excess niacin levels
    C. Increased HDL cholesterol
    D. All of the above
16. Yellow discoloration of palm and soles can occur with high doses of:
    A. Provitamin A B. Vitamin K
    C. Vitamin D D. Vitamin C
17. Which of the following is fat soluble vitamin:
    A. Vitamin A B. Vitamin B_1
    C. Vitamin C D. Vitamin B_{12}
18. Wernicke's encephalopathy occur due to deficiency of:
    A. Vitamin A B. Vitamin C
    C. Vitamin B_1 D. Vitamin E
19. Cardiomyopathy and congestive heart failure can occur due to deficiency of:

- A. Vitamin K
- B. Vitamin B_1
- C. Vitamin D
- D. Niacin

20. **Anaphylaxis has been reported with parenteral use of:**
    - A. Thiamine
    - B. Niacin
    - C. Pyridoxine
    - D. Vitamin D

21. **People who consume rice as a staple diet are prone to develop deficiency of:**
    - A. Ascorbic acid
    - B. Riboflavin
    - C. Pyridoxine
    - D. Niacin

22. **Dark and scaly lesions in sun exposed areas such as neck (Casal's necklace) can occur in deficiency of:**
    - A. Cyanocobalamin
    - B. Vitamin C
    - C. Folate
    - D. Niacin

23. **Flushing can occur with use of high doses of:**
    - A. Choline
    - B. Pantothenic acid
    - C. Niacin
    - D. Pyridoxine

24. **Use of isoniazid can cause deficiency of:**
    - A. Vitamin B_1
    - B. Vitamin B_2
    - C. Vitamin B_6
    - D. Vitamin B_{12}

25. **High dose of vitamin B_6 (pyridoxine) can cause:**
    - A. Raised intracranial tension
    - B. Excessive bleeding
    - C. Sensory neuropathy
    - D. Osteoporosis

26. **Which of the following is required for synthesis of collagen:**
    - A. Vitamin C
    - B. Vitamin A
    - C. Vitamin K
    - D. Vitamin B_1

27. **High doses of vitamin C can cause:**
    - A. Hyperuricemia
    - B. Hyperlipidemia
    - C. Hyperkalemia
    - D. Hypercholesterolemia

28. **Raised intracranial tension can occur with prolonged use of:**
    - A. Vitamin A
    - B. Vitamin K
    - C. Vitamin C
    - D. Vitamin E

29. **Vitamin K is required for the synthesis of:**
    - A. Facror II, VII, X, XI
    - B. Factor II, V, Xi, XII
    - C. Protein C, Protein S
    - D. Factor VII, VIII, IX, X

30. **Vitamin K deficiency can cause:**
    - A. Increased bleeding time
    - B. Increased prothrombin time
    - C. Increased clot lysis time
    - D. Increased reaction time

Fill in the Blanks

1. Diarrhea, dementia and dermatitis are due to _____ deficiency.
2. Wernicke's encephalopathy is due to the deficiency of _____ vitamin.
3. Night blindness is a feature of _____ deficiency.
4. Bitot's spot is seen in _____.
5. Osteomalcia is due to deficiency of _____.
6. Vitamin _____ is required for synthesis of clotting factors.
7. Subacute combined degeneration of spinal cord can occur in _____ deficiency.
8. Deficiency of vitamin B_1 is more common with _____ based diet.
9. Corneal vascularization can occur in _____ deficiency.
10. _____ is used to prevent isoniazid-induced neuropathy.
11. People who eat corn based diet are prone to develop _____ deficiency.

CHAPTER 15

Preoperative Evaluation

Patients must be thoroughly assessed preoperatively for their fitness for anesthesia and surgery. Preanesthesia evaluation refers to the process of clinical assessment that is usually done prior to the delivery of anesthesia services for both surgical and nonsurgical procedures. Preanesthetic clinic or PAC is a clinic where patients are evaluated before surgery by the anesthesiologists to establish a baseline report upon which risk assessment and perioperative management decisions can be done.

The focus during the preanesthesia evaluation should be to gain relevant information regarding the patients health by medical history, general physical and systemic examinations, past medical records, laboratory tests and radiological imaging.

Preoperative assessment gives a unique opportunity to the anesthesiologist to educate and individualize the perioperative needs of the patients in terms of intraoperative care, better pain control, postoperative recovery and lesser duration of hospital stay.

Goals achieved by preoperative evaluation:
- Helps in improving doctor-patient relationship, with reduced anxiety levels during perioperative period.
- Helps achieving the target of optimized patient before anesthesia, with help of relevant investigations and specialized consultations if needed.
- Better management of comorbid conditions and preexisting pathologies.
- Reduces the overall cost of perioperative care and avoidance of last minute operating room (OR) cancellations.
- Better documentation and ideal time for Informed Consent.
- Provide opportunity for behavioral modification intervention (e.g., smoking cessation, alcohol abstinence, and lifestyle modification).

The *ultimate goal* of preoperative anesthesia evaluation is to *mitigate the risk of perioperative morbidity and mortality* and to return the patient to his/her routine work as early as possible.

The appropriate time of preanesthesia evaluation should be decided on factors like general health status of the patient, urgency for the surgical/nonsurgical procedure, optimization of the comorbid diseases and the risk associated with the required procedure. Healthy patients with low risk procedures can be evaluated a day before or on the day of procedure. Patients with high risk should be evaluated well in advance for better work up and to provide time for any medical intervention before the required procedure.

American Society of Anesthesiologists (ASA) Practice Advisory for *Preanesthesia Evaluation should include, at a minimum*, the following:
- Patients medical history with review of medical records
- General examination and focused systemic examination (most important are airway, lungs and heart)
- Indicated preoperative tests
- Consultation with specialists if deemed necessary.

MEDICAL HISTORY

Extremely necessary to identify (Name, age, sex, registration number) and take a detailed patient history, which should include the following components:
- **History of present illness:** Concise history behind the current medical condition leading up to the surgical intervention and what is the type of surgical intervention.
- **Past medical history:** Document comorbidities, especially those involving heart, lungs, liver, and kidneys, with special attention to hypertension, diabetes, coronary artery disease, reactive airway disease, recent pulmonary infections, and history of stroke or myocardial infarction.
- **Past surgical history:** Type of surgery, type of anesthesia received [regional, monitored anesthetic care (MAC), or general anesthesia].

- **Any complications from anesthesia:** Difficult intubation, prolonged wake up, difficulty with ventilation, postoperative nausea and vomiting, review of any prior anesthetic records available.
- **Allergies** (including specific reaction).
- **Current medications:** Particular attention to the dosages and last administration of blood pressure medications, anti-platelet medications, diabetic medications (oral and parenteral) and steroids, any herbal or home medications.
- **Family medical history:** Family member having problems with general anesthesia like malignant hyperthermia or pseudocholinesterase deficiency.
- **Social history:** Tobacco use, alcohol consumption, and illicit drugs.
- **Obstetric history** and menstrual history are important for females.
- **Birth history,** birth weight, immunization and history of recent upper respiratory tract infections are important for pediatric age group patients.

PHYSICAL EXAMINATION

The physical examination should be based on relevant information gathered during the patients history.

At a minimum, a focused preanesthetic physical examination should include an assessment of the airway, lungs, and heart, with documentation of vital signs as per ASA practice advisory.

- **General examination:** Height, weight, BMI, pallor, cyanosis, icterus, lymphadenopathy, edema, etc.
- **Vital signs:** Noninvasive blood pressure (NIBP), heart rate (HR), respiratory rate, oxygen saturation (SpO_2) and examination of peripheral pulses.
- **Pulmonary system examination:** Auscultation of breath sounds to identify any rhonchi, wheeze, crepts or other sounds of lung pathology.
- **Cardiovascular system examination:** Auscultation of heart sounds and identification of any irregular rhythms, murmurs or any adventitious sounds.
- **CNS examination:** Motor and sensory function assessment and cognitive functions, document any signs of peripheral neuropathy before planning spinal/epidural blocks/peripheral nerve blocks.
- If regional anesthesia (Neuraxial blocks/peripheral nerve blocks) is planned then the regional anesthesia site should be identified and examined to rule out any local infection or technical difficulty.

AIRWAY EXAMINATION

Airway management is the most important aspect of patient care during sedation or general anesthesia, and examination of the patient's airway is an essential component of the preoperative assessment. Airway should be assessed on following points:
- Neck mobility
- Mouth opening/Modified Mallampati score (simple scoring system that relates the amount of mouth opening to the size of the tongue, and provides an estimate of space available for oral intubation by direct laryngoscopy)
- Teeth: Artificial dentures, loose tooths and dental caps, temporomandibular joint mobility
- Thyromental distance
- Alignment of mandibular and maxillary incisors
- Tongue size
- Presence of beard and facial hair.

MODIFIED MALLAMPATI CLASSIFICATION

Examination is done in sitting position with head in neutral position, with mouth widely open and tongue protruded to the maximum. Classified as per the pharyngeal structures being visible **(Fig. 15.1)**.

Class I: Pillars, uvula, soft palate and hard palate visible
Class II: Uvula, soft palate and hard palate visible
Class III: Soft palate and hard palate visible
Class IV: Only hard palate is visible.

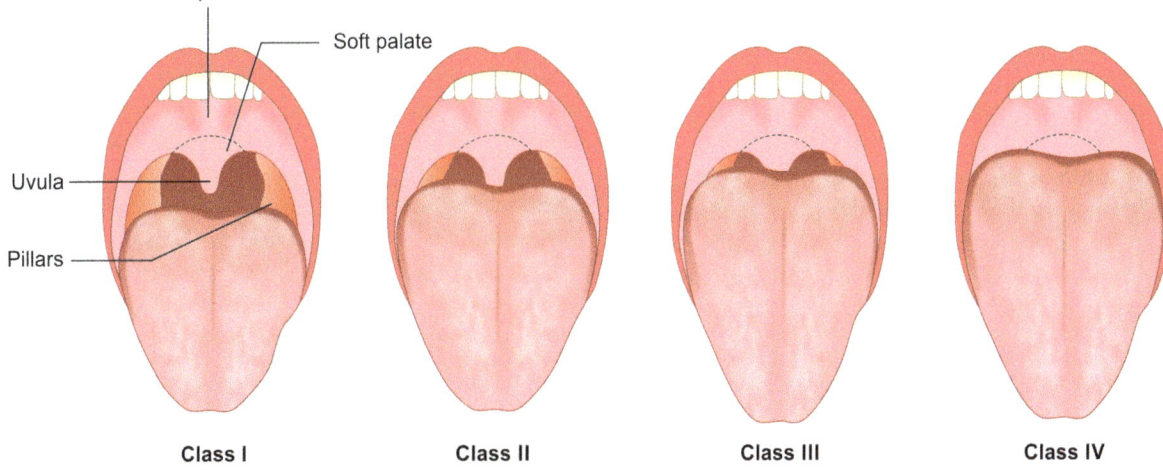

Fig. 15.1: Preanesthetic evaluation of oral cavity.

Patients with higher modified Mallampati scores are more difficult to intubate.

PREOPERATIVE LABORATORY TESTS

The indications for preoperative testing should be based on information obtained from medical records, patient's history, physical examination, and type and invasiveness of the planned procedure.

Routine preoperative laboratory tests in patients who are apparently healthy on clinical examination and history are not beneficial or cost effective **(Table 15.1)**.

RISK ASSESSMENT

Perioperative risk is cumulative and represents the risk associated with planned procedure, the risks associated with patients medical conditions and the type of anesthesia administered.

Risk assessment is vital for planning and execution of anesthesia for safety and comfort of the patient. Elevated risk may suggest the need for preoperative interventions, in-hospital care under specialists and enhanced postoperative monitoring and care in ICU set up.

ASA Physical Status

The American Society of Anesthesiologists physical status (ASA-PS) defines the overall health of the patient and is used extensively around the globe. ASA-PS is subjective and may vary among clinicians. Higher ASA-PS is associated with increased mortality **(Table 15.2)**.

Functional Status

Exercise tolerance is a major determinant of perioperative risk. It is usually evaluated by the estimated energy requirement for various activities and graded in metabolic equivalents (MET) on a scale defined by the Duke Activity Status Index **(Table 15.3)**. One MET represents the oxygen consumption of a resting adult (3.5 mL/kg/min). MET score of <4 represents poor exercise tolerance and increased perioperative risk **(Table 15.3)**.

Surgical Risk Assessment

Surgical procedures can be stratified into three categories, according to their level of perioperative physiological stress (risk of death or major adverse events) as per ACC/AHA 2007 guidelines on perioperative cardiovascular evaluation for noncardiac surgery **(Table 15.4)**.

Risk Mitigation Strategies

Risk mitigation strategies should be done to optimize the patient to a good clinical condition as possible. Factors that can be reversed like, anemia, smoking and substance abuse should be rectified at least before the elective procedure. The relative risk of pulmonary complications among smokers as compared with nonsmokers ranges from 1.4 to 4.3. Stopping smoking even 6 hours before surgery may allow the carbon monoxide levels in the blood to drop. It takes 8 weeks of smoking cessation to allow the mucociliary transport mechanism to recover and the secretions to decrease.

Adequate fasting orders before surgery **(Table 15.5)**, anxiety correction, antibiotic prophylaxis with prior sensitivity, local anesthesia sensitivity, optimum pain control and postoperative nausea and vomiting prophylaxis are few steps in risk mitigation.

Table 15.1: Indications for preoperative testing.	
Complete blood counts (Hemoglobin, Hematocrit, Total Leucocyte Count, Differential Leucocyte Count, Platelet Counts)	Major surgery, Chronic cardiovascular, pulmonary, renal or hepatic disease, Malignancy, Known or suspected anemia, bleeding diasthesis, myelosuppression, age <1
Coagulation studies (Prothrombin Time, Activated Partial Thromboplastin Time, International Normalized Ratio, Platelet Counts)	Liver diseases, Chronic renal diseases, Trauma, Bleeding tendencies, Anticoagulant therapy
Serum Electrolytes, Creatinine and Blood Urea Nitrogen	Hypertension, Heart failure, Diabetes, Renal disease, Pituitary or adrenal disease, Gastrointestinal disease (Vomiting, Diarrhea, long term parenteral diet) Diuretic therapy, Digoxin, ACE inhibitors, Angiotensin receptor blocker, NSAIDS, etc.
Random blood sugar and HbA1c	Diabetes, Steroids therapy, Obesity
Albumin, Liver function tests	Anasarca, Alcohol abuse, Liver disease,
Chest radiograph	Cardiovascular diseases, Hypertension, Pulmonary diseases, Tuberculosis, COPD, Cough, Dyspnea Radiotherapy to chest, lungs, breast and thorax
ECG	Cardiovascular diseases, palpitations, arrhythmia, chest pain, Dyspnea, Digoxin, Amiodarone, pacemakers
Urine analysis	Suspected urinary tract infections, surgical implantation of foreign materials (Joint prosthesis etc)
Arterial or venous blood gases (ABG/VBG)	Useful in assessing the oxygenation, ventilation, lactate levels, acid base balance, electrolytes. Benefits of being bed side and quick test
Pregnancy test	Should be considered for females of child bearing age

Table 15.2: ASA physical status.

ASA Physical Status	Definition	Example
ASA-PS I	A normal healthy patient	Healthy, non-smoker, non-alcoholic or minimal use
ASA-PS II	A patient with mild systemic disease (Mild diseases only without substantive functional limitations)	Current smoker, social alcohol drinker, pregnancy, obesity (BMI = 30–40), well-controlled DM/HTN, mild lung disease, normal pregnancy, well controlled gestational hypertension, controlled preeclampsia
ASA-PS III	A patient with severe systemic disease (With substantive functional limitations)	Poorly controlled DM or HTN, COPD, morbid obesity (BMI ≥40), active hepatitis, alcohol dependence or abuse, implanted pacemaker, moderate reduction of ejection fraction, ESRD undergoing regularly scheduled dialysis, premature infant PCA<60 weeks, history (>3 months) of MI, CVA, TIA, or CAD/stents. Severe preeclampsia
ASA-PS IV	A patient with severe systemic disease that is a constant threat to life	Recent (<3 months) MI, CVA, TIA, or CAD/stents, ongoing cardiac ischemia or severe valve dysfunction, severe reduction of ejection fraction, sepsis, DIC, ARDS, or ESRD not undergoing regularly scheduled dialysis
ASA-PS V	A moribund patient who is not expected to survive without the operation	Ruptured abdominal/thoracic aneurysm, massive trauma, intracranial bleed with mass effect, ischemic bowel in the face of significant cardiac pathology or multiple organ/system dysfunctions
ASA-PS VI	A declared brain-dead patient whose organs are being removed for donor purposes	

The addition of "E" to the numerical status denotes Emergency surgery (Example: IE, IIE, etc.)
(BMI: body mass index; DM: diabetes mellitus; HTN: hypertension; COPD: chronic obstructive pulmonary disease; ESRD: end-stage renal disease; PCA: post-conceptual age; MI: myocardial infarction; CVA: cerebrovascular accident; TIA: transient ischemic attack; CAD: coronary artery disease; DIC: disseminated intravascular coagulation; ARDS: acute respiratory distress syndrome)

Table 15.3: Evaluation of functional status.

1-4 MET's	Standard light home activities, walk around the house, walk on level ground for 1–2 blocks at 3–5 km/hr
5-9 MET's	Climb a flight of stairs, walk on level ground @ 6 km/hr walk up a hill, run short distance, moderate activities (playing golf, dancing, etc.)
>10 MET's	Strenuous activity (swimming, tennis, football, bicycle) Heavy professional work

Table 15.4: Surgical risk assessment.

High risk (Cardiac complication >5%)	Intermediate risk (Cardiac complication 1–5%)	Low risk (Cardiac complication <1%)
Emergency surgery	Abdominal or thoracic surgeries	Breast surgery
Aortic or major vascular surgery	Neurosurgery ENT surgery	Superficial surgery, eye surgery, ambulatory surgery
Surgery with large fluid shifts	Minor vascular surgery	Endoscopic surgery
Unstable hemodynamics	Orthopedic	Plastic and reconstructive surgery

Table 15.5: Recommended fasting guidelines to prevent aspiration.

Type of meal	Minimum fasting period
Clear liquids (water, no pulp juices, tea without milk, black coffee)	2 hours
Breast milk	4 hours
Nonhuman milk, infant formula feed	6 hours
Light meal (no fats) like toast	6 hours
Heavy meal (good fatty content)	8 hours

Clinical Pearls for Few Conditions

Hypertension

- Anxiety is common cause of hypertension in dental setup and anxiolytic should be administered.
- Asymptomatic patients on regular treatment with BP of <160/100 mm of Hg can undergo planned procedure.
- BP> 180/110 mm of Hg is a contraindication for elective procedure.
- Antihypertensive agents to be continued up to and including the day of surgery, except Angiotensin-converting enzyme (ACE) inhibitors and angiotensin II receptor blockers (ARBs).

Previous Myocardial Infarction

- Any event in the coronary circulation (ischemia, infarction, or revascularization), induces a high (within 6 weeks) to intermediate risk period (till 3 months).
- 3-month minimum delay is therefore indicated before elective procedure.

Informed Consent

Last process during preoperative evaluation is an informed consent by the patient or his guardian. Obtaining consent is a patient centric process that balances risks and benefits, while taking into account the patient's informed requirements. Communications of the risks, benefits and the available alternatives between the surgeon, anesthesiologists and the patient is a must. Maintenance of preoperative evaluation records is absolutely mandatory and documentation should never be missed.

- Emergency surgical procedure if required with proper consultation with a cardiologist and under the protection of beta-blockers, which reduces the cardiac complication rate in such patients.
- When possible, beta-blockers should be started days or weeks before elective surgery, with a target heart rate between 50 and 60 beats per minute.

Diabetes Mellitus

- Levels of HbA1c < 8% (long term glycemic control) should be the target for optimization before planned elective procedure.
- Adequate control of blood glucose concentration (< 180 mg/dL) must be established perioperative period and maintained until oral feeding is resumed after operation.
- Oral hypoglycemic agents are withheld the day of surgery for an agent with a short half-life and up to 48 hours preoperatively for a long acting agent.
- Hypoglycemia (glucose < 50 mg/dL in adults and < 40 mg/dL in children) may develop postoperatively due to residual effects of long-acting oral hypoglycemic agents.

Bronchial Asthma

- Asthma should be under control and the patient should be free of wheezing for elective procedure.
- Patients on regular medications should continue therapy; steroids supplement may be required during anesthesia.
- Avoid use of NSAIDs for pain, as patient may have aspirin-induced asthma.
- Inhalers should be handy and readily available during anesthesia.

Patients on Anticoagulant

- Warfarin is advised to be discontinued at least 5 days before surgery. Invasive elective surgery is generally safe (from major hemorrhagic complication) when the INR is ~1.5.
- If the surgery is emergent, the anticoagulation can rapidly be reversed through the administration of fresh frozen plasma, vitamin K, or prothrombin complex concentrate.
- Clopidogrel to be stopped 7 days prior to surgery, Ticlopidin should be discontinued 14 days prior to surgery.
- Most minor oral surgical procedures can be easily and safely performed while the patients continue their low dose aspirin therapy. There is very low risk of post-surgical bleeding.

Renal Insufficiency

- Patients with compensated renal disease can easily undergo day care oral surgery and dental extraction under local anesthesia.
- Patients on hemodialysis should undergo surgery on non-dialysis day to avoid problems with anticoagulation.
- In emergent situations heparin free dialysis can be asked to avoid problems with anticoagulation.
- Arterial blood gases (ABG) analysis is always helpful.

Test Paper

1. Which of the following clinical features is indicative of left ventricular failure?
   A. Neck vein distension B. Ascites
   C. Orthopnea D. Edema
2. Which of the following is a sign of aortic stenosis?
   A. Diastolic rumble
   B. An opening snap
   C. Loud second heart sound
   D. Harsh systolic murmur
3. All the following are cardiac risk factors, *except*:
   A. Hypertension B. Family history of CAD
   C. High levels of HDL D. Diabetes mellitus
4. All of the following features are seen in patients with pulmonary embolism, *except*:
   A. Cyanosis B. Hypoxia
   C. Bradycardia D. Right heart failure
5. A reduced one second forced expiratory volume to forced vital capacity is present in all the following, *except*:
   A. Allergic asthma B. Chronic bronchitis
   C. Emphysema D. Lung abscess
6. Match the following:
   A. VSD 1. Absent femoral pulses
   B. ASD 2. Continuous murmur
   C. PDA 3. Fixed, wide second heart sound
   D. Coarctation of aorta 4. Holosystolic murmur
7. Match the following:
   A. AS 1. Loud first heart sound
   B. MS 2. Parvus et tardus
   C. MR 3. Austin flint murmur
   D. AR 4. Pansystolic murmur
8. Match the following:
   A. Pulsus alternans 1. Cardiac tamponade
   B. Pulsus paradoxus 2. LVF
   C. Water-Hammer pulse 3. AF
   D. Irregularly irregular pulse 4. AR

9. Following are the features of iron deficiency anemia, *except*:
   A. Low serum ferritin
   B. Hypochromic microcytic
   C. Absent marrow iron on biopsy stain
   D. Decreased total iron binding capacity
10. All are true regarding idiopathic thrombocytopenic purpura, *except*:
    A. Steroids are used in treatment
    B. Splenomegaly is usually present
    C. Bone marrow reveals increased megakaryocytes
    D. Splenectomy can be effective therapy
11. All of the following patients may have DIC, *except*:
    A. Patients with gram-negative infections
    B. Patients with multiple trauma
    C. Patients with administered thrombolytic agents
    D. Patients with retained dead fetus
12. Hemolysis is indicated by all of the following, *except*:
    A. Increased LDH levels
    B. Shortened red blood cell survival
    C. Decreased number of reticulocytes
    D. Reduced serum haptoglobin
13. All the following can cause inflammatory bloody diarrhea, *except*:
    A. *Entamoeba histolytica* B. *Giardia lamblia*
    C. *Campylobacter jejuni* D. *Shigella* species
14. Following is not true regarding Plummer-Vinson syndrome:
    A. Esophageal webs are present
    B. Webs may be associated with iron deficiency anemia
    C. Also known as Paterson-Kelly syndrome
    D. Lesions are not premalignant
15. Therapy of ascites includes all the following, *except*:
    A. Diuretics
    B. Paracentesis
    C. Unrestricted salt intake
    D. Bedrest

16. **Rifampicin is used in:**
    A. Treatment of tuberculosis
    B. Prevention of meningococcal meningitis
    C. Treatment of staphylococcal endocarditis
    D. All of the above

17. **Match the following:**
    A. Cough   1. Calcium channel blockers
    B. Gingival hyperplasia   2. Beta blockers
    C. Precipitation of   3. ACE inhibitors
       asthma
    D. Hypokalemia   4. Diuretics

18. **Limb edema can occur with the use of following drug:**
    A. Beta blockers   B. Calcium channel blockers
    C. Diuretics   D. Nitrates

19. **Following is a cause of secondary hypertension:**
    A. Eclampsia   B. Renovascular
    C. Coarctation of aorta D. All of the above

20. **Which of the following is given to prevent isoniazid induced neuropathy?**
    A. Steroids   B. Folic acid
    C. Vitamin B_{12} D. Pyridoxine

21. **Match the following:**
    A. Rheumatic fever   1. H. infuenzae
    B. Subacute endocarditis   2. S. aureus
    C. Nosocomial   3. Group A Sreptococcus pneumoniae
    D. Meningitis in children 4. Streptococcos viridans

22. **Match the following:**
    A. Rifampicin   1. Optic neuritis
    B. Ethambutol   2. Ototoxicity
    C. Streptomycin   3. Neuropathy
    D. Isoniazid   4. Thrombocytopenia

23. **The most common organism for lobar pneumonia is:**
    A. S. aureus
    B. S. pneumoniae
    C. Mycoplasma pneumoniae
    D. Gram-negative bacteria

24. **Which of the following should be avoided in treatment of tuberculosis in mild-to-moderate renal failure?**
    A. Rifampicin   B. Pyrazinamide
    C. Isoniazid   D. Streptomycin

25. **All the following can cause hypercalcemia, *except*:**
    A. Sarcoidosis
    B. Multiple myeloma
    C. Tumor lysis syndrome
    D. Prolonged immobilization

26. **A 52-year-old female with type 2 diabetes is found to have 24-hour urinary proteinuria of 280 mg. Which of the following drug should be used to retard progression of renal disease?**
    A. Aspirin   B. Thiazide
    C. Ramipril   D. Amiloride

27. **In a patient of *Listeria meningitis* who is allergic to penicillin, the antimicrobial of choice is:**
    A. Gentamicin
    B. Ceftriaxone
    C. Trimethoprim-sulphamethoxazole
    D. Vancomycin

28. **All the following can cause megakaryocytic thrombocytopenia, *except*:**
    A. Aplastic anemia
    B. Systemic lupus erythematosus
    C. Disseminated intravascular coagulation
    D. Idiopathic thrombocytopenic purpura

29. **The following tests may be abnormal in disseminated intravascular coagulation, *except*:**
    A. D-dimer level
    B. Clot solubility
    C. Prothrombin time (PT)
    D. Activated partial thromboplastin time (APTT)

30. **A patient of acute leukemia is admitted with febrile neutropenia. On day four of being treated with broad spectrum antibiotics, his fever increases. Which of the following should be most appropriate next step in the management?**
    A. Add antiviral therapy   B. Add antifungal therapy
    C. Add cotrimoxazole   D. Continue chemotherapy

31. **A 28-year-old man is noted to have blood pressure of 180/104 mmHg. He has prominent ejection click in aortic area and murmurs heard over the ribs on both sides anteriorly and posteriorly. In addition, the pulses in the lower extremities are feeble and he complains of mild claudication with exertion. The most likely diagnosis is:**
    A. Cardiomyopathy   B. Atrial septal defect
    C. Coarctation of aorta D. Aortic stenosis

32. **All the following are true about therapy for tuberculosis, *except*:**
    A. Hyperuricemia is a side effect of pyrazinamide
    B. Red-green color impairment is a sign of ethambutol toxicity
    C. Ethambutol accumulates in renal failure
    D. 'Flu-like syndrome' is usually seen in people taking rifampicin on daily basis

33. **Which of the following organisms, when isolated in blood, requires the synergistic activity of penicillin plus an aminoglycoside for appropriate therapy?**
    A. Enterococcus faecalis
    B. S. aureus
    C. Streptococcus pneumoniae
    D. Bacteroides fragilis

34. **All the following can cause DIC, *except*:**
    A. Amniotic fluid embolism
    B. Intrauterine fetal death
    C. Diabetes mellitus
    D. Abruptio placentae

35. **Epstein-Barr virus is associated with:**
    A. Carcinoma larynx
    B. Carcinoma bladder
    C. Carcinoma nasopharynx
    D. Carcinoma maxilla

36. **A 12-year-old girl has history of recurrent bulky stools and abdominal pain since 3 years of age. She has pallor and her weight and height are below the third percentile. Which of the following is the most appropriate investigation to make a specific diagnosis?**
    A. Barium studies
    B. D-xylose test

C. 24-hour fecal fat estimation
D. Endoscopy and small intestinal biopsy

37. A child underwent a tonsillectomy at 6 years of age with no complications. He underwent a preoperative screening for bleeding at the age of 12 years before an elective laparotomy and was found to have a prolonged partial thromboplastin time but normal prothrombin time. There was no family history of bleeding. The patient is likely to have:
    A. Acquired liver disease
    B. Acquired vitamin K deficiency
    C. Mild hemophilia A
    D. Factor XII deficiency

38. Endosopic biopsy from a case of *H. pylori* related early chronic gastritis is most likely to reveal:
    A. Multifocal atrophic gastritis
    B. Erosive gastritis
    C. Antral predominant gastritis
    D. Gastric atrophy

39. All the following diseases cause massive splenomegaly, *except*:
    A. Malaria
    B. Kala azar
    C. Idiopathic myelofibrosis
    D. Infective endocarditis

40. A 10-day-old neonate is posted for pyloric stenosis surgery. The investigations report shows a serum calcium level of 6.0 mg/dL. What information would you like to know before you supplement calcium to this neonate?
    A. Blood glucose
    B. Serum bilirubin
    C. Serum albumin
    D. Oxygen saturation

41. All the following drugs are used in the management of status epilepticus, *except*:
    A. Phenytoin
    B. Thiopentone sodium
    C. Carbamazepine
    D. Diazepam

42. Urgent reversal of warfarin therapy can be done by administration of:
    A. Platelet concentrates
    B. Cryoprecipitate
    C. Fresh frozen plasma
    D. Packed red blood cell

43. Which of the following is generally not seen in idiopathic thrombocytopenic purpura (ITP)?
    A. Petechiae, ecchymosis and bleeding
    B. Palpable splenomegaly
    C. More common in females
    D. Increased megakaryocytes in the bone marrow

44. A young patient presenting with massive hematemesis was found to have splenomegaly. In this case, the most likely source of bleeding is:
    A. Duodenal ulcer
    B. Esophageal varices
    C. Erosive gastritis
    D. Gastric ulcer

45. Following resuscitation, a patient with bleeding esophageal varices should be treated initially with:
    A. Sclerotherapy
    B. Sengstaken-Blackmore tube
    C. Propranolol
    D. Surgery

46. In which of the States in India the maximum number of AIDS cases have been reported till now:
    A. Delhi
    B. Kerala
    C. Tamil Nadu
    D. Bihar

47. Most sensitive test to detect hypothyroidism is:
    A. T_3
    B. T_4
    C. TSH
    D. Radioactive iodine uptake

48. Following is not an anterior pituitary hormone:
    A. FSH
    B. TSH
    C. ACTH
    D. ADH

49. HIV positive patients usually have:
    A. Low CD_4, low CD_8
    B. High CD_4, low CD_8
    C. Low CD_4, high CD_8
    D. High CD_4, high CD_8

50. Which of the following mediators is released during late phase reaction of anaphylactic reaction?
    A. Eosinophil chemotactic factor (ECF-A)
    B. Histamine
    C. Leukotriene B_4
    D. Angiotensinogen

51. IgE-mediated hypersensitivity is implicated in all of the following reactions, *except*:
    A. Serum sickness
    B. Latex anaphylaxis
    C. Systemic reaction to insect sting
    D. Asthma

52. Following are indications of surgery in endocarditis, *except*:
    A. Congestive heart failure
    B. Fungal endocarditis
    C. History of injection drug use
    D. Failure to respond to antibiotic therapy

53. Generalized lymphadenopathy is found in all, *except*:
    A. Infectious mononucleosis
    B. HIV-1
    C. Malaria
    D. Syphilis

54. Bacterial and viral meningitis are characterized by all, *except*:
    A. Neck rigidity
    B. Increased protein in CSF
    C. Increased cells in CSF
    D. Decreased CSF glucose

55. Which of the following hormones is given in cases of hypothyroidism?
    A. TSH
    B. T_3
    C. T_4
    D. Thyroglobulin

56. All the following are features of diabetic ketoacidosis, *except*:
    A. Glycosuria
    B. Decreased peripheral utilization of glucose
    C. Decreased lipolysis
    D. Increased protein catabolism

57. A 37-year-old patient presented with generalized repetitive convulsions for 35 minutes. He is given 10 mg of diazepam intravenously. The next appropriate step would be to administer:
    A. Carbamazepine orally
    B. Phenytoin intravenously
    C. Phenobarbitone intravenously
    D. Conazepam orally

58. Chronic type A gastritis is characterized by all the following clinical findings, *except*:
    A. Pernicious anemia
    B. Presence of parietal cell antibody
    C. Antral involvement
    D. Associated other autoimmune disorder

59. A person vaccinated against hepatitis B will have following serologic finding:
    A. Hepatitis B surface antigen (HBsAg)
    B. Hepatitis B surface antibody (anti-HBs)
    C. Both HBsAg and anti-HBs
    D. Hepatitis Be antibody
60. All the following can precipitate hepatic encephalopathy in patients of cirrhosis:
    A. Gastrointestinal bleeding
    B. SBP
    C. Ampicillin therapy
    D. Sedatives
61. A positive Chovstek's sign is found in:
    A. Hyperkalemia   B. Hypocalcemia
    C. Acidosis   D. Hypoglycemia
62. In pseudohypoparathyroidism the lab test reveal:
    A. Low calcium and high PTH (parathyroid hormone)
    B. High calcium and low PTH
    C. High calcium and high PTH
    D. Low calcium and low PTH
63. All the following features may be in hyperthyroidism, *except*:
    A. Atrial fibrillation   B. Pretibial myxedema
    C. Constipation   D. Lid lag
64. Crackles are present in which of the following condition:
    A. Pleural effusion   B. Pneumothorax
    C. Left ventricular failure D. Emphysema
65. A 50-year-old asymptomatic patient has fasting blood glucose of 132 mg% on routine examination, he has:
    A. Normal report
    B. Diabetes mellitus
    C. Impaired fasting glucose
    D. Impaired glucose tolerance
66. Which of the following tests is most appropriate to know glucose control in diabetic patients?
    A. Fasting glucose   B. Postprandial glucose
    C. Urinary glucose   D. Glycated hemoglobin
67. A patient with lung malignancy has presented with nausea, vomiting, weakness and serum calcium value of 14.5 mg%. First line step would be to administer:
    A. Oral prednisolone
    B. Mithramycin
    C. Insulin
    D. Intravenous saline and frusemide
68. The definitive diagnosis of pulmonary embolism is best made by:
    A. ABG analysis   B. Chest X-ray
    C. Ventilation perfusion scan
    D. Pulmonary angiography
69. Clubbing may be seen in all the following conditions, *except*:
    A. Fallot's tetralogy   B. Eisenmenger syndrome
    C. Infective endocarditis D. Constrictive pericarditis
70. A female patient has presented with a history of menorrhagia and easy bruising. Lab studies show a normal PT, a prolonged APTT and prolonged bleeding time. The most likely diagnosis is:
    A. Hemophilia
    B. Factor IX deficiency
    C. von Willebrand's disease
    D. Severe hepatic dysfunction
71. A patient has serum calcium of 13.5 mg% on routine examination. Which of the following would be most appropriate test to diagnose primary hyperparathyroidism?
    A. Serum phosphate
    B. Ultrasound of the neck
    C. Serum parathyroid levels
    D. Serum ionized calcium
72. The side effects of thiazide diuretic therapy is:
    A. Hypoglycemia   B. Hyperuricemia
    C. Cough   D. Bronchospasm
73. All the following are causes of eosinophilia, *except*:
    A. Ascaris infestation
    B. Nitrofurantoin therapy
    C. Enteric fever
    D. Allergic bronchopulmonary aspergilosis (ABPA)
74. Following are features of enteric fever, *except*:
    A. Splenomegaly   B. Rose spots
    C. Relative tachycardia D. Leukopenia
75. A patient has fasting blood sugar level of 98 mg/dL and has 182 mg% blood sugar level 2 hour after glucose load (GTT). A patient is having:
    A. Diabetes mellitus
    B. Impaired fasting glucose
    C. Impaired glucose tolerance
    D. Diabetic ketoacidosis
76. A patient has purpura with a platelet count of 2 lacs/mm³. Following may be the possibilities, *except*:
    A. Henoch-Schönlein purpura
    B. Uremia
    C. ITP
    D. Vasculitis
77. Cryoprecipitate is rich in:
    A. All coagulation factors
    B. All coagulation factors and platelets
    C. Factor VIII, vWF and fibrinogen
    D. Platelets and leukocytes
78. Serum creatinine is generally normal in:
    A. Acute renal failure
    B. Nephrotic syndrome
    C. End-stage renal disease
    D. Nephritic syndrome
79. Following is true in Gilbert's syndrome:
    A. Raised alkaline phosphates
    B. Unconjugated hyperbilirubinemia
    C. High ALT and AST
    D. Tender hepatomegaly
80. Which of the following is not an oral manifestation of HIV?
    A. Hairy leukoplakia   B. Papillomavirus (warts)
    C. Candidiasis   D. *P. carinii*
81. Which of the following is not matched properly?
    A. Primary syphilis – chancre
    B. Tertiary syphilis – gumma
    C. Secondary syphilis – mulberry molars
    D. Congenital syphilis – Hutchinson's teeth
82. HIV can be confirmed and detected by:
    A. Polymerase chain reaction (PCR)
    B. Reverse transcriptase – PCR (RT-PCR)

C. Real-time PCR
D. Mimic PCR

83. Patients infected with HIV may have:
    A. Elevated blastogenesis
    B. Depressed serum immunoglobulin levels
    C. High T4-T8 ratio
    D. Thrombocytopenia

84. AIDS is associated with depletion of:
    A. T4 lymphocytes   B. T8 Lymphocytes
    C. B lymphocytes   D. Monocytes

85. AIDS is frequently complicated by opportunistic infections, notably pneumonia due to:
    A. *Klebsiella pneumoniae*
    B. *Pneumocystis carinii*
    C. *Streptococcus pneumoniae*
    D. *Mycoplasma pneumoniae*

86. Diagnosis of typhoid fever in the first week is made by following test:
    A. Widal test   B. Stool culture
    C. Urine culture   D. Blood culture

87. Causes of chest pain include all, *except*:
    A. Prinzmetal's angina   B. Pericarditis
    C. Aortic stenosis   D. Mitral stenosis

88. Which of the following is used in hypertensive crisis?
    A. Atenolol
    B. Thiazides
    C. Enalapril
    D. Nitroglycerine or nitroprusside

89. Multiple myeloma is commonly associated with all, *except*:
    A. Anemia
    B. High serum calcium
    C. High serum alkaline phosphatase
    D. High ESR

90. Following type of insulin has longest duration of action:
    A. Regular   B. Lispro
    C. Aspart   D. Glargine

91. Hypoglycemia may occur in:
    A. Insulin overdose   B. Insulinoma
    C. Severe hepatitis   D. All of the above

92. Polyurea is seen with:
    A. Diabetes mellitus   B. Diabetes insipidus
    C. Hyperparathyroidism   D. All of the above

93. Earliest indication of diabetic nephropathy is:
    A. Hematuria   B. Oliguria
    C. Proteinuria   D. Raised serum creatinine

94. Hypovolemic shock occurs when intravenous volume is decreased by:
    A. 5%   B. 15%
    C. 25%   D. 40%

95. Which of the following drugs is bacteriostatic?
    A. Rifampicin   B. Pyrazinamide
    C. Isoniazid   D. Ethambutol

96. Dressler syndrome is a complication of:
    A. Hypertension   B. Pericarditis
    C. Mitral stenosis D. Myocardial infarction

97. Most sensitive marker of MI is:
    A. Troponin T   B. CPK
    C. SGOT   D. LDH

98. All the following are true for hemophilia A, *except*:
    A. Increased PT   B. Increased APTT
    C. Soft tissue hematoma D. Decreased factor VIII

99. Which of the following is not used in the treatment of peptic ulcer?
    A. Omeprazole   B. Itraconazole
    C. Rabeprazole   D. Pantaprazole

100. Which of the following is used in CML?
    A. Cyclophosphamide   B. Imatinib mesylate
    C. Prednisolone   D. Chlorambucil

101. Normal daily excretion of protein in urine is:
    A. <150 mg   B. <300 mg
    C. <500 mg   D. <1000 mg

102. Carbamazepine is used to treat the following, *except*:
    A. Partial seizures
    B. Trigeminal neuralgia
    C. Postherpetic neuralgia
    D. Tension headache

103. Déjà vu phenomenon is associated with:
    A. Absence seizures
    B. Grand mal seizures
    C. Simple partial seizures
    D. Complex partial seizures

104. Recently identified liver protein which regulates iron metabolism is:
    A. Hepadna   B. Haptoglobin
    C. Hepcidin   D. Transferrin receptor

105. Iron therapy is not indicated in:
    A. Chronic blood loss   B. Pregnancy
    C. CRF   D. Thalassemia minor

106. Anemia of chronic inflammation has following features, *except*:
    A. Low ferritin   B. Normal bone marrow iron
    C. Low serum iron   D. Low TIBC

107. Infective endocarditis is least likely to occur in:
    A. VSD   B. Fallot's tetralogy
    C. ASD   D. Coarctation of aorta

108. Infective endocarditis is suggested by all, *except*:
    A. Clubbing   B. Splenomegaly
    C. Osler's node   D. Berry's aneurysm

109. The cardiac valve affected in the infective endocarditis in IV drug abusers is:
    A. Mitral   B. Tricuspid
    C. Aortic   D. Pulmonary

110. Black water fever is a feature of:
    A. Kala azar   B. Malaria
    C. Enteric fever   D. Dengue fever

111. Which of the antitubercular drugs mostly interferes with antiretroviral therapy?
    A. INH   B. Rifampicin
    C. PAS   D. Streptomycin

112. Which of the following drugs can precipitate hemolysis in G6PD deficiency?
    A. Chloroquine   B. Primaquine
    C. Mefloquine   D. Quinine

113. Type of malaria generally not found in India:
    A. *P. ovale*   B. *P. vivax*
    C. *P. malariae*   D. *P. falciparum*

114. 'P' wave is absent in:
    A. Atrial flutter   B. Atrial fibrillation
    C. Complete heart block D. Second degree heart block
115. Indicator of active replication of hepatitis B virus is:
    A. HBsAg   B. HBcAg
    C. HBeAg   D. Anti-HBe
116. Austin Flint murmur may be mistaken for:
    A. MR   B. MS
    C. TS   D. PR
117. Match the following:
    A. Graham Steel murmur   1. AR
    B. Mid-diastolic murmur 2. VSD
    C. Pansystolic murmur   3. PR
    D. Early diastolic murmur 4. MS
118. Collapsing pulse may be present in all the following, *except*:
    A. AR   B. PDA
    C. Severe anemia D. AS
119. Following drugs cause bronchodilatation, *except*:
    A. Salbutamol B. Terbutaline
    C. Corticosteroids D. Ipratropium bromide
120. Clopidogrel is a following agent:
    A. Antiplatelet B. Throbolytic
    C. Fibrinolytic D. Anticoagulant
121. Following are causes of hypocalcemia, *except*:
    A. Hypomagnesemia B. Acute pancreatitis
    C. Milk alkali syndrome D. Hypoparathyroidism
122. Following is associated with high mortality if it occurs during pregnancy:
    A. Hepatitis A B. Hepatitis B
    C. Hepatitis C D. Hepatitis E
123. Drug of choice in trigeminal neuralgia is:
    A. Carbamazepine B. Phenobarbitone
    C. Beta blockers D. Verapamil
124. Pulmonary oligemia is characteristically seen in:
    A. ASD   B. VSD
    C. PDA   D. Fallot's tetralogy
125. All the following are associated with infranuclear facial palsy, *except*:
    A. Bell's palsy B. Acoustic neuroma
    C. Cerebral infarction D. Middle ear disease
126. In adults, the spinal cord normally ends at:
    A. Lower border of L_1 B. Lower border of L_3
    C. Lower border of S_1 D. Lower border of L_5
127. Iron is present in all the following, *except*:
    A. Myoglobin   B. Cytochrome
    C. Catalase   D. Pyruvate kinase
128. The National AIDS Control Program has the following components, *except*:
    A. Serosurveillance.
    B. Health education and information
    C. Screening of blood and blood products
    D. Banning of sexual contact with foreigners
129. The antibiotic cover is mandatory before extraction in the following condition of the heart:
    A. Ischemic heart disease (IHD)
    B. Hypertension
    C. Congestive cardiac failure
    D. Congenital heart disease
130. Blue sclera is characteristic of:
    A. Amelogenesis imperfecta
    B. Tetracycline hypoplasia
    C. Fluorosis
    D. Osteogenesis imperfecta
131. Bence Jones protein found in the urine may be suggestive of:
    A. Hyperparathyroidim B. Hodgkin's disease
    C. Multiple myeloma D. Christian's syndrome
132. The syndrome which is associated with predisposition to the development of carcinoma of oral mucous membrane is:
    A. Gardner's syndrome
    B. Osler-Rendu-Weber syndrome
    C. Sturge-Weber syndrome
    D. Plummer-Vinson syndrome
133. The most preferred approach for pituitary surgery at present is:
    A. Transcranial B. Transethmoidal
    C. Transphenoidal D. Transcallosal
134. The normal range of serum osmolality (in mOsm/kg H_2O) is:
    A. 275–295   B. 310–330
    C. 350–375   D. 200–250
135. Afferent component of corneal reflex is mediated by:
    A. Vagus nerve
    B. Facial nerve
    C. Trigeminal nerve
    D. Glossopharyngeal nerve
136. Ground glass appearance in bone is seen in:
    A. Hyperparathyroidism
    B. Fibrous dysplasia
    C. Condensing osteitis
    D. Osteopetrosis
137. An affected male infant born to normal parents could be an example of all the following, *except*:
    A. An autosomal dominant disorder
    B. An autosomal recessive disorder
    C. A polygenic disorder
    D. A vertically transmitted disorder
138. Nevirapine is a:
    A. Protease inhibitor
    B. Nucleoside reverse transcriptase inhibitor
    C. Non-nucleoside reverse transcriptase inhibitor
    D. Fusion inhibitor
139. All the following are the known causes of osteoporosis, *except*:
    A. Fluorosis   B. Hypogonadism
    C. Hyperthyroidism D. Hyperparathyroidism
140. All the following are risk factors for atherosclerosis, *except*:
    A. Increased waist-hip ratio
    B. Hyperhomocysteinemia
    C. Decreased fibrinogen levels
    D. Decreased HDL levels
141. All the following antibacterial agents act by inhibiting cell wall synthesis, *except*:
    A. Carbapenems B. Monobactams
    C. Cephamycins D. Nitrofurantoin

142. A diabetic patient developed cellutitis due to *Staphylococcus aureus*, which was found to be methicillin resistant on the antibiotic sensitivity testing. All the following antibiotics will be appropriate, *except*:
    A. Vancomycin
    B. Imipenem
    C. Teicoplanin
    D. Linezolid

143. Calcitonin is secreted by:
    A. Thyroid gland
    B. Parathyroid gland
    C. Adrenal glands
    D. Ovaries

144. Bisphosphonates act by:
    A. Increasing the osteoid formation
    B. Increasing the mineralization of osteoid
    C. Decreasing the osteoclast-mediated resorption of bone
    D. Decreasing the parathyroid hormone secretion

145. Brown tumors are seen in:
    A. Hyperparathyroidism
    B. Pigmented villonodular synovitis
    C. Osteomalacia
    D. Neurofibromatosis

146. Megaloblastic anemia due to folic acid deficiency is commonly due to:
    A. Inadequate dietary intake
    B. Defective intestinal absorption
    C. Absence of folic acid binding protein in serum
    D. Absence of glutamic acid in the intestine

147. Which one of the following drugs is an antipseudomonal penicillin?
    A. Cephalexin
    B. Cloxacillin
    C. Piperacillin
    D. Dicloxacillin

148. All of the following are therapeutic uses of penicillin G, *except*:
    A. Bacterial meningitis
    B. Rickettsial infection
    C. Syphillis
    D. Anthrax

149. Which of the following organs is not involved in calcium homeostasis?
    A. Kidneys
    B. Skin
    C. Intestines
    D. Lungs

150. Mycotic aneurysm is due to:
    A. Bacterial infection
    B. Fungal infection
    C. Viral infection
    D. Mixed infection

Answers

CHAPTER 1: CLINICAL METHODS

Multiple Choice Questions

1. B   2. B   3. C   4. C   5. C   6. B
7. C   8. E   9. D   10. B   11. C   12. B
13. C   14. C   15. B   16. C   17. B   18. B
19. A   20. C   21. D   22. D   23. D   24. D
25. A   26. A   27. B   28. C   29. A

Fill in the Blanks

1. Coarctation of aorta
2. Left ventricular failure
3. 4
4. Kussmaul's breathing
5. Tricuspid regurgitation
6. <60
7. >100
8. 12 –16
9. Frequent ectopics
10. Hepatic failure
11. Carbon monoxide poisoning
12. Cheyne-Stokes respiration
13. Enteric fever
14. Hodgkin's lymphoma

CHAPTER 2: GASTROINTESTINAL SYSTEM

Multiple Choice Questions

1. B   2. D   3. C   4. C   5. D   6. A
7. B   8. A   9. A   10. D   11. D   12. A
13. B   14. D   15. C   16. A   17. A   18. A
19. C   20. C

Fill in the Blanks

1. Hematemesis
2. Malabsorption (steatorrhea)
3. Ascites
4. Cushing's ulcer
5. Curling's ulcer
6. Proximal small intestine

CHAPTER 3: HEPATOBILIARY SYSTEM

Multiple Choice Questions

1. C   2. A   3. B   4. D   5. C   6. D
7. D   8. D   9. B   10. D   11. D   12. C
13. C   14. D   15. C   16. D   17. B   18. A
19. B   20. D   21. D   22. C   23. C   24. D
25. D   26. C   27. C   28. B   29. C   30. A
31. D   32. A   33. D   34. B

Fill in the Blanks

1. 10–12 mmHg
2. Caput medusae
3. 0.3-1 mg/dL
4. Liver
5. II, VII, IX, X
6. Alcoholic hepatitis
7. Liver
8. Fetor hepaticus

9. Ascites
10. Cirrhosis of liver

CHAPTER 4: HEMATOLOGICAL SYSTEM

Multiple Choice Questions

1. C   2. C   3. A   4. D   5. C   6. D
7. A   8. B   9. D   10. A   11. B   12. B
13. C   14. B   15. C   16. B   17. A   18. A
19. B   20. B   21. D   22. B   23. C   24. D
25. B   26. D   27. C   28. B   29. C   30. D
31. C   32. B   33. A

Fill in the Blanks

1. ALL
2. CML
3. PT
4. Heparin
5. Iron deficiency anemia
6. Low
7. CML
8. 10,000/µL
9. Hodgkin's disease
10. Hemolytic
11. vWD
12. Metastasis
13. Left supraclavicular LN due to metastasis
14. Vitamin B_{12}
15. Vitamin B_{12}
16. More than 8 cm from left costal margin
17. Cervical
18. Tuberculosis
19. Ferrous sulfate 200 mg tds
20. Raised
21. Iron deficiency anemia
22. 40–440/µL
23. 120 days
24. Megaloblastic
25. Malabsorption of vitamin B_{12}

CHAPTER 5: CARDIOVASCULAR SYSTEM

Multiple Choice Questions

1. B   2. C   3. B   4. C   5. B   6. A
7. A   8. C   9. C   10. A   11. D   12. C
13. D   14. D   15. B   16. B   17. B   18. B
19. B   20. C   21. A   22. A   23. D   24. C
25. A

Fill in the Blanks

1. PDA
2. AR
3. Acute rheumatic fever
4. Eisenmenger syndrome
5. Pulmonary hypertension
6. VSD
7. PDA
8. Ostium secundum
9. Calcium channel blocker
10. Heart failure
11. 120–139 and 80–89 mm Hg
12. No
13. SABE
14. Coarctation of aorta
15. SABE
16. AR
17. ASD
18. Loud
19. Left
20. Penicillin V, sulfadiazine, benzathine penicillin

CHAPTER 6: RESPIRATORY DISEASES

Multiple Choice Questions

1. D   2. C   3. D   4. C   5. A   6. A
7. D   8. C   9. A   10. D   11. C   12. C
13. C   14. D   15. C   16. B   17. C   18. C
19. D   20. D   21. C   22. B   23. D   24. B
25. B   26. A   27. D   28. A   29. D   30. A
31. A   32. B   33. A   34. A   35. C   36. A
37. D   38. D   39. D   40. A   41. A   42. C
43. D   44. D   45. A   46. D   47. A   48. D

Fill in the Blanks

1. Right ventricle
2. Anaerobic
3. Pulmonary edema
4. *S. pneumoniae*
5. Gram-negative bacteria
6. Emphysema
7. Decreased
8. Crackles
9. Wheeze
10. Stridor
11. Ghon's lesion
12. Chyene-Stokes breathing
13. COPD
14. Diethylcarbamazine
15. Emphysema
16. Pleuritis
17. Egophony
18. PaO_2 80–100 mm Hg
19. $PaCO_2$ 35–45 mm Hg
20. pH 7.38–7.44
21. Triglycerides, cholesterol
22. Isoniazid, Rifampici

23. Calcification, Fibrosis
24. 12, 200
25. Resistant Asthma
26. LAMA
27. Adeno
28. Small Cell
29. Exudative, Transudative

CHAPTER 7: RENAL DISEASES

Multiple Choice Questions

1. B 2. B 3. C 4. D 5. C 6. B
7. D 8. C 9. B 10. B 11. A 12. D
13. C 14. C 15. D 16. A 17. D 18. A
19. B 20. C 21. D 22. A 23. D 24. C
25. B 26. B 27. C 28. B

Fill in the Blanks

1. 3.5 g
2. 400 mL
3. Azotemia
4. 20–40 mg/dL
5. <1.5 mg/dL
6. 5.5–8 g/dL and 3.5–5.5 g/dL
7. 10–15

CHAPTER 8: NERVOUS SYSTEM

Multiple Choice Questions

1. A 2. A 3. A 4. A 5. C 6. A
7. D 8. B 9. C 10. C 11. D 12. D
13. D 14. C 15. C 16. A 17. C 18. B
19. A 20. A 21. D 22. D 23. C 24. D
25. C 26. C 27. C 28. D 29. A 30. A
31. B 32. D

Fill in the Blanks

1. Todd's palsy
2. Trigeminal neuralgia
3. Complication of injection therapy in trigeminal neuralgia
4. Common migraine
5. <5/mm³ lymphoytes
6. Tuberculous
7. Cryptococcal
8. Stapedius
9. Chorda tympani
10. Temporal and frontal lobes
11. Meningococcal meningitis
12. Meningococcal meningitis
13. Inhalation of 100% oxygen
14. Coronary artery disease and uncontrolled hypertension
15. Cribriform plate

CHAPTER 9: ENDOCRINE AND METABOLIC DISORDERS

Multiple Choice Questions

1. B 2. D 3. A 4. C 5. C 6. B
7. C 8. C 9. B 10. C 11. A 12. C
13. A 14. B 15. B 16. D 17. D 18. D
19. B 20. D 21. D 22. D 23. D 24. C
25. C 26. A 27. D 28. B 29. B 30. B
31. C

Fill in the Blanks

1. Cushing's syndrome
2. T_3
3. Hypocalcemia
4. 9–10.5 mg/dL
5. Hypocalcemic tetany
6. Graves' disease
7. Pseudohypoparathyroidism
8. Parathyroid adenoma
9. Chronic hypocalcemia due to hypoparathyroidism
10. >126 mg/dL
11. 100, 126 mg/dL
12. Kussmaul's breathing
13. 30–300 mg
14. ACE inhibitors
15. Regular insulin

CHAPTER 10: INFECTIONS

Multiple Choice Questions

1. B 2. B 3. B 4. C 5. C 6. C
7. A 8. B 9. C 10. C 11. B 12. B
13. B 14. C 15. B 16. C 17. C 18. B
19. B 20. C 21. C 22. B 23. B 24. C
25. D 26. B 27. B 28. D 29. C 30. D
31. C 32. D 33. C 34. C 35. B 36. C
37. D 38. A 39. D 40. D

Fill in the Blanks

1. Rubella
2. Congenital syphilis
3. Tertiary syphilis
4. Benzathine penicillin G
5. *Treponema pallidum*
6. Falciparum
7. Malaria
8. *Entamoeba histolytica*

9. Amoebic liver abscess
10. Diphtheria
11. <90%, > 30/Min

CHAPTER 11: MEDICAL EMERGENCIES IN DENTAL PRACTICE

Multiple Choice Questions

1. A   2. B   3. A   4. C   5. B   6. D
7. C   8. C   9. B

Fill in the Blanks

1. Vasovagal syncope
2. > 20 mm Hg, > 10 mm Hg
3. Frusemide
4. Sublingual nitroglycerine
5. Intravenous diazepam or lorazepam

CHAPTER 12: CRITICAL CARE

Multiple Choice Questions

1. D   2. C   3. C   4. C   5. C   6. C
7. D   8. D   9. C   10. C

Fill in the Blanks

1. > 20%
2. Leukocytohosis and leukopeni
3. Acute myocardial infarction
4. <60
5. 2 minutes

CHAPTER 13: ANAPHYLAXIS AND DRUG ALLERGY

Multiple Choice Questions

1. B   2. B   3. D   4. B   5. D   6. A
7. D   8. A   9. C   10. B

Fill in the Blanks

1. IgE
2. Anaphylactoid reactions
3. Adrenaline
4. >30%
5. Histamine, prostaglandin (PGD2)

CHAPTER 14: NUTRITION

Multiple Choice Questions

1. B   2. D   3. D   4. B   5. A   6. D
7. D   8. B   9. C   10. B   11. C   12. A

13. A   14. A   15. A   16. A   17. A   18. C
19. B   20. A   21. B   22. B   23. C   24. C
25. C   26. A   27. A   28. A   29. C   30. B

Fill in the Blanks

1. Niacin
2. Thiamine
3. Vitamin A
4. Vitamin A
5. Vitamin D
6. Vitamin K
7. Vitamin B_{12}
8. Polished rice
9. Riboflavin
10. Pyridoxine
11. Niacin

ANSWERS TO TEST PAPER

1. C   2. D   3. C   4. C   5. D
6. A-4, B-3, C-2, D-1   7. A-2, B-1, C-4, D-3
8. A-2, B-1, C-4, D-3   9. D   10. B   11. C
12. C   13. B   14. D   15. C   16. D
17. A-3, B-1, C-2, D-4   18. B   19. D   20. D
21. A-3, B-4, C-2, D-1   22. A-4, B-1, C-2, D-3
23. B   24. D   25. C   26. C   27. C   28. A
29. B   30. B   31. C
32. D (Flu-like syndrome is usually seen in intermittent regime)
33. A   34. C   35. C
36. D (biopsy can tell the specific cause of malabsorption)
37. D   38. C   39. D   40. C   41. C   42. C
43. B   44. B   45. B   46. C   47. C   48. D
49. C   50. C   51. A   52. C   53. C   54. D
55. C   56. C   57. B   58. C   59. B   60. C
61. B   62. A   63. C   64. C   65. B   66. D
67. D   68. D   69. D   70. C   71. C   72. B
73. C   74. C   75. C   76. C   77. C   78. B
79. C   80. D   81. C   82. B   83. D   84. A
85. B   86. D   87. D   88. D   89. C   90. D
91. D   92. D   93. C   94. D   95. D   96. D
97. A   98. A   99. B   100. B   101. A   102. D
103. D   104. C   105. D   106. D   107. C   108. D
109. B   110. B   111. B   112. B   113. C   114. B
115. C   116. B   117. A-3, B-4, C-2, D-1
118. D   119. C   120. A   121. C   122. D   123. A
124. D   125. C   126. C   127. D   128. C   129. D
130. D   131. C   132. D   133. C   134. A   135. C
136. D   137. A   138. C   139. A   140. C   141. D
142. B   143. A   144. C   145. A   146. A   147. C
148. B   149. D   150. A

Reference Laboratory Values

CHEMICAL CONSTITUENTS OF BLOOD

Albumin (s)	3.5–5.5 g/dL
Aminotransferases (s)	
-Alanine (ALT, SGPT)	0–35 U/L
-Aspartate (AST, SGOT)	0–35 U/L
Amylase (s)	60–180 U/L
Arterial blood gases (p)	
-HCO_3^-	21–30 mEq/L
-PCO_2	35–45 mmHg
-PO_2	80–100 mmHg
-pH	7.38–7.44
Bilirubin, total (s)	0.3–1.0 mg/dL
-Direct	0.1–0.3 mg/dL
-Indirect	0.2–0.7 mg/dL
Calcium, ionized (p)	4.5–5.6 mg/dL
Calcium total	9.0–10.5 mg/dL
Creatine kinase (s)	
-Females	20–170 U/L
-Males	30–200 U/L
Creatine kinase MB isoenzyme	<6% of total CK
Creatinine (s)	<1.5 mg/dL
Ferritin (s)	
-Female	10–200 ng/mL
-Male	15–400 ng/mL
-Folate (s)	3.1–17.5 mg/mL
Glucose (Fasting) (p)	
-Normal	75–100 mg/dL
-Impaired	100–125 mg/dL
-Diabetes mellitus	≥126 mg/dL
Glucose, 2 hour postprandial (p)	
Normal	<140 mg/dL
Impaired glucose tolerance	140–199 mg/dL
Diabetes mellitus	≥200 mg/dL
Hemoglobin A1c	up to 6% of total Hb
Iron (s)	50–150 mg/dL
Iron binding capacity (s)	250–370 mg/dL

Transferrin saturation	20-45%
Lactate dehydrogenase (LDH) (s)	100-190 U/L
Lipase (s)	0-160 U/L
Osmolality (p)	285-295 mosmol/Kg serum water
Phosphatase, acid (s) (ACP)	0-5.5 U/L
Phosphatase, alkaline (ALP) (s)	30-120 U/L
Phosphorous, inorganic (s)	3.0-4.5 mg/dL
Potassium (s)	3.5-5.0 mEq/L
Sodium (s)	136-145 mEq/L
Protein, total (s)	5.5-8.0 g/dL
Protein, fractions	
-Albumin	3.5-5.5 g/dL (50-60%)
-Globulin	2.0-3.5 g/dL (40-50%)
-$\alpha 1$	0.2-0.4 g/dL
-$\alpha 2$	0.5-0.9 g/dL
-β	0.6-1.1 g/dL
-γ	0.7-1.7 g/dL (13-23%)
Troponin I (s)	0-0.4 ng/mL
Troponin T (s)	0-0.1 ng/mL
Urea Nitrogen (s)	10-20 mg/dL
Urea (s)	20-40 mg/dL
Uric acid (s)	
-Female	1.5-6.0 mg/dL
-Male	2.5-8.0 mg/dL
Vitamin B_{12}	250-900 ng/mL

HEMATOLOGICAL EVALUATION

Hemoglobin (p)	
-Female	12-15 g/dL
-Male	13-16 g/dL
Hematocrit (p)	
-Male	42-52%
-Female	37-48%
TLC	4000-11000/mm^3
DLC	
-Neutrophils	45-74%
-Lymphocytes	16-45%
-Monocytes	4-10%
-Eosinophils	0-7%
-Basophils	0-2%
Platelets	1.5-4.0 lacs/mm^3
ESR	
Westergren <50 years	
-Male	0-15 mm for 1st hour
-Female	0-20 mm for 1st hour
Westergren >50 years	
-Male	0-20 mm for 1st hour
-Female	0-30 mm for 1st hour
Bleeding time	<7 minute
Prothrombin time (PT)	control ± 1 second
Partial thromboplastin time	comparable to control (Activated PTT)
Thrombin time	control ± 3 seconds
Mean corpuscular Hb (MCH)	27-33 pg
Mean corpuscular Hb concentration (MCHC)	31-35%
Mean corpuscular volume (MCV)	82-98 fL

Osmotic Fragility
    -Slight hemolysis   0.45–0.39%
    -Complete hemolysis   0.33–0.3%
Reticulocyte
    -Adults   0.5–1.5%
    -Children   2.5–6.5%

CEREBROSPINAL FLUID

CSF Pressure	50–180 mmHg
CSF Volume	~150 mL
Glucose	40–70 mg/dL
Protein	20–50 mg/dL
Cells total	<5 per mm^3
DLC	
-Lymphocyte	60–70%
-Monocyte	30–50%
-Neutrophils	None

ATP 3 (ADULT TREATMENT PANEL) CLASSIFICATION OF LDL, TOTAL AND HDL CHOLESTEROL (mg/dL)

LDL Cholesterol	
-Optimal	< 100
-Near normal	100–129
-Borderline high	130–159
-high	160–189
-Very high	≥ 190
Total Cholesterol	
-Desirable	<200
-Borderline high	200–234
-High	≥ 240
HDL Cholesterol	
-Low	<40
-High	>60

TRIGLYCERIDES

Normal	<150 mg/dL
Borderline high	150–199 mg/dL
High	200–499 mg/dL
Very high	>500 mg/dL

AVERAGE VALUES IN PULMONARY PHYSIOLOGY

Parameters	Male	Female
Forced vital capacity (FVC)	4.8 L	3.3 L
Forced expiratory volume in 1 second (FEV$_1$)	3.8 L	2.8 L
FEV$_1$/FVC	76%	77%
Maximal expiratory flow rate	9.4 L/second	6.1 L/second
Total lung capacity (TLC)	6.4 L	4.9 L
Functional residual capacity (FRC)	2.2 L	2.6 L
Residual volume (RV)	1.5 L	1.2 L
Inspiratory capacity (IC)	4.8 L	3.7 L
Expiratory reserve volume	3.2 L	2.3 L
Vital capacity	1.7 L	1.4 L

Index

Page numbers followed by *f* refer to figure and *t* refer to table.

A

Abacavir 264, 265
Abciximab 111
Abdomen
   pain in 2
   shape of 19
Abducens nerve 192
Abortion 3
Abscess
   multiple 256*f*
   solitary 255*f*
Acarbose 233
Accessory nerve 193
   spinal part of 194
Accommodation reflex 189
Acetminophen 206
Achalasia 24
Acid-fast bacilli 165
Acidosis 7, 259, 290
Acquired immunodeficiency syndrome 225, 259, 261
Actinobacillus 97
Activated partial thromboplastin time 281
Acute blood loss 64, 229
Acute coronary syndrome 110, 111*t*, 277, 292
Acute kidney injury 176, 179, 181, 182, 268
   causes of 182*t*
   treatment of 183*t*
Acute leukemia 64, 66*t*
   classification of 64*t*
Acute massive pulmonary embolism 154
Acute myeloid leukemia 64, 65, 65*f*, 66, 66*t*
Acute myocardial infarction
   investigations 112
   management 113
Acute nephritic syndrome 180
   etiology of 180*t*
Acute pulmonary edema 93, 115-117, 119, 276
   management of 276
Acute respiratory distress syndrome 133, 134, 140, 259, 268, 288, 313
Acyclovir 245, 247
Addison's disease 224, 226*f*, 228
   causes of 225
   features of 225*f*
   maintenance therapy 226
Adefovir dipivoxil 44, 45
Adenocarcinoma 31

Adenosine 125
   deaminase 165
Adenoviruses 139
Adie pupil 190
Adjunctive therapy 203
Adrenal androgens 224
Adrenal crisis, precipitating factors for 281
Adrenal disease 312
Adrenal disorders 224
Adrenal failure, cause of 225
Adrenalectomy, bilateral 225
Adrenaline 274, 280
Adrenocortical insufficiency, causes of 288
Adrenocorticotropic hormone deficiency 223
Adrenomedullin 118
Advanced cardiac life support 281, 291
Ageusia 192, 192*t*
Agranulocytosis 80, 253
   causes 81
   investigations 81
   management 81
   manifestations 81
Air pollution 147
Airway 291
   examination 311
   obstruction 151, 248, 249, 278
      prevention of 278
Alanine aminotransferase 40, 45, 270
Albumin 312
   excretion rate 184
Albuminuria stages 184
Alcohol
   abuse 312
   ingestion, acute 128
   related liver disease 44
   use 279
   withdrawal 198, 279
Aldosterone 224
   antagonist 106, 118
   excess 107
Alirocumab 114
Aliskiren 106
Alisprovir 46
Alkaline phosphatase 36
Alkalosis 50, 220
Allergic contact dermatitis 295
Allergic reactions, history of 2
Allergy 311
   tests 145
Almotrptan 206

Alogliptin 233
Alpha-glucosidase inhibitors 233
Alpha-thalassemia 62
Alteplase 111, 113
Ambu bag 274
Ambulatory blood pressure monitoring 101
   indications of 102
   recording 102*f*, 103*f*
Amebiasis 255
Ameboma 255
Amenorrhea 216, 218
American Society of Anesthesiologists
   Physical Status 312
Amikacin 162, 163
Amiloride 105, 106, 227
Aminocaproic acid 83
Aminotransferases 36
Amiodarone 125, 215, 218, 312
Amitriptyline 207
Amlodipine 24, 106, 111, 112
Amnesia 302
Amoxicillin 98, 99, 141
Amphotericin 98
Ampicillin 98, 99, 192, 202
Amprenavir 265
Amrinone 117, 118, 277
Amylin analog 233
Amyloidosis 115, 126, 215, 225
Anal fissure 17
Analgesia 111, 112*t*
Anaphylactic reaction
   causes of 294
   diagnosis of 294
   management of 294
Anaphylaxis 119, 280, 293, 295
   clinical features of 294
   management of 280
   mechanism of 293*f*
Anaplastic lymphoma kinase 170
Anasarca 312
Anchovy sauce 255
Ancylostoma duodenale 57
Anemia 5, 7, 55, 64, 66, 86-88, 101, 229
   chronic 115
   classification of 56, 56*t*
   clinical presentations 55
   hemorrhagic 56
   severe 62, 257, 259
   symptomatic 73
Anesthesia, general 281

Angina 95, 124
    atypical 109
    pectoris 108
Anginal chest pain 218
Angioedema 131, 294f
    treatment of 295
Angiography, coronary 91
Angiotensin 112
    converting enzyme 134, 182
        inhibitors 106, 107, 118, 232, 312, 313
    receptor blocker 105-107, 118, 232, 312, 313
    receptor-neprilysin inhibitor 118
Anorexia 2, 19, 58, 59
Anosmia, causes of 188, 188t
Antacids 28
Anti-arrhythmic drugs 124
    classification of 125t
Anti-arrhythmic therapy 119
Antibacterial drugs 286
Antibiotic 150
    prophylaxis 99
Antibody cocktail drug 271
Anticoagulant 112t, 155t, 281
    therapy 111, 112, 114, 119, 135, 312
Anticoagulation 155
Anticonvulsants 81
Antidepressants 300
Anti-diabetic drugs 233
Anti-diuretic hormone deficiency 223
Antiepileptic drug 199t
    therapy 199
Antigen detection methods 257
Antihypertensive drugs, side effects of 107t
Anti-ischemic therapy 111, 112t
Antimicrobial agents 30
Antimotility 30
Anti-neutrophil-cytoplasmic-antibody 180
Antinuclear antibodies 179
Antioxidants 151
Antiparkinsonism 192
Antiphospholipids antibody syndrome 153
Antiplatelet 281
    agents 110, 113, 277
        doses of 111t
    therapy 111
Anti-P-selectin monoclonal antibody 64
Antipsychotics 192, 300
Antiretroviral drugs 264, 265
    toxicity of 264f
Antiretroviral therapy 264
Antisecretory agents 30
Antithyroid drugs 219
Antitubercular drugs 159, 160t
Antiviral therapy 244, 245
Antral ulcers 27f
Anuria 2, 176
Anxiety 3-5, 122, 152
Aorta 121
Aortic aneurysm 24
    rupture of 283
Aortic dissection 96
Aortic regurgitation 90, 96, 101
    causes of 96t
    clinical manifestations 96
    clinical signs of 96t
    investigations 96
    pathophysiology 96
    peripheral signs of 96
    treatment 96
Aortic root disease 96
Aortic stenosis 87, 90, 95, 290
    causes of 95t
    clinical manifestations 95
    clinical signs of 95t
    pathophysiology 95
    treatment 95
Aortic valve replacement 97
Aplastic anemia 61, 61f
    clinical features 61
    investigations 61
    pathogenesis 61
    treatment of 61
    types of 61t
Appendicitis 16, 17
Appetite, loss of 16
Aqueous penicillin G 254
Argyll Robertson pupil 190
Arrhythmia 87, 108, 114, 122, 124, 312
    cardiac 124, 200
    classification of 124, 124t
Artemether plus lumefantrine 258, 259
Artemisinin-based combination therapy 258, 259
Arterial blood gas analysis 137, 145, 149, 154, 285f
Arterial pulse 4, 87, 88
Artery, hepatic 35
Artesunate plus
    amodiaquine 258, 259
    mefloquine 258, 259
    sulfadoxine-pyrimethamine 258, 259
Arthritis 242, 244, 251
Ascites 10, 21, 47, 51
    causes of 51t
    clinical features 51
    management 52
    pathogenesis 51
Ascitic fluid 52
Aspartate aminotransferase 40
Aspergillosis, allergic bronchopulmonary 153
Aspergillus 81
Aspiration 134, 138
Aspirin 25, 111, 113, 179, 206, 274
Asterixis 50
Asthma 144t, 301
    acute severe 144, 146, 151
    anti-inflammatory drugs used in 146t
    bronchodilator drugs used in 146t
    cardiac 116, 117
    chronic persistent 145
    control 145t
    management of acute severe 277
    provoke 144t
    severe 133
    symptoms 146
Asystole 290
Ataxia 211
Atazanavir 265
Atenolol 106, 111, 112, 125
Atheroma 108
Atheromatous plaque 109f
Atherosclerosis 108, 109t
    coronary 108
Atherosclerotic cardiovascular disease 236
Atorvastatin 111, 112
Atrial fibrillation 93, 127, 128f, 211
    causes of 128t
    management of 128
Atrial flutter 127, 127f
Atrial septal defect 120
    clinical manifestations 121
    investigations 121
    treatment 121
Atrioventricular re-entrant tachycardia 129
Atrophic lingual papillae 300
Atropine 125
    sulphate 125
Attack
    acute 206
    asthmatic 277
Auscultation 21, 90, 136
Autoimmune 225
    diabetes 228
    gastritis 26
    hemolytic anemia 63, 248, 249
    hepatitis 44, 46, 47
    hypothyroidism 216
    thrombocytopenic purpura 76, 281
    thyroiditis 216
Automatic external defibrillator 290f
Autosplenectomy 82
Azathioprine 46
Azilsartan 106
Azithromycin 99, 141, 250-252, 254, 264, 270
Azotemia 32, 176
Aztreonam 286

B

Bacillary dysentery 29
Bacillus Calmette-Guerin vaccine 241
Backache 301
Bacteria, anaerobic 12
Balloon tamponade 49
Bariotic surgery 301
Baroreflex pathway, normal 123f
Basal energy expenditure 298
Basedow's disease 217
Basic life support 281, 290
Beau's lines 11
Beclomethasone 146, 150
Bedaquiline 162, 163
Behcet's syndrome 253
Bell's palsy 210, 213, 246
Bendamustine 73
Benfotiamine 302
Benralizumab 146
Benzathine penicillin G 254
Berapamil 125
Beri-beri 5, 115
Bernard-Soulier syndrome 78
Best motor response 195
Best verbal response 195
Beta-adrenergic antagonists 106, 107
Beta-agonists, long-acting 150
Beta-blockers 5, 110, 111, 118, 125, 126, 300
Bictegravir 265
Bicuspid aortic valve, congenital 96
Biguanides 233
Bile acid
    reduced 31
    sequestrant 233
Biliary tract obstruction 52

Bilirubin
   conjugated 37
   metabolism 37, 37*f*
   overproduction of 38
   unconjugated 62
Biomass fuel smoke exposure 147
Biotin 299, 304
Bisferiens pulse 5, 89
Bismuth 28
Bisoprolol 106, 111, 112, 117, 118
Bitot's spots 306, 306*f*
Bivalirudin 111
Bleeding 2, 257
   excessive 281
   gums 300, 305*f*
   tendencies 312
   time 281
   treatment of 28
Bleomycin 72
Block sodium channels 125
Blood
   culture 98
   examination 241
   glucoses, self-monitoring of 230
   investigations 269
   loss of 283
   pressure 5, 89
      classification of 6*t*, 100*t*
      control of 179, 232
      measurement of 6*f*, 101
      noninvasive 311
      reduces 233
      systolic 280
   tests 141, 229
   transfusion 229
      multiple 220, 288
   urea nitrogen 312
   vomiting of 2
Boceprevir 46
Body mass index 4*t*, 300, 313
Bodyache 2
Bolus fibrinolytics 113
Bone marrow 58, 61*f*, 73
   transplantation 61, 64
Bosutinib 69
Botulinum toxin A 207
Bowel habits 16, 17
Bowman's capsule 175
Brachial artery, localization of 6*f*
Bradyarrhythmias 115, 124
Bradycardia 5, 89, 122, 201, 216
Bradykinin 118
Brain
   death 196
   infarction 212*f*
   natriuretic peptide 117
Brainstem 196
Breast
   atrophy 47
   cancer 301
Breath sound 137*f*
   type of 136
Breathing 291
Breathlessness 112, 115
Bretylium 125
Bright red glossitis 303
Brivaracetam 199
Bromocriptine mesylate 233

Bronchi 134, 262
Bronchial asthma 143, 314
   clinical features 144
   investigations 144
   management 145
   pathophysiology 143
Bronchial breath sounds 136
Bronchial provocation tests 144
Bronchiectasis 135, 142, 143*f*, 152
   causes of 142*t*
   clinical manifestations 142
   complications 143
   lung abscess, empyema 135
   treatment 143
Bronchitis, chronic 135, 137, 147, 151
Bronchodilators 149
Bronchopneumonia 139
Bronchoscopy 138
Brown tumors 222
Brudzinski's sign 201, 202
Brugada syndrome 290
Bruit
   abdominal 89, 104
   over thyroid gland 218
Bruton tyrosine kinase inhibitors 73
Budd-Chiari syndrome 48
Budesonide 150
Buffalo hump 226
Bull neck 249
Bumetanide 106, 118
Bundle branch block 124
Burkitt's lymphoma 73, 247, 249
Burns 283, 288

C

Cabotegravir 265
Calcium 299
   antagonists 110
   channel blockers 107, 111, 112, 125
   metabolism 219
      regulation of 219
Caloric stimulation test 195
Canagliflozin 233
Cancers
   colon 301
   endometrial 301
Candesartan 106, 118, 207
Candida 81, 97
   albicans 22
Candidal leukoplakia 23
Candidiasis 267
   esophageal 25*f*, 262
Cangrelor 111
Canker sore 21
Capreomycin 162
Captopril 106, 111, 118
Caput medusae 19, 48
Carbamazapine 81, 199, 208
Carbimazole 215, 219
Carbohydrate 298
Carcinoma 142
   bronchogenic 135, 168
   esophagus 24*f*
   hepatocellular 44, 50
   rectum 18*f*
   right lung 169*f*

Cardiac
   arrest 290
   cachexia 116
   diseases 7, 9
   failure, congestive 165
   injury 268
   tamponade 292
Cardiobacterium 97
Cardiomyopathy 115
   hypertrophic 115, 290
Cardiovascular diseases 152, 236, 312
   chronic 312
   signs of 86
   symptoms of 86
Cardiovascular system 2, 86
   examination 311
Carditis 92
Carey Coombs' murmur 92
Carotenemia 8
Carotenoderma 8, 37
Carotid
   artery, palpation of left 5*f*
   sinus 129
Carotidynia 205
Carpal tunnel syndrome 216, 301
Carvedilol 106, 111, 112, 117, 118
Casal's necklace 303
Casirivimab 271
Cataract 230
Cavitary lung disease, causes of 142*t*
Cefazolin 98, 99
Cefepime 202, 286
Cefixime 251, 252
Cefotaxime 202
Cefpodoxime 141
Ceftazidime 202
Ceftriaxone 52, 98, 99, 202, 251, 252, 254
Cefuroxime axetil 141
Central nervous system 56, 104
   complications 248
   examination 311
   lymphoma 249
   toxoplasmosis 262
Cephalexin 99
Cerebellar ataxia 244, 302
Cerebellopontine angle 210
Cerebral malaria 257, 259
Cerebrospinal fluid 242
Cerebrovascular
   accident 128, 211, 279, 313
   disease 211, 230
Cervical
   lymph node 83*f*
   lymphadenopathy 71*f*, 83*f*, 267
   spine, disease of 205
Cervix 301
Chaga's disease 126
Cheilitis, angular 23, 262
Cheilosis 21, 23, 56, 300
Chemiluminescence immunoassay 254
Chemoprophylaxis 161
Chest
   barrel-shaped 136
   deformities 87
   emphysematous 148*f*
   imaging 288
   inspection of 136*t*
   pain 2, 86, 135, 277, 312

causes of 87t
  management of 277
  radiograph 312
  X-ray 169f, 269, 269f
Cheyne-Stokes
  breathing 195
  respiration 8, 136, 136f
Chiasma 189
Chickenpox 243
Chlamydia 97, 141
  pneumoniae 139
  psittaci 72
  trachomatis 252
Chloramphenicol 81
Chloride 299
Chloroquine 258
Chlorpheniramine 274
Chlorthalidone 106
Chlorthiazide 117
Cholecystitis 16, 17, 87, 251
Choline 299, 305
Chorea 92
Chromium 299
Chronic kidney disease 107, 176, 178, 184-186, 186t
  etiology of 184t
  pathophysiology of 184f
  stages of 184t
Chronic obstructive pulmonary disease 134, 137, 147, 148, 313
  complications of 151
Chvostek's sign 220
Chylothorax 165
Ciclesonide 146, 150
Ciguatoxin 30
Cilastatin 162, 286
Ciprofloxacin 52, 251, 252, 286
Circulation 291
Circulatory failure, acute 250, 287
Cirrhosis 44, 46, 47, 242
  cardiac 47
  causes of 47t
  clinical features of 47t
  complications of 48t
Clarithromycin 99, 141, 250, 264
Clevidipine 108
Clindamycin 99
Clobazam 199
Clofazimine 162, 163
Clonal plasma cell 73
Clonazepam 199, 200
Clonidine 106
Clopidogrel 111, 113
Clostridium perfringens 29
Clot formation 75
Clotrimazole lozenges 23
Clubbing 218
Clutton's joint 254
Coagulation disorders 78, 80
Coarctation of aorta 104, 107, 121
  clinical features 121
  investigations 121
  management 121
Cobalamin 59
  causes of 59t
  deficiency 60
  causes of 59
Coccidiomycosis 262

Cold intolerance 216
Colesevelam 233
Colicky pain 1
Colonic obstruction 17
Color vision 189
Coma 3
  causes of 194t
  hepatic 50
  pathophysiology of 194
Combination therapy 150
Complete blood count 281
Confusional state 3, 194
Congenital heart disease 115, 120, 128
  classification 120
Consciousness 194
Constipation 2, 16, 50, 216
  causes of 17t
Contact dermatitis 296
Continuous blood glucose monitoring system 230
Continuous subcutaneous insulin infusion 236
Convalescent plasma therapy 270
Convulsions 257
Cooley's anemia 62
Coombs' test 63
Copper 299
Cor pulmonale 115, 151, 301
Corneal reflex 192
Corneal xerosis 306
Corona virus disease 19 268
Coronary artery
  bypass grating 110
  disease 3, 107, 108, 230, 290, 301, 313
Corticosteroids 100, 150, 153, 300
Corynebacterium diphtheriae 249
Cotrimoxazole 264
Cough 2, 86, 87, 134, 181, 312
  causes of 134t
  characteristics of 134t
  productive 134
Covaxin 271
COVID-19 268, 270
  clinical categories of 269
Covishield 271
Cranial fossa, middle 191
Cranial nerve 193, 209f
  examination of 188
  palsies 248
  pathway of 209f
Cretinism 217f
Cribriform 213
Criggler-Najjar syndromes 38
Crizanlizumab 64
Crocodile tears 210
Crohn's disease 31
Cryptococcal disease 267
Cryptosporidiosis, chronic 262
Cushing's disease 104, 226
  features of 227f
Cushing's reflex 201
Cushing's syndrome 100, 104, 226, 237, 300
Cushing's ulcer 25
Cyanosis 9, 10f, 87, 88, 121, 135, 148
  cardiac causes of 88
  causes of 10t
  central 9f, 10, 10f, 88, 116, 120
Cyclophosphamide 73, 180

Cycloserine 162, 163
Cyclosporine 61, 83, 180
Cystitis 16
Cytarabine 67
Cytokines 47
  monocyte-mediated 108
Cytomegalovirus 31, 84, 184, 248, 246, 264, 267
  infection 262
Cytosine arabinoside 66

D

Dacarbazine 72
Daclatasvir 44, 46
Dapagliflozin 233
Dapsone 264
Dark-field microscopic examination 254
Darunavir 265
Dasabuvir 46
Dasatinib 67, 69
Daunorubicin 66, 67
D-dimer test 154
Deep reflexes, delayed relaxation of 216
Defibrillation 274, 290
Delamanid 159, 162, 163
Delavirdine 265
Delerium 3
Dementia 3
Dental
  diseases 205
  trauma 206
  treatment 275
Depression 3, 4, 17, 152, 205, 301
Dermopathy 217, 218
Dexamethasone 67, 203, 204, 270
Dextrocardia 120
Dextromethorphan 269
Dextrose 274
Diabetes insipidus 226
  causes of 227
  central 226
Diabetes mellitus 3, 4, 17, 31, 104, 107, 184, 227, 242, 312-314
  classification of 228
  complications of 230
  diagnosis of 229
  gestational 228, 229
  history of 3
  management of 232, 236
  type 1 228, 229
  type 2 228, 229, 301
Diabetic retinopathy, non-proliferative 231f
Diarrhea 2, 16, 28, 32, 59, 218, 230, 283, 312
  acute 29
  causes of 29t, 31t
  chronic 31
  factitious 31
  secretory 31, 32
Diathesis, hemorrhagic 80
Diazepam 114, 200, 274
Didanosine 265
Diffuse infiltrative lymphocytosis syndrome 267, 268, 268f
DiGeorge syndrome 222
Digitalis 118
Digoxin 5, 118, 125, 126, 312

Dihydroartemisinin plus piperaquine 258
Dihydroergotamine 206
Dihydropyridine 106
Diltiazem 24, 106, 111, 112, 125
Diphtheria 192, 249
    antitoxin, dose of 250
        clinical manifestations of 250
        tetanus, pertussis 241
Direct renin inhibitor 106
Directly observed treatment short course 160
Disopyramide 125
Disseminated intravascular coagulation 76, 80, 251, 257, 313
    clinical features 80
    investigation 80
    management 80
Disseminated nontuberculous mycobacterial infection 262
Diuretics 50, 114
    therapy 179, 312
Dizziness 211
Dobutamine 117-119, 277
Dofetilide 125
Dolutegravir 264, 265, 267
Domperidone 206
Dopamine 117-119, 277
    antagonists 206
    receptor agonist 233
Doravirine 265
Doripenem 286
Dothiepin 207
Down's syndrome 120
Doxazosin 106
Doxorubicin 72
Doxycycline 141, 252, 254, 270
Dressler's syndrome 114
Drowsiness 194
Drug-induced hypersensitivity syndrome 295, 296
Drugs 218, 225, 242, 281, 294
    allergy 293, 295
        management of 297
    contraindication of 270
    reaction 295
    resistant tuberculosis 161
    therapy 105, 117, 119, 145, 277
    toxicity 198
Drumstick appearance 9f
Dry beriberi 302
Dry coarse skin 216
Dry powder inhaler 150
D-sotalol 125
Dubin-Johnson syndromes 38
Duke's criteria 98
Dulaglutide 233, 234
Duncan's disease 249
Duodenal ulcer 26, 27f
Dupilumab, subcutaneous 146
D-xylose test 32
Dysarthria 211
Dysentery 28, 29
    amebic 29, 255
Dysgeusia 33
Dyshormonogenesis 215
Dyslipidemia 104, 233, 301
Dyspepsia 19, 26
Dysphagia 2, 16, 19, 23, 56, 193
    classification 23

Dyspnea 2, 7, 86, 115, 116, 133, 312
    acute 134, 154
    cardiac 86
    causes of 134t
    chronic 134
Dysuria 2, 251

E

Ecchymosis 77
Eclampsia 107
    treatment of 108
Ectopic pregnancy rupture 283
Edema 2, 10, 86-88, 135
    acute noncardiogenic pulmonary 257
    cardiogenic pulmonary 119, 277
    localized 11
    origin of 289
    unilateral 10
Efavirenz 265
Egophony 137
Ehlers-Danlos syndrome 76
Eisenmenger's syndrome 88, 120, 121
Elbasvir 46
Electrolyte
    abnormalities 290
    management 30
Eletriptan 206
Elvitegravir 265
Embolectomy 155
Embolism, chronic pulmonary 154
Empagliflozin 233
Emphysema 137, 147
    diffuse 149f
    surgical 167
Emtricitabine 265
Enalapril 105, 106, 111, 114, 117, 118
Enalaprilat 108
Encephalitis 242, 244, 248
Encephalopathy, hepatic 47, 49, 50, 50t
Endocarditis 96, 97
Endocrine disorders 100, 215
Endomyocardial diseases 115
Endoscopic retrograde cholangiopancreatography 36
Endoscopic therapy 25
Endothelial cells 35
Endotracheal tube 274
Endovascular mechanical embolectomy 212
Energy 298
Enfuvirtide 265
Entacavir 45
Entamoeba histolytica 29, 255
Entecavir 44, 45
Enteric fever 250
    antibiotics for 251
    complications of 251
Enterocytozoon bieneusi 31
Enzyme immunoassay 254
Eosinophilia 152, 153, 295, 296
    tropical 152
Epilepsia partialis continua 197
Epilepsy 196
    classification 196
    diagnosis of 199
    type of 199
Epinephrine 130, 280, 295
Episodic asthma 144

Epistaxis 77
Eplerenone 106, 118
Epstein-Barr virus 71, 246, 247, 249
Eptifibatide 111
Erectile dysfunction 230
Ergotamine 206
Ertugliflozin 233
Erythema marginatum 92
Erythromycin 92, 141
Erythropoiesis, normal 55f
Erythropoietin 175, 185
Esmolol 108, 111, 112, 125
Esomeprazole 25
Esophageal dysphagia 19, 24
    causes of 24t
Esophageal mucosal ring, lower 24
Esophageal varices 18f, 48, 57
Esophagitis 87
Estimated glomerular filtration rate 232, 270
Ethambutol 159, 160, 162, 163, 204
Ethionamide 162, 163
Ethosuximide 199
Etomidate 225
Etoposide 66
Etravirine 265
Evolocumab 114
Exacerbation, acute 151
Exanthematous pustulosis, acute generalized 295
Exenatide 233, 234
Exercise 5, 232
Exophthalmos 217
Extracorporeal lung support 289
Eyes 13
    involvement 246

F

Fabry's syndrome 24
Facial diplegia 209
Facial expression 4
Facial migraine 205
Facial nerve 192
    palsy 209, 209f
        causes of 209
        features of 209
Facial pain 207
    atypical 208
    causes of 207t
Facial palsy
    infranuclear 210
    ipsilateral 244
Facial puffiness 216f
Falciparum malaria
    complications of 257
    severe 257
Fallot's tetralogy 88
Famciclovir 245, 247
Famotidine 25
Fasting glucose, impaired 229
Fasting plasma glucose 229
Fat 298
    deposition 264f
Fatigue 86, 87, 115, 279
Fatty acids, polyunsaturated 298
Fatty liver 244
    disease, nonalcoholic 301
Febrile mucocutaneous syndromes 296

Fecal fat estimation 32
Felbamate 199
Fetor hepaticus 50
Fever 2, 5
    acute rheumatic 91
    mild 250
Fibrin
    degradation products 80
    deposition 75
Fibrinolytic agent 113
Fibroblast influx 181
Fibrosis 115
Fine finger tremors 218
Fistula
    arteriovenous 101, 115
    bronchopleural 167
Fixed drug eruptions 295, 296
Flecainide 125, 128
Fluid
    management 30
    thrill 21
Flunarizine 207
Fluorescent treponemal antibody-absorbed test 254
Fluoride 299
Fluoroquinolones 141
Fluticasone 146, 150
Folate 299, 304
    deficiency 60
Folic acid deficiency, causes of 59, 59t
Follicle stimulating hormone 223
Follicular lymphoma 73
Fondaparinux 111
Food poisoning 28, 30
    causes of 30t
Foot, diabetic 230, 230f
Forced expiratory volume 138
Forced vital capacity 138
Formoterol 150
Fosamprenavir 265
Fosinopril 118
Fosphenytoin 200
Fractional inactivated polio vaccine 241
Fracture long bones 283
Frank hemoptysis 134
Fresh frozen plasma 80
Frovatriptan 206
Frusemide 119, 277
Functional platelet disorders 77
    causes of 78t
Fungal 267
    infections 142
    meningitis 204
    nail infections 262
Furosemide 105, 106, 118
Fusion inhibitor 265

G

Gabapentin 199, 207, 300
Galactorrhea 216
Gallbladder
    cancer 301
    diseases 16
Gallstone 16, 301
Gancyclovir 264
Gastric
    adenocarcinoma 26
    carcinoma 19
    contents, aspiration of 288
    erosions, multiple 25f
    malignancy 49
    varices 48
Gastritis 25, 26, 57
    acute 25
    chronic 26
    erosive 49
    hemorrhagic 25
    treatment of acute 25
    types of 26
Gastroenteritis 17
Gastroesophageal reflux 117, 152, 301
Gastrointestinal bleeding 50, 283
Gastrointestinal disease 9, 312
    signs of 16
    symptoms of 16
Gastrointestinal system 2, 16
Gastroparesis 17, 230
Gatifloxacin 141
Gaucher's disease 81, 82
Genetic
    disorders, history of 3
    enzyme defects 215
Genital herpes 246
Genitalia 20
Gentamicin 98
Germ cell tumor 169f
German measles 242
Ghon's lesion 156f
Giant cell arteritis 205
Giardia lamblia 29
Giemsa's stain 247
Gigantism 4
Gilbert's syndrome 38
Gingival growth 213
Gingival hyperplasia 23
    causes of 24t
Gingivostomatitis 22
Glanzmann's thrombasthenia 78
Glasgow Coma Scale 195t
Glaucoma 205, 230
Glecaprevir 46
Glibenclamide 233
Gliclazide 233
Glimepiride 233
Glipizide 233
Glomerular basement membrane 180
Glomerular filtration rate 184
Glomerulonephritis 179, 181
    chronic 184
    rapidly progressive 180
Glomerulosclerosis 301
    focal segmental 184
Glossitis 23, 56, 300, 305f
Glossopharyngeal nerve 193
Glucagon 274
Glucocorticoid 224
    therapy 249
Glucometers 230
Glucose
    dependent insulinotropic polypeptide 234
    lowering agents 233, 233t
    powder 274
    tolerance, impaired 229
Glutamic acid decarboxylase 228
Glutamine 64
Glyburide 233
Glyceryl trinitrate 274
Glycoprotein 111, 171
Glycopyrronium 150
    bromide 150
Goiter 216, 218
Gonadotropin
    deficiency 223
    releasing hormone 223
Gonorrhea 251
    treatment of uncomplicated 252
Goodpasture's syndrome 135
Gout 301
Granulocytopenia 248
Grave's disease 4, 217, 218
    hyperthyroidism of 218
Grazoprevir 46
Growth hormone 223
    releasing hormone 223
Guillain-Barré syndrome 242
Gum
    bleeding 77
    hyperplasia 65, 65f
Gynecological diseases 16
Gynecomastia 47

H

Haemophilus influenzae 139, 241
Hair loss 216
Halitophobia 12
Halitosis 12
    causes of 12t
    pathophysiology of 12
    tests for 12
    types of 12
Hartnup's disease 303
Hashimoto's thyroiditis 215, 216
Headache 2, 204, 207
    acute severe 204
    causes of 205t
    cluster 207
    hemicranial 205
    pathological basis of 204
    secondary 205
Hearing, tests of 193
Heart
    beat 129
    block
        complete 126, 126f
        congenital complete 120
        first-degree 125
    burn 2, 16, 17
    disease 129
        classification of congenital 120t
        cyanotic 88f
        cyanotic congenital 290
        hypertensive 115
        ischemic 108, 108t, 115, 128, 216
    failure 86, 107, 108, 114, 118t, 127, 312
        acute 116
        backward 116
        biventricular 116
        causes of 115, 115t
        chronic 116
        clinical features of 116t
        congestive 165, 211
        control of 117

diastolic 116
drugs in 117t
high output 116
low output 116
pathophysiology 115
signs of 115, 115t
symptoms of 115, 115t
systolic 116
treatment 117
types of 116
rate 311
Heat intolerance 218
Helicobacter pylori 72
    gastritis 26
Hemagglutinin 171
Hematemesis 2, 17, 48, 135, 135t
Hematochezia 2
Hematological diseases 23
Hematological system 55
Hematopoiesis, normal 55
Hematuria 2, 79, 176
Hemiplegia 210
Hemochromatosis 115, 225
Hemodialysis 119
Hemoglobin, normal 62
Hemoglobinopathies 229
Hemoglobinuria 62, 259
Hemolysis 38, 63t
Hemolytic anemia 56, 62, 63t
    classification of 62t
    clinical features 62
    Coomb's positive 248
    hemoglobinopathy 62
    treatment 63
Hemoperitoneum 283
Hemophilia 78
    A 76, 78, 281
    B 76, 78, 281
        therapy of 80
        genetics of 79f
Hemoptysis 2, 87, 116, 134, 135, 135t, 181
    causes of 135t
Hemorrhage
    intestinal 251
    intra-adrenal 25
    intracerebral 212f, 212t
    petechial 88
    subarachnoid 205
Hemorrhagic disorders 135
Hemorrhoids 48
    painful 17
Hemosiderinuria 62
Hemostasis
    disorders of 76
    normal 74
    secondary 75
Hemostatic disorders 76t, 281
Hemothorax 165, 283
Henoch-Schönlein purpura 76
Heparins 111, 155
Hepatic vein thrombosis 48
Hepatitis 16, 17, 242, 244, 248
    A 39, 42
        serology 40t
    acute 39, 40f, 41
    B 40, 43, 43t, 84, 181, 185, 241
        chronic 44
        core antigen 40

        serology 40t
        surface antigen 40
        vaccination 43t
    B E antigen 40
    C 41, 46t, 84, 185
        chronic 44
        serology 41t
    causes of 39t, 44t
    chronic 43, 44
    complications of 42t
    D 41
    E 41
        serology 41t
    tests for 44t
    viruses 39
Hepatobiliary system 35
Hepatocellular diseases 39
Hepatocytes 35
Hepatorenal syndrome 50
Hernia, umbilical 217
Herpes
    congenital 246
    labialis 23f
    simplex 245, 246, 253, 267
        infection, treatment of 247
        labialis 246f
        virus 25
    virus hominis 246
    zoster 243, 244, 245f, 262, 263f, 267
        multidermatomal 245f
Herpetic stomatitis 22
High arched palate 254
Histamine 144
Histoplasmosis 225, 267
    extrapulmonary 262
Hodgkin's disease 247
Hodgkin's lymphoma 70-72, 72f, 249
Hormone 223
Horner's syndrome 190
Human herpes virus 72, 246, 247
Human immunodeficiency virus 178, 225, 260f
    disease
        clinical stages of 261
        pathogenesis of 261f
    encephalopathy 262
    infection
        diagnosis of 262
        management of 263
        oral manifestations in 267
        prevention of 267
        primary 253
    syndrome, acute 260, 261
Hutchinson's teeth 254
Hydralazine 106, 108, 117
Hydrocephalus 204f
Hydrochlorothiazide 106
Hydrocortisone 67
    sodium succinate 274
Hydrothorax 10
Hydroxocobalamin 60
Hydroxychloroquine 270
Hydroxyurea 64
Hyperbilirubinemia 37, 38
    conjugated 38
    unconjugated 38
Hypercalcemia 17, 221
    causes of 221

Hypercapnia, clinical features of 163t
Hypercapnic respiratory failure 163, 289
Hypereosinophilic syndrome 153
Hyperkalemia 129, 183, 292
Hyperkinetic pulse 5, 89
Hypermagnesemia 183
Hyperosmolar states 283
Hyperparathyroidism 185, 222
    secondary 222
    types of 222
Hyperphosphatemia 183, 220
Hyperplasia 81
    congenital adrenal 225
Hyperpyrexia 4, 257
Hyper-reflexia 218
Hypersensitivity reactions, history of 2
Hypersplenism 82
Hypertension 3, 96, 100, 105, 107, 115, 117, 128, 184, 201, 216, 301, 312, 313
    accelerated 100
    causes of secondary 100t
    diagnosis, thresholds for 101
    effects of 104
    essential 100
    history of 3
    malignant 100
    masked 103, 104
    resistant 107
    secondary 100
Hypertensive crisis 107, 276
Hyperthyroidism 31, 128, 129, 215, 217, 218, 221
Hypertriglyceridemia 105
Hyperuricemia 105, 183
Hyperventilation
    causes of 278
    management of 278
Hypervolemia 183
Hypnotics 50
Hypoalbuminemia 179, 220
Hypocalcemia 183, 219, 220
    causes of 220
    laboratory findings in 220
Hypogeusia 300
Hypoglossal nerve 194
Hypoglycemia 122, 198, 237, 257, 280
    symptoms of 280
Hypokalemia 50, 129, 292
Hypomagnesemia 129, 220
Hyponatremia 183, 198
Hypoparathyroidism 31, 220, 222
Hypopituitarism 215, 223
Hypotension 32, 129, 182, 257, 259, 280
    persistent 155
Hypothalamus, disorders of 215
Hypothermia 4, 216, 292
    causes of 4
Hypothyroidism 17, 215, 216f, 217, 300
    causes of 215
    congenital 217
    secondary 215, 216, 218
Hypotonia 217
Hypovolemia 182, 292
    mild 283
    moderate 283
    severe 284
Hypoxemia 163, 292
    clinical features of 163t

Hypoxemic respiratory failure 163
Hypoxia 290

I

Ibalizumab 265
Ibuprofen 206
Ibutilide 125
    intravenous 128
Icterus 37
Idiopathic thrombocytopenic purpura 76, 281
    clinical features 77
    diagnosis 77
    treatment 77
Imatinib 69
Imdevimab 271
Imepenem 286, 162
Immobilization 221
Immunization
    active 42
    passive 43
Immunosuppressive therapy 61
Indacaterol 150
Indapamide 106
Indinavir 265
Indomethacin 227
Infections 39, 147, 240, 267, 281
    bacterial 244
    prevention of 81, 263
    source of 246, 247
Infective endocarditis 97, 97t, 98t, 115, 211
    clinical manifestations 97
    investigations 98
    pathology 97
    peripheral signs of 88
    signs of 87
    subacute 97
    treatment 98
Infertility 216
Inflammation 58, 300
    acute 58
    chronic 58
Inflammatory lesions 24
Influenza 139
Infranuclear facial nerve palsy, causes of 210t
Insane, general paresis of 253
Insect bites 294
Insomnia 3
Insulin 233, 235, 300
    preparations 235
    regimens 235
    secretagogues 233
    types of 235
Insulinoma 300
Interstitial lung disease 167, 167f
    classification 167
    clinical features of 167, 167t
    common causes of 167
    pathogenesis 167
    treatment 168
Intracranial pressure 207
Intramuscular benzathine penicillin G 92
Intrinsic acute kidney injury 182
Invasive cervical carcinoma 262
Iodine 215, 299
    deficiency 215
    ingestion, excessive 218

Ionotropic agents 118, 119, 277
Ipratropium bromide 146, 150
Irbesartan 106, 118
Iron 19, 57, 299
    deficiency anemia 57, 57f
        causes of 57, 57t
        differential diagnosis of 58
Irritable bowel syndrome 17
Ischemic acute kidney injury,
        pathophysiology of 183f
Ishihara plate 190f
Isoniazid 39, 158-160, 204, 264
Isosorbide
    dinitrate 111, 112, 117
    mononitrate 110, 112
Isosporiasis, chronic 262
Ivabradine 118
Ivermectin 270

J

Jacksonian march 197
Janeway's lesions 88, 97
Japanese encephalitis vaccine 241
Jarisch Herxheimer reaction 254
Jaundice 2, 8, 37, 47
    acholuric 38
    cholestatic 39
    hepatocellular 39t
    obstructive 19, 39
    physiologic neonatal 38
    prolonged 217
    types of 38, 38t
    visible over sclera 8f
Jaw, cysts of 222
Jod-Basedow disease 218
Jugular venous
    pressure 148, 165
    prominent 6f
    pulse 6, 89
        wave forms of 7f

K

Kala azar 81, 82
Kanamycin 162
Kaposi's sarcoma 261, 262, 267
Keratomalacia 306, 306f
Kernicterus 38
Kernig's sign 201, 202f
Ketoacidosis, diabetic 230
Ketoconazole 23, 225
Kidney
    biopsy 179, 183
    functions of normal 175, 176t
    palpable 104
Knee
    effusion, bilateral 254
    hemarthrosis of 79f
Koilonychia 11, 57
Koplik spot 240f
Korsakoff's syndrome 302
Kupfer cells 35, 47
Kussmaul's breathing 136, 195
Kussmaul's sign 7, 89
Kwashiorkor 299, 300, 300f
Kyphosis 136

L

Labetalol 106, 108
Labyrinthitis 17
Lacosamide 199, 200
Lactate dehydrogenase 60, 164, 165
Laennec's cirrhosis 47
Lamivudine 44, 45, 264, 265, 267
Lamotrigine 199
Lansoprazole 28
Laryngeal edema 133
Laryngeal paralysis 193, 250
Laryngoscope 274
Larynx 134, 250
    innervation of 194t
L-asparaginase 66
Latex rubber products 294
Ledipasvir 44, 46
Left heart failure 116
    clinical features of 116t
Legionella pneumonia 141
Leishmaniasis, atypical disseminated 262
Leukemia 64, 81, 221
    acute lymphoblastic 64, 66, 67t
    chronic lymphocytic 69, 72
    chronic myeloid 67, 82
Leukocytosis 241
Leukoencephalopathy, progressive multifocal 262
Leukonychia 11
Leukopenia 241
Levator palpebrae superioris 192
Levetiracetam 199, 200
Levofloxacin 141, 162, 163, 251, 252, 286
Lexisenatide 234
Lid lag retraction 218
Lidocaine 125
Linagliptin 233
Linezolid 162, 163
Lipid lowering drugs 179
Lipodystrophy 264f
Lipoprotein, low-density 178
Liraglutide 233, 234
Lisinopril 105, 106, 117, 118
Listeria monocytogenes 201, 203
Lithium 215, 221
Liver 35
    abscess 16
        amebic 255, 255f
    biopsy 37
    cancer 46
    cell dysfunction 47
    cirrhosis of 47
    disease 38, 50, 80, 281, 312
    enlarged 20
    function tests 35, 35t, 312
    palpation of 20f
Lixisenatide 233
Lobar pneumonia, respiratory signs in 139t
Loeffler syndrome 152
Lopinavir 265
Lorazepam 114, 200
Losartan 106, 117, 118
Lower limbs 13, 211
Lower motor neuron
    lesion 191
    type 209

Lower respiratory tract 133
Lung 26, 134, 262
    anterior aspects of 133*f*
    capacity, total 138
    disease, chronic obstructive 26
    fibrosis of 158*f*
    malignancy of 221
    parenchyma 134
    posterior aspects of 133*f*
    transplant 149
    volumes 138*f*
Lung abscess 141, 142, 142*f*
    causative organisms 141
    clinical features 142
    diagnosis 142
    risk factors 141
    treatment 142
Lung cancers 148, 152, 168, 170
    classification 168
    clinical features 168
    etiology of 168
    investigations 168
    sign of 168
    symptoms 168
Lung injury
    direct 288
    indirect 288
Lupus amyloidosis 192
Lupus nephritis 180
Luteinizing hormone 223
Lutembacher's syndrome 120
Lyell syndrome 296
Lyme disease 126
Lymph gland enlargement 2
Lymph node
    enlargement 135
    inguinal 82
    palpation of 11
Lymphadenitis 157
Lymphadenopathy
    causes of 82*t*
    diagnosis 82
Lymphatic obstruction 31
Lymphohistiocytosis, hemophagocytic 249
Lymphoma 31, 70, 73, 73*t*, 81, 221, 225, 262, 267, 268
    classification of 70*t*
    staging of 70, 71*t*
    type of 73
Lymphopenia 269

M

Macrovascular complications 232
Macular lesions 97
Maculopapular eruptions 295
Magnesium 299
Malabsorption 31, 222
    blood tests in 32*t*
    causes of 31*t*
    syndromes 31
Maladie de Roger's murmur 120
Malar rash 181
Malaria 81, 82, 84, 256
    chronic complications of 257
    clinical criteria for severe 259
    drugs for severe 258
    in pregnancy 259
    severe 259
    transmission of 256
    uncomplicated 259
Malarial parasite, life cycle of 257*f*
Maldigestion, intraluminal 31
Mallampati classification, modified 311
Mallory-Weiss tear 49
Malnutrition 2
Mantle cell lymphoma 73
Marasmic kwashiorkor 299
Marasmus 299, 300, 300*f*
Marfan's syndrome 4, 94, 96
Marginal zone lymphoma 73
Marrow disorder 77
Massive ascites 18*f*
Massive splenomegaly, causes of 82*t*
Maxillary hypoplasia 254
Measles 240, 240*f*, 241
Mechanical ventilation 289
Medulla 196
Mefloquine 258
Megaloblastic anemia 59, 60*f*
Melkersson-Rosenthal syndrome 209
Membranoproliferative glomerulonephritis 184
Meningeal irritation, signs of 201, 203
Meningitis 200, 241, 244, 248, 251, 262
    acute 200
        bacterial 201, 202
    aseptic 242
    bacterial 201, 201*t*, 202*t*, 203*t*
    chronic 200, 203
    signs of 201*t*
    subacute 200, 203
    types of 200*t*
Meningococcal infection, prevention of 203
Meningovascular syphilis 253
Menorrhagia 77, 216
Menstrual abnormalities 47
Menstrual history 3
Mental and emotional status 3
Mental impairment 302
Mental retardation 217
Mental stress 198
Meperidine 206
Mepolizumab 146
Mercaptopurine 66
Meropenem 162, 163, 202, 286
Merozoites 256
Mesenteric ischemia 16
Metabolic acidosis 183, 185, 257, 285*f*, 292
Metabolic causes 46
Metabolic disorders 185, 215
Metabolic equivalents 312
Metabolic functions 35
Metabolic syndrome 152, 236, 236, 301
Metaprolol 207
Metastatic carcinoma 225
Metered dose inhaler 150
Metformin 233
Methemoglobinemia 9
Methimazole 215, 219
Methotrexate 66, 67
Methyl prednisolone 146
Methylcobalamin 60
Methyldopa 39, 106, 108
Methylmalonic acid 60
Methylprednisolone 147, 270
Methylxanthines 146
Methysergide 207
Metoclopramide 206
Metolazone 106, 111, 112, 117, 118, 125
Metoprolol succinate 118
Metronidazole 192, 202
Metyrapone 225
Mexiletine 125
Microalbuminuria 176
Microcytic hypochromic anemia 58*f*
    differential diagnosis of 59*t*
Midazolam 200
Middle East respiratory syndrome 268
Miglitol 233
Migraine
    basilar 205
    classical 205
    common 205
    complicated 205
    equivalent 205
    familial hemiplegic 205
    ophthalmoplegic 205
    pathophysiology of 206
    prophylactic therapy of 207*t*
    treatment of acute 206*t*
    variants of 205
Migrainous neuralgia 207
Miliary pneumonia 139
Miliary tuberculosis 157, 157*f*, 288
Milk alkali syndrome 221
Milrinone 117-119, 277
Mineral bone disorder 185
Mineralocorticoids 224
Minoxidil 106
Misoprostol 28
Mitiglinide 233
Mitral regurgitation 86, 90, 94
    causes of 94*t*
    clinical manifestations 94
    clinical signs of 94*t*
    pathophysiology 94
    treatment 94
Mitral stenosis 90, 93, 120, 135
    causes of 93*t*
    clinical manifestations 93
    clinical signs of 93*t*
    investigations 93
    pathophysiology 93
    treatment 93
Mitral valve 92, 93
    repair 95
    replacement 95, 94
Mitral valvotomy 94
Moist warm skin 218
Molecular abnormalities 66
Molecular test 170
Mollaret's meningitis 247
Molluscum contagiosum 261, 263*f*
Mometasone 146
Monoclonal antibody 180
Mononucleosis, infectious 81, 247-249, 253
Monospot test 248
Montelukast 146
Moon face 226
Morphine 113
    intravenous 119, 277
    sulphate 111, 112
Motility disorders 31

Motion sickness 17
Mouth wash 13
Moxifloxacin 141, 162
Mucolytics 151
Mucosal defects 31
Mucosal protective agents 28
Mulberry molars 254
Multinodular goiter 218
Multiorgan failure 269
Multiple antral ulcers 27f
Multiple osteolytic lesions 74f
Multiple trauma 119
Mumps 241, 242f
    complications of 242
Murmur, types of 90t
Murphy's sign 21
Muscle
    cramps 218
    mass, maintain 233
Mycobacterium
    avium complex 264
    genome 161
    tuberculosis 203
Mycophenolate mofetil 46, 180
Mycoplasma pneumoniae 139
Mycosis, disseminated 262
Myelitis, acute transverse 248
Myelofibrosis 82
Myeloid sarcoma 65
Myeloma, multiple 24, 73
Myeloproliferative
    disorders 81
    neoplasms 67t
Myocardial infarction 17, 87, 91, 94, 108, 112f, 113f, 211, 313
    initial management of 277
Myocardial perfusion scanning 109
Myocarditis 115, 242, 244, 248, 250, 251
Myopathy, proximal 218
Myxedema 216
    coma 217
Myxoma, atrial 290

N

Nafcillin 98
Nails 11
Naproxen 206
Naratriptan 206
Narcotic analgesics 206
Nasal cavity 250
Nasopharyngeal airway 274
Nasopharyngeal carcinoma 247, 249
Natiglinide 233
Natriuretic peptides 115, 118
Nausea 2, 17, 56, 205, 211
    causes of 17t
Near drowning 288
Nebivolol 106, 111, 112
Nebulizer 147, 274
    therapy 147f
Necator americanus 57
Neck rigidity 201, 201f
Necrotizing stomatitis 267
Necrotizing ulcerative
    gingivitis 267
    stomatitis 22
Nedocromil 146

Neisseria gonorrhoeae 251
Nelfinavir 265
Nephritic syndrome 180t
Nephritis 176, 242, 244, 251
    acute 176, 180
    interstitial 248
Nephrogenic diabetes insipidus 226
Nephrolithiasis 176
Nephrology, syndromes in 175
Nephron, structure of 175f
Nephropathy, diabetic 231
Nephrotic syndrome 176, 178, 178f, 178t, 179f, 180t, 257
    idiopathic 178
    primary 178
    secondary 178
    treatment of 179
Nerve palsy 192f
Nervous system 2, 188, 216
Nesiritide 118
Neuralgia, glossopharyngeal 208
Neurally mediated syncope 122
Neuraminidase 171
Neuritis 251
Neurologic complications 185
Neurological dysfunctions 205
Neurological manifestations 59
Neuromodulation 207
Neuropathy 230
    diabetic 232
Neurosyphilis 253
Neutropenia
    causes of 81t
    cyclic 81
Nevirapine 265
Niacin 299, 303
Nicardipine 108
Nicorandil 110
Nicotinamide adenine dinucleotide 303
Niemann-Pick disease 81
Nifedipine 24, 106, 112
Night blindness 306
Nilotinib 67, 69
Nitrates 110, 111
Nitric oxide 144
Nitroglycerine 108, 111, 112
    intravenous 119, 277
Noctural dyspnea 116, 133
Nocturia 176
Nonbacterial thrombotic endocarditis 97
Noncardiac causes 87
Noncardiac chest pain 109
Noncardiogenic pulmonary edema 119t
Nonconvulsive status epilepticus 199
Non-dihydropyridine 106
Non-falciparum malaria 259
Non-Hodgkin lymphoma 70, 72, 249
Noninvasive ventilation, long-term 149
Non-ketotic hyperosmolar diabetic coma 231
Non-pollen extracts 294
Non-pruritic erythematous maculopapular rashes 240
Nonsteroidal anti-inflammatory drugs 25, 178, 182, 184, 249
Non-treponemal antibody tests 254
Non-typhoidal salmonella 262
Non-viral chronic hepatitis, treatment of 46t
Normocytic normochromic anemia 257

Nortryptiline 207
Nucleic acid amplification test 269
Nutrition 183, 298
Nutritional deficiency 23
Nystagmus 302
Nystatin 23

O

Obesity 300, 312
    complications of 300
    treatable causes of 300
Obstruction, intestinal 16
Obstructive jaundice 38
    causes of 39, 39t
Obstructive lung disease 138f
Ocular complications 231
Oculocephalic test 195
Oculomotor nerve 190
Odynophagia 16, 19, 24
Office blood pressure measurement 101
Ofloxacin 251, 252
Olfactory nerve 188
Oligomenorrhea 218
Oliguria 2, 176
Olmesartan 106, 118
Omalizumab 146
Ombitasvir 46
Omeprazole 28
Onycholysis 11
Oophoritis 241, 242
Ophthalmic division 191
Ophthalmopathy 218
Ophthalmoplegia 302
Opportunistic infection 263, 264
    management of 263
Optic chiasma 189
Optic nerve 188, 188f
Optic neuritis 205
Optimal glycemic control 232
Oral anticoagulant 94, 155
Oral aphthous ulcers, idiopathic 267
Oral candidiasis 22, 23, 23f, 263f, 267
Oral cavity 13
Oral contraceptives 100
Oral glucose tolerance test 229
Oral hairy leukoplakia 249, 249f, 267
Oral infection 83
Oral iron therapy 58
Oral lesions, differential diagnosis of 253
Oral mucosa
    hyperpigmentaion of 60f
    pigmentation of 226f
Oral penicillin 92
Oral polio 241
Oral rehydration solutions 30
Oral sulphadiazine 92
Oral ulcer 21, 22f, 23
    causes of 22t
    recurrent 262
Orchitis 241, 242
Oropharyngeal airway 274
Oropharyngeal dysphagia 23
    causes of 23, 24t
Oropharyngeal tumors 24
Orthopnea 2, 7, 86, 93, 115, 116
Orthostatic hypotension 122, 123, 275
Oseltamivir 171

Osler's nodes 88
Osmotic diarrhea 31, 32
Osteitis fibrosa cystica 222
Osteoarthritis 301
Osteoarthropathy
    hypertrophic 9, 88
        pulmonary 135
Osteomalacia 220, 222, 308
Osteomyelitis 251
Osteoporosis 152
Ostium
    primum 120
    secundum 120
Otitis media 241, 262
Ovarian teratoma 218
Oxacillin 98
Oxcarbazepine 199, 208
Oxygen
    saturation 311
    source 274
    therapy 113, 149, 151, 277
        long-term 149
    toxicity 288

P

Pacemakers 312
Paget's disease 5
Pain
    cardiac 1
    relief of 113, 277
Palatal paralysis 193, 250
Palatal reflex 193
Pallor 2, 8, 216
    visible over face 57*f*
Palm, pallor of 8*f*
Palpation 20, 136
Palpebral conjunctiva 8*f*
Palpitation 2, 86, 218, 312
Pancreatic enzyme deficiency 31
Pancreatic exocrine functions 33
Pancreatitis 16, 17, 87, 241, 242, 283, 288
    acute 119, 220
Pancytopenia 248
Pantoprazole 28
Pantothenic acid 299, 305
Papanicolaou's stain 247
Papilledema 201
Papilloma virus infection 267
Papular pruritic eruptions 262
Paracetamol 39, 206, 269
Paradoxical pulse 5, 89
Paraproteinemia 76
Parathyroid
    adenoma 221, 222
    carcinoma 221, 222
    disorders 221
    hormone 219
    hyperplasia 221, 222
Parenteral iron therapy 58
Paritaprevir 46
Parosmia 188
Parotid cyst 241
Parotid duct, stone in 242
Parotid swelling, causes of 242
Parotitis 251
Paroxysmal atrial tachycardia 127
Paroxysmal nocturnal dyspnea 7, 86, 93, 115, 116

Parvovirus 84
Patent ductus arteriosus 120, 121
    clinical manifestations 121
    investigations 121
    management 121
Patterson-Kelly syndrome 57
Paul-Bunnell test 248
Pedal edema
    bilateral 10, 10*f*, 87*f*
    causes of 10*t*
Pelvic inflammatory disease 16, 251
Penicillin
    allergy 99
    G 98, 202
Pentamidine 264
Peptic ulcer 16, 26, 28, 57, 87
    clinical features 27
    complications of 27, 27*t*
    disease 16, 49
        risk factors for 27*t*
    etiology 26
    treatment 27
Peptides 118
Percutaneous transhepatic cholangiography 36
Pericardial disease 117, 128
Pericardial effusion 216
Pericarditis 185, 248, 251
    constrictive 115
Perinatal varicella 244
Perindopril 105, 106
Periodontal infections 267
Peripheral blood 60*f*, 61*f*
Peripheral cyanosis 10, 88
Peripheral neuropathy 250
Peripheral vascular disease 230
Peritoneum 51
Peritonitis 17
Pernicious anemia 26, 60, 228
Persistent bradyarrhythmias 290
Petechiae 77
Petit mal 197
Pharyngitis 262
Pharynx 13, 134
Phenothiazine 242
Phenytoin 39, 125, 127, 199, 200, 208
    equivalents 200
Pheochromocytoma 100, 104
Philadelphia chromosome 68*f*
Phlebotomy 149
Phlegmonus gastritis 25
Phonophobia 205
Phosphodiesterase inhibitors 150, 277
Phosphorus 299
Photodermatitis 296
Photophobia 205
Phylloquinone 306
Physical stress 279
Physiologic bad breath 12
Physique 135
Pibrentasvir 46
Pink frothy sputum 115
Pink puffers 148
Pioglitazone 233, 300
Piperacillin-tazobactum 286
Piperazine derivative 110
Pituitary gland 222
Pituitary hormones 223*f*
Pituitary tumor 215

Pizotifen 207
Plaque stabilization therapy 111
Plasma glucose, lowers 233
Plasmodium vivax 256
Platelet
    count 281
    disorders 76
    plug formation 74, 75*f*
Pleomorphic rash 243
Pleural biopsy 138
Pleural diseases 164
Pleural effusion 116, 137, 164, 165*t*, 216
    causes of 164*t*
Pleural origin 135
Pleural rub 137
Pleurisy, causes of 164
Pleurodesis 165, 166
Plummer-Vinson syndrome 24
Pneumococcal conjugate vaccine 241
Pneumocystis
    carinii 261, 264
    jiroveci 261
    pneumonia 262
Pneumonia 133-135, 138, 139, 140*f*, 151, 244, 261, 269*f*, 288
    acute eosinophilic 152
    bilateral interstitial 140*f*
    chronic eosinophilic 153
    clinical manifestations 139
    community acquired 139*t*
    complications of 140, 140*t*
    etiology 138
    interstitial 139, 248
    lobar 139
    nosocomial 138
    pathology 139
    route of infection 139
    treatment 141
Pneumonitis, hypersensitivity 3
Pneumothorax 133, 137, 151, 165, 166*f*
    classification 165
    complication of 167
    primary spontaneous 166
    secondary spontaneous 166
    signs of 166*t*
    spontaneous 165
    symptoms of 166
    tension 166
    traumatic 165, 166
    types of 165
Pollakiuria 176
Pollen extracts 294
Polyarthritis 92
Polychromasia 56
Polycyclic aromatic 168
Polycystic kidneys 104
Polycystic ovary syndrome 301
Polycythemia 149
Polydipsia 226, 228
Polyneuritis 248
Polyuria 2, 176
Ponatinib 69
Poor memory 216
Porphyria 17, 192
Portacaval shunt surgery 52
Portal hypertension 47, 48, 82
    causes of 48, 48*t*
Portal vein obstruction 48
Portal venous pressure, reduction in 49

Postherpetic neuralgia 208
Postnecrotic cirrhosis 47
Postresuscitation care 290
Post-splenectomy 229
Poststreptococcal glomerulonephritis 181
Post-thyroidectomy 215
Post-transplant lymphoproliferative disease 249
Post-tubercular fibrobronchiectasis 143f
Postural hypotension 123, 275
    causes of 123, 275
Postural syncope 123
Potassium 299
Pramlintide 233, 235
Prasugrel 111
Prazosin 106
Precipitate dysarrhythmias 130
Prediabetes 229
Prednisolone 46, 67, 73, 146
    primarily 179
Pregabalin 300
Premonitory symptoms 123
Primaquine 258
Primary adrenal
    failure 224
    insufficiency, tests for 225
Primary headache disorders 205
Primary herpes simplex virus 247
Primary hyperaldosteronism 100
Primary hypothyroidism 215, 216, 218
Primidone 199
Prinzmetal's angina 111
Probenecid 254
Procainamide 125
Procaine penicillin G 254
Prochlorperazine 206
Proliferative diabetic retinopathy 231f
Prominent veins 19
    over abdomen 19f
Propafenone 125, 128
Prophylactic antibiotics 63
Prophylactic therapy 207
    primary 263
Prophylaxis 94, 99
    pre-exposure 43
    primary 264
Propofol 200
Propranolol 106, 207, 219
Propylthiouracil 215, 219, 242
Prosthetic valve endocarditis 99
Protease inhibitors 265
Protein energy malnutrition 299
Proteinuria 176
Prothrombin 75
Proton pump inhibitor 28
Pruritus 295
Pseudohypoparathyroidism 220
Pseudomonas aeruginosa 139
Pseudotumor
    cerebri 301
    syndrome 79
Psychiatric illnesses 17
Psychosis 251
Pteroylmonoglutamic acid 59
Puffy face 216
Pulmonary angiography 137, 155
Pulmonary artery 121
Pulmonary capillary pressure, signs of 93, 94

Pulmonary complications 161
Pulmonary contusion 288
Pulmonary disease 128, 312
Pulmonary edema 119, 129, 134
Pulmonary embolism 115, 133, 134, 151, 153, 301
    causes of 154t
    clinical syndromes 154
    diagnosis 155
    differential diagnosis 154
    differential diagnosis of 154t
    investigations 154
    prevention of 156
    treatment 155
Pulmonary eosinophilia 152
Pulmonary eosinophilic
    disease, causes of 152t
    syndromes 152
Pulmonary function tests 144, 148
Pulmonary hypertension, signs of 93, 94, 154
Pulmonary infarction 135, 142
Pulmonary insult 288
Pulmonary rehabilitation 149, 151
Pulmonary secretion examination 141
Pulmonary stenosis 290
Pulmonary syndromes 297
Pulmonary system examination 311
Pulmonary thromboembolism 292
Pulmonary tuberculosis 156
    complications of 160, 161t
    post-primary 157
    primary 156
Pulse 4
    pressure 5, 101
    rate abnormalities, causes of 5t
Pulseless electrical activity 290, 292
Pulsus alternans 116
Pump failure 114
Pupils, causes of smaller or larger 190t
Pupillary examination 189
Purple striae 20f
Pyelonephritis 16
Pyloric obstructions 17
Pyogenic liver abscess 256f
Pyopneumothorax 167
Pyrazinamide 159, 160, 162, 163, 204
Pyridoxine 204, 303
Pyrimethamine 258

Q

Quadrantanopia 189
Quartan malaria 256
Quinapril 106, 118
Quinidine 125
Quinine 258
Quinolones 192

R

Rabeprazole 28
Radial artery, palpation of 4f, 88f
Radioactive iodine 219
Radio-femoral delay 89
Raltegravir 265
Ramipril 105, 106, 111, 114, 117, 118
Ramsay-Hunt syndrome 209, 244
Random blood sugar 312

Random donor platelets 66
Ranitidine 25
Ranolazine 110
Rapid antigen test 269
Rapid plasma reagin test 254
Rare complications 248
Recurrent anaphylaxis, prevention of 295
Red blood cell 178
    indices 56t
    transfusion 58
Red cell aplasia 248
Reed-Sternberg cell 72f
Reflex, hepatojugular 7
Reiter's syndrome 253
Remedesivir 270
Remogliflozin 233
Renal artery stenosis 89, 107
Renal autoregulation 182
Renal biopsy 176
Renal denervation therapy 107
Renal disease 77, 175, 176, 178, 312
    chronic 312
    end-stage 186f, 313
Renal disorders 77
Renal failure 257, 259
    chronic 220, 222
    rapidly progressive 176
    symptoms of 185
Renal function tests 71
Renal impairment 117
Renal insufficiency 314
Renal replacement therapy 186
Renal stones 16
Renal sympathetic nerves 107
Renal syndromes 176t, 296
Renin-angiotensin system inhibition 179
Renin-angiotensin-aldosterone
    inhibitors 107
    system 184
Repaglinide 233
Reperfusion therapy 113
Resistant malaria, treatment of 259
Reslizumab 146
Respiration 7
Respiratory causes 134
Respiratory diseases 7, 9, 133, 135
    symptoms 133
Respiratory distress 294
Respiratory failure 163, 164
Respiratory muscle 86
Respiratory obstruction 250
Respiratory rate 311
Respiratory syncytial viruses 139
Respiratory system 2, 133
    diseases of 133
    examination 135
Respiratory tract infections, recurrent 262
Restrictive cardiomyopathy 115
Resuscitation, cardiopulmonary 281, 290, 291
Reteplase 111, 113
Reticulocyte 64
    count, correction of 56
Reticuloendothelial organ 81
Retinitis 262
Retinol 306
Retinopathy 230
Retropharyngeal abscess 24
Reye's syndrome 244

INDEX

Rhagades 254
Rheumatic fever 96
Rheumatic valvular heart disease 90*t*, 92
Rhinitis 181
Rhythm 5, 89
    control 128
Riboflavin 207, 299, 303
Rickets 222, 307, 307*f*
Rickettsia 97
Riedel's thyroiditis 215
Rifabutin 264
Rifampicin 39, 98, 158, 159, 160, 162, 203, 204
Rifaximin 30, 50
Right heart failure 116
    clinical features of 116*t*
    signs of 93, 94
Rilpivirine 265
Rinne test 193
Ritonavir 265
Rituximab 73, 77, 180, 249
    chemotherapy 73
Rizatriptan 206
Rosuvastatin 111
Rotavirus 241
Roth's spots 88
Rotor syndromes 38
Rubella 242
    congenital 243
Rubeola 240
Rufinamide 199

S

Sacubitril 118
Saddle nose 254
Salbutamol 146, 150
    solution 274
Salicylates 92
Salivary gland disease 267
Salivary secretion, lack of 192
Salmeterol 150
Salmonella
    paratyphi 250
    typhi 250
Salt restriction 105
Saquinavir 265
Sarcoidosis 48, 115, 126, 215, 221, 242
SARS-COV-2 variants 268
Saxagliptin 233
Schamroth's window test 9, 88
Schatzki's ring 24
Schilling test 32
Scleroderma 24
Scoliosis 136
Scombotoxin 30
Scotoma 189
Scurvy 305*f*
Seborrheic dermatitis 262
Second line drugs 159
Sedatives 50
Segmental glomerulosclerosis 180
Seizure 2, 122, 123, 123*t*, 196, 278
    absence 197
    causes of 197, 198*t*
    classification of 196*t*
    complex partial 197
    emergency management of 279
    immediate care of 198

    partial 196
    precipitating factors for 279
    repeated 259
Selenium 299
Semaglutide 233, 234
Sensory, special 196
Sepsis 288
Septic shock 284, 286
    causes of 284
Septicaemia, recurrent 262
Sequential organ failure assessment 284
Serological tests 141, 254
Serology 269
Serum
    albumin 35, 36
        low 220
    alpha-1 antitrypsin 149
    ascites albumin gradient 51
    bilirubin 35
    biochemistry 176
    cobalamin 60
    electrolytes 312
    enzymes 35, 36
    fructosamine measurement 229
    protein albumin 72
    sickness 295
Severe disease
    risk factors for 268
    treatment of 270
Sexual route
    heterosexual 260
    homosexual 260
Sheehan's syndrome 215, 223
Shifting dullness 21
Shock 201, 257, 283, 287
    cardiogenic 114, 286, 287
    causes of obstructive 284
    classification of 283
    hypoadrenal 288
    hypovolemic 283
    neurogenic 288
    obstructive 284
        treatment of 284
Short stature 217
Shunt, without 120
Sick sinus syndrome 124, 125
Sickle cell
    anemia 62, 63*f*
    disease, management of 63, 64*t*
Simeprevir 46
Simple partial seizures 196
Simple pulmonary eosinophilia 152
Simvastatin 111
Sinus
    arrhythmia 124
    bradycardia 124
        causes of 125
    rhythm 124
        restoration of 127
    tachycardia 124, 127
    venosus 120
Sinusitis 181, 205, 262
Sitagliptin 233
Sjögren's syndrome 242, 268
Skin 20
    lesions 294
    rashes 201
Skipped meal 279

Sleep 194
    apnea 107, 216
        obstructive 152, 301
    deprivation 279
Slide test 248
Smell sense 188
Smoking 26
    cessation 149
Snellen's chart 189*f*
Sodium
    nitroprusside 108, 118
    valproate 207, 300
Sofosbuvir 44, 46
Solitary nodule 218
Somatosensory 196
Sore throat 250
Spectinomycin 252
Sphygmomanometer 274
Spinal cord injury 17
Spirometry 138, 138*f*
Spironolactone 105-107, 118
Spleen
    infiltration of 81
    palpation of 20*f*
Splenic infarction 16
Splenic rupture 248
Splenic sequestration 77
Splenomegaly 53, 81
    causes of 81, 81*t*
    clinical manifestations 81
    diagnosis 82
Splinter hemorrhages 11
Spondylitis, ankylosing 96
Spontaneous bacterial peritonitis 52
Sputnik V 271
Sputum 2, 134, 141
    examination 137
Sreptomycin 204
Stable angina 109
    chest pain in 2*t*
    clinical features 109
    treatment 110
Staphylococcus aureus 97, 139, 244
Statins 112
Status asthmaticus 144
Status epilepticus 199, 200, 279
    complications of 200
    drugs used in 200*t*
Stavudine 265
Steatohepatitis, nonalcoholic 44, 46
Stellate cells 35
Stem cell transplant 67
Stensen's duct 241
Stercobilin 37
Stercobilinogen 37
Steroid 92, 146
    therapy 312
    withdrawal 281
Stethoscope 274
Stevens-Johnson syndrome 253, 295, 296*f*
Stokes-Adams attack 87, 122, 127
Stomatitis 21, 58
    angular 21, 300
Storage disorders 82
Strawberry gums 24
Streptococci, eradication of 92
Streptococcus
    pneumoniae 139

pyogenes 244
viridans 97
Streptokinase 111, 113
Streptomycin 160
Stress 3
　echocardiography 109
　embolic 279
　relief of 105
　testing 109
Stria, abdominal 20*f*
Stridor 135
Stroke 2, 211, 279
　causes of 211*t*
　embolic 128
　hemorrhagic 212
　ischemic 211, 212
　risk factors for 211*t*
Stupor 3
Sturge-Weber angiomatosis 24
Subarachnoid hemorrhage, management of 213*t*
Subcutaneous mepolizumab 146
Subcutaneous nodules 92
Subendocardial ischemia 112
Sublingual nitroglycerine 113
Submandibular lymph nodes, palpation of 11*f*
Substitution therapy 223
Sucralfate 28
Suction machine 274
Sudden cardiac death 108, 290
　causes of 290
Sudden death 108
Sulfadoxine 258
Sulfhemoglobinemia 9
Sulfonylureas 233
Sulphonamides 81
Sulphonylureas 300
Sumatriptan 206
Superinfection, bacterial 248
Supraclavicular lymphadenopathy, left 82*f*
Supranuclear facial palsy 210, 210*t*
Sweating 218
Swine flu 171
　antiviral drugs for 171*t*
Swine influenza A 171
Sympathetic inhibition 123
Sympathomimetic amines 118
Sympathomimetic drugs 100
Symptomatic disease, mildly 260, 261
Syncope 86, 87, 122, 123, 123*t*, 275, 276
　cardiac 122
　causes of 122, 122*f*, 122*t*
　resemble 122
Synpharyngitic hematuria 181
Synthetic function 35, 36
Syphilis 84, 96, 252
　benign tertiary 253
　cardiovascular 253
　congenital 253
　drugs in 254
　early 252-254
　endocarditis 97
　late latent 253
　primary 252
　secondary 253
　serological tests for 254
　treatment of late 254

Systemic antifibrinolytic agents 83
Systemic disorders 2*t*
Systemic inflammatory response syndrome 284, 286
Systemic lupus erythematous 184
Systemic steroids 147, 278
Systolic flow murmur 121

T

Tabes dorsalis 253
Tachyarrhythmia 122, 124, 127
　atrial 124
　chronic 115
Tachycardia 5, 117, 127, 250
　atrial 127
　narrow complex 127
Tachypnea, causes of 7*t*
Tacrolimus 180
Tactile vocal fremitus 136
Takayasu's disease 121
Taste
　alteration in 192*t*
　causes of loss of 192*t*
　sensation examination 192
Telaprevir 46
Telbivudine 44, 45
Telmisartan 106
Temporal arteritis 205
Temporal bone 210
Temporomandibular joint disease 205
Tender hepatomegaly 89
Tenecteplase 111, 113
Teneligliptin 233
Tenofovir 44, 267
　alafenamide 45, 264, 265
　disoproxil fumarate 45, 264, 265
Tension
　headache 207
　pneumothorax 292
Terazosin 106
Terbutaline 146
Terizidone 163
Tertian malaria 256
Tertiary hyperparathyroidism 222
Tertiary syphilis 253
Testicular atrophy 47
Tetracycline 192, 254
Tetralogy of Fallot 122
　investigations 122
　management 122
Thalassemias 62
Theophylline 128
Therapeutic pleural aspiration 165
Thiamine 299, 302
　pyrophosphate 302
Thiazide 106, 221, 227
　diuretics 117, 118
Thiazolidinediones 233, 234
Thrombocytopenia 76, 80, 242, 248
　causes of 76, 77*t*
　severe 249
Thromboembolism, prevention of 128
Thrombolysis 212
Thrombolytic therapy 111, 113*t*, 155
Thrombosis, coronary 292
Thyroid
　carcinoma metastasis 218

　crisis 219
　disorders 24, 215
　surgery 219
Thyroid function tests
　clinical features of 216*t*
　interpretation of 216*t*
Thyroid gland
　anatomy of 215
　enlarged 218*f*
Thyroid hormone
　feedback control of 215*f*
　secretion, regulation of 215
Thyroidectomy, subtotal 219
Thyroiditis 242
　subacute 218
Thyroid-stimulating hormone 223
Thyrotoxicosis 4, 5, 86, 101, 104, 115, 218
　causes of 218
　clinical features of 218
　factitia 218
　primary 216
　secondary 216
Thyrotropin-releasing hormone 223
Tiagabine 199
Ticagrelor 111
Tiotropium 150
Tipranavir 265
Tirofiban 111
Tissue plasminogen activator 113
Tobramycin 286
Tocilizumab 270
Todd's paralysis 197
Tongue
　and bad breath 12
　enlarged 217
　fissuring 300
　innervation of 192*t*
　large 216
Tonic pupil 190
Tonic-clonic seizures 197
Tonsillitis 262
Tonsils 250
Topiramate 199, 207
Torsemide 105, 106, 118
Tourniquet 274
Toxic adenoma 218
Toxic epidermal necrolysis 295, 296*f*
Toxic inhalation 288
Toxicity 302, 304-307
　chronic 306
Toxin 29, 292
　production 29
Toxoplasmosis 264
Trachea 134, 136
　candidiasis of 262
Trail sign 136
Trandolapril 118
Tranexamic acid 83
Transdermal nitroglycerine 112
Transient ischemic attack 197, 211, 313
Transitory bad breath 12
Traube's sign 96
Trauma 281, 283, 300, 312
　severe 288
Treatable disease 147
Treponema pallidum 203, 252, 253
Treponemal antibody tests 254
Triamterene 106

Tricuspid valve 97
Trigeminal nerve 191, 208*f*
   different divisions of 191*f*
Trigeminal neuralgia 207
Trimethoprim-sulfamethoxazole 251
Trochlear nerve 191
Trophoblastic tumors 218
Trousseau's sign, elicitation of 220*f*
Tubercular effusion 165
Tubercular meningitis, treatment of 204*t*
Tuberculin skin test 158
Tuberculoma 198*f*
Tuberculosis 4, 81, 135, 142, 156, 157, 225, 264, 312
   causative organism 156
   extensively drug resistant 161
   extrapulmonary 156, 157, 157*t*, 262
   history of 3
   infection 161
   isoniazid-resistant 161
   mono-resistant 161
   multidrug resistant 161
   poly-drug resistant 161
   preventive treatment 161
   primary 156
   rifampicin resistant 161
   treatment of 159, 264
Tuberculous meningitis 203
Tuberous sclerosis 24
Tubulointerstitial nephritis, chronic 184
Tumor 300
Turner's syndrome 78, 120
Typhoid 81
   fever 250
Typical angina 109
Tyrosine kinase inhibitor 69
Tzanck preparation 247

U

Ulcer
   aphthous 21, 22, 253
   perforation of 16
   trophic 192
Ulcerative colitis 31
Ulcerative stomatitis 21, 22
Umbilical hernia 18*f*
Unstable angina 110
   pathophysiology of 111
Upper abdomen discomfort, right 86, 87
Upper gastrointestinal
   bleeding 49
   endoscopy 50*f*
Upper limbs 13
Upper respiratory tract 133
   infection 134
Uremia 50, 176
Ureteric colic 17
Ureteric obstruction 16
Urinary sediments 184
Urinary stress incontinence 301
Urinary system 2
Urinary tract
   infection 178, 312
   obstruction 176
Urine 38, 62
   analysis 312
   bilirubin 35

   examination 176, 183
   output 86, 87
   test 229
Urticaria 294*f*, 295, 296
   treatment of 295
Uterine cervix 301

V

Vaccine 149, 271
   preservative 294
Vagal afferent fibers 123
Vagus nerve 193
Valacyclovir 245, 247
Valproate 200
Valproic acid 199
Valsartan 106, 117, 118
Valvular heart disease 115, 128
Vancomycin 98, 202, 286
Variceal bleeding, prevention of 49
Variceal hemorrhage, treatment of 49
Varicella
   congenital 244
   infection, complications of 244
   pneumonia 244
Varicella-zoster 267
   immunoglobulin 244
   virus 243, 246
Varicose veins 301
Vasculitis 76, 295
Vasovagal syncope 123, 275
Velpatasvir 44, 46
Venlafaxine 207
Venous blood gases 312
Ventricular fibrillation 130, 130*f*, 290
Ventricular premature beats 129
Ventricular septal defect 97, 120
Ventricular tachyarrhythmias 86, 124, 129
Ventricular tachycardia 129, 130*f*, 290
Verapamil 5, 24, 106, 111, 112, 125, 207
Vertebrobasilar strokes 211
Vertigo 211
Vessel wall abnormalities 76
Vestibular functions, tests of 193
Vestibulocochlear nerve 193
Vigorous
   diuresis 52
   paracentesis 50
Vildagliptin 233
Vinblastine 72
Vincent's infection 22
Vincristine 66, 73
Vinyl chloride 48
Viral hepatitis 44, 46, 47
   causes of 39*t*
   prevention of 42
Viral meningitis 203
Virchow's node 82, 82*f*, 153
Vision, loss of 189
Visual acuity 189
Visual field 189
Vital signs 311
Vitamin 298, 299, 301, 302
   A 299, 302, 306
      deficiency 306
   B_1 302
   B_{12} 59, 299, 304
      deficiency 2, 59, 60*f*

   B_2 302, 303
   B_3 302, 303
   B_6 299, 302-304
   C 229, 269, 299, 302, 305
   D 175, 219, 299, 302, 307
      deficiency 220
      excess 221
   D_3 269
      deficiency 19, 302, 304*f*
   E 229, 299, 302, 305
      deficiency 306
      fat-soluble 301
   K 36, 50, 75, 299, 302, 306, 307
      antagonist 155
      deficiency of 36, 307
Vitiligo 228
Vocal resonance 137
Voglibose 233
Voice, hoarseness of 250
Vomiting 2, 17, 205, 211, 283, 312
   causes of 17*t*
von Willebrand disease 76, 78, 281
Voxilaprevir 46

W

Waist circumference 300
Warfarin 94, 97
Water soluble vitamins 298, 301
Waterhouse-Friderichsen syndrome 201, 225
Weakness 2, 115, 216
Weber test 193
Wegener's disease 24
Wegener's granulomatosis 135, 142
Weight gain 2, 216
Weight loss 2, 4, 19, 59, 218, 233
   unexplained moderate 262
Weight reduction 105
Weil's disease 39
Wernicke's encephalopathy 302
Westermark's sign 154
Wet beriberi 302
Wheezes 136
White blood cell 64, 178
White coat hypertension 101, 103, 104
Wilson's disease 44, 46, 47
Wolf-Parkinson-White syndrome 129, 290

X

Xerosis, conjunctival 306

Y

Yersinia enterocolitica 29

Z

Zafirlukast 146
Zenker's diverticulum 24
Zidovudine 264, 265
Zileuton 146
Zinc 269, 299
   transporter 8 228
Zolmitriptan 206
Zonisamide 199

EU GSPR Authorised Reprsentative
Logos Europe, 9 rue Nicolas Poussin
1700, La Rochelle, France
Phone: +33 (0) 6 67 93 73 78
E-mail: contact@logoseurope.eu

www.ingramcontent.com/pod-product-compliance
Ingram Content Group UK Ltd.
Pitfield, Milton Keynes, MK11 3LW, UK
UKHW050431150426
5217IPUK00019B/1331